Illustrated Guide to Orthopedic Nursing

Third Edition

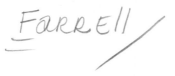

Acquisitions Editor: Diana Intenzo
Developmental Editor: Jeanne Wallace
Manuscript Editor: Patrick O'Kane
Indexer: Elizabeth Herr Hallinger
Design Director: Tracy Baldwin
Design Coordinator: Don Shenkle
Designer: Katharine Nichols
Compositor: Progressive Typographers
Printer/Binder: The Murray Printing Company

3rd Edition

Library of Congress Cataloging-in-Publication Data

Farrell, Jane.
  Illustrated guide to orthopedic nursing.

  Includes bibliographies and index.
  1. Orthopedic nursing.   I. Title. [DNLM:
1. Orthopedics — nursing. WY 157.6 F245i]
RD753.F37 1986   610.73'677   86-118
ISBN 0-397-54596-7

The author and publisher have exerted every effort to ensure that drug
selection and dosage set forth in this text are in accord with current
recommendations and practice at the time of publication. However, in view
of ongoing research, changes in government regulations, and the constant
flow of information relating to drug therapy and drug reactions, the reader
is urged to check the package insert for each drug for any change in
indications and dosage and for added warnings and precautions. This is
particularly important when the recommended agent is a new or infrequently employed drug.

This edition belongs to
my husband and family,
who lived through all of it

Contents

Preface

Although the content of this book deals with the facts of orthopedic nursing care, the presentation of those facts also reflects a personal philosophy. I believe that orthopedic nursing has a unique responsibility within a rehabilitation team effort and *should* and *can* be as creative and constructive as the specialty of orthopedics itself. However, this is only possible if the nurse recognizes that everyone involved in the care of the patient, including the patient and the family, has a valuable contribution to make in the planning and delivery of that care. Therefore, while the book draws extensively on knowledge and insights acquired from clinical nursing and interactions with patients after discharge, it utilizes the input of other nurses, orthopedic surgeons, physical therapists, and x-ray technologists, as well as representatives of community rehabilitation resources, and those people engaged in the manufacture of orthopedic appliances and equipment.

This book focuses on the nursing care of the adult orthopedic patient in the hospital environment, on those factors that influence the patient's adjustment, behavior, and recovery, and on practical suggestions for fitting the patient back into the home environment. Basic information on conditions and disorders is also presented.

The pages that follow are heavily peopled with specific examples from patient care experiences, so that the nurse or nursing student can more readily identify his or her patient's problems with what is written.

Hopefully this approach to orthopedic nursing will be helpful to the nurse who desires to make an effective contribution that is practical, creative, enthusiastic, and loving.

Jane Farrell

Acknowledgments

As I finish the second revision of this book, I realize that in the middle of a successful professional life, I have managed with the help of a good and loyal husband, Mike, who became my photographer, to raise three children and maintain a home and marriage. Sheila and Gary were young children and Bill was 15 when they first posed for my photographs. Now Bill is married, Gary is in the U.S. Navy, and Sheila was my chief typist.

In searching for words to write my acknowledgments I also realize I have just found the correct word for everyone: loyal.

I look back through the years and the loyal support of George E. McGuire, M.D., orthopedic surgeon and knee specialist, my friend and mentor, and Carla Cain, R.N., patient care manager and close friend, stands out in my mind. The loyalty, friendship, and support of Daniel R. Smith, President of Bellin Memorial Hospital, and the entire staff have always been invaluable, from top to bottom and corner to corner, Dorothy Martin, manager in surgery, to Dick Esser, manager in central supply. There is Cindy Reinl in the library, Jim Odau in radiology, Fred Monthei in media services across the street, and Lolly Amble in general stores even farther away.

The entire excellent staff in the physical therapy and occupational therapy departments deserve credit for much valuable input through the years. A special "thank you" is in order for Wanda Gindt and Sue Sutrick, both physical therapists, for consulting assignments for this revision.

There are not enough words for the nursing staff on 2 North. Without them, nothing I have ever accomplished in orthopedics would have been possible. I acknowledge the continuing help and moral support of Julie Guilette, my other typist, model, and dearest friend, and the expertise (as my first photographer) of her husband and my friend, Gale Guilette.

The willingness of the orthopedic surgeons to contribute input and to care about me is summed up in a prescription I received with a slide I had requested:

To: Jane Farrell

    Slides as included.
    Use as directed.
    Cheers.

      Rolf S. Lulloff, M.D.

Along with Dr. Lulloff are HA Tressler, RD Horak, WS Mohr, WF Schneider, WD Jones, TG Kempken, JA Hinckley, and MD O'Reilly. They have been friends and colleagues and are special to me. Dr. Kempken, with whom I spent the most time learning, is my family's friend, too. To the neurosurgeons and other physicians who have answered my questions when appropriate, I say "thank you."

Another special "thank you" goes to Connie Korger, Nursing Instructor at Bellin College of Nursing, who served as a sounding board and gave me much-appreciated constructive criticism. My thanks to Ray Gustin at Wisconsin Orthopedic Appliance Company, who posed for my amputee chapter and advised his staff that I was the "girl you don't say no to." Thank you Richard Jubert, of Green Bay Orthopedic Supply Company, and James and Diane Tyo of Tyo and Tyo Ltd., Orthotists. Diane did some work on my scoliosis content. Then there are the many sales representatives from various orthopedic supply companies who supply me with brochures and contacts, especially Max Sherman at Zimmer, for whom I served as an orthopedic nursing consultant.

I wish to extend my gratitude to the health care personnel from all over this country and Canada whom I have met in the past 15 years, who have shared their experiences and expertise with me.

To Diana Intenzo, my editor at the J.B. Lippincott Company, whose help and friendship have become a natural part of my life, I say "thanks." I believe we still have a long way to go together in providing books for health care personnel.

As I have said so many times during my career, I sincerely hope I have forgotten no one.

1

The Orthopedic Patient: Nursing Assessment and Diagnosis

Orthopedic nursing is primarily the care of patients with disorders of the musculoskeletal system. Because these disorders affect body mechanics, it is important for anyone practicing in this specialized field to have an understanding of normal body movement and posture, as well as of the theoretical basis of orthopedic problems. Such a knowledge base is imperative in making intelligent assessments and diagnoses, and in planning effective care. For this reason, Chapter 1 reviews nursing assessment in general, with emphasis on physical assessment of the extremities and the spine. It also presents some guidelines for assessing orthopedic patients in a variety of situations, including the emergency room (ER) and admission to the hospital, and as an ongoing process.

Nursing Assessment: Review and Purpose

Nursing assessment, as the first step in the nursing process, may be defined as the systematic collection of data concerning the patient, gleaned through interview, physical examination, a review of reports and records, and accurate monitoring of responses.

Data are both subjective and objective. *Subjective data* are experienced by the person and, as such, are unique to the individual patient. Feelings of pain fall into this category. *Objective data* refer to those data that can be observed and measured by another person, such as vital signs. Collecting data is a continuous process; it includes the patient, the family, other significant persons, and those responsible for or concerned with the patient's welfare.

The purpose of nursing assessment is to provide the baseline for planning independent and individualized nursing care. An initial assessment results in a tremendous amount of information that must be validated, analyzed, and interpreted to identify patient problems that demand nursing actions. Formal summary statements of these problems are called *nursing diagnoses*.

The nursing diagnosis differs from the medical diagnosis. "Rheumatoid arthritis," for example, is a medical

diagnosis, whereas "frustration related to dependency" is a nursing diagnosis based on an assessment of a patient with rheumatoid arthritis. The medical diagnosis identifies pathology, whereas the nursing diagnosis is designed to identify potential health problems or the patient's responses to an altered health state. Diagnoses of the potential for health problems take into account the physiologic, psychological, and socioeconomic factors related to overall health. For example, a patient who is immobilized for a long time has the potential for alterations in physiologic functions, such as muscle weakness and constipation. This patient may also develop boredom, depression, frustration, and fear. These problems may be caused by lack of diversion, lack of knowledge, or concern over finances, relationships, body image, and lifestyle.

Because assessment is a continuous process, nursing diagnoses change as the patient's problems change or are resolved. Thus, when a patient with rheumatoid arthritis learns how to use adaptive equipment and is preparing for discharge, the nursing diagnosis of "frustration related to dependency" may be inaccurate and a nursing diagnosis of "anxiety over home environment" may become appropriate.

The terms *goal* and *expected outcome* are used interchangeably and identify the basis for evaluating results of nursing intervention. There are nursing goals as well as patient goals.

Making nursing diagnoses requires a balance between knowledge of theory and assessment skills and actual practice. The student or beginning practitioner may be more comfortable with the nursing diagnosis list from the 5th National Conference on the Classification of Nursing Diagnoses (p. 2).* However the process of standardizing nursing diagnoses is still in its infancy. The orthopedic nurse has a professional responsibility to test these diagnoses and formulate new ones.

Physical Assessment of the Extremities and Spine

In nursing, physical assessment of the extremities and spine should be confined to recognizing the normal and describing the abnormal. When describing the abnormal, the nurse should consider

- Pain
- Limitation of motion
- Paresthesia
- Pulses
- Loss of sensation
- Swelling

* The National Group for the Classification of Nursing Diagnosis, which developed this list, is now known as the North American Nursing Diagnosis Association (NANDA).

- Temperature and color (if different in opposite extremities)

In each instance, the description must be as specific as possible.

Methods and Tools of Assessment

The primary methods of assessment include the following:

1. Inspection — looking at the part
2. Palpation — feeling the part
3. Movement and observation of movement
4. Comparison. This is essential when examining the

extremities. *The upper extremities must be compared with each other during all aspects of assessment, as must the lower extremities.* Any discrepancy must be noted carefully.

A *percussion hammer* for testing reflexes is a necessary tool in the physical examination of the extremities. A *safety pin* may also be used to test patient response to stimulus at any point on an extremity. Measuring the circumference or length of an extremity with a *tape measure* may be part of the comparison process. The *goniometer*, which measures the angle of a joint, is a sophisticated tool for determining limitation of movement.

ACCEPTED NURSING DIAGNOSES FROM THE 5th NATIONAL CONFERENCE ON THE CLASSIFICATION OF NURSING DIAGNOSES

Activity intolerance
Airway clearance, Ineffective
Anxiety
Bowel elimination, Alteration in, Constipation
Bowel elimination, Alteration in, Diarrhea
Bowel elimination, Alteration in, Incontinence
Breathing patterns, Ineffective
Cardiac output, Alteration in, Decreased
Comfort, Alteration in, Pain
Communication, Impaired verbal
Coping, Ineffective individual
Coping, Ineffective family, Compromised
Coping, Ineffective family, Disabling
Coping, Family, Potential for growth
Diversional activity deficit
Family processes, Alteration in
Fear (specify)
Fluid volume deficit, Actual
Fluid volume deficit, Potential
Fluid volume excess
Gas exchange, Impaired
Grieving, Anticipatory
Grieving, Dysfunctional
Health maintenance, Alteration in
Home maintenance management, Impaired
Injury, Potential for (specify):
   Poisoning
   Suffocation
   Trauma
Knowledge deficit (specify)
Mobility, Impaired physical
Noncompliance (specify)
Nutrition, Alteration in, Less than body requirements
Nutrition, Alteration in, More than body requirements

Nutrition, Alteration in, Potential for more than body requirements
Oral mucous membrane, Alteration in
Parenting, Alteration in, Actual
Parenting, Alteration in, Potential
Powerlessness
Rape-trauma syndrome
Self-care deficit:
   Total
   Feeding
   Bathing/hygiene
   Dressing/grooming
   Toileting
Self-concept, Disturbance in
Sensory perceptual alteration:
   Visual
   Auditory
   Kinesthetic
   Gustatory
   Tactile
   Olfactory
Sexual dysfunction
Skin integrity, Impairment in, Actual
Skin integrity, Impairment in, Potential
Sleep pattern disturbance
Social isolation
Spiritual distress
Thought processes, Alteration in
Tissue perfusion, Alteration in:
   Cerebral
   Cardiopulmonary
   Renal
   Gastrointestinal
   Peripheral
Urinary elimination, Alteration in patterns of
Violence, Potential for

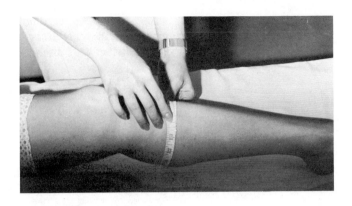

Range-of-Motion Terminology

The following terms are used in describing range of motion in a joint.

Abduction—movement away from the midline of the body

Adduction—movement toward the midline of the body

Flexion—bending a joint

Dorsiflexion—bending the wrist backward, or bending the foot up toward the shin

Plantar flexion—bending the wrist forward, or pushing the foot down away from the front of the leg

Extension—straightening a joint

Hyperextension—extending the joint beyond ordinary range

Rotation—turning around an axis

Internal rotation—turning a part inward toward its center

External rotation—turning a part outward away from its center

Eversion—turning the foot outward toward the little toe

Inversion—turning the foot inward toward the midline of the body

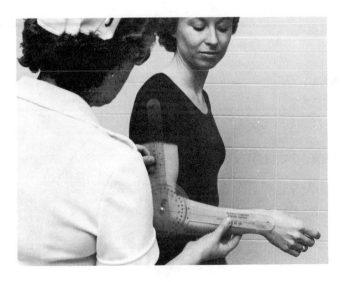

The terms *varus* and *valgus* are used to describe deviations. *Varus* refers to a joint that is angled away from the midline of the body (bowlegs). *Valgus* refers to a joint that is angled toward the midline of the body (knock-knees).

A Guide for Physical Assessment

Physical assessment of the extremities and spine involves activity by the patient and the nurse. One method is described in the illustrated guide on the following pages.

Assessment of Orthopedic Patients: Initial Phase

Orthopedic patients in the hospital may be categorized in two ways: as emergencies or as elective, planned admissions. The *emergency orthopedic patient* is the patient who comes to the emergency department with musculoskeletal trauma and other possible injuries. Such a patient does not necessarily require admission. The *elective orthopedic admission* is admission either of a medical patient, such as one who has arthritis, or of a patient who is about to undergo surgery such as a total hip replacement. In both emergency and routine hospital admissions, a thorough nursing assessment with accurate and detailed documentation is essential in planning and implementing initial nursing care.

THE EMERGENCY ORTHOPEDIC PATIENT

Priority

Any life-threatening condition in the injured patient must be considered before a detailed assessment can be made. Treatment of respiratory, circulatory, or cardiac derangements (such as an obstructed airway, obvious hemorrhage, or cardiac arrest) has priority. Once the emergency-room nurse has established that the patient is "living and breathing," an assessment can be carried out.

Guidelines for Assessment

When there are multiple injuries, a rapid and systematic assessment of the total patient is indicated once any life-threatening situation has been addressed, because the most obvious injury is not always the most serious. This assessment will be facilitated if the patient is undressed. *Each nurse should develop a particular system of assessment and adhere to it* to decrease the chance of overlooking hidden injuries. (See outline for total assessment, pp. 24–26 and sample assessment of orthopedic injury, p. 27.)

Mental Status

Immediate evaluation of the patient's mental status is critical in establishing a basis for determining the significance

(Text continued on p. 24)

ASSESSMENT OF EXTREMITIES AND SPINE

I. Upper Extremities

A. SHOULDER AND UPPER ARM

Position/Patient Activity	Nursing Activity	Description/Action	Describe Discrepancy
1. Standing, arms at sides	Inspect.	Shoulder is rounded in appearance.	
2. Standing, arms at sides	Palpate upper arms and shoulders	Muscle mass is firm in upper arm and shoulder. Clavicle, acromion process, and head of humerus are palpable.	
3. Flex lower arm and contract muscles in upper arm.	Palpate biceps and triceps in both arms.	They should be taut.	
4. Raise arms sideways until they point to ceiling.	Observe.	Abduction	

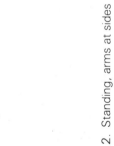
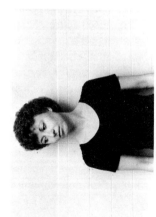
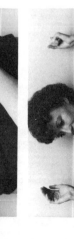
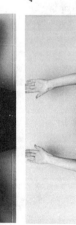
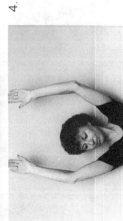

(continued)

5. Cross arms in front of body, touch right shoulder with left hand and left shoulder with right hand.

Observe.

Adduction

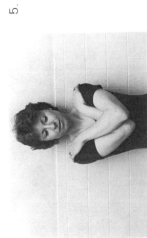

6. Move arms behind body.

Observe.

Internal rotation

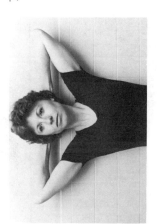

7. Touch the back of the neck while holding elbows well back.

Observe.

External rotation

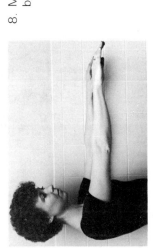

8. Move arms forward and back.

Observe.

Flexion and extension

ASSESSMENT OF EXTREMITIES AND SPINE

A. SHOULDER AND UPPER ARM

	Position/Patient Activity	Nursing Activity	Description/Action	Describe Discrepancy
	9. Move arms forward and back.	Apply resistance.	Any difference in strength should be minimal.	

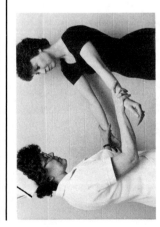

B. ELBOW AND LOWER ARM

	Position/Patient Activity	Nursing Activity	Description/Action	Describe Discrepancy
	1. Arms alongside body, palms forward	Inspect.	Arms should be straight. Contours of lower arm should appear even and taper toward wrist.	
	2. Same as in 1	Palpate.	Muscle groups on lateral, medial aspects of arms are firm, coming to a V-shaped antecubital space at elbow.	
	3. Elbows at right angles	Palpate.	Medial and lateral epicondyles and olecranon process are palpable.	

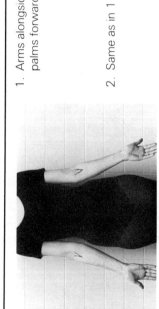

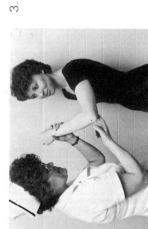

(continued)

4. Hold arms along-side body, palms forward. Bring lower arms up, touch shoulders with palms. Then bring lower arms down straight.	Observe.	Flexion and Extension of elbow
5. With elbows tucked into the sides of the body, flexed to 90 degrees, lower arm should demonstrate a rotary motion at radioulnar joints (elbow and wrist).	Observe.	Supination and pronation of the hand
6. Move lower arms up and down.	Apply resistance to forearms.	Any difference in strength should be minimal.

C. WRIST, HANDS, FINGERS

| 1. Hold arms close to sides with elbows at right angles, palms down. | Inspect. | On back of wrist, styloid process of ulna is visible. |
| 2. Same as in 1 | Palpate. | Styloid processes of radius and ulna are palpable. A radial pulse is obtainable, regular, and can be counted. |

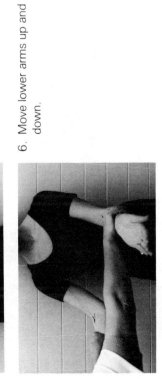
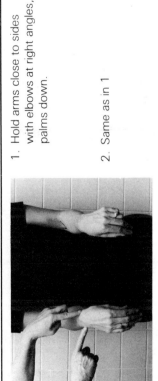

ASSESSMENT OF EXTREMITIES AND SPINE

C. ANKLE AND FOOT

	Position/Patient Activity	Nursing Activity	Description/Action	Describe Discrepancy
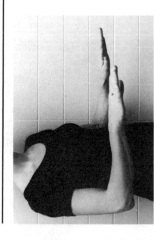	3. Same as in 1. After bending hands down at wrist, straighten them out.	Observe.	Plantar flexion and extension of wrist	
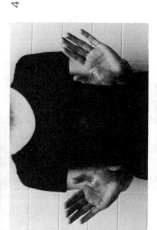	4. Same as in 1. Then bend hands at wrist, back toward body.	Observe.	Dorsiflexion of wrist	
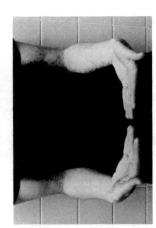	5. Tuck elbows in at waist, at right angles, palms up. At wrists, move hands toward radial (thumb) side; then toward ulnar (little finger) side.	Observe.	Ulnar deviation is more than twice radial deviation.	

(continued)

6. Elbows at right angles, palms down. Bend hands down, then straighten them out.

Apply resistance.

Any difference in strength should be minimal.

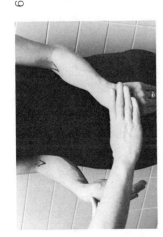

7. Lay hand down, palm up, in a resting, relaxed position.

Inspect.

Each finger is in slightly more flexion than the next, moving from little finger to thumb. Nail beds should be pink in color.

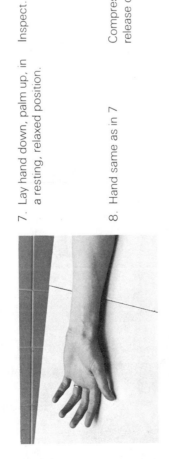

8. Hand same as in 7

Compress each nail and release quickly. Observe.

The blanching sign: as each nail is compressed, it turns white; as it is released, it returns to a pink color immediately.

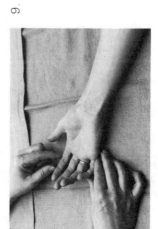

9. Hand same as in 7

Palpate fingers and thumbs.

Interphalangeal joints and metacarpophalangeal joints are palpable.

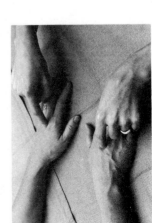

ASSESSMENT OF EXTREMITIES AND SPINE

C. ANKLE AND FOOT

Position/Patient Activity	Nursing Activity	Description/Action	Describe Discrepancy
10. Make tight fists and then open hands completely.	Observe.	Abduction and adduction	
11. Spread fingers wide (including thumb) and then bring them back together.	Observe.	Abduction and adduction	
12. Hold thumb to index finger as if writing with a pencil.	Observe.	*Motor Functions* Pincer action	

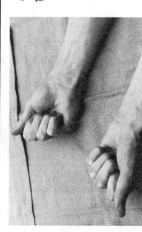

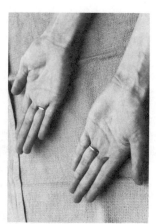

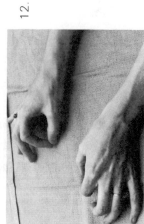

13.	Grasp a finger of the nurse's hand as if holding a hammer.	Observe.	Vise grip
14.	Tap each finger on back of nurse's hand.	Observe.	Movement
15.	Grasp the nurse's two hands tightly in your hands.		Grasps should be equal.

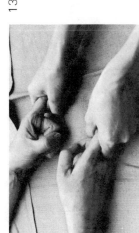
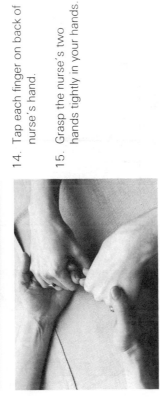

D. REFLEXES, SENSATION, TEMPERATURE, AND COLOR

| 1. | Support patient's lower arm (palm up, elbow flexed) in relaxed position with your arm. Place thumb over biceps tendon and tap thumb with reflex hammer. Observe biceps. | *Biceps Reflex* Biceps muscle should contract. |
| 2. | Holding arm in same position, tap triceps tendon above olecranon process and observe triceps muscle. | *Triceps Reflex* Triceps muscle should contract. |

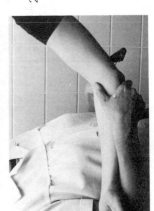
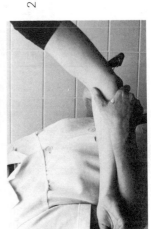

(continued)

ASSESSMENT OF EXTREMITIES AND SPINE

D. REFLEXES, SENSATIONS, TEMPERATURE, AND COLOR

Position/Patient Activity	Nursing Activity	Description/Action	Describe Discrepancy
3.	Hold arm as in 1. Tap styloid process of radius and observe action of forearm.	*Brachoradialis Reflex* Slight flexion of elbow and pronation of forearm	
4.	Prick patient lightly with safety pin on various locations on both upper extremities.	Sensation should be present equally on both.	
5.	With both hands, grasp patient's arms and hands lightly in several locations. Observe color of skin on both extremities.	In general, the skin on both extremities should "feel" the same temperature and be the same color.	

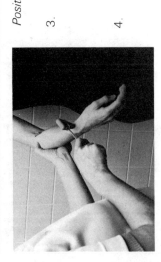

II. Lower Extremities

A. HIP AND THIGH

1. Stand with back to nurse. Lift each leg by flexing hip and knee.	Inspect.	Each hip bears one-half of body weight when in standing position. When one leg is lifted in this manner entire weight of body is transferred through the other leg. This causes trunk to incline toward weight-bearing leg.	
2. Lying on back	Inspect.	Contours of thighs appear smooth and taper to knee.	

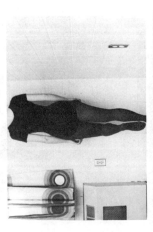

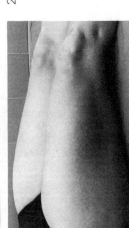

3. Lying on back

Palpate. Anchor thumb against anterior superior iliac spine.

Head of trochanter can be palpated by middle finger.

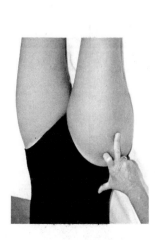

4. Lie on back; press knees down onto bed or table.

Palpate.

Quadriceps should be tightened and firm.

5. Lying relaxed

Palpate.

Femoral pulses are present and regular.

6. Flex each hip, one at a time; hold 5 seconds against abdomen.

Inspect.

As each hip is flexed and held in flexion, the other hip remains in extension.

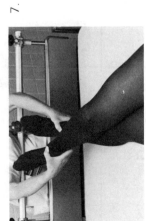

7. Lying on back

Move patient's legs in a scissors motion.

Amount of abduction and adduction should be the same in both hips.

(continued)

ASSESSMENT OF EXTREMITIES AND SPINE

A. HIP AND THIGH

Position/Patient Activity	Nursing Activity	Description/Action	Describe Discrepancy
8. Lying on back	Hold both ankles and turn entire leg inward and then outward.	Internal and external rotation	
9. Lying on abdomen	Inspect.	Gluteal muscles appear firm.	
10. Lying on abdomen; lift one leg at a time.	Observe.	Hip extension should be equal.	

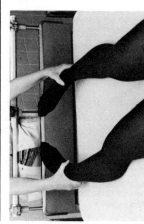
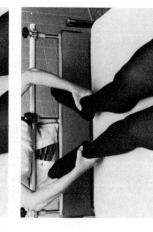
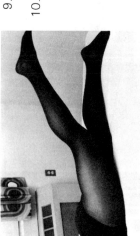

B. KNEE AND LOWER LEG

1. Lying on back, legs flat against a surface.	Inspect.	Lower leg tapers to ankle. Front of knee joint (with patella) appears rounded. Knees meet at medial aspects.	

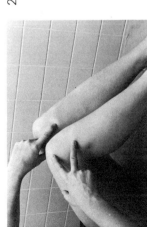

2. Knees in about 90 degrees of flexion

   Palpate.

   Bony prominences, femoral and tibial condyles, joint line, and patella are palpated with thumbs. Anterior tibias are palpable down length of lower legs.

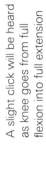

3. Tighten calf muscle on request.

   Palpate.

   Gastrocnemius muscle is taut in both legs.

4. Lying on back, bend knee until muscles in back of leg meet, and then straighten leg.

   Observe and listen.

   A slight click will be heard as knee goes from full flexion into full extension

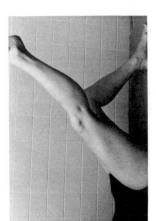

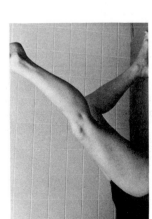

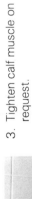

(continued)

[15]

ASSESSMENT OF EXTREMITIES AND SPINE

B. KNEE AND LOWER LEG

Position/Patient Activity	Nursing Activity	Description/Action	Describe Discrepancy
5. Lying on back, knees straight	With one hand steadying the knee, and in various degrees of flexion, move lower leg inward and outward.	Internal and external rotation	
6. Flex hips 45 degrees and knees 90 degrees.	Stabilize patient by sitting on the feet and with both hands attempt to move tibia backwards and forwards.	Movement should be absent, signifying stable cruciates.	
7. Lying, knees flat	Flex knee with one hand, and push patella laterally with the other hand.	Patient should not resist this movement (apprehension test).	
8. Lying, knees flat	Hold lower leg by the foot; place one hand behind knee and attempt lateral movements.	No abduction or adduction should be possible.	

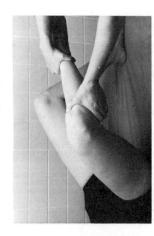
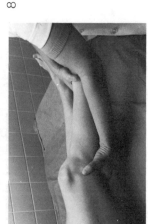

9. Flex and extend knees.

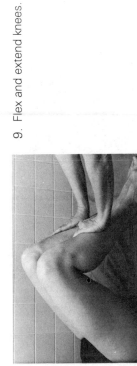

Apply resistance.

Any difference in strength should be minimal.

C. ANKLE AND FOOT

1. Standing

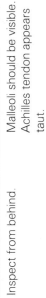

Inspect from behind.

Malleoli should be visible. Achilles tendon appears taut.

2. Standing

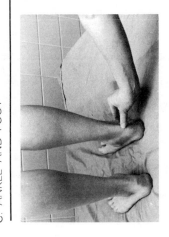

Inspect from the front.

The toes become shorter in length from great toe to fifth toe. Nail beds are pink.

3. Lying on back

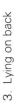

Compress each nail; release quickly and observe.

Blanching sign: as each nail is compressed it turns white, and as pressure is released it becomes pink again immediately.

(continued)

ASSESSMENT OF EXTREMITIES AND SPINE

C. ANKLE AND FOOT

Position/Patient Activity	Nursing Activity	Description/Action	Describe Discrepancy
4. Lying on back	Palpate.	The malleoli are palpable. Achilles tendon is firm. Dorsalis pedis pulse and tibial pulse are present and regular.	
5. Bend foot up toward shin and then down toward bed or table.	Observe.	Dorsiflexion and plantar flexion	
6. Turn the feet outward and then inward.	Observe.	Inversion and eversion should be equal.	

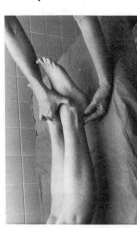

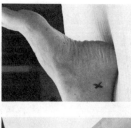

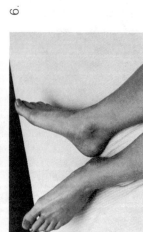

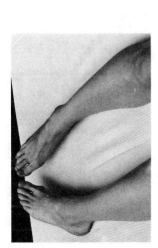

7. Lying on back   Palpate toes.   Metatarsophalangeal and interphalangeal joints are palpable.

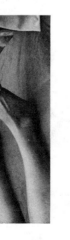

8. Move toes back and forth.   Observe.   Flexion and extension

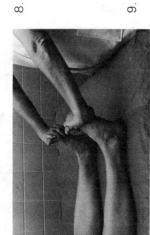

9. Bend feet up and then down.   Apply resistance.   Any difference in strength should be minimal.

D. REFLEXES, SENSATION, TEMPERATURE, AND COLOR

1. Lying on abdomen   Stroke skin in gluteal area.   *Superficial Reflex*
Skin becomes taut.

(continued)

ASSESSMENT OF EXTREMITIES AND SPINE

D. REFLEXES, SENSATIONS, TEMPERATURE, AND COLOR

Position/Patient Activity	Nursing Activity	Description/Action	Describe Discrepancy
2. Sitting on edge of bed or table, feet not touching floor	Tap patellar tendon with reflex hammer and observe.	*Patellar Reflex* Extension of knee	
3. Sitting as in 2	Tap Achilles tendon with reflex hammer and observe.	*Achilles Reflex* Plantar flexion of foot	
4. Sitting as in 2	Stroke plantar surface of foot.	*Superficial Reflex, Plantar* Toes will flex.	
5. Sitting as in 2	Prick patient lightly with safety pin on various locations on both lower extremities.	Sensation should be present equally on both.	

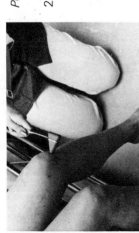

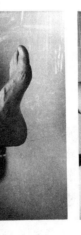

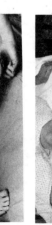

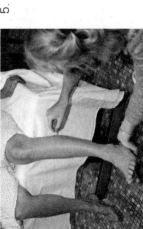

6. Sitting on edge of bed or table, feet not touching floor.

With both hands, grasp patient's legs and feet lightly in several locations. Observe color of skin on both extremities.

In general, skin on both extremities should "feel" the same temperature and be the same color.

III. Gait and Motion of the Spine

A. STANDING AND WALKING

1. Stand on both tiptoes, then on heels.

Observe.

Patient is standing evenly on toes and then on heels.

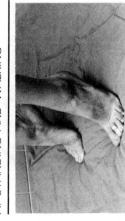

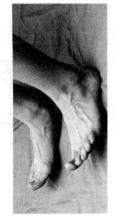

2. Walk straight ahead.

Observe.

Toes point straight ahead and weight appears to be taken equally, first on heels and then on balls of feet. Shoulders are straight across.

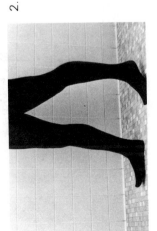

(continued)

ASSESSMENT OF EXTREMITIES AND SPINE

B. MOTION: HEAD, NECK, AND TRUNK

Position/Patient Activity	Nursing Activity	Description/Action	Describe Discrepancy
1. Standing, bend head forward	Observe.	Head and neck flexion, chin touching chest	
2. Hold head straight.	Observe.	Extension of head and neck.	
3. Bend head backward.	Observe.	Hyperextension, head and neck	
4. Bend head to right side, ear to shoulder; then to left side.	Observe.	Lateral flexion of head	

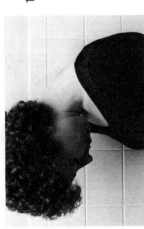

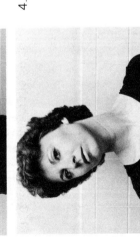

5. Turn head to look over right shoulder, then over left shoulder.

Observe.

Rotation of head

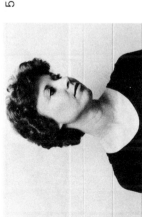

6. Bend forward from waist.

Observe

Flexion of trunk

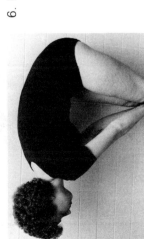

7. Stand with trunk straight.

Observe.

Extension of trunk

8. Bend backward from waist.

Observe.

Hyperextension of trunk

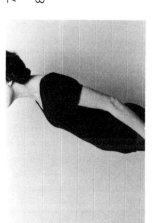

9. Bend sideways from waist, to right and left.

Observe.

Lateral trunk flexion

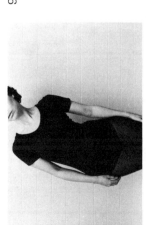

of later responses. Any evidence of drug or alcohol ingestion should be noted at this point, along with reference to medical history that may contribute to mental aberration.

Head, Neck, and Torso

Assessment of the head, neck, and torso should be the next consideration. Fractures of the ribs and pelvis are often associated with serious internal injuries. Vertebral fractures frequently mean spinal-cord injury and must be detected in early assessment.

Once the nurse has established the fact that there is no other serious trauma, attention can be paid to any injured extremity and a more comprehensive examination can be carried out.

Obviously, every patient who is brought into the emergency room with an orthopedic injury does not require total assessment. In each instance, assessment is based on the circumstances surrounding the accident. Therefore, whenever possible the nurse should know the history of the accident and the mechanism of injury before beginning any examination. Since the emergency patient experiences a certain degree of apprehension and fear, it is imperative to explain the procedures that are being carried out and to implement the assessment in as careful a manner as possible.

The Injured Extremity

The assessment of an injured extremity involves the following steps:

1. Observe the type of bleeding that is present.
   - Arterial blood spurts.
   - Venous bleeding is steady.
   - Blood from a bone oozes and is oily.
2. At this point it may be necessary to apply direct pressure to bleeding areas.
   - If bleeding persists, apply direct pressure over the main artery (*i.e.*, the brachial artery in the upper extremity and the femoral artery in the lower extremity).
3. Check for apparent deformities, such as unusual "bends" and "bumps" in the bone, because these are signs of fracture or dislocation.
   - Deformity near a joint, accompanied by inability to move the extremity, is a sign of a dislocation. *Dislocations are always considered emergencies* because of the tension on or compression of nerves and blood vessels; they need immediate medical attention.
4. Carefully examine the distal end of the extremity

(Text continued on p. 27)

OUTLINE FOR TOTAL ASSESSMENT

I. *Head and Neck*
  A. Level of consciousness: an index of neurologic status
    1. Does the patient open his eyes
      - Spontaneously?
      - In response to speech?
      - In response to painful stimuli?
    2. Verbal response: is the patient
      - Oriented to time and place?
      - Disoriented but able to converse appropriately?
      - Inappropriate in response?
      - Incomprehensible?
      - Incapable of any verbal response?
    3. Motor response
      - Can the patient obey a command?
      - What is his response to a painful stimulus?
  B. Head
    1. Palpate and examine scalp for lacerations, tenderness, and depressed fractures.
    2. Examine ear canals and nose for any drainage and record whether it is clear or bloody.
    3. Examine the eyes for periorbital bruising or obvious fracture of the orbital rim, position, and pupil size.
    4. Smell the patient's breath for evidence of odors.
    5. Palpate and move the mandible for flail.
    6. Observe for expectoration or vomiting and describe.
    7. Examine mouth for dentures, missing or broken teeth.

OUTLINE FOR TOTAL ASSESSMENT *(continued)*

C. Neck
  1. Examine trachea for displacement, movement, and crepitus.
  2. Palpate carotid pulses.

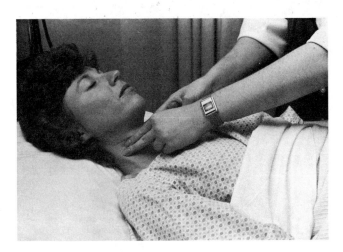

  3. Check for neck vein distention.
  4. When checking the back of the neck, assume that the patient has a cervical spine injury until proven otherwise in all head injuries, motor vehicle accidents, diving accidents, and falls. If the patient is conscious, gently palpate the back of the neck for any tenderness.

II. *Chest*
  A. Observe for difficulties in breathing.
  B. Examine the chest for external signs of trauma, such as sucking wounds or rib deformities.
  C. Percuss and auscultate the chest wall for signs of fluid, decreased aeration, hyperresonance, or asymmetry.

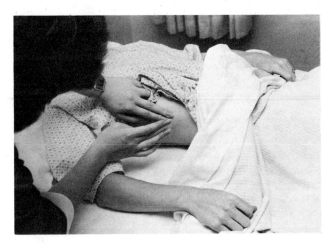

  D. Do heart-sound auscultation for changes in rhythm.
III. *Abdomen*
  A. Inspect abdomen for swelling, ecchymosis, or open wounds.
  B. Palpate all quadrants for tenderness or distention.

OUTLINE FOR TOTAL ASSESSMENT *(continued)*

    C. Auscultate bowel sounds.

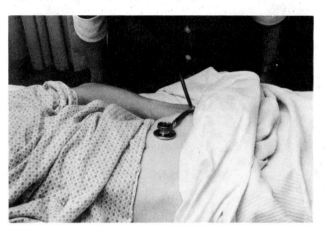

 IV. *Pelvis*
    A. Patients with pelvic fractures may bleed into the retroperitoneal area. Consider this as cause of undiagnosed shock.
    B. Palpate iliac crest. Check for movement or pain on one side.

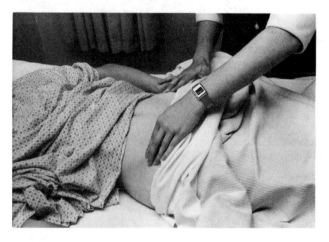

    C. Assess for bruising in flank area.
    D. Consider bladder injury with pelvic trauma.
  V. *Extremities*
    A. Inspect each extremity for visible deformities indicative of fracture or dislocation.
    B. Take joints through range of motion only if there is no evidence of fracture or dislocation.
    C. Assess neurovascular (NV) function of each finger and toe.
       1. Color
       2. Temperature
       3. Motion
       4. Sensation
    D. Determine if patient can move and feel each extremity.
       1. Suspect nerve damage with lack of sensation only.
       2. Suspect spinal-cord injury if patient can neither move nor feel the extremity.
    E. Compare extremities.
 VI. *Thoracic and Lumbosacral Spine* — Log-roll patient and palpate thoracic and lumbosacral spine.
VII. *Blood Pressure* — Check the blood pressure last.

SAMPLE ASSESSMENT: ORTHOPEDIC INJURY

Reason for Admission

10:30 A.M.: 22-year-old female patient admitted from emergency room per wheelchair. States she was in a car accident on way to work at bank. Skidded into back of a parked car. Was wearing a seatbelt loosely around waist. Hit both knees on "something" when she went forward. Also fell onto steering wheel on chest and face. Did not lose consciousness. Was seen by ER physician and had x-ray films of both knees. Given codeine gr i.

Initial Assessment

1. Pupils equal, react to light. States she was never unconscious.
2. No drainage from eyes, ears, nose.
3. Has small abrasion across bridge of nose. Says it "smarts."
4. No complaints of headache.
5. No other marks noted on head, neck, or face.
6. No problem swallowing or speaking. Teeth intact.
7. Respirations 16-regular.
8. Points to sternum as area of chest she "may have hit on steering wheel."
9. No marks on chest and has no pain in sternum unless pressure is applied.
10. Breath sounds normal on auscultation.
11. Complaints of tenderness mid to lower abdomen: no abrasions or contusions noted.
12. Bowel sounds present. Abdomen firm, flat. Unable to void at present.
13. Upper extremity and spinal exam normal.
14. Lower extremities: small abrasion across right knee. Right knee moderately swollen when compared to left. Complains of aching in both knees, more severe in right. Left knee does not appear swollen. Can flex and extend left knee. Right knee in about 20 degrees of flexion, states she cannot extend it without severe pain.
15. Color, motion, temperature, sensation (CMTS) both feet satisfactory and equal.
16. Pedal pulses present, strong, and equal.
17. Slightly tearful, states it was her "brand new car."

Immediate Intervention

1. Bed rest
2. Elevate both legs and apply ice to both knees.
3. Keep NPO until seen by own MD. Explain to patient this is routine until MD decides what medical treatment is necessary.
4. Inform staff to check color and measure urine when patient voids.
5. Evaluate effect of narcotics.

Priorities in First Reassessment

   12 noon

1–6. Inspect face and neck for developing bruises or swelling. Ask the following:
   - Do you have any headache or neck pain now?
   - Can you still swallow without difficulty?
   Examine abrasion on nose for drainage.
   Check pupils and level of consciousness.

7–10. Examine sternum for developing bruises or other marks. Palpate gently. Ask the following questions:
   - Is this more or less painful than before? Where?
   - Do you have any other pain in your chest or any difficulty breathing?
   Check respirations.

11–12. Examine mid to lower abdomen and palpate. Ask these questions:
   - Does this feel more tender or any different than before? Where?
   - Have you used the bedpan? If not, will you try now?

14–16. Evaluate NV status of both feet and compare with each other and with previous findings. Inspect both knees. Evaluate swelling, discoloration and compare with previous findings. Ask the following:
   - Will you describe the pain in your knees now?
   - Can you move your left leg as before?
   - Will you try, carefully, to move your right lower leg?
   Check abrasion on knee for evidence of drainage.

17. Assess emotional state.

---

that is fractured or has a dislocated joint for signs of neurovascular disturbance.
- Recheck the color, motion, temperature, and sensation (CMTS) of each toe or finger and *compare with that of the opposite extremity.*

- Compress each toenail or fingernail and release it quickly. The nail should become white as it is compressed and should return immediately to a pink color as pressure is released. This is the *blanching sign* and a test of capillary filling.

5. Check the pulses and note presence and quality or absence.
   - On the upper extremity, check the brachial, radial, and ulnar pulses.
   - On the lower extremity, assess the femoral, popliteal, tibial, and dorsalis pedis pulses.
   - Compare affected with unaffected extremity.
6. Carefully note the overall color of the hand or foot on an injured extremity and then compare it with that of the opposite extremity.
   - A white hand or foot indicates inadequate arterial blood flow, whereas one that is bluish has a problem with venous return.
7. Examine the injured extremity for swelling and bruises.
8. Look for open wounds and abrasions. If any are present, note the extent and cover them with sterile dressings.
9. Ask the patient to describe the type of feeling present in the injured extremity.
   - Is it burning, tingling, prickling?
   - If the patient complains of numbness, be certain he does not mean *cold.*
10. Ask the patient to describe feelings of pain and whether or not pain is increased or decreased upon movement.
    - It is important to remember that dressings, bandages, or makeshift splints that have been applied hastily at the time of injury may be the cause of pain. For this reason, and to facilitate assessment, such applications should be removed.
    - When splints and bandages are removed, the extremity must be supported until treatment is begun.
11. Elevate and support all injured extremities.

CLOSER ASSESSMENT OF THE SURROUNDING ANATOMY

Since the forces required to produce skeletal injury are often violent enough to cause damage to the surrounding structures and soft tissue, the nurse must make frequent assessments of such areas. This is particularly important in the case of a fractured femur or pelvis, with which internal bleeding may occur to such an extent that shock is the result.

- When multiple fractures are present, observations for signs of internal injuries and hidden hemorrhage must continue for at least 48 hours.

When trauma patients are taken to the x-ray department, the nurse is responsible for telling the technologist what observations are ongoing and crucial. For example, if the patient has a fractured hip or pelvis, the x-ray technologist should be asked to watch for signs of shock and abdominal distention.

Documentation

All data collected on initial assessment of the emergency orthopedic patient must be recorded accurately in every detail. Not only is this critical in terms of planning treatment and care and evaluating results, but it is also critical from a legal standpoint.

Important points to remember in documentation are as follows:

1. Record time of observations and actions accurately and frequently.
2. When recording the description of injury or mechanism of injury, do not draw conclusions that may have legal implications. For example, in describing gunshot wounds, the nurse should not differentiate between where the missile entered the extremity and where it exited.
3. Whenever possible, use the patient's own account of exactly what happened and how he is feeling.

THE ELECTIVE ADMISSION

The procedure and forms that are used in the nursing assessment of any patient should reflect a holistic approach. That is, the patient should be viewed as a biological, psychological, social, and spiritual being. Therefore, the orthopedic patient who enters the hospital for surgery or other treatment must be interviewed for the purpose of collecting data in the following areas:

1. History of present condition (reason for admission)
2. General health status
3. Family history
4. Patient profile
5. Mental and emotional status
6. Social history and observations
7. Spiritual considerations

A thorough examination of the involved extremity or body part is an assessment priority and is based on the information presented in the preceding sections. A systems review, with emphasis on examination of those areas in which problems are identified, is a minimal requirement of the admission procedure.

GUIDELINES FOR AN ADMISSION INTERVIEW

Once the patient has been settled in his surroundings and the "routine admission" procedure completed, data collection can begin. (See sample orthopedic admission data base charts pp. 29–32.)

(Text continued on p. 33)

ORTHOPEDIC ADMISSION DATA BASE

Louise Smith
Age: 55   Married
Religion: Catholic

Date _5/6/86_ Time _4_ AM/(PM) Mode of admission _Ambulatory_
Ht (Stated/Actual) _5'2"_ Stated Wt _____ Hospital scale weight _160_
T–P–R _98 76 16_ B/P _140/86_ UA _X_ Chest x-ray _X_ CBC _X_
Identiband on: Yes _X_ No _____ General consent form signed: Yes _____ No _____
Oriented to:

Electric bed _X_	A. Cafeteria hours for visitors _X_
Beside console _X_	B. Placing local/long-distance calls _X_
TV _X_	C. Visiting hours. _X_
Patient ed. (Channel 7) _X_	D. Children's visiting (if appropriate) _X_
Smoking regulations _X_	E. Newspapers _X_
Smoker _No_	F. Check-out time _X_
	G. Dentures _None_
	H. Glasses _Yes_
	I. Prosthesis _No_

Description and disposition of valuables (be specific) _None—sent money home with husband_

Completed by: _R. Nelson, LPN_

TO BE COMPLETED BY REGISTERED NURSE:

1. Information obtained from _patient_
2. Reason for admission _painful right hip—may have surgery_
3. History of present condition _States she has been having pain in her rt. hip for past 3 years. Fell down flight of stairs almost 4 years ago. At that time had bruises on both hips and buttocks. Pain worse after walking any distance. Sometimes wakes up with pain at night._

4. Other health problems (include history of surgeries and other medical problems, like diabetes, hypertension, etc.)
   Ovarian cyst removed 1980
   T & A and appendectomy when a "child"
   Gallbladder x-ray films 2 years ago were negative
   Has "stomach spasms when nervous"

5. Family history of health problems _Mother died of Ca. larnyx 10 years ago._
   Father living and well. Sister died at 28 Ca. of spine.

6. Medications: Collected _X_ Not collected _____

Name	Dosage Frequency	Reason for Taking	Last Dose
Donnatol	tab ii p.r.n.	when "stomach spasms starts"	2 days ago
ASA	tab ii p.r.n.	for hip pain	last night

(Continued)

ORTHOPEDIC ADMISSION DATA BASE   *(continued)*

7. Allergies, include food intolerances (describe symptoms)_____
   Intolerence to fatty foods
   "Feels full"

   Allergy band on ___*X*___   Chart/Kardex labeled for allergy   *X*_____

8. Patient profile of activities of daily living (ADL)
   A. Current diet and meal schedule _*Low fat*_____
   B. Hygiene _*Showers daily about noon*_____
   C. Ambulation _*Slight limp on right*_____
   D. Sleep pattern_*6 – 7 hours — watches TV late*_____
   E. Bladder health_*No problem*_____
   F. Bowel habits_*Regular*_____

9. Will your family (close person) be able to visit you? _*Yes*_____
   If no, explain._____

10. Mental/emotional state (briefly state patient's social history)
    This patient is pleasant, cooperative, but expresses some anxiety about possibility of surgery on hip. "I hope surgery
    won't be necessary." She is not employed. She has a married daughter who lives 20 miles from town, plus 2 sons,
    age 15 to 19, at home. The 19-year-old works 4 – 9 P.M. as a carryout boy in supermarket and goes to the university. Her
    husband works 3 – 11 P.M. at the papermill. She plays bridge one night a week, watches a lot of TV, and reads "some."
    She also knits and crochets.

R.N. Signature: ___*J. Doe, R.N.*_____

REVIEW OF SYSTEMS

Skin	
_____ Dryness	
_____ Eruptions	
_____ Pruritus	
_____ Decubiti	
_____ Jaundice	__*X*__ No apparent abnormalities

Head/Neck	
__*X*__ Impairment in seeing *Has glasses*	
_____ Impairment in hearing	
_____ Nasal bleeding	
_____ Ear drainage	
_____ Mouth lesions	
_____ Hoarseness	
_____ Throat soreness	
_____ Difficulty swallowing	
_____ Neck pain	
_____ Neck swelling	_____ No apparent abnormalities

Cardiorespiratory	
_____ Chest pain	
_____ Palpitations	
_____ Dyspnea	
_____ Leg edema	
_____ Orthopnea	
_____ Cough	
_____ Hemoptysis	
_____ Rales	
_____ Paroxysmal nocturnal dyspnea	
_____ Sleeps with more than one pillow or in a chair	__*X*__ No apparent abnormalities

Gastrointestinal/ Nutritional	Amount of weight loss (5 — 10 — 15 — 20 — 25 — 30 + — pounds)*(circle one)* Within the last week — month — 3 months — 6 months *(circle one)* Reasons for weight loss or possible poor nutritional status (be specific as to duration and severity): _____ Lack of appetite _____ Increased appetite __*X*__ Food intolerances and allergies *"full" feeling from fatty foods* _____ Vomiting _____ Nausea __*X*__ Abdominal pain *gastric — stomach spasms when nervous or excited* _____ Diarrhea _____ Constipation __*X*__ Alcohol consumption (describe quantity and frequency) *occasional gin and sour* _____ No apparent abnormalities
Circulatory/ Hematologic	_____ Abnormal color of extremities _____ Bleeding tendencies _____ Petechiae _____ Bruises _____ Pallor _____ Varicose veins __*X*__ No apparent abnormalities
Genito- Urinary	_____ Change in frequency _____ Nocturia _____ Dysuria _____ Hematuria _____ Incontinence __*X*__ No apparent abnormalities
Reproductive Female	_____ Vaginal discharge _____ Bleeding between periods _____ Breast abnormalities _____ Irregular periods Last menstrual period _____ Last Pap smear results *1 year ago, negative* Last self-breast exam (SBE) *doesn't do* SBE teaching pamphlet given *X* Instructed to watch SBE on Channel 7 *X* _____ No apparent abnormalities
Reproductive Male	_____ Penile discharge _____ Lesion _____ Testicular pain _____ Testicular swelling _____ No apparent abnormalities
Musculoskeletal	__*X*__ CMTS *both feet — satisfactory and equal* __*X*__ Deformities *cannot abduct rt. hip as far as lt. without pain* *rt.hip* Joint pain or stiffness *see (3) first page* _____ Growths _____ Fractures _____ Muscle pain or cramps *denies* Arthritis *knowledge* _____ No apparent abnormalities *in upper extremities*

REVIEW OF SYSTEMS *(continued)*

Neurologic	_____ Weakness _____ Spasms __X__ Change in gait *has a slight limp "when tired"—favors rt. side* _____ Loss of sensation _____ Fainting _____ Headaches _____ Seizures _____ Vertigo	_____ No apparent abnormalities
Endocrine	_____ Enlarged thyroid _____ Polyuria _____ Polydipsia _____ Polyphagia _____ Hirsutism	__X__ No apparent abnormalities

Signature __*J. Doe, R.N.*_____

NURSING DIAGNOSES

1. Alteration in comfort: pain, related to hip pathology
2. Anxiety, related to possible surgery
3. Potential stomach discomfort, related to anxiety
4. Knowledge deficit, SBE
5. Potential disturbance in self-concept, related to obesity

NURSING ORDERS/INTERVENTIONS

1. Back care q 3 hr while awake
2. Investigate patient's H.S. routine and follow as much as possible.
3. Offer ASA q 3–4 hr.
4. Assess patient's knowledge of her hip pathology and her understanding of what the surgeon has told her about possible surgery or treatment. Clarify p.r.n.
5. Encourage patient to verbalize feelings about self, condition, and the effect her hospitalization may have on youngest son who will be home alone evenings.
6. Identify other potential causes of anxiety.
7. Discuss SBE film after patient has seen it.
8. Assess needs relative to further cancer teaching.
9. Ask dietitian to see patient about low-fat diet as well as to explore patient's feelings about a weight-reduction diet.

PATIENT GOALS*

1. Hip pain not increased and fairly well controlled with medications and nursing measures
2. Sleeping well most of night
3. Understands hip pathology and possible treatments
4. Can do breast self-examination
5. "Comfortable stomach"

* Patient goals are formulated with patient. Additional goals may be added as patient and nurse identify needs. Nursing goals may be desirable after the nurse has carried out initial interventions. For example, after the dietitian has seen the patient, the nurse may want to help the patient make a decision about a weight-reduction diet. Assessment of learning needs regarding cancer may result in a goal that might be stated: "Patient can list warning signs of cancer."

History of Present Condition

What is the reason for admission? Careful attention to how the patient talks about the problem offers clues to his feelings and fears about hospitalization. The patient who has "put off" a total hip replacement for 6 months after having visited an orthopedic surgeon has had ample time to think about every possible outcome. Now that a decision has been made, the immediate need may be emotional support. The history, therefore, provides the nurse with a baseline for establishing rapport that will help in using the nursing process effectively.

General Health Status

Specific details must be recorded in answer to these questions:

- Does the patient have any chronic disease?
- What is the medical history?
- Is the patient on medications?
- Does he have any allergies?

Such information is vital for the nurse in planning actions to help the patient maintain or improve his general health, to identify instructional needs, and to prevent complications.

An overweight diabetic may need some instruction about diet and eating habits. The patient who has undergone a vein stripping and has contracted pneumonia in the last year is more prone to pulmonary embolism than the patient who has been active and in good health. Therefore, the nursing-care plan includes observations for signs of respiratory distress and thrombophlebitis.

Family History

The most significant data from the family medical history are those that might affect the patient's physical or emotional well-being while he is hospitalized. A 36-year-old male patient who enters the hospital to have knee surgery informs the nurse during his admission interview that his father died of a "heart attack" when he was 39. The nurse must ask this patient if he has concerns about his own cardiac status and make him aware of the available instructional material about maintaining a healthy heart.

Patient Profile

The extent to which patient care is individualized to take account of unique needs partly depends on the completeness of the information contained in the patient profile. Nursing problems are often resolved by referring to and using the data that describe the patient as a person. For example, the patient who is not very responsive to or cooperative during a daily assessment at 8 A.M. may be accustomed to sleeping late in the morning. This fact, along with information about his eating patterns, hygiene routines, and use of glasses, hearing aid, or dentures, should be part of his patient pro-

file. Vital statistics and vital signs are also noted in this section of an admission interview. In the assessment of the elderly patient, the nurse must obtain specific information on bowel and bladder habits. Along with the more obvious advantages of having this information, it will be easier to differentiate, in the postoperative patient, retention with overflow from frequent voiding in small amounts.

Mental/Emotional State

An observation should be made about the patient's orientation and mental acuity. Beyond that, the nurse must be careful in describing this aspect of patient behavior in order to avoid the pitfall of labeling the patient. A patient who is described as "uncooperative" may in fact be fearful. Validation of emotional states aids the planning of supportive care.

Many factors besides the medical condition influence the mental and emotional state of the newly admitted patient. These include the reason for admission, past experience in the hospital, and first impressions of the hospital staff.

Social History and Observations

Where and with whom the patient resides becomes important in communicating information about his care and ultimate discharge. At the same time, the nurse can acquire insights into how the patient feels about himself if she explores how he feels about his occupation or how he spends his time.

Information about hobbies and interests is useful in planning diversion and giving supportive care. The long-term traction patient who likes sports but not television or reading will become bored very fast. This fact should be considered in the patient's initial-care plan even though he is in too much discomfort to be concerned about diversion, because it will take some time and effort to find activities that are acceptable to him.

The nurse should observe interactions between the patient and the person who accompanied him to the hospital, in order to learn more about the way he relates to others. A patient who allows his wife to answer every question for him may need encouragement to ask for what he needs when he is in a dependent state.

Spiritual Considerations

As far as spiritual needs are concerned, religious affiliation is usually noted on the admission sheet. The nurse's responsibility during the interview is to acquaint the patient with the services available in the hospital and the type of outside spiritual support that may be obtained.

Orthopedic Assessment

The extent of physical assessment performed by the nurse is determined by nursing service policies within an institution. However, the section on methods of examining an injured extremity (p. 24) and the outline for physical assessment of the extremities and spine (p. 4) present guidelines for total orthopedic nursing assessment. In general, the following data are considered part of the baseline for assessing the medical or surgical problem of the orthopedic patient.

1. *Location and type of pain.* All descriptions of pain are recorded in the patient's own words. Factors that precipitate pain, such as body position or activity, are included.
2. *Weakness.* Comparison of extremities is helpful when describing weakness.
3. *Paresthesias.* The exact location of any numbness, tingling, or prickling must be determined.
4. *Limitation of motion.* The patient should be asked to demonstrate any limitations of movement in the affected extremity and to show movement in the opposite extremity for comparison. When the patient has a

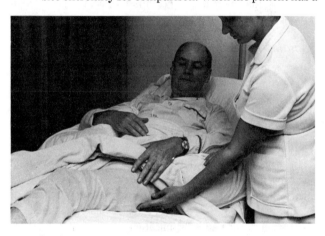

back problem, the nurse can go through movements such as forward bending with the patient or estimate the degree to which the patient can move.

5. *Appearance.* Visible evidence of the condition or disease must be noted.
6. *Ambulation.* The nurse should describe the patient's gait and mention the use of any assistive devices.
7. *Neurovascular status.* Each digit on the hand or foot of an affected extremity must be assessed for color, motion, temperature, and sensation and then compared with that of the unaffected extremity. Pulses in the extremities should be taken, compared, and recorded.

Validation of Observations

When data are collected, the observations should be validated while the assessment is in progress. One way to do this is to clarify and repeat the patient's statements with one's own observations. It is also important to phrase questions so as to uncover pertinent information missed by the patient. Patients often feel that some data are unimportant

because they "happened so long ago." For example, a 65-year-old female patient may not mention that she had thrombophlebitis with every pregnancy. Yet such information is vital in planning nursing care for such a patient. The emotional impact of hospitalization may also affect the patient's ability to recall facts that could be very important. Therefore, allowing the patient ample time to relax, think, and answer questions, and then reviewing the entire assessment with the patient, is invaluable.

As a final step in compiling the data base, the nurse should confer with a family member or significant other person to obtain additional pertinent information. Obviously, there are times when the patient may have difficulty in communicating because of an impaired mental status or a visual, hearing, or speech impairment. Then, too, the patient may neglect to mention such things as common afflictions because they are not "serious." Yet a recent case of influenza or an upper-respiratory infection may leave residual effects, such as a tendency to tire easily, that could affect the patient's rehabilitation and puzzle the surgeon, the nursing staff, and the physical therapist.

Sometimes another person may contribute information that the patient is reluctant to provide—information that can be very significant in terms of evaluating treatment and planning care. For instance, an active, independent 73-year-old woman is admitted to the hospital to have a bunionectomy. She is accompanied by her granddaughter who tells the nurse when she leaves that her grandmother "throws up every time she gets nervous, which is a lot!" The nursing implications are clear. The first action should be to analyze the information obtained in the initial assessment to determine if the grandmother has mentioned this problem. Perhaps the patient will verify the fact that she has a "nervous stomach" if the nurse spends a few extra minutes establishing rapport. At any rate, because vomiting due to nervousness has been identified as a potential problem, the nurse will want to prepare the patient psychologically for surgery as soon as possible to relieve any anxiety she may be experiencing.

ONGOING ASSESSMENT OF THE ORTHOPEDIC PATIENT

The first nursing reassessment of the newly admitted orthopedic patient may take place in minutes or hours, depending on the condition of the patient and the situation. There are times, shortly after admitting the patient, when the nurse may want to go back and reaffirm an observation. For example, a patient who is admitted with back pain appears to have great difficulty in getting out of the chair. He is also slow in moving and grimaces when he gets into bed. His behavior seems to verify his complaint of severe pain, and the nurse notes this observation at the admission interview.

However, shortly after admission and before any treatment has been started, a team member tells the nurse that the patient is asking to visit a friend on another floor. Clearly some reassessment is necessary.

When pain medications are administered or some form of treatment, such as traction, is initiated on a newly admitted patient, the nurse should evaluate the results within 1 hour.

General Factors in Reassessment of the Preoperative Patient

Patients forget what they have been taught just as quickly as any other learners. For this reason, the nurse who sees the patient shortly before surgery should evaluate what the patient has retained in the way of instruction about postoperative routines, the scheduled operative procedure, and any tests that may have been ordered.

The results of laboratory tests must be checked as soon as they are completed, and appropriate assessments and actions must be taken when there are abnormalities. For instance, an elevated leukocyte count may be indication of infection. The nurse should begin by rechecking the data base to note whether the patient has reported any recent illnesses. Then the nurse should question the patient about minor symptoms that he may have neglected to mention, such as a "slight sore throat." Urinary frequency is associated with anxiety. Therefore, the patient who is having this symptom may consider it normal when it could be an early sign of infection. The urinalysis on such a patient may show a moderate amount of bacteria and white blood cells. In this instance, the nurse needs to collect more data and notify the surgeon immediately in the event that surgery has to be postponed.

In the instance of a patient with an electrolyte imbalance, an intravenous solution with potassium may need to be started before surgery. On the other hand, a patient who has an elevated triglyceride level would be a candidate for further medical evaluation after his ankle has been fused.

The orthopedic nurse should know what labortory findings are compatible with the patient's orthopedic problem. Table 1-1 lists laboratory values that may be increased or decreased in certain orthopedic disorders and diseases. Specific tests that frequently are ordered to aid in the diagnosis of specific diseases are discussed in Chapter 10.

The effects of drug therapy must also be taken into consideration when evaluating the results of laboratory studies. For example, aspirin in large doses, a common treatment for arthritis, increases the prothrombin time.

The nurse who understands the significance of laboratory test results can identify priorities when reporting to the physician. In all cases, the physician correlates laboratory findings with the results of other diagnostic tests and clinical signs and symptoms in making a diagnosis.

In nursing assessment, the ability to interpret x-ray film reports is probably most helpful in evaluating the patient's complaints of pain and loss of function. For example, when an x-ray film report notes that the patient has a compression of a lumbar vertebra, the nurse may expect the patient to have symptoms related to pressure on a nerve root.

General Assessment: The Orthopedic Problem

In order to do an accurate and comprehensive orthopedic assessment, the nurse must have an understanding of what is "normal" for the situation. This knowledge provides a baseline for ongoing assessments after the plan of care has been initiated. The nature and extent of an orthopedic injury, surgical procedure, or disease determines the normal or anticipated condition of the patient's extremity or body part.

Therefore, it may be stated that the nurse must be able to recognize the following:

1. When the neurovascular status of an extremity is satisfactory
2. When any bleeding or other drainage is characteristic in both type and amount
3. When the limitation of motion is at an appropriate level
4. When the degree, kind, and location of pain is an expected outcome or diagnostic symptom
5. When an elevation of body temperature is no cause for alarm

For example, a patient who has undergone extensive surgery on his foot will have edematous toes. This edema, in turn, will affect the neurovascular status of the toes. They will be whiter and cooler than the toes on the unaffected foot. Motion will be restricted. The patient may state that he "can hardly feel" a pinprick on any toe of the operated foot. However, at this point in time, his responses are normal.

For this patient, nursing intervention is planned to prevent the neurovascular status from deteriorating and to promote a gradual lessening of edema in the toes of the operated foot. Other considerations for this patient relate to the type of surgery and any possible complications. An extensive surgical procedure means that bleeding through the dressing or cast is expected for about 24 hours. Bleeding that persists to any degree after 24 hours should be reported to the surgeon. Any other kind of drainage that is noted after the bleeding has ceased may be indicative of infection and is also reported. The patient is likely to have severe pain in his entire foot for the first few days. Complaints of severe pain 4 days postoperatively are not anticipated; when such complaints occur, assessment to identify a developing complication is required. (Pain assessment is discussed in detail in the following section.)

Although the patient with extensive surgery on his foot

Table 1-1. Common Screening Tests and Orthopedic Implications

Laboratory Test	Change in Value	Significance
Serum Chemistries		
Serum calcium	Increased	Malignant bone tumor with or without metastases
		Multiple myeloma
	Decreased	Osteomalacia (sometimes)
Serum phosphorus	Increased	Multiple myeloma
	Decreased	Osteomalacia
		Advanced metastatic disease
Uric acid	Increased	Gout
		Multiple myeloma
Serum creatinine	Increased	Large muscle mass
Serum protein electrophoresis	Increased	Multiple myeloma
Alkaline phosphatase	Increased	Paget's disease
		Metastatic bone cancer
		Osteogenic sarcoma
	Mild to moderate increase	Osteomalacia
	Slight increase	Elevated in young during growth period: also during pregnancy
Serum lactic dehydrogenase (LDH)	Slight increase	Pulmonary embolism
		Malignancies of skeletal muscle
Serum glutamic oxaloacetic transaminase (SGOT)	Increased	Skeletal muscle damage
	Slight increase	Skeletal muscle disease
Creatine phosphokinase (CPK)	Increased	Skeletal muscle disease
		Unusually large muscle mass
		Following vigorous exercise
		Post IM injections and muscle biopsies (elevation lasts about 1 day)
Total protein/AG ratio	Decreased albumin: increased globulin	Multiple myeloma
Electrolytes		
Serum potassium	Increased	Massive destruction of muscle tissue
Hematology		
Neutrophilic leukocytosis	Increased	Rheumatoid arthritis
		Gout
Urinalysis		
Calcium	Increased	Metastatic bone tumors
		Multiple myeloma
	Decreased	Osteomalacia

would have that foot immobilized in a rigid dressing or cast, movement of the lower part of the extremity should be possible and should become easier as the general status of the foot returns to normal.

After the operation, it is normal for an orthopedic patient to have a temperature elevation for 24 to 48 hours. How high a temperature must be before action is taken depends on the extent of the surgical procedure and the surgeon.

Pain: Causes, Nature, Patient Perception

Because pain is unique to the patient who complains of it, he is the only one who knows exactly how it feels. Meaningful assessment of pain in an orthopedic patient demands knowledge of the nature and causes of pain, as well as comprehension of the many factors that affect a patient's perception of pain.

Pain is an unpleasant sensation that is generally classified as acute, chronic, or intermittent–chronic. There are three types of pain normally associated with the orthopedic conditions: localized, referred, and phantom. *Localized pain* is confined to a specific area, such as an injured knee. *Referred pain* extends from an original site of discomfort, such as may occur in a patient with an arthritic hip who experiences pain along the anterior and medial aspect of the thigh as far down as the knee. *Phantom pain* is the sensation or pain experienced in an area of a limb that has been amputated.

Orthopedic patients may have pain due to trauma, surgery, treatment, or bone and joint disease. Another significant cause of pain is an impending complication. For this reason, it is essential that the nurse pinpoint the exact location of pain, especially when the patient's complaints appear to be out of proportion to his problem. For instance, the patient who has a total knee replacement (p. 244) should not have severe pain in his knee 7 days postoperatively. Moderate soreness and swelling are to be expected if he is "working hard" in physical therapy. However, this type of pain should be relieved with oral pain medication and should not persist to any significant degree when the patient is at rest. When the patient continues to complain of a "sore leg" or "aching behind my knee," the nurse should assess the leg carefully for signs of thrombophlebitis. Pain behind the knee could be pain in the calf.

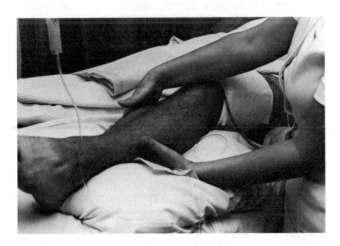

Much has been written on the subject of pain tolerance of people based on race, socioeconomic status, education, sex, and age, but there are a number of other factors that affect an individual's response to pain. To understand these, the nurse must collect data that will provide answers to a number of questions:

What was the patient's past experience with pain?

The 74-year-old woman with a fractured or broken hip who has never been in the hospital may make a statement such as, "I don't know why that hurts me so much when I turn." Obviously, this patient has learned to tolerate pain and accept it as part of living, because it is inconceivable that she has never experienced pain at her age. The patient's statement should alert the nurse to the fact that this patient's postoperative behavior will need to be watched closely, because she may not complain of pain even if it is severe. Pain could render her tense, apprehensive, and difficult to position.

What does this hospitalization mean to the patient?

The professional football player with torn knee ligaments who is anxious about his future may at first have a problem coping with his pain because "it shouldn't have happened." Once he has had surgery and can look forward to rehabilitation, he may tend to minimize his discomfort in an effort to be discharged as soon as possible.

What are the patient's fears about what is happening to him?

Fear and anxiety intensify pain. "First-time" routines are frightening. A patient with an injured or operated lower extremity may be afraid of falling when he is helped out of bed the first time and may complain of increased pain.

How does the patient feel about having pain?

There are patients who deny pain because they do not like injections. Some individuals are reluctant to admit that they have pain because they believe pain is private and as such must be endured without complaint. Others have been conditioned to believe that "big boys" never cry. Or a person who survived an accident that took the life of another person may feel too guilty to complain of pain.

What effect do other people have on the patient's pain?

Psychologically, pain may be caused by the actions or reactions of persons with whom the patient comes in contact. A patient may become too stimulated and active when he has visitors and consequently may have more pain after they leave. Patients become apprehensive when they hear noises from other patients that suggest pain or crises, and this apprehension may heighten their own discomfort. Finally, patients sometimes become so compatible as roommates that they have episodes of pain at the same time.

Pain: Assessment Process

As has been stated previously , knowing what is normal for a patient with a specific condition is the baseline for examining the painful area. The nurse must determine if the extremity or body part is correctly positioned. This also includes evaluating whether a dressing is too tight and checking general body alignment. Any equipment, such as traction, should be inspected to make certain that it is functioning properly.

Close attention must be given to complaints that may indicate complications or problems associated with the orthopedic condition.

The patient should be asked to describe his pain. What is it? Where is it? How long has it been there? The nurse should accept the patient's explanation of how the pain feels because this can be important in deciding the cause. A burning pain under a tight dressing may be indicative of skin irritation, whereas a throbbing pain is probably due to the operation. The patient's complaints should be recorded in his own words.

The nurse should question the patient about factors or events that precipitate pain.

In all orthopedic patients, pain is aggravated to some degree by enforced immobility. Movement and repositioning are also causes of pain. A patient who has had surgery on his hip or leg may have more pain after an attempt to sit on a bedpan. The nurse must be aware of the patient who does not follow instructions, such as keeping the operated leg elevated on pillows. All of this information may be valuable in identifying the cause of unexpected discomfort.

Validating observations with a patient is important because it is sometimes difficult for a patient to give the information that is needed to evaluate his pain. For instance, the patient with multiple injuries may not be able to indicate exactly where in his leg he is having pain at any particular time. The nurse should ask specific questions and touch the areas on his leg gently in an effort to decide if the pain is at the site of injury or if it is suggestive of another problem.

In going through the process of assessment, the nurse watches for nonverbal signs of pain such as clenched fists, grimacing, rigidity, or restlessness. Some patients become unusually quiet but appear tense or apprehensive when they are having severe pain.

While inspecting, observing, asking questions, and palpating, the nurse should explain her actions to the patient in an effort to help him understand why she must know what his pain is all about. Although it is possible to evaluate pain to some degree on the basis of experience with similar treatments or problems, the patient's individual responses must always be the first and most important consideration. Finally, the nurse must refrain from allowing personal feelings about pain or concern about drug abuse to interfere with assessment.

General Condition of the Patient

The priority in an ongoing assessment may not be directly related to the patient's orthopedic problem. For example, when a patient's temperature is considered abnormally elevated, systemic infection and wound infection must be ruled out.

Immobility may be causing anorexia, constipation, difficulties in the urinary tract, circulatory problems, skin irritation, muscle contractures, and boredom.

Patients with injuries of or surgery on the lower extremities or pelvis are most susceptible to pulmonary embolism (p. 49). The slightest complaint of chest pain or "shoulder pain" must be investigated immediately. The nurse should check vital signs on the patient and obtain the following information.

- What is the pain like?
- Where exactly is it located?
- Has the patient had this kind of pain before? (This is important because it is not uncommon for elderly orthopedic patients to have a history of cardiac problems.)
- Does the pain increase on deep inspiration?
- Is the pain accompanied by nausea or vomiting or a feeling of fullness in the epigastric region?
- What activity preceded the pain? For instance, did the patient just return from physical therapy (PT)?
- Does that patient have any symptoms of respiratory distress? Thrombophlebitis?
- What is the patient's medical history?

Because the signs and symptoms of pulmonary embolism depend on the size of the embolus, the patient may have only vague complaints of feeling as if he is catching the "flu." He may have a complaint similar to the following, "I have a catch in my ribs, like I pulled a muscle in PT."

Although any patient may develop this complication, the nurse must be especially alert for signs of pulmonary embolism in orthopedic patients who have been relatively immobile for a week or longer, especially if they are elderly.

Any chronic disease or condition that the patient may have must enter into nursing assessment at all times. A patient who develops nausea and vomiting 24 hours postoperatively may need a different pain medication or antibiotic. However, if the patient is a diabetic this factor must be considered in assessment.

In the orthopedic patient who is confused, the nurse must consider electrolyte imbalance, the kind of medications being administered (narcotics, sedatives, tranquilizers), and fat-embolism syndrome (p. 49).

A lethargic patient may be bored or depressed, or he may be receiving a sedative or narcotic that his system is unable to tolerate. He may not be sleeping well, or he may be exercising too strenuously in physical therapy. Anemia must always be considered when a patient becomes listless.

Psychological Aspects

Fear and anxiety have been discussed to some degree in the section dealing with pain. These emotional states are manifested in a variety of behaviors, perhaps as numerous as the patients who experience them.

The "pesty" patient who asks every nurse the same question about his condition or treatment may be fearful or anxious about the outcome. For instance, an accident victim often regains consciousness in a hospital under the care of a physician he does not know. This may be a source of concern to him, particularly if his pain is unremitting. A typical question for such a patient to ask over and over again might be, "Why does my leg hurt as much now as it did before he fixed it?" In a situation like this, the nurse should assess the patient's knowledge about what has happened to him at the same time as evaluating his pain.

When orthopedic patients are in the physical-therapy department, they compare problems and treatments. In some cases, such interaction generates anxiety. The patient who suddenly becomes pessimistic or depressed over his progress may have met a patient in physical therapy with a condition similar to his who seems to be recovering at a more rapid rate. For this reason, an orthopedic nurse must take the time periodically to observe interactions between patients and to evaluate how these interactions influence patient behavior.

When an older orthopedic patient is alert and communicative, moves easily in bed, and is "young for his age," the nurse may expect him to progress steadily once he begins his physical-therapy program. However, orientation in the elderly is no guarantee of physical stamina. Even though this patient may not express fear of falling or fear of failure, the nurse must recognize that he may have both and should encourage him to verbalize his feelings about the plans for his rehabilitation.

Frustration may be mistaken for depression in the long-term orthopedic patient because the symptoms are often the same. A frustrated patient and one who is depressed may both be quiet and appear to be on the verge of tears. In assessing these patients, the nurse must ask questions or make statements that allow her to make the distinction between these emotional states. To convey the message that crying and the verbalization of feelings is acceptable behavior, the nurse might say, "You must feel sometimes like the day (or night) will never end."

In searching for a way to help and be supportive the nurse might ask, "Do some things about being so helpless bother you more than others? We don't know and would like to understand so that we are better able to give you the help you need."

Because patients are essentially the same people when they are ill as they are when they are well, the time of day may be very important in evaluating a patient's response to nursing care or medical treatment. People who cannot function cheerfully much before noon do not automatically become cooperative in the morning when they are hospital patients. Some patients are more responsive to nursing actions and physical therapy in the afternoon simply because they are "afternoon people."

In all phases of nursing assessment, the total life-style of a patient is an important consideration.

Discussion Questions

1. What nursing assessment is necessary on the following patients?

    a. A 22-year-old male who rolled over his motorcycle is admitted to the emergency room. He has an injured right lower arm that is swollen and appears deformed. He complains of severe pain in his right side and abdomen. He is conscious.

Consider: His mental state. What orthopedic assessment is necessary? What gastrointestinal symptoms might he have?

    b. A 13-year-old male is transferred from another hospital's emergency room 4 hours after an accident in which he collided with another bicyclist head on. He was thrown forward, caught his chin on the handlebars, and then tumbled to the ground. He complains of pain in his neck. He has a splint on his left lower extremity and abrasions on his right knee.

Consider: His mental state. What orthopedic assessment is necessary? What should you look for in assessing his neck?

2. What are the implications for nursing assessment besides orthopedic considerations when admitting a 37-year-old male with an injured back who states that his father died of a heart attack when he was only 45?

Consider: The significance of his age. His occupation. What is his present health status? What are his educational needs relative to heart disease?

Bibliography

Aish A, Brown A: How to use risk factors and assessment skills to individualize patient care. Can Nurs 78(11):46, Dec 1982

Alagaratnam WJ: Pain and the nature of the placebo effect. Nurs Times 77:1883, Oct 28, 1981

Allan D: Glasgow coma scale. Nurs Mirror 158(23):32, Jun 1984

Armitage P: Strategies for dealing with discomfort . . . how nurses can help to reduce the patient's anxiety and pain. Nurs Mirror 156(13):23, Mar 30, 1983

Assessment. Nurse's Reference Library. Springhouse, PA, Intermed Communications, Inc., 1982

Assessment tips: performing palpation. Nursing (Horsham) 13(1):68, Jan 1983

Baer CL: Nursing diagnosis: A futuristic process for nursing practice. Top Clin Nurs 5(4):89, Jan 1984

Barnett DE: Planning patient care: A problem-oriented approach to identifying patients' problems. Nurs Times 78(30):suppl, Jul 28, 1982

Bashor PH: A nursing communication assessment guide. Rehab Nurs 8(1):20, Jan–Feb 1983

Bechtel SL: Anatomy and assessment of the foot and ankle. Assessment and Fracture Management of the Lower Extremities, p. 6, Oct 1984

Bobb J: What happens when your patient goes into shock? RN 47(3):26, Mar 1984

Booker JE: Pain: It's all in your patient's head (or is it?). Nursing (Horsham) 12:31, Mar 1982

Bourbonnais F: Pain assessment: Development of a tool for the nurse and the patient. J Adv Nurs 6:277, July 1981

Brodoff AS: Teaching as therapy for chronic pain. Patient Care 13:127, Jan 15, 1979

Brown MS, Hudak C: Student Manual of Physical Examination, 2nd ed. Philadelphia, JB Lippincott, 1984

Brunner NA: Orthopedic Nursing, 4th ed. St. Louis, CV Mosby, 1983

Bubela N: Is your client at risk for respiratory complications? Can Nurs 79(3):46, Mar 1983

Buckwalter KC, et al: Pain assessment and management in the patient with a fracture. J Nurs Care 14:17, July 1981

Budassi SA: Trauma flow sheet. JEN 9(1):61, Jan–Feb 1983

Cardona VD: Trauma postop: The real nursing challenge. RN 25:22, Mar 1982

Carl L: Assessment of injury severity with the trauma score. JEN 10(5):242, Sep–Oct 1984

Carpenito LJ: Is the problem a nursing diagnosis? Am J Nurs 84(11):1418, Nov 1984

Cohen S: Patient assessment: Examining joints of the upper and lower extremities. Am J Nurs 81:763, Apr 1981

Connell MJ: Therapeutic touch: A natural potential for nurses. New Zealand Nurs J 74:19, Dec 1981

Cookson JC: Orthopedic manual therapy. An overview. Part 1 — The extremities, Part 2 — The spine. Phys Ther, 59:136, Feb 1979; 59:259–67, Mar 1979

Crutchley C: Trends in orthopedic surgery. Today's OR Nurse, 6(12):22, Dec 1984

Cyriax J, Cyriax P: Illustrated Manual of Orthopaedic Medicine. London, Butterworth, 1983

Danis DM: Fear in ED patients. J Emerg Nurs, 10(3):151, May–June 1984

Davitz L, et al: Suffering as viewed in six different cultures. Am J Nurs 76:1296, Aug 1976

DeCrosta T: What the experts say. Relieving pain: four noninvasive ways you should know more about. Nurs Life 4(2):28, Mar–Apr 1984

Dickinson GR, Gorman TK: Adult arthritis: The assessment. Am J Nurs, 83(2):262, Feb 1983

Dolan MB: Controlling pain in a personal way. Nursing (Horsham) 12:144, Jan 1982

Donahoo CA, Dimon JH: Orthopedic Nursing. Boston, Little, Brown and Co, 1977

Drain CB: Managing postoperative pain . . . it's a matter of sighs. Nursing (Horsham) 14(8):52, Aug 1984

Dunn BH: Gait assessment. Assessment and Fracture Management of the Lower Extremities, p. 34, Oct 1984

Dunn BH: Components of musculoskeletal examination. Orthop Nurs 1(6):33, Nov–Dec 1982

Dunn BH: Musculoskeletal assessment: Gait assessment. Orthop Nurs 1(3):33, May–June 1982

Fadden TC, Seiser GK: Nursing diagnosis: A Matter of form. Am J Nurs, 84(4):470, Apr 1984

Farrell J: The human side of assessment. Nursing '80 80:10, Apr 1980

Farrell, J: Orthopedic pain: What does it mean? Am J Nurs 84(4):466, Apr 1984

Fay MF: Controlling pain. Today's OR Nurse, 5(10):10, Dec 1983

Fiedman HR: Psychological differentiation and the phenomenon of pain. ANS 6(2):50, Jan 1984

Frampton VM: Pain control with the aid of transcutaneous nerve stimulation. Physiotherapy 68:77–81, Mar 1982

Fray CP: An accountability-classification instrument for orthopedic patients. J Nurs Adm 14(7–8):32, Jul–Aug 1984

Hackett C: Limbering up your neurovascular assessment technique. Nursing (Horsham) 13(3):40, Mar 1983

Hewitt D: Don't forget your preop patient's fears. RN 47(10):63, Oct 1984

Hilt N, Cogburn S: Manual of Orthopedics. St. Louis, CV Mosby, 1980

Hoppenfeld S: Physical Examination of the Spine and Extremities. New York, Appleton-Century-Crofts, 1976

Hosking KJ: Postoperative pain: Preoperative preparation, part 1. Nurs Mirror 155(4):25, Oct 6, 1982

King RC: Refining your assessment techniques. RN 46(2):43, Feb 1983

Laughlin R, Clancy G: Musculoskeletal assessment: Neurovascular examination of the injured extremity. Orthop Nurs 1:43, Jan–Feb 1982

Lerner R: Sleep loss in the aged: Implications for nursing practice. J Gerontol Nurs 8(6):323, June 1982

Levin RF: Choice of injection site, locus of control, and the perception of momentary pain. Image 14:26, Feb–Mar 1982

Light RR, et al: Diagnosis and management of fractures in the multiply-injured patient. Surg Clin North Am 60(5):1121, Oct 1980

Lockstone C: Pain: It's what the patient says it is. Nurs Mirror 154:ii–iv, Feb 17, 1982

Macleod J: Clinical Examination. New York, Churchill Livingstone, 1976

Malasanos L, et al: Health Assessment. St. Louis, CV Mosby, 1977

Malkiewicz J: A pragmatic approach to musculoskeletal assessment. RN 45(11):57, Nov 1982

Mardlin R: Pain: A nurse's perspective. CONA J, 5(2):4, Apr 1983

Marks-Maran D: Can nurses diagnose? Nurs Times, 79(4):68, Jan 26, 1983

Mayfield P: Health Assessment: A Modular Approach. New York, McGraw-Hill, 1980

McCaffrey M: Relieve your patient's pain fast and effectively with oral analgesics. Nursing '80 10(11):58, Nov 1980

McCaffrey M: Understanding your patient's pain. Nursing '80 10(9):26, Sept 1980

McCarthy KP: Anatomy and assessment of the hip. Assessment & Fracture Management of the Lower Extremities, p. 22, Oct 1984

McGuire DB: The measurement of clinical pain. Nurs Res 33(3):152, May–June 1984

McGuire L: Seven myths about pain relief. RN 46(12):30–1, Dec 1983

McGuire L: A short simple tool for assessing your patient's pain, part 7. Nursing (Horsham), 11:48–9, Mar 1981

McGuire L, Dizard S: Managing pain in the young patient. Nursing (Horsham), 12(8):52, Aug 1982

McGuire MA: A "minor" hand injury? Use these simple tests just to make sure. RN 45(1):28, Jan 1982

McMahon RH: Orthopedic implications for anesthesia in the ambulatory care setting. Orthop Nurs 2(3):41, May–June 1983

Mercier LR: Practical Orthopedics. Chicago, Year Book Medical Publishers, 1980

Miller CA: PRN drugs . . . to give or not to give? Geriatr Nurs (New York) 3(1):37, Jan–Feb 1982

Mourad L: Nursing Care of Adults with Orthopedic Conditions. New York, John Wiley & Sons, 1980

Myers SJ, et al: A model of clinical pain. Am J Phys Med 61:1, Feb 1982

Ogden L: Stopping the pain. Home Health Nurs 2(2):6, Mar–Apr 1984

Panayotoff K: Managing pain . . . in the elderly patient. Nursing (Horsham) 12(8):53, Aug 1982

Patterson DC: Musculoskeletal examination. Occup Health Nurs 32(7):356, Jul 1984

Pepmiller EG: The patient in chronic pain. J Pract Nurs 32:21, Jan 1982

Perdue P: Abdominal injuries and dangerous fractures. RN 44(7):34, July 1981

Performing percussion. Nursing (Horsham) 12(2):63, Feb 1983

Quinlan M: Would you recognize this dangerous electrolyte imbalance? RN 46(3):50, Mar 1983

Raiman J: Responding to pain. Nursing (Oxford) 1:1362, Nov 1981

Rankin EJ: Endorphins and pain: A comparative study of injured athletes and non-athletes. CONA J, 5(5):7, Dec 1983

Richards M: Osteoporosis. Geriatr Nurs (New York), 3(2):98, Mar–Apr 1982

Richardson J: The manipulative patient spells trouble. Nursing '81 11:48, Jan 1981

Richlin DM, et al: The use of oral analgesics for chronic pain. Hosp Formulary, 17:32, Jan 1982

Roberts A: Systems of life No. 95. Systems and signs: Locomotor system—1. Head, neck and shoulders. Nurs Times 78(44), suppl 1–4, Nov 1982

Rodts MF: An orthopedic assessment you can do in 15 minutes. Nursing '83 13:66, May 1983

Ross DG: Anatomy and assessment of the knee. Assessment and Fracture Management of the Lower Extremities. NAON monograph, pp. 14–21, Oct 1984

Ross DG: Musculoskeletal assessment: Range of motion of the fingers and hand. Orthop Nurs 1(5):11, Sep–Oct 1982

Ross DG: Musculoskeletal assessment: The knee. Orthop Nurs, 2(5):23, Sept–Oct 1983

Rothrock JC: Nursing diagnosis in the days of Florence Nightingale. AORN J 40(2):189, Aug 1984

Salmond SW: Trauma and fractures: Meeting your patient's nutritional needs. Orthop Nurs 3(4):27, July–Aug 1984

Schaffner MH, Jelenko C: Rapid orthopedic and neurologic evaluation. Ann Emerg Med 9(2):103, Feb 1980

Sheredy C: Factors to consider when assessing responses to pain. MCN 9(4):250, July–Aug 1984

Sigmon HD: Trauma: This patient needs your expert help. Nursing (Horsham) 13(1):33, Jan 1983

Signor G, Del Bueno DJ: A sinfully easy way to interpret ABGs. RN 45(9):45, Sept 1982

Simon A: Nursing diagnosis: Its implications for the future. Imprint 31(2):47, Apr–May 1984

Skillcheck: On assessing shock. Nursing (Horsham) 12(1):90, Jan 1982

Sofaer B: Pain relief—The core of nursing practice. Nurs Times 79(47):38, Nov 23, 1983

Sofaer B: Pain relief—The importance of communication. Nurs Times 79(49):32, Dec 7, 1983

Strong AG: Teaching TENS. Va Nurse 51(4):228, Winter 1983

Stuhler-Schlag, MK: Pre-and postoperative fluids and electrolytes: Nursing assessment and intervention. Today's OR Nurs, 4(7):11, Sept 1982

Tait A, et al: Improving communication skills. Nurs Times 78(51):2181, Dec 22, 1982

Taylor SL: Musculoskeletal assessment. Low back pain assessment, part 1: History taking. Orthop Nurs 2(4):11, July–Aug 1983

Taylor SL: Musculoskeletal assessment. Low back pain assessment, part 2: Defining range of motion and terminology. Orthop Nurs 2(5):39, Sept–Oct 1983

Taylor SL: Musculoskeletal assessment. Low back pain assessment, part 3: The physical exmination. Orthop Nurs 2(6):21, Nov–Dec 1983

Test your knowledge of nursing assessment and intervention, part 1. Nursing (Horsham) 14(11):89, Nov 1984

Thorpe DM: Neurovascular assessment of the lower extremity. Assessment and Fracture Management of the Lower Extremities, a monograph published by NAON—National Assoc. of Ortho Nurses, p. 29, Oct 1984

Turner PS: Test your knowledge of the multiple trauma patient. Nursing (Horsham) 12(2):129, Feb 1982

Vanderbeck KA: Getting the facts: A guide to orthopaedic assessment. Orthop Nurs 3(5):31, Sep–Oct 1984

Wainwright P: Information and the surgical patient . . . the relation of postoperative pain. Nurs Times 78(35):1480, Sept 1, 1982

Wallace KG, Hays J: Nursing management of chronic pain. J Neurosurg Nurs 14:185–91, Aug 1982

Wallach J: Interpretation of Diagnostic Tests, 3rd ed. Boston, Little, Brown & Co, 1978

Walleck CA: A neurologic assessment procedure that won't make you nervous. Nursing (Horsham) 12(12):50, Dec 1982

Wassel A: Symposium on orthopedic nursing assessment of injuries to the lower extremity. Nurs Clin North Am, 16:739, Dec 1981

Webb KJ: Early assessment of orthopedic injuries. Am J Nurs 74:1048, June 1974

Wells N: Responses to acute pain and the nursing implications. J Adv Nurs 9(1):51, Jan 1984

Westfall UE: Nursing diagnosis: Its use in quality assurance. Top Clin Nurs, 5(4):78–88, Jan 1984

Witt JR: Relieving chronic pain. Nurse Pract 9(1):36, Jan 1984

Yoder ME: Nursing diagnosis—applications in perioperative practice. AORN J 40(2):183, Aug 1984

2

Care of the Patient With a Fracture and Cast

Since most fractures are the result of trauma, anyone who acquires a fracture has to make rapid and often long-range adjustments in his pattern of daily activities, besides accepting the discomfort and limitations of his condition. Although fracture patients do not always appear "sick," they require specialized nursing care based on scientific principles about fractures and how they are treated. The nurse should be familiar with these principles and should have an understanding of human adaptation to the emotional stress caused by fractures, treatment, and rehabilitation. On this premise, Chapter 2 is concerned with the physical and psychological care of the fracture patient in a cast.

Fractures

DEFINITION AND CAUSES

A fracture is a break in the continuity of a bone. In adults this break is usually complete, in that the periosteum and cortical tissue on both sides of the bone are completely severed. An incomplete break, or *"greenstick" fracture,* is more common in children, since bone tissue in children is relatively soft. A fracture-separation at the epiphysis in a long bone may also be considered a pediatric fracture.

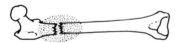

Complete fracture—Periosteum and cortical tissue completely severed on both sides of bone

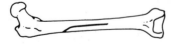

Greenstick fracture—Bone broken, bent, but still securely hinged at one side

In normal bone, fractures occur when more stress is placed upon a bone than it is able to absorb, such as from a direct blow or a crushing force. Other forces responsible for such stress can be indirect, such as a twisting motion (tor-

sion) or an extreme muscle contraction. Bones that have been weakened by disease or tumors are subject to pathologic fractures. For example, bone cancer causes bone to become like "dry toast" and to crumble under little or no stress.

CLASSIFICATION AND DESCRIPTION

Fractures are placed in two broad classifications—closed and open—and are further described as to pattern or appearance and location. When there is no communication between the bone and the outside, the fracture is *closed* or *simple.* When bone ends come through the skin, the fracture is known as *open* or *compound.*

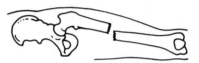

Closed (simple) fracture—No open wound

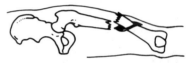

Open (compound) fracture—Wound in skin communicates with fracture

The designation of "simple" to describe fractures that do not come through the skin is usually omitted from x-ray reports and surgical discussions and is only mentioned here to emphasize the point that it is misleading. Fractures could only be "simple" if they caused no problems. This is hardly possible. In a casted fracture, for example, the cast itself creates problems of adjustment for the individual who is confined in it.

The direction of the force responsible for a fracture determines its pattern. These patterns are *transverse, oblique,* or *spiral.*

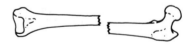

Transverse fracture—Break runs across bone

Oblique fracture—Break runs in slanting direction on bone

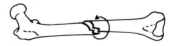

Spiral fracture—Break coils around bone

If there are three or more fragments, the fracture is termed *comminuted*. When the fractured ends of a bone are pushed into each other, the fracture is called *impacted*.

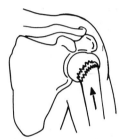

Comminuted fracture—Bone splintered into fragments

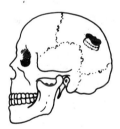

Impacted fracture—Bone broken and wedged into other break

A *compression* fracture is one in which bone, typically a vertebra, collapses on itself. A *depressed* fracture usually occurs in the skull, with the broken bone being driven inward. A *longitudinal* fracture line is one that is parallel with the bone.

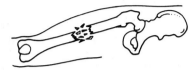

Depressed fracture—Broken skull bone driven inward

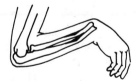

Longitudinal fracture—Break runs parallel with bone. (The preceding fracture drawings, courtesy Ethicon Corp)

When a fracture is accompanied by a bone out of joint, it is called a *fracture dislocation.*

In relation to the joint, fractures are described as *intracapsular* (within the capsule), *extracapsular* (outside the capsule), or *intra-articular* (in the joint).

A *supracondylar* fracture is above the condyle or condyles.

The kind of bone tissue being subjected to stress is also significant in fracture patterns. Cancellous or spongy bone, such as that found near the ends of long bones, in the vertebrae, or in the os calcis, is subject to crushing, comminuted fractures. The compact, hard, or cortical tissue found in the shafts of long bones fractures under force into transverse, oblique, and spiral patterns and the fracture may or may not be comminuted.

Fracture description and diagnosis includes the location and the displacement, if any, of bone fragments. In long bones, fractures are described as being *proximal, distal,* or *midshaft,* depending on their location on the bone.

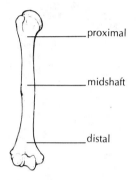

Displacement of fracture ends depends on the causative force and the strength of surrounding muscle attachments. As is shown below, fragments may be displaced sideways (*A*), or may override (*B*), angulate (*C*), or rotate (*D*).

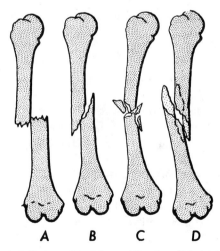

(Rhoads, et al: Surgery: Principles and Practice. Philadelphia, Lippincott)

Implications for Nursing Care

Many aspects of independent nursing care in fracture patients are based on knowledge of fracture classification, patterns, and methods of treatment.

For example, an x-ray film report that describes a spiral fracture of the humerus as *angulated* indicates that the end of a fragment may have entered a muscle mass. The nurse can visualize an x-ray film such as the one that follows (on the left), and know that the patient will have much swelling and pain.

For a comminuted fracture of the distal femur with overriding and posterior displacement of the distal fragment, the nurse can visualize the x-ray film on the right and know that the patient may have a great deal of muscle spasm, in addition to pain, during the initial phase of treatment as the fragments are being pulled into alignment.

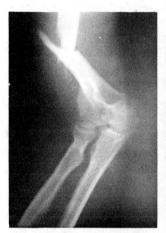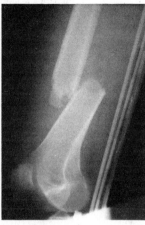

(Left) Spiral fracture of humerus with angulation. *(Right)* Comminuted fracture of distal femur with overriding and posterior displacement of fragments.

When the location of a fracture is given as supracondylar or intra-articular, a nurse realizes that there could be interference with joint motion.

Likewise, any compound fracture requires observation for signs of infection. Besides being open and contaminated, compound fractures are usually accompanied by a fair amount of damage to the soft tissues. This condition increases the chance of infection, the development of osteomyelitis, and nonunion of the fracture. Therefore, these wounds are thoroughly cleansed and debrided and are often left open for as long as 6 days. In some cases the physician will choose to suture drainage tubes into the wound and initiate irrigation with antibiotics for a specific period of time. Prophylactic antibiotic therapy and tetanus immune globulin or toxoid are usually indicated in treatment of compound fractures.

With this kind of knowledge, patient needs and physician's orders can be anticipated and nursing care can be efficiently planned and effectively given. (For a brief discussion of fractures of specific bones and their treatment refer to the Appendix, pp. 360–366.)

SIGNS AND SYMPTOMS

Signs and symptoms of fractures vary, depending on whether the fracture is compound or closed, displaced or undisplaced, transverse or comminuted, located in the shaft of a long bone or in a joint, and so on. For example, in a closed transverse fracture caused by a direct force, there is more observable evidence of soft-tissue damage in the area than there would be in a fracture caused by a twisting motion. The skin itself appears damaged in the first.

Signs and symptoms of a fracture include the following:

1. Pain (especially at the time of injury)
2. Tenderness at the site
3. Swelling
4. Loss of function
5. Deformity
6. Crepitus (grating sensation either heard or felt as bone ends rub together)
7. Discoloration
8. Bleeding from an open wound with protrusion of bone ends

TREATMENT

There are three principles of fracture treatment.

1. Reduction or realignment of bone fragments
2. Maintenance of realignment by immobilization
3. Restoration of function

Reduction

Reduction is accomplished (1) by closed manipulation in which a cast or sling is used, (2) by internal fixation in surgery (open reduction) in which various types of holding devices are used, (3) by external fixation, also in surgery, in which pins are inserted into the bone above and below the fracture and held in place by a clamping device, and (4) by traction.

Immobilization

The single most important element in obtaining union of fracture fragments is immobilization. In *closed reductions,* this is often accomplished by application of a plaster cast, once the fracture ends have been manipulated into alignment with or without the use of anesthesia. For proper immobilization, plaster casts are applied to include the joint above and below the fracture line.

In *open reduction,* the work of immobilization is done by the nails, screws, pins, wires, or rods that are inserted with or without plates. Such devices usually stay in the patient indefinitely unless they produce symptoms after healing has taken place.

The x-ray film on the left shows internal fixation of the tibia by means of a compression plate. A compression plate with screws is often used to reduce tibial fractures when closed reduction is not possible. The compression force helps stimulate bone growth and healing. The fractured fibula,

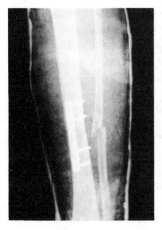
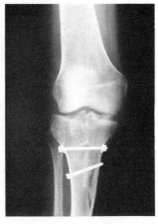

(Left) Internal fixation of tibia with compression plate. *(Right)* Internal fixation of intra-articular fracture of upper tibia with screw and bolt.

also seen on the x-ray film, is not reduced. Should the fibula heal out of alignment, no serious problem would develop because the fibula is not a weightbearing bone.

The x-ray film on the right shows an intra-articular fracture of the upper tibia that was reduced by surgical fixation by means of a screw and a tibial bolt.

Common internal fixation methods for selected femoral shaft fractures are shown in the following illustrations. The x-ray film on the left shows an intramedullary rod in place,

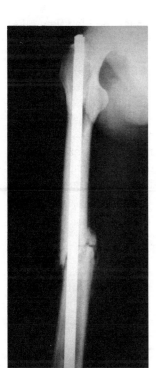
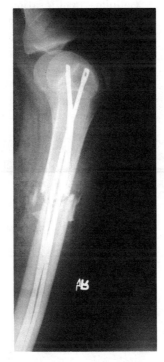

(Left) From a point in the trochanteric region, an intramedullary rod is driven down through the medullary canal to stabilize the fracture fragments. *(Right)* Multiple Enders rods are inserted through the distal femur along the medullary canal to stabilize the fracture.

and the film on the right demonstrates internal fixation with several rods. The method chosen is a matter of surgeon preference.

Since surgery entails a risk of infection and delayed union, open reduction is indicated only if closed manipulation and traction would be unsatisfactory or if the surgeon wishes to shorten the period of hospitalization.

External fixation is indicated for fractures that are difficult if not impossible to immobilize by other methods. The best example of such a fracture is a severe open or compound fracture in which bone and tissue damage is so extensive that amputation of the limb is a consideration.

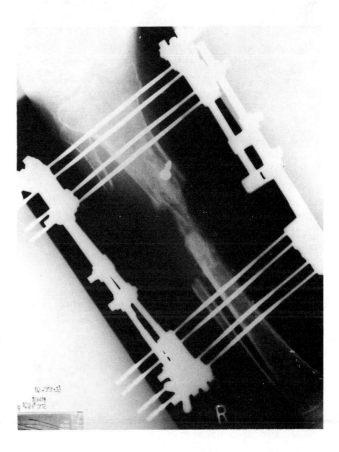

(*Traction*, the application of a pulling force, is discussed in Chapter 3.)

The type and location of the fracture are factors in deciding on the method of reduction. For example, if fracture fragments are angulated into the surrounding tissue in such a way that damage to nerves or blood vessels would occur with closed manipulation, then open reduction is indicated. The same is true in fractures involving the tibial condyles, where position of fragments could interfere with restoration of joint motion.

Functional bracing is a method of fracture treatment in which a semiflexible brace is used to apply firm equal pressure on the soft tissues surrounding a fractured long bone in

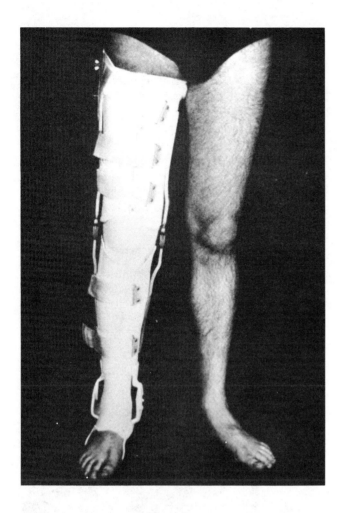

order to achieve a stable reduction. Functional braces have hinges incorporated to permit motion of adjacent joints.

Restoration of Function

Restoration of function actually begins with the *maintenance* of function of the unaffected joints and extremities. Healing of the fractured part will be faster if normal circulation in the rest of the body is maintained. If the fracture has been reduced and immobilized adequately and if damage to the surrounding tissues has not been so severe as to cause extensive scarring, rehabilitation of the fractured part will have a headstart, once it is begun. (Specific rehabilitation exercises are discussed in later sections of this chapter.)

FRACTURE HEALING

Stages of Healing

The repair of a fracture takes place in an orderly sequence: (1) formation of a hematoma, (2) cellular proliferation, (3) callus formation, (4) ossification, and (5) consolidation and remodeling. Obviously, some of the same physiologic pro-

cesses necessary for healing of soft-tissue wounds are active in fracture repair. The healing sequence is conditioned by the fact that bone is rigid; thus, when it is fractured, its fragments require a long time and strict immobilization to establish a "perfect union."

1. Hematoma Formation. When a bone is fractured, blood extravasates into the area between and around the fragments and the bone marrow. The formation of a hematoma or clot begins 24 hours after the fracture occurs. Through this fibrin network, young fibroblasts and new capillaries invade the clot, and granulation tissue is formed to replace the hematoma.

1. HEMATOMA STAGE

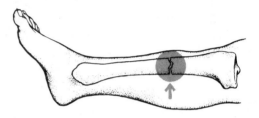

The local clot serves as a fibrin network for subsequent cellular invasion

2. Cellular Proliferation. Cellular proliferation takes place at the fracture site, where torn ends of periosteum, endosteum, and bone marrow supply the cells that proliferate and differentiate into fibrocartilage, hyaline cartilage, and fibrous connective tissue. The tearing away of periosteum by the injury stimulates its deep layers so that proliferation of osteoblasts, the bone-forming cells, also takes place. Osteogenesis is rapid. The fibrous layer of periosteum is elevated away from the bone. After several days the combination of periosteal elevation and the granulation tissue forms a collar around the end of each fragment. These collars eventually advance, unite, and form a bridge across the fracture site.

2. CELLULAR PROLIFERATION STAGE

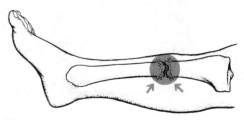

Fibroblastic and endothelial cells invade and colonize the fibrin scaffolding of the cast

3. Callus Formation. The fibroblasts in the newly formed granulation tissue differentiate into cartilage or bone, depending on where they are located in relation to capillary circulation. Those adjacent to the surface of the shaft, especially where the periosteum is reflected from the shaft, form a cancellous bone. Those internal fibroblasts at the level of the fracture and more removed from capillary circulation tend to form cartilage. Cartilage formation at this site may also be due to motion during healing.

This large mass of differentiated tissue bridging the fracture is called *callus*. The osteoid matrix, or young uncalcified bone, calcifies as mineral salts are deposited. Gradual development of cancellous bone occurs near the fracture site in the marrow cavities of the fragments. Cartilage callus also undergoes changes to become bone. The size and shape of callus is in direct proportion to the amount of bone damage and displacement that has taken place.

3. CALLUS FORMATION STAGE

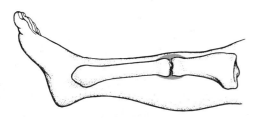

Osteoblasts are derived from mesenchymal cells to produce an osteoid matrix

4. Ossification. Ossification, or the final laying down of bone, is the stage in which the fracture ends knit together.

4. CALLUS OSSIFICATION OR UNION STAGE

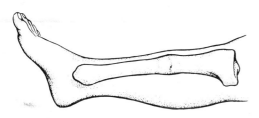

Ossification of callus occurs

5. Consolidation and Remodeling. The primary cancellous bone is remodeled, compact bone being formed according to stress patterns. Remodeling continues according to Wolff's law, which says that bone is formed in relation to its function.

5. CONSOLIDATION AND REMODELING

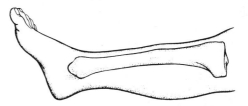

(The preceding figures of stages of bone healing are from Moe JH: Delayed union and nonunion of long bone fractures. Hosp Med 9:35, Feb 1970)

Healing Time

Different fractures heal at different rates. Impacted fractures heal in several weeks, while displaced fractures may take months or years to heal completely. Different bones also heal at different rates. The bones of the arm may heal in 3 months, while the tibia and femur require 6 months or longer. The more surface area the fracture fragments have, the faster they unite. For example, spiral fractures heal more rapidly than transverse fractures. Occasionally fractures unite after 8 months, although they are usually united 6 months after the date of injury.

As far as function is concerned, most function returns in 6 months after bony union takes place, but complete function may not be regained for a year or so. A fracture that has healed in excellent position may still be followed by some limitation of joint motion.

Complications in Healing

Interruptions in the sequence of fracture healing may be caused by any of the following:

1. The original injury
2. Debridement
3. Loss of bone substance
4. Soft tissue interposed between bone ends
5. Infection
6. Loss of circulation
7. Interrupted or improper immobilization
8. Inadequate fixation
9. Necrosis due to fixation devices
10. Metabolic disturbances

These interruptions prevent or delay bony union. *Delayed union* implies that the fracture is not forming a bony union in the usual amount of time. *Nonunion* is the complete failure of healing to take place. In nonunion there may be motion at the site of the fracture due to *pseudoarthrosis* (false joint). The bone ends may be sclerotic with molding of the fracture surfaces, and the medullary canal may be sealed with compact bone. Bone grafting is one form of treatment for this problem.

Nonunion can also be treated by the use of electromagnetic stimulation to induce osteogenesis. This stimulation can be internal or external. Internal stimulation is accomplished by inserting cathodes or implanting a stimulator. In external stimulation, coils are placed on opposite sides of the limb at the fracture site.

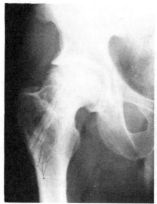

Avascular necrosis   Nonunion

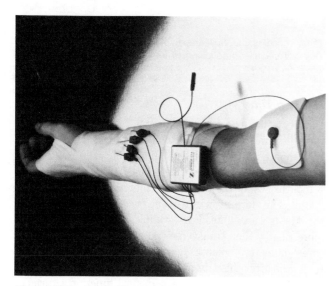

(Courtesy Zimmer Co, Warsaw, Ind)

Aseptic or *avascular necrosis* is death of the bone that is due to loss of blood supply. The most common locations are the femoral head, carpal navicular, astragalus, or any fragment that is separated from its source of circulation.

Sometimes inaccurate reduction or inadequate immobilization causes a *malunion* of fracture fragments. Depending on the severity and location of the malunion, surgery may be required.

Serious Complications of Fracture Conditions

The complications that are most threatening to the life of a fracture patient are also the ones that can hardly be prevented. These are pulmonary embolism, fat embolism, gas gangrene, and tetanus. Table 2-1 shows the *early* clinical features in each of these complications and is a guide to prompt nursing action. An understanding of the cause and treatment of serious fracture complications is also necessary.

Table 2-1.   Possible Complications from Fractures

Complication	Early Clinical Features	Recommended Nursing Intervention	Most Common Fracture Type—Location
Pulmonary embolism (may occur *without* clinical symptoms)	*Substernal pain,* dyspnea; rapid weak pulse	Administer oxygen. Notify physician immediately about pain and vital signs.	Lower extremities
Fat embolism	*Mental confusion,* apprehension, restlessness due to hypoxia; then fever, tachycardia, tachypnea, dyspnea	It is advisable to have a standing order to draw blood gases at the first sign of mental confusion. Notify physician immediately. Administer oxygen.	Lower extremities or multiple fractures
Gas gangrene	*Mental aberration* followed by signs of infection	Notify physician immediately of mental status, vital signs, and appearance of wound.	Compound (especially with small open area)
Tetanus	*May be none* until patient has tonic twitchings and difficulty opening mouth	Notify physician immediately. Check to see if patient is getting prochlorperazine (Compazine).*	Compound

* One of the side effects of the normal therapeutic dose of Compazine *is* hypertonia.

Pulmonary Embolism

The occlusion of a pulmonary artery (or arteries) by a thrombus may be secondary to thrombophlebitis or may occur by itself. Patients with fractures of the lower extremities are most susceptible to pulmonary embolism because they are relatively inactive.

Assessment. Pulmonary embolism can occur *with* or *without* clinical symptoms. If symptoms are present, they are dependent on the area and size of the affected vessel or vessels. Therefore, symptoms range from those of bronchopneumonia to sudden acute, substernal pain with dyspnea and a rapid, weak pulse, shock, or death. In orthopedic patient care, any sudden chest pain or related medical emergency should be considered a pulmonary embolism until proven otherwise.

Management. Since pulmonary embolism may be asymptomatic, some physicians prescribe prophylactic anticoagulation agents based both on the type of injury and on factors that contribute to venous stasis and thrombophlebitis, such as obesity and varicose veins.

Women who are using oral contraceptives are more susceptible to thrombophlebitis and should be told to use an alternative method of birth control while recuperating from a fracture of the lower extremity. Along with the administration of prophylactic anticoagulation agents, other well-known preventive measures are carried out, such as early ambulation, exercises, and use of elastic stockings.

Once pulmonary embolism has been diagnosed, the treatment is symptomatic, along with anticoagulation agents to prevent further formation of emboli.

Fat Embolism

The origin of fat emboli is still a matter of debate. The mechanical theory states that fracture (especially of the femur) allows release of fat from the bone marrow into the circulation. The physiochemical theory holds that the alteration of fat in the bloodstream, due to trauma, results in the formation of large droplets. Other authorities agree that many factors are involved, including that of traumatic shock.

The typical patient with a fat-embolism syndrome is a young adult with multiple fractures, including those of the long bones.

The pathologic effect of fat embolism is pulmonary effusion caused by fat droplets occluding the capillaries in the pulmonary circulation. This results in defective gas transfer across the alveolar or arteriolar membrane causing *hypoxia* and tissue death.

Assessment. The *first* clinical sign of fat embolism, is mental disturbance due to hypoxia in the brain, and it may occur within 12 to 72 hours after the initial injury. *Early* diagnosis is made by arterial blood gas analysis, which shows a low pO_2 content.

Other possible manifestations include progressive dyspnea, respiratory distress, tachycardia, tachypnea, and fever. Although petechiae are a classic symptom, it could be detrimental to the patient to wait for them to appear before making a definite diagnosis and instituting treatment. Petechiae are usually found on the upper chest, axillae, and conjunctiva.

Other diagnostic findings that may be present are fat globules in the urine or sputum, elevated serum lipase, electrocardiographic changes due to myocardial ischemia, and a decreased platelet count. A chest x-ray film would show a pulmonary infiltrate that looks like a "snowstorm."

Management. The most effective form of treatment is the administration of oxygen in concentrations of up to 10 liters per minute. Restoration of normal blood volume is important. Steroids are sometimes used to reduce tissue damage in the lungs. Patients who do not respond to treatment progress to respiratory failure and neurologic dysfunction.

Preventive measures include early immobilization of the fracture, a minimal amount of manipulation of the fragments, replacement of lost blood, and prevention of hypotension.

Gas Gangrene

The possibility of gas gangrene is a prime consideration when a compound fracture has been sustained with a relatively small open wound area. Gas gangrene is caused by anaerobic saprophytic bacteria, *Clostridium welchii.* This organism grows well in deep wounds in which there is a decreased supply of oxygen due to muscle trauma. *Gas gangrene* is a rapid decomposition of tissue with the formation of gas bubbles and edema.

Assessment. Gas gangrene is characterized by the onset of an acute fulminating infection without any other apparent symptoms. In susceptible patients, therefore, the nurse must be watchful for signs of apprehension or mental aberration. The patient would have an abrupt fever, chills, a fall in blood pressure, an increased pulse and respiratory rate, and prostration. The wound is painful, and edema may mask the crepitus of gas bubbles.

In advanced stages, the skin becomes bronze-colored, and profuse drainage with a characteristic fruity odor is present. The muscles are reddish-purple or black. When the condition is unchecked, other systemic features occur such as anorexia, vomiting, diarrhea, and shock. Death may result from toxemia.

Management. *Treatment* includes opening the wound for debridement, irrigating the area with antiseptics, initiating hyperbaric oxygen therapy, and administering antibiotics.

Parenteral fluids are given for supportive treatment. The effect of anti–gas-gangrene serum is questionable. Amputation of the affected limb is sometimes necessary.

Tetanus

Like gas gangrene, tetanus occurs in compound fractures, especially puncture wounds. It, too, is caused by an anaerobic organism.

Symptoms may be absent until the occurrence of tonic muscular twitchings and spasms. The patient would have difficulty opening his mouth.

Treatment is similar to that for gas gangrene, with the added use of sedatives when convulsions occur.

Casts in Fracture Treatment

TYPES OF CASTS

In immobilization of a fracture, the cast is applied to include the joint above and below the fracture. The type of cast used is determined by the type of fracture. Some of the more common types of casts used on extremities are pictured in the following pages. Potential pressure points for each extremity are shown.

Short Arm Casts

Short arm casts are used in the treatment of *stable* fractures of the metacarpals, carpals, or distal radius. Arm casts should not extend any farther on the hand than is necessary to maintain stabilization of the fracture. Finger motion should be as free as possible. As indicated in the following figure, pressure points of concern are located at the radial styloid *(cross)* and the ulnar styloid *(arrow)*.

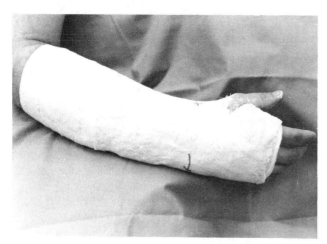

Short arm cast

Long Arm Casts

Long arm casts immobilize unstable fractures of the carpals, stable fractures of the distal humerus, and fractures of

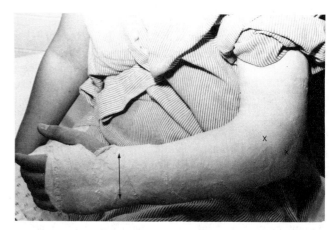

Long arm cast

the radius, ulna, or both. Possible pressure points are the styloid processes *(arrows)* and the olecranon and lateral epicondyle *(crosses)*.

Hanging Arm Casts

A hanging arm cast is applied when the weight of the arm is not sufficient to correct displacement on a fracture of the humerus. It may be heavier than a long arm cast because its purpose is to exert light traction on the humerus when the patient is upright. The patient is usually instructed to stay in this position even while sleeping. However, if the patient is allowed to lie flat in bed, traction may be applied. A 5-lb weight is attached to a rope that is tied to a loop just below the elbow of the cast and drawn through a pulley at the foot of the bed.

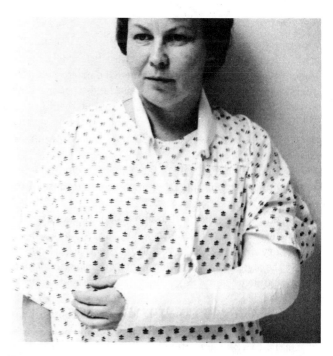

Hanging arm cast

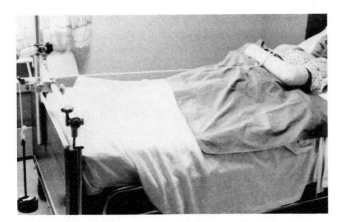

Traction applied to a hanging arm cast

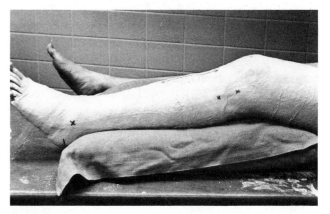

Long leg cast

Short Leg Casts

Short leg or boot casts are used in the treatment of stable fractures of the ankle or metatarsals, and fractures of the calcaneus, talus, navicular, cuboid, and cuneiform bones. Toes should always be visible and the knee joint should be freely movable. Pressure areas include the heel *(arrow)* and malleolus *(cross)*. Pressure on the peroneal nerve may also be a problem if the cast extends to that point.

The ankle joint may or may not be flexed at 90 degrees. The type of fracture and position of fragments necessary for immobilization are also factors in determining the position of the foot. Often an orthopedist casts the foot in slight plantar flexion, because this is the position normally assumed when the foot is off the floor. A foot casted at a right angle is more prone to develop pressure sores on the heel.

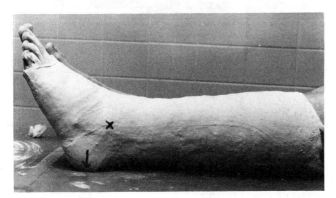

Short leg cast

Long Leg Casts

Long leg casts extend above the knee and are used in treatment of fractures of the tibia, fibula, and ankle joint. Pressure points in this instance are located at the heel *(small arrow)*, malleolus *(cross at angle)*, and the peroneal nerve *(crosses to the side of the knee)*. The shinbone may also be subject to pressure.

Weight bearing in leg casts is made possible by the attachment of a walking iron or heel to the cast after it has set.

The use of either of these devices is a physician's preference and is often determined by the position of the foot in the cast or by how weight should be distributed when the patient is walking.

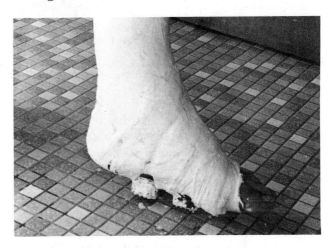

Walking heel on leg cast

Spica Cast

A spica cast is a spiral reverse that goes between an appendage and the main part of the body or extremity, thereby immobilizing the joint between the two. In a *hip spica*, for example, the bandage goes around the femur and then the trunk in a figure-of-eight fashion. Hip spicas are applied most often for fractures of the femur and are of three varieties: (1) a single spica, which covers the lower trunk and the affected leg; (2) one and one-half hip spica, which covers the

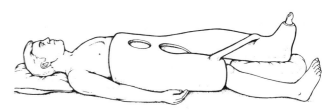

1 1/2 hip spica cast. (Brunner and Suddarth: Textbook of Medical-Surgical Nursing. Philadelphia, Lippincott)

lower trunk and the affected leg and extends to above the knee on the unaffected leg; and (3) a double spica, which covers the lower trunk and includes both extremities.

Thumb spicas (gauntlet) immobilize fractures of the carpal navicular, thumb metacarpal, and phalanges. Pressure points to watch are the radial styloid and ulnar styloid at the wrist and the metacarpophalangeal joint at the base of the thumb.

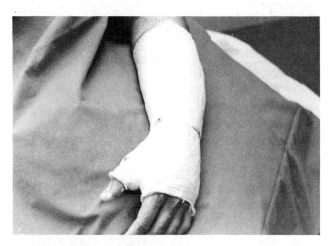

Thumb spica cast

Some casts are infrequently used in the treatment of fractures. These include the shoulder spica, which may be indicated in the treatment of unstable fractures of the shoulder girdle and humerus when other methods of immobilization are not suitable. The patellar tendon bearing (PTB) cast is applied by some orthopedic surgeons in the treatment of tibial shaft fractures. The cast is indented over the patellar tendon and molded around the patella. In full extension, pressure is exerted over the tendon. The proximal tibia is prevented from rotating by the shape of the cast.

Selected severely displaced and closed fractures may be treated by applying a traction pull (see Chapter 3) under anesthesia and realigning the fragments with pins on either side of the fracture site. A cast is applied over the pins, and the arrangement is referred to as "pins and plaster."

Body casts are not applied for fractures; the conditions for which they are used are identified in a later chapter.

Application of a Cast

Materials

Casting materials include plaster of Paris and the synthetics: fiberglass, thermoplastic, and polyester/cotton knit.

Because it is cheap and durable, *plaster of Paris* is the material most widely used for casting. It is a chalky white powder, anhydrous calcium sulfate, made from gypsum

crystals. As the crystals are heated, the water in them is given off, and they are reduced to powder. This powder is incorporated into mesh rolled bandages or strips (splints) of varying widths and lengths. When these plaster bandages or splints are placed in water, an opposite chemical reaction takes place. The water reacts with the powder to form crystals, and in doing so gives off heat. The strength of the plaster depends on how closely the crystals interlock as they dry.

Casting equipment is frequently maintained on a cart, or at least kept in one place such as a "cast room." The equipment consists of plaster rolls and splints, sheet wadding, stockinette, waxed disposable or metal buckets, and plastic bags for lining buckets. The purpose of lining the bucket with plastic bags is to make it easier to dispose of the water without pouring the plaster sediment down a drain.

The tools used for trimming and cutting may be on the cart also. They are a cast knife or knives, a large bandage scissors, and a "duckbilled" cast bender. Additional material may include heavy felt or foam rubber, which is used in padding bony prominences in the application of body or hip spica casts, and aluminum and wooden splints, which are frequently incorporated into the cast for additional strength. All of these supplies should be readily accessible during a casting procedure.

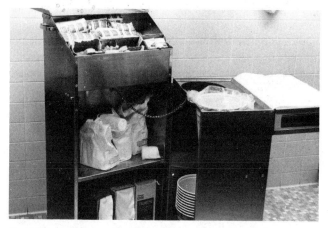

Cast cart

Patient Preparation

The amount of skin preparation before cast application depends on the degree of pain in the fracture, whether or not there are abrasions to be cleansed, and the cause of the fracture. A patient with gravel clinging to his broken leg after a motorcycle accident needs to have more extensive cleansing than the patient who fractured his leg at home. If he is undergoing reduction under general anesthesia, cleansing can wait until he is anesthetized. If this is not the case, he needs an analgesic and an extremely gentle nurse to do the necessary procedure.

The skin should be dried completely with a towel. Some sources recommend using alcohol or a powder. Powders containing zinc oxide, purified talc, cornstarch, and magnesium stearate should be used because they do not cake. *Thorough inspection* of the skin for open or bruised areas is the most essential aspect of skin preparation. It is as important for the nurse to do this as it is for the physician, because inspection helps later in evaluating patient complaints of pain or tenderness under the cast.

At this time, the patient should be informed about what happens during cast application. He should know specifically that the cast will be added weight. How heavy a cast is will depend on the material used (a fiberglass cast is lighter than plaster) and the extent of the coverage. He must also know that as the cast dries it gives off heat and becomes lighter.

Pain and apprehension need to be relieved as much as possible before cast application. If the limb has been splinted or otherwise immobilized for 24 to 48 hours to allow the swelling to subside, a patient will fear the prospect of having that painful limb exposed and handled again. A combination of pain medication, instruction, and reassurance are the most helpful in this situation.

Steps in Application of a Plaster Cast

1. A plastic-lined bucket is filled with tepid water, unless otherwise specified. Hot water in combination with the recrystallization that takes place in the plaster could burn the patient's skin. Cold water is sometimes used for very large casts to prevent them from setting before they have been completely applied and molded. Assistance in this procedure is required in proportion to the size and location of the cast and the condition of the patient. Maintaining the extremity in the position in which it is being casted is the priority. One nurse may be required to help hold the limb and another to "dip" and perhaps aid in the wrapping.

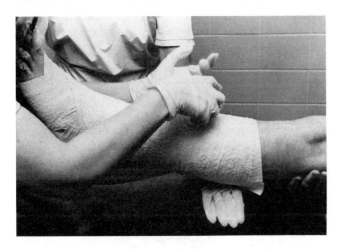

2. Disposable rubber gloves and plastic aprons should be worn by those involved with the wet plaster. Plaster is almost abrasive to the hands, and the effort required to rub plaster out of clothing is enough to make an apron worthwhile.

3. If stockinette is used, a long enough piece is cut so that there is plenty left over to be secured in place over the cast edges. It is rolled up in a doughnut shape and applied over the limb. Stockinette is not always used because the process of applying this material over a severely fractured extremity is extremely difficult as well as painful for the patient. In addition, stockinette stretches and may wrinkle if the cast loosens around the limb.

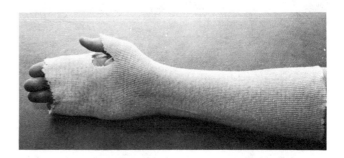

4. Rolls of sheet wadding material are used directly over the skin or stockinette to wrap the extremity. This material clings and molds to the contours of the limb.

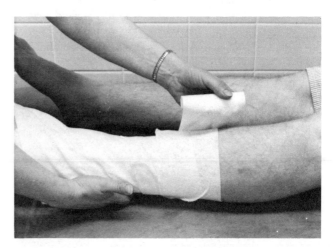

5. The plaster rolls and splints take only seconds to prepare. The corner of a roll should be turned back and the roll dropped into the bucket. The roll should not be held while it is bubbling, to allow it to become evenly soaked and to avoid any "dry" spots made by pressure of the fingers. When it has stopped bubbling, the roll should be taken out of the water and the ends should be pushed gently toward the middle. Excess water is thus removed without loss of plaster. The roll

should not be "wrung out" and should be a little sloppy. It is handed immediately to the person applying the cast. The corner of the roll, which was folded back when the roll was placed in the bucket, is separated so that it can be grasped and used as a starting point for unrolling and wrapping.

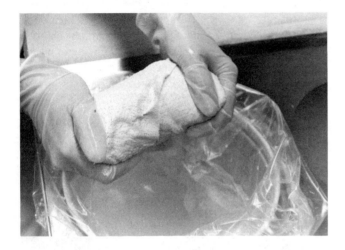

Seconds count in cast application; the plaster must be applied promptly once the strips are wet. As soon as the fragments are in alignment, they should be immobilized quickly to maintain that position. Plaster sets very fast, and movement during this process interferes with the interlocking of crystals. As mentioned previously, it is this formation that gives plaster its strength. The nurse who has wasted several seconds in locating the beginning of a wet roll of plaster soon learns the importance of correct dipping.

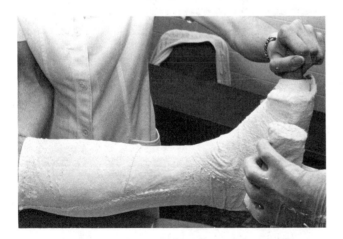

6. When plaster splints are requested they should be held in the water, one end in each hand, until they are ready. They are then pushed together in "accordion" fashion to remove most of the water. To remove any wrinkles and remaining excess water, one end of the splint should be held over the bucket and run between two fingers of the other hand.

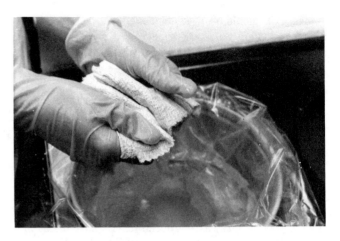

After the cast is applied, it is placed immediately on pillows. A wet edge may be trimmed here or there, but the cast is not completely finished as to padding and petals (pp. 56–57) until it is set, or perhaps dry, and until patient needs are established in this area. Before the patient is returned to his room, the plaster that dripped on his skin should be removed with warm water and a washcloth.

SYNTHETIC CASTS

Synthetic casting materials come in rolls and splints and require specific padding. These materials are moistened and then applied; the method of application varies according to their composition. Since most synthetics are still in a state of change and improvement, the nurse should carefully read the instructions that come with *any* such casting material. This will save time and trouble. For example, some fiberglass casting materials contain polyurethane, which is activated by the dipping prior to cast application. This substance is colorless and adheres to instruments (bandage scissors), skin, furniture, and the floor. Nail polish remover, applied as soon as possible to the affected area, will help remove this polyurethane.

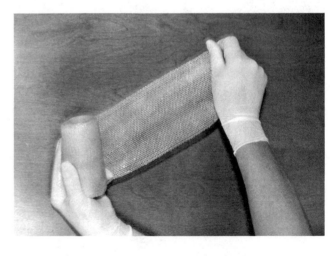

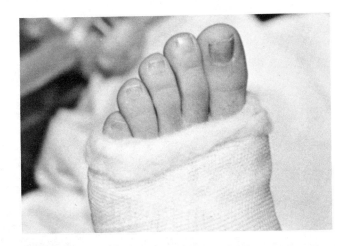

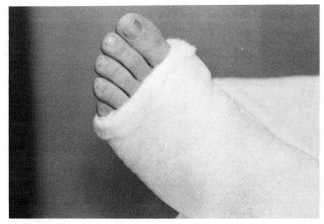

Uses

Although synthetics are more expensive than plaster they have advantages that make them appropriate cast materials for certain patients. Since synthetic casts are generally lighter and shed water, they may be indicated for the active patient who needs to wear a cast for a long period. Because they are easy to clean, they may be indicated for the very young child or the elderly patient with problems of bladder and bowel incontinence. Because synthetic casting materials are costly, they are most often used in the application of a second long-term cast after the initial edema subsides in a plaster cast or splint with dressing. They are not as easily shaped or molded as plaster and therefore may not be as useful in the immobilization of grossly displaced or unstable fractures.

Specific Care Considerations

The synthetics are stronger than plaster, so that less material is required in casting, making these casts lightweight. They dry and harden in minutes and are less susceptible than plaster to flat spots and dents. Although they are easier to clean they can be difficult to petal (p. 57), since most standard taping materials do not adhere to the dried cast surface. Moleskin, which is also expensive, is an exception. Liquid adhesives under tape petals may aid in keeping

rough edges covered. Rough edges must be cut or filed before petals can be applied. In discharge planning, the patient must be cautioned that if he bathes or swims, or if he washes the cast, he must dry it thoroughly as soon as possible to avoid skin breakdown. Towels should be used to dry off the exterior of the cast and then the cast may be dried under a portable hair dryer on a cool setting. Although the following nursing care is concerned with plaster casts, any suggestions related to the care of the extremity or the patient are applicable to the fracture patient in a synthetic cast.

General Care of the Patient in a Cast

Immediate Care and Patient Teaching

Once the cast is on, the patient may have some questions about its size or appearance. Answers are more easily given if the nurse remembers that plaster has no therapeutic effects beyond the points at which it is molded to hold fracture fragments in alignment. For example, for a fractured wrist, the points of immobilization are on the back of the wrist and on the top and bottom surfaces of the forearm. A patient will be more satisfied with an answer to his question about the length of the cast if this explanation is given rather than a vague statement about "holding it in place."

A patient with a fractured ankle may be alarmed if he notices that his foot is casted in a slightly inverted position. Again, he needs reassurance that the physician knows what he is doing, especially if the patient has a neighbor who recently had a leg cast that was set at a right angle. A simple statement pointing out that all leg casts cannot look alike since they immobilize different types of fractures is all that is needed.

While settling a patient with a new cast, the nurse should explain that frequent checks will be made of the neurovascular status. The patient should be aware that a warm pink finger or toe that can feel a pinch and can be moved in

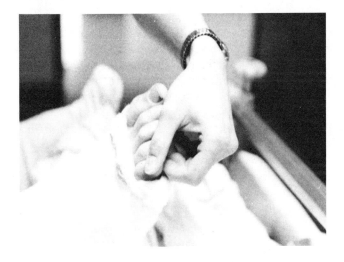

response to a request indicates to the nurse that the cast is not too tight and confirms for the physician the fact that the fracture and its reduction have not interfered with the blood supply or innervation.

Nursing Management While the Cast Dries

A *green* cast is one that is "set" but still contains water. The pockets left by evaporation of this water make the cast lighter and porous. The entire drying process takes about 48 hours, although large casts such as hip spicas may require longer. As a cast dries, it becomes white, shiny, and odorless as opposed to being gray, dull and musty-smelling when damp.

Nursing measures need to be taken at once to combat the heat from the drying cast and also to prevent excessive swelling, which causes circulatory and pressure problems. These measures include the application of icebags and elevation of the cast (the higher, the better). Icebags should be placed on the sides of the cast, so they will not cause pressure and make dents. The position of the icebag needs to be checked frequently; if it does not lean slightly against the cast, it will not stay in place. Icebags can be removed in 48 hours.

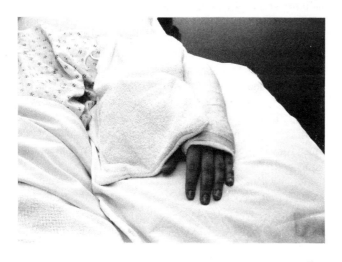

Regular pillows, rather than those that are covered with rubber or plastic, are advised for elevation right from the beginning, because the combined heat of the drying cast and airtight material on a pillow may burn the skin. Casts on extremities should always be elevated when the patient is in bed to reduce the amount of swelling. Patients accept and cooperate in these routines if they know why they are important.

While the cast dries, special attention must be given to the prevention of dents and flat spots that may cause pressure problems. A damp cast needs to be handled with the palms of the hands. When lifting it to check the underside, or when supporting it in patient-turning procedures, the

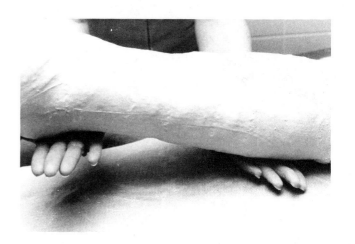

nurse should place the palms of the hand against the cast surface with the fingers extended so the fingertips do not touch the plaster.

Flat spots are further prevented by the use of pillows for elevation. Repositioning on those pillows every 3 hours, along with visual inspection of the entire cast, is essential.

The patient in a hip spica may be turned every 3 hours by the evening of the day the cast is applied (p. 75). Besides its physiologic benefits, frequent turning helps the cast to dry faster.

A cast should be dried from the inside out. Hair dryers, heat lamps, light cradles, and fans facilitate cast drying but are rarely necessary. One of these methods may be indicated if the patient is to be discharged from the hospital early. However, they are to be used with caution. A cast that dries too rapidly will crack or may burn the skin. Lamps and lights should be 15 to 18 inches (38–46 cm) from the cast; heat cradles should not be covered, so that the moisture can escape. A fan frequently cools the patient more than he would like, and so its use is discouraged.

Finishing Cast Edges

Once a cast has dried and swelling in the digits has begun to subside, the nurse and the patient should check for rough edges that need to be covered by adhesive petals. As the patient settles into his cast and moves about, troublesome edges will become apparent. If there is a stockinette under the cast, it will have pulled out over the edge, making petals unnecessary. Likewise, an arm or leg cast may be left without petals if enough sheet wadding extends from under the plaster to provide protection for the skin. However, the patient should be instructed to watch for the appearance of rough edges and should be shown what to do if they develop.

Applying petals to a cast edge around fingers, toes, or arms is frustrating and not always successful, because of the lack of working space. A binding of tape applied just along the edge may be workable, because wrinkling will occur on the *out*side.

A simple way of making petals from adhesive tape is to

cut 2- to 3-inch strips of tape and then round the corners on one end. The rounded end is tucked just inside the cast edge; then the tape is pulled over the edge and secured down onto the cast. The width of tape used is a matter of preference and often depends on how much cast edge there is to cover. It is expedient to use wider tape when there is a lot of edge that must be covered.

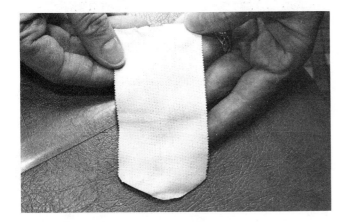

The only purposes in rounding the corners of the tape strip are to make it easier to handle once it is inside the cast edge and to reduce the chance of having it wrinkle. If the tape next to the skin is not smooth, it defeats its own purpose. There is no reason to round the corners on the end of the tape that is attached to the cast surface, unless it is to make it appear neater. Other sources recommend different ways of cutting petals, but the one described here is effective and *fast*.

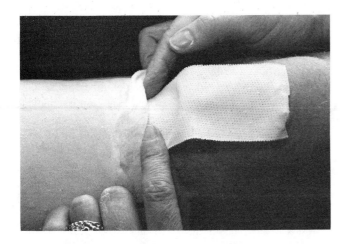

Edges that are extremely rough to begin with should be trimmed or smoothed very slightly with a cast knife. Care should be taken to avoid wrinkling of any of the material under the edges of the cast, be it the petals or padding. Wrinkles press into the skin and cause irritation and breakdown.

Keeping a Cast Clean

There really is no way to keep a cast clean. It cannot be washed, although a damp rag with cleanser may be used. The best way to clean up a cast before discharge is with more wet plaster. The nurse may apply another plaster roll over the soiled area or rub it with a wet plaster splint. A think layer of white shoe polish may be used to cover soiled spots. Care must be taken not to saturate, and thereby soften, the cast. A cast should not be sprayed or painted with any compound that will make it waterproof or easy to clean. Covering the cast surface in this manner prevents evaporation of body moisture and causes maceration of the skin.

Pain and Pressure

When a cast is too tight, it causes symptoms due to compression of blood vessels and nerves. Ongoing assessment of the fracture patient is important in preventing complications and providing optimal care. (See sample nursing-care plan, p. 58.) Swelling in the fracture area is the main cause of tightness, although sometimes a cast is applied too snugly. Orthopedic personnel must remember never to ignore *any* complaints of pain or pressure. (See guidelines for the assessment and management of pain, p. 60.) Serious complications arise in the space of several hours, and irreparable damage can be done to any extremity overnight. Consequently, a nurse may find herself constantly checking the patient who complains endlessly about his cast. If he does complain continuously, measures need to be taken to relieve his symptoms, because if that same patient stops complaining, it may be too late. An arm that "ached" all night and ceases to do so in the morning may have an ischemic muscle, one with a decreased supply of oxygenated blood. A nurse's thoughfulness in allowing the physician to sleep until morning will not be appreciated.

Compartment Syndrome

Compartment syndrome, or progressive vascular compromise, may occur in an extremity as a complication of some types of fractures or injuries. Most commonly, the fractures that precede compartment syndrome are as follows: (1) a supracondylar fracture in the elbow, (2) a fracture of the forearm, or (3) a proximal fracture in the tibia.

A compartment consists of a muscle group enveloped by a tough inelastic fascial tissue. Usually the entry and exit points from the compartment are only large enough to accommodate the route of major arteries and nerves and tendons. Therefore, there is little room for swelling in the muscles of that compartment. The compartments most commonly involved in the forearm are the superficial flexor and deep flexor, with the extensor sustaining secondary involvement. In the leg, the compartments that are involved are the anterior, the lateral and the posterior compartments.

FRACTURE PATIENT: ONGOING ASSESSMENT AND UPDATING OF NURSING-CARE PLAN

Data Collection: 7:00 A.M. Shift Report

Mrs. S., 36 years old, open reduction of a right tibial plateau fracture, 2 days postoperative. She is in a long leg cast. This morning she complains of "tightness" across her knee. She also complains of discomfort at the top of her cast on her posterior thigh. Her toes on the affected leg are slightly swollen. She can dorsiflex all five toes, although she complains that they are all numb. She says she is "tired already" of being in bed.

Nursing Assessment: 8:00 A.M.	*Data Collected*
Was the tightness in the knee a problem before now?	"Not as much."
Is the pain in the knee becoming more severe?	"Not really."
Check amount and method of leg elevation	Two pillows under knee and calf
Check neurovascular (NV) status of toes	Slightly dusky, cool to touch, swollen; "numb" only to touch at distal ends of toes
Check posterior edge and underlying skin in thigh part of cast	Skin not reddened; edge covered with padding, but digging into skin
What kind of activity does the patient feel ready for? Will someone bring diversion in, and how can we help?	Will call home to have husband bring magazines; will "just watch TV"

Nursing Diagnoses

1. Potential impairment of neurovascular status related to pressure of cast.
2. Potential impairment of skin integrity related to pressure of cast on skin surface
3. Alteration in comfort: Discomfort related to fracture and cast
4. Diversional activity deficit related to boredom and inability to perform usual recreational activities

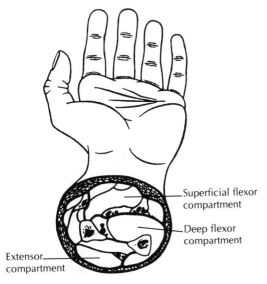

Cross-section of forearm showing compartments outlined by heavy lines

Superficial flexor compartment

Deep flexor compartment

Extensor compartment

Initial ischemia may result from (1) *compression* of blood vessels in the muscle due to swelling associated with trauma or to a cast that is too tight, or (2) an *interruption* of the blood supply to a muscle group when an artery is compressed or severed, as, for example, in a supracondylar fracture of the elbow.

Histamine is released in an ischemic muscle and dilates the capillaries. This allows transudation of plasma into the muscle mass and, consequently, further swelling. Since a compartment is enclosed in an envelope of fascia, swelling is intramuscular, and the pressure exerted compresses small veins and arteries within the muscle. The result is ostensibly a reflex spasm that is an occlusion of the larger arteries entering the muscle compartment. The blood flow is further reduced and more muscle ischemia occurs. The vicious cycle repeats itself and the muscle ischemia is progressive.

If the condition is left untreated, motor and sensory components of the peripheral nerve, which passes through the muscle compartment, also become ischemic and begin to

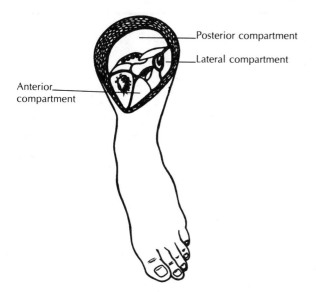

Cross-section of leg showing compartments outlined by heavy lines

lose their functions. Irreversible damage to the muscle group and nerves begins after 6 hours. In 24 to 48 hours the extremity is rendered useless because of scarring, contractures, paralysis, and loss of sensation. One classic example of such deformity is Volkmann's contracture of the hand.

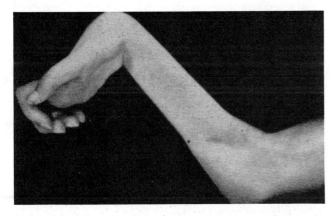

Volkmann's contracture (Boyes: Bunnell's Surgery of the Hand. Philadelphia, Lippincott)

Assessment of Symptoms. The symptoms of compartment syndrome all begin with "P." *Pain* is the most important, because it occurs *first*. This pain is increased on *passive motion*. The remaining symptoms include *paralysis* as evidenced by lack of ability to flex or extend toes or fingers, *paresthesias* with numbness and tingling, and *pulselessness*. Different sources list these in different order. Some authorities consider pulselessness an unreliable sign. Others include *polar*, to indicate coldness. However, *all* are symptoms; and if the nurse is alert to the initial symptom of

pain (especially *pain on passive motion*) and takes measures to relieve it, the order in which she remembers the other symptoms is unimportant. Special devices have been designed to measure compartment pressure. However, they are not in common use.

Other Nursing Responsibilities. The patient who is a candidate for vascular compromise must be instructed in the importance of keeping the involved extremity properly elevated and of reporting symptoms promptly.

The nurse must understand the importance of frequent assessment of the extremity and accurate documentation of all nursing actions and patient responses, both for the patient's welfare and for her own legal protection. For instance, if the patient does not keep his fractured leg elevated as instructed, this fact should be recorded.

Management. Treatment of compartment syndrome begins with elevation of the extremity and removal of the cast. If signs and symptoms are not reduced in at least 1 hour, surgical decompression or *fasciotomy* is indicated.

If fasciotomy is necessary, the surgeon makes an incision in the skin over the involved compartment and then incises the fascia in order to allow the muscle to swell freely. The area is covered with a sterile dressing and left open until swelling has subsided and the skin can be closed or skin grafts applied. Performing a fasciotomy early enough prevents permanent disability.

Neurovascular Assessment

An understanding of what has occurred under the cast in terms of injury or surgery helps the nurse to know what to expect in the way of edema and discoloration. For example, the patient who has had extensive open reduction of a severely comminuted fracture of the ankle would have more edema and discoloration of his toes than the patient with a less extensive operation.

In all casted patients, color, motion, and temperature and sensation of toes or fingers should be observed every 30 minutes for several hours after cast application (longer if there is much edema) and then regularly every 3 hours.

Circulatory impairment results in symptoms of coldness, edema, pallor or cyanosis, pain, and finally numbness in the toes or fingers. The blanching sign in a patient with a casted limb indicates whether or not there is adequate circulation. When the nail of the thumb or great toe is compressed and immediately released, the color should go from white to pink with the same speed as in the uncasted limb. If not, the circulation is slow and the toes or fingers need closer observation. Peripheral pulses in the casted and uncasted extremity should be compared, whenever it is possible to get at them. A casted foot or hand does not leave much room for finding pulses.

GUIDELINES FOR ASSESSING AND MANAGING PAIN IN THE PATIENT WITH A FRACTURED FEMUR OR TIBIA*

Fractured Femur

Expected Pain	Nursing Interventions
Patients with comminuted, compound, or displaced fractures may have severe pain with muscle spasm for at least 7–10 days; unable to tolerate anyone touching any part of thigh	Offer analgesics on schedule. Have enough help when moving patient to do nursing routines. Do them *carefully.* Explain every step that involves patient movement. Check traction q 6 hr. Make certain sling is comfortable and leg is in alignment. Evaluate need for muscle relaxant.
By end of second week, only mild discomfort	Allow patient control over own movements during care routines.

Signs of Complications	Nursing Interventions
Compound fracture: pain that increases or does not seem to be decreasing 1 week post injury	Check for signs of infection.
Early post injury; pain in thigh associated with increasing pressure	Suspect bleeding. Check thigh for swelling ecchymosis. Apply ice. Notify physician.

Fractured Tibia

Expected Pain	Nursing Interventions
Patients with comminuted, compound, or displaced fractures may have severe pain 3–7 days; variable	Offer analgesics on schedule. Elevate leg high. Give adequate support to thigh to maintain position of cast on pillows. Apply ice. Evaluate NV status on schedule. Frequency depends on extent of injury and complaints. In severe fractures, may be every hour for 24 hr and then q 3–6 hr.

Signs of Complications	Nursing Interventions
Pain and pressure unrelieved by analgesics early post injury, localized in area of fracture	Suspect swelling. Elevate higher. Evaluate NV status of toes more frequently. If unsatisfactory, notify physician.
Pain, unrelieved by analgesics, down length of tibia, increased on dorsiflexion of toes. Patient may have paresthesias in toes; 1–3 days post injury	Suspect developing compartment syndrome. Elevate higher. Evaluate NV status and ability of patient to dorsiflex toes. Notify physician immediately. If patient has lost active dorsiflexion, bivalve cast before calling physician, or have someone else notify him while you are doing bivalving.
"Burning" pain, localized, under cast at any time	Suspect skin irritation from pressure spot. Try different positions of casted leg. If problem area is near cast edge, bend edge out slightly. Call problem to attention of physician on rounds.

* These are very general guidelines and in all cases the total patient situation must be considered.

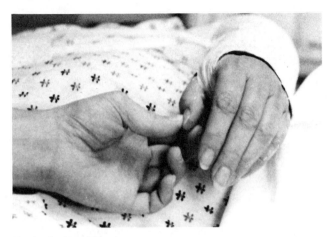

Testing for blanching sign

Patients in arm and leg casts should be able to *move* and *feel* each toe or finger, because the same nerve does not innervate each one. It is not sufficient to pinch the great toe or one or two fingers lightly and conclude that sensation is "good" if the patient responds. All fingers or toes should be checked. This is also true in regard to motion. The patient

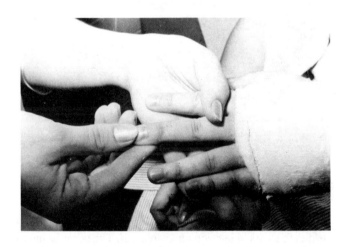

should be able to flex and extend, fully, all of his fingers or toes. A compressed nerve causes localized and constant pain, with numbness of increasing depth until it finaly results in paralysis. Nerves especially subject to compression lie over the bony prominences. Therefore, when a nurse suspects compression of a nerve, the first action should be to check the position of the casted extremity. Table 2-2 illustrates some tests for nerve function.

Skin over bony prominences is also prone to problems due to pressure, such as necrosis and formation of decubitus ulcers. The surface of the cast should be felt over the areas where pain has been reported. If necrosis or infection is developing the cast will feel warm. For patients in leg casts, other places to watch for signs of pain and pressure are the heel and Achilles tendon.

Table 2-2. Assessment of Nerve Function

Nerve	Action By the Nurse: Test for Sensory Function	Action by the Patient: Test for Motor Function
Radial	Prick web space between thumb and index finger	Hyperextend thumb or wrist
Median	Prick distal surface of index finger	Oppose thumb and little finger; flex wrist
Ulnar	Prick distal end of small finger	Abduct all fingers
Peroneal	Prick lateral surface of great toe and medial surface of second toe	Dorsiflex ankle; extend toes
Tibial	Prick medial and lateral surfaces of sole of foot	Plantarflex ankle and flex toes

Mention should be made of the fact that severe edema often causes blisters and adds to complaints of discomfort in fractures in which there is not much tissue over and around the area to absorb fluid. Specific locations for fracture blisters are on the ankle or the skin over the tibia.

Location and description of *all* pain should be clear in the nurse's mind before analgesics are given. Is it discomfort in the fracture area? Does it run along a nerve? Is it over a bony prominence? Is the cast green or has it been on 3 days and is the pain therefore a new one? The answers to questions such as these determine the need for further assessment.

Nursing Interventions. Basic to the care of a patient with a cast is recognizing and *teaching the patient to recognize* that added discomfort in the form of *pain*, tingling, and numbness *at any time* after application may be due to pressure on nerves or blood vessels and must be reported to the physician.

Because of this danger, it is routine, especially after an open reduction, for many orthopedic surgeons to mark a cast where it could be split should it prove to be too tight in the first day or two postoperatively. This then becomes a nursing judgment, when circulation to fingers or toes becomes obviously constricted and swelling is not decreased by elevation or ice. In general, a cast should be split *all the way*, including the padding, if this procedure is done to relieve edema. Nurses are sometimes reluctant to do this, but it is far better to ruin a cast unnecessarily than to risk serious damage to an extremity.

Cutting a cast is best done by using an oscillating saw (cast cutter) and then separating the edges slightly with a spreader. The split can be taped temporarily with adhesive. Later the surgeon may apply additional plaster rolls to cover the opened area and ensure proper immobilization. If the cast is to be *bivalved*, it is split down both sides so that half of it can be removed. This becomes necessary if a large area (such as a surgical incision) needs inspection or if the patient

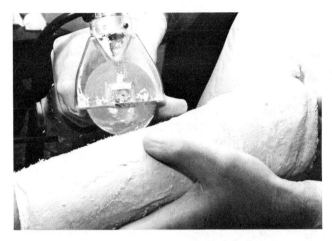

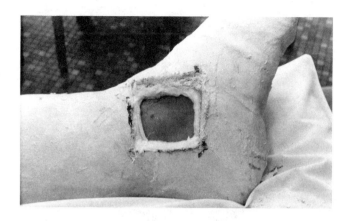

continues to complain after one split has been made and the problem seems extensive. The physician should do this procedure. The limb is left elevated in the bottom half of the cast until swelling is diminished. Then the top half is replaced and secured with new plaster rolls.

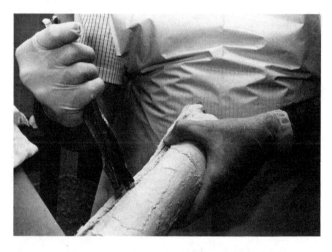

At times a window is cut in a cast to inspect a surgical dressing or to apply one, or to relieve pressure on a tender area (usually the heel or ankle). The danger in this procedure is that the exposed area might swell quickly and add

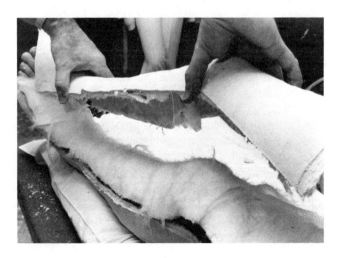

another problem. As with bivalving, the surgeon should cut such windows. If the nurse is instructed to do so, a pad should be placed over the windowed area and an ace bandage applied to reduce the chance of excessive edema. The piece of the cast that was removed should be saved in case the physician decides to put it back in place.

A simple method of relieving localized pressure is to cut slits in the cast over the affected area.

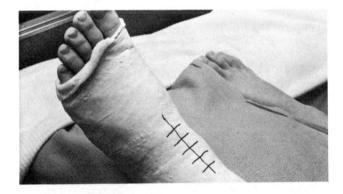

Assessing Damage

Two types of drainage occur in casted fracture patients. One is due to surgical incision and is normal. The other is due to infection or the sloughing away of tissues and is not normal.

In patients who have undergone open reductions, drainage occurs through the cast in proportion to the extent of surgery and the number of blood vessels in the operative area. Drainage, if profuse, may seep down and discolor the back of the cast, so it is important to check this area also.

The drainage appears to increase for 24 to 48 hours and is bright red, gradually turning brown as it decreases and stops. During this period the color and amount should be observed, recorded every 3 hours, and brought to the attention of the surgeon daily. "New" drainage should be recorded in a unit of measurement, "two inches by one inch," or as compared with an object, "the size of an egg," rather than circled on the cast. Since measurement of drainage must be recorded on the chart, drawing circles on a cast is superfluous, calls the patient's attention to the fact that he has drainage, and may cause him unnecessary alarm.

There is also some risk of *infection* when an open reduction is done. Drainage from an infection or necrotic area may be preceded by complaints of pain, pressure, and warm area on the cast. Smelling the cast by getting the nose down next to the edge is the only way to detect the musty, offensive odor from necrosis or infection that has not begun to drain through the cast. This should be done daily.

Cast odors, exclusive of perspiration or those from large casts caused by soilage from elimination, are abnormal and should be considered danger signals. Drainage over an open reduction is also abnormal if it is any color but red or reddish brown. All such drainage needs to be reported promptly to the physician, along with any systemic symptoms of infection.

Improving Observations

An excellent way for the orthopedic nurse to appreciate the postoperative complaints of the patient and the concerns of the surgeon after an open reduction, or any other orthopedic operation for that matter, is to observe or participate, if possible, in such a procedure. It is easy for a nurse, once removed from the surgical experience of a nursing education and absorbed in the role at hand, to become less aware of the trauma and manipulation of body tissues that must take place during surgery. Becoming part of an orthopedic surgery team for an open reduction is an excellent opportunity to review the vascular structure of bones and the proximity of the bones to muscles, nerves, and blood vessels. This type of experience is also a reminder of the skill, knowledge, and time involved in putting fractured bones back together by *any* method. The routines, such as those established for cast observations, take on more meaning.

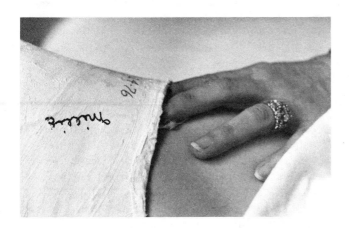

Skin Care

The skin near and under cast edges should be inspected each time neurovascular checks are done. At this time loose crumbs should be removed from under the edge as well as brushed away from the area, so they will not cause irritation. Alcohol rubbed lightly under the edges will keep the skin dry. Lotion should not be used as it builds up and feels

"sticky." The cast edges themselves need to be felt to see if petals or other protection are in need of repair. Chances of skin breakdown at these edges lessen as edema subsides. Instruct the patient to report irritated spots under cast edges, rather than pull out or insert more padding on his own initiative.

The padding under the posterior edge of the cast should be inspected when the patient is turned. If the padding has been pushed down into the cast, it should be pulled up carefully, and the edge should be petaled at that time. Explain that the purpose of padding and stockinette is the protection of the skin and proper fit of the cast. The temptation to scratch under a cast is almost irresistible, especially when it is warm and itchy. Patients should be told that anything stuck inside a cast to scratch may (1) damage the skin and promote infection and (2) cause the lining of the cast to become wrinkled, possibly intensifying the itching.

Should irritation develop at any point under the cast edge, every effort should be made to remove the cause. When an extremity is not elevated properly, cast edges press into the skin and cause pain. A common complaint of the patient in a long leg cast is pain at the top and back of the cast. In this instance, the nurse should further elevate the

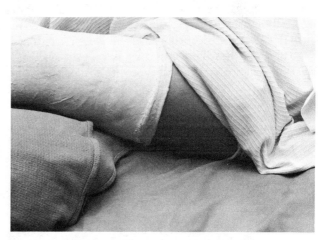

distal end of the cast to allow the top posterior edge of the cast to drop away from the skin. If irritation along a cast edge persists, the nurse should bend that edge *slightly* (unless it is a cast brace) with a duckbilled cast bender. Exces-

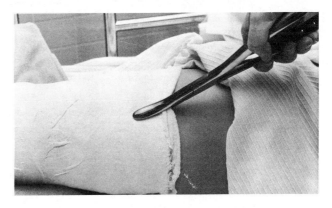

sive bending or any trimming of the cast should not be done without a physician's order. A scarcely noticeable alteration in a cast edge or pillow position often affords the patient instant relief.

Exposing a reddened or sore spot a little so that air will circulate over it is more desirable than applying emollient ointments. Using a mirror and flashlight to see inside a cast is *not* successful if a cast is tight. If the cast is not tight, such investigation is probably not necessary.

Rubbing may occur at the edges of a cast. The sheet wadding used in plaster cast application is useful in these situations. The nurse should tuck a length of sheet wadding inside the cast edge until the patient notes relief, and then tear the sheet wadding off so that several inches hang over and outside the cast. This allows for adjustment, removal, and a means of securing the padding in place, since the end can be taped to the cast.

Many nurses have their own "tricks of the trade" in identifying and solving problems, and they do whatever works for them. Even the best ideas work only if put into practice, and observed, on a regular schedule.

Toes and fingers on a casted extremity need to be cleaned daily. Soap and water should be used if it is possible to do so without getting the cast wet. The use of alcohol on an applicator is suggested to ensure that the skin between the fingers and toes is dry. Lotions or oils soften skin that is becoming dry. Cracking of the skin is to be avoided as an added precaution against irritation and infection.

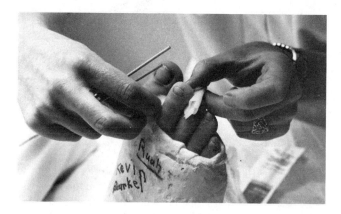

Patients in casts, especially long leg casts, body casts, and hip spicas, do not move easily in bed. Even an arm cast makes movement in bed awkward or slow. Pressure areas may develop on the buttocks, back, iliac crests, elbows, heels, ears, or any body part that rests on the bed. *All* potential pressure areas on the body need to be inspected twice daily. Skin care for the entire body is important. Bathing, careful drying, and lotion rubs keep the skin in good condition and provide opportunities for inspection and patient teaching. Include the patient in his plan as much as possible, since he will be caring for himself a long time in his cast. Many times he learns to do things better himself. For instance, he may be able to reach areas under cast edges

more easily because he knows how far he can go without it hurting.

Seeing that the patient changes position frequently and that the bed linen is free from wrinkles and plaster crumbs is part of complete skin care.

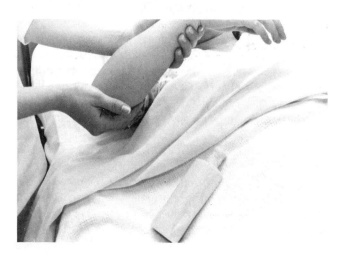

Exercise

With the emphasis on immobilization in fracture treatment, casted patients need exercise if they are to maintain muscle strength and prevent the complications of immobility. Joints above and below the cast are exercised to minimize stiffness, unless otherwise ordered. In addition, the patient should be encouraged to flex, extend, and generally keep his unaffected limbs active so that three limbs can more easily do the work of four. Teaching him what full range of motion is, gives him a routine to follow. He should also be instructed that using the trapeze strengthens a left arm that needs to perform the tasks of the right, or prepares both arms for supporting body weight on crutches. As indicated earlier, the patient should be aware that moving the fingers or toes of a casted extremity increases circulation.

Muscle-setting or isometric exercises should be taught on the uninvolved extremity so that they can be done on the fractured extremity under the cast. The physician should be consulted as to how much of this exercise is appropriate. For example, if the quadriceps mechanism has been involved in the fracture or its repair, the surgeon would want to proceed very cautiously with any exercising. However, if and when exercise is permitted, it should be done faithfully. Without exercise, the quadriceps begins to atrophy in about a week.

There are simple ways to explain this exercise to a patient. One way is to tell him to push the back of his knee as far down as possible against the mattress. Another method of teaching quadriceps setting is to ask the patient to tighten his unaffected anterior thigh muscle, or quadriceps, so that he pulls his kneecap up into the muscle. If possible, have him place his hand on the thigh while doing this exercise so that he can feel the change that occurs in contraction and relaxation of the quadriceps.

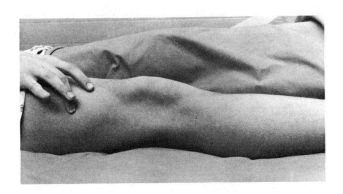

An alert, properly instructed and guided patient is his own best source of prevention in the case of contractures.

General Discomfort

In the care of the casted patient, a few insights may help develop what might be called "common nursing sense." Aside from the irritation that a cast causes because of its specific location, sleeping with any body part in a new cast is often like sleeping in cracker crumbs. Even conscientious removal of crumbs from under the cast edges and the bottom sheet is relatively futile for the first few days at least. Added problems arise from the awkwardness and weight of the cast. Moving suddenly at night may mean a bump or a clunk on the head. A jerk into wakefulness is the result when a heavy leg slides off a pillow. Because a patient has not required a pain pill for 8 hours does not necessarily mean he or she had a good night's sleep. A whole day's behavior may reflect the effects of a restless, uncomfortable night that is never verbalized by the patient.

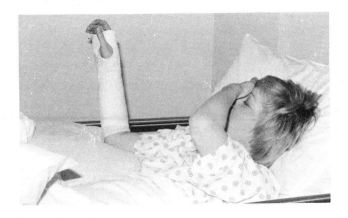

Psychological Considerations

Some authorities claim that a properly fitting cast is very comfortable. While this may be true, it is also true that casts frequently make patients feel insecure when making moves that are not routine. For instance, transferring a patient with a long leg cast onto a stretcher for a trip to the x-ray department may be awkward. To relieve the patient's apprehension during this procedure, see that pillows are properly placed for support, make sure the siderails are up, and

take a moment to question the patient and make certain she feels secure.

Since a cast is a relatively common sight, it may be difficult for those outside of it to believe that some people are embarrassed by having to wear one, since it subjects them to quizzical glances from strangers and questions from friends. An understanding of this makes a nurse more sensitive to the emotional needs of the patient.

Many people take wearing a cast in stride, whereas others are constantly at odds with the limitations and discomforts imposed on them. In some purely mechanical ways, life in a cast is the same for everyone. However, the psychological problems that present themselves to "cast dwellers" are unique for each individual.

Cast-Care Instruction

All patients in casts should be taught that swelling of the fingers or toes lingers for a long time, requiring periods of elevation for relief. However, any change in neurovascular status, as well as any odor not associated with soiling from elimination, should be reported.

It is unwise to try to give the patient any advice about bathing, except to tell him to avoid wetting the cast. Otherwise, a patient may misunderstand the directions and fall into the bathtub, incurring additional injury to himself, and creating a few problems for the person who gave him the advice.

As for general instructions, the "tips" outlined on page 66 might be written in pamphlet form and sent home with all casted patients.

The nurse can still offer psychological support to the long-term casted patient and his family if she maintains contact with them after the patient leaves the hospital.

When an active individual has been in a cast for a prolonged period and the cast is beginning to show signs of wear, it becomes a nuisance both to him and to those with whom he lives. The patient is tired of the cast and tired of explaining how he came to be in it. His family may be tired of accommodating him. In addition, casts take their toll on furniture. Very likely, everyone in the household has noticed that old casts become "smelly." This patient would benefit emotionally from being able to communicate with those who cared for him in the hospital. In return, the nurse will gain insight into possible problems and solutions that might help in discharge planning for other casted patients.

Care of the Patient in an Arm Cast

Patient Education

A woman who stepped out of her car onto ice and fell, fracturing her forearm, may have undergone closed reduction and cast application in the emergency room before reaching the orthopedic ward. In this type of situation, it is

IMPORTANT THINGS TO WATCH FOR AND DO WHILE YOU ARE WEARING YOUR CAST

Caring for Your Cast

- If it becomes soiled, clean it with a damp cloth with dry cleanser. If it is still soiled, use white shoe polish, but sparingly; too much may saturate and soften the cast.
- Avoid getting water on or in your cast. If it becomes damp, use a hair dryer to dry the affected area.
- Plastic bags are good covering in wet weather.
- If the cast edges become rough, cover the rough area with tape.
- Arm casts are most comfortable with a sling support.

Caring for Your Skin

- Wash the skin area around cast, taking care not to saturate the cast in the process.
- Rub the areas around the cast frequently with alcohol. Lotion has a tendency to build up on the inside of the cast and become sticky, so it should never be used around the cast or under it.
- If edges are causing irritation to the skin, pad with soft materials such as cotton or foam. Be sure the padding is well anchored to the cast; loose material slipping into the cast causes even more irritation.

Important Things to Watch for

Twice a day check your fingers, if the cast is on your arm; toes, if the cast is on your leg.

- Are they pink in color? Squeeze the nail till white; when released, pink color should return immediately. If return is slow, call your doctor.
- Do not be alarmed if your foot appears darker when it is down. This is normal.
- Watch for swelling. Compare it to the other hand or foot. Are they about the same?
- Move fingers or toes. DO NOT JUST WIGGLE — fully extend the fingers or toes. If there is any loss of motion or any increased pain, call your doctor.
- Make sure there is feeling on all surfaces of the hand and fingers, or foot and toes. If any numbness, tingling, or pinprick pain develops, call your doctor.
- Check around cast for any odors other than those that may be from something spilled on or around the cast. Ordinarily, casts won't smell. Be especially conscious of odors if there are stitches under the cast. If you notice any smell, don't delay; call your doctor. Also watch for any staining of, or discharge from, the cast.
- If you notice swelling after activity, elevate the extremity — the higher the better.

If Your Doctor Permits, Then

- If you are wearing an arm cast, to keep shoulder from becoming stiff, *each day,* four times a day, remove the sling and exercise the arm by putting it through its full range of motion. In other words, move it the way it normally goes.
- For the leg in a cast, if possible, work at "*setting,*" that is, tightening then relaxing, the thigh muscles, doing this frequently, or every 2 hours while awake. You should discuss this with your doctor *first,* but some exercise is essential.
- If skin under the cast begins to itch, *do not* try to stick anything inside the cast to scratch, especially if there is an area with stitches. Parents, be especially alert to children sticking forks, sticks, or other ingenious objects inside the cast.

Remember:
Cast Care Must Continue as Long as Your Cast is on.

wise to assume nothing as far as previous patient teaching is concerned, because no matter what instruction has taken place, the emotional atmosphere of an emergency room is not an ideal setting for learning. Because of the demands of the job, an emergency-room nurse does not always have time to evaluate how effective efforts to teach patients about their casts have been. Therefore, the nurse on the orthopedic ward may realize in the course of an admission interview that the patient heard nothing anyone told her about her cast because she was preoccupied with the pain and shock of her injury, the absurdity of the accident that brought her here, and, most important, concern about the alterations she will have to make in her pattern of daily living. Therefore, one of the first priorities for the nurse is to plan *with* the patient and to discuss the type of care and observations necessary for successful treatment, comfort, and prevention of complications.

Assessing for Compression Complications

In an arm fracture near the elbow, trauma to the blood vessels or edema in that area may cause ischemia in the forearm muscles and could result in Volkmann's contracture. The essential observation in checking for the onset of this complication is finger movement. When checking fingers for motion, it is not sufficient to request the patient to "wiggle" them. She must be able to extend them fully. If she cannot, or if this action causes her more pain, the surgeon should be notified immediately. As is shown below, deformity results in a claw-shaped hand with flexed wrist and fingers and some atrophy in the forearm.

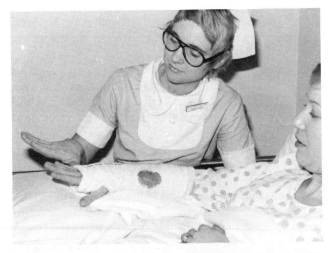

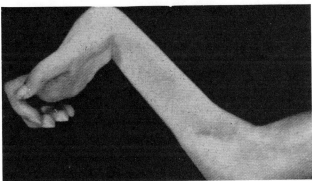

Volkmann's contracture (Boyes: Bunnell's Surgery of the Hand. Philadelphia, Lippincott)

Swelling around or injury to the median nerve causes loss of or delayed sensation in the index and middle finger, and in the case of the ulnar nerve, in the ring and little finger. The condyles and olecranon process at the elbow and the radial and styloid processes at the wrist are the bony prominences where compression problems or skin breakdown might occur. Fingers should be checked closely for color, motion, temperature, and sensation.

As was emphasized earlier, the type of fracture helps determine the specific observations. In the very common Colles' wrist fracture, the end of the radius is fractured and displaced backward. The styloid process of the ulna may also be broken off. After reduction, it becomes important to check the fingers for motion, not only because of possible blood vessel and nerve damage, but also because there are at least 24 tendons in the wrist.

The nurse must also be familiar with complications resulting from fractures of the humerus. The radial nerve more or less wraps itself around the humerus on its journey down the arm, and injury or edema in the proximity of this nerve causes wristdrop.

If a hanging cast is used in treatment, it immobilizes the wrist, making evaluation of wrist movement impossible. However, if the radial nerve has been damaged, the first phalange will not be able to offer resistance to pressure, nor will extension of the thumb be possible.

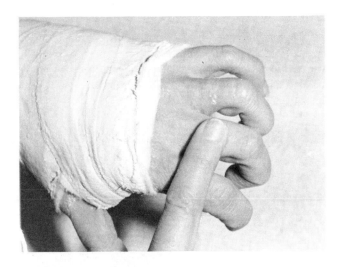

Hanging Cast

When a hanging cast is applied for fractures of the humerus, two factors must be taken into consideration. A hanging cast is heavier than an arm cast. In addition, patients requiring such a cast are usually in the older age group. This combination produces a patient with a greater feeling of helplessness than is normally encountered in fracture patients.

Although the strap that goes around the neck and is attached to the cast at the wrist is usually padded with felt or foam, it is still a source of pressure and irritation. A woman wearing such a cast is prone to skin irritation and breakdown from the pressure of the cast on her ribs and breasts because of her inability (due to fracture location) or reluctance to move her arm. If a woman has large breasts, she may complain of discomfort caused by the casted arm pressing against them. All of these areas that are prone to irritation require meticulous skin care and observation. Padding the axilla with a thick dressing keeps the cast edge on the arm's medial side from irritating the skin.

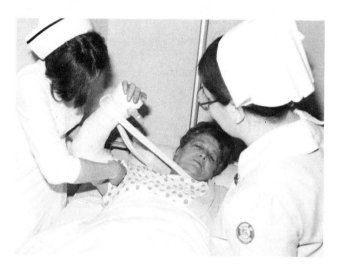

Sling

Usually the patient with an arm cast is up and about, during which time a sling should be used to support the weight of the cast as well as the hand and wrist. A casted arm should be placed in a sling slightly flexed position to prevent strain on the shoulder muscles.

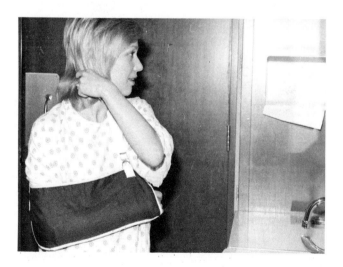

Orthopedic supply companies manufacture various types of slings, but they all share basic design principles. That is, they are made to give comfort and support by spreading the weight of the extremity evenly across the neck and shoulders. Materials used permit circulation of air in and around the cast and arm. These slings are generally most comfortable for long-term use.

The triangular sling, when used, should be pinned at both sides of the back of the neck rather than knotted over the cervical spine. This allows the stress of weight to be distributed and avoids pressure on the spine.

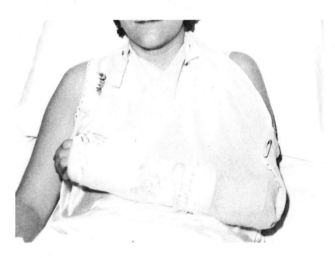

Exercise

Range-of-motion exercises for the shoulder are a priority for the patient in an arm cast. Since there are patients who react as if the best way to heal a fractured arm is to hold it still, the nurse must encourage and supervise arm exercises. Location of the fracture determines the extent of exercise allowed. The patient with a fractured humerus may also have severe tissue injury in the shoulder area and may be very reluctant to exercise. A stiff or "frozen" shoulder due to contractures is a real danger when motion is limited; a patient must be taught and encouraged to keep this joint as active as possible. Fingers on the affected hand also need exercise. Whatever exercise is indicated, active or passive, should be explained to the patient.

Since the unaffected arm is the "worker," muscle fatigue is common in a patient who is striving for independence by

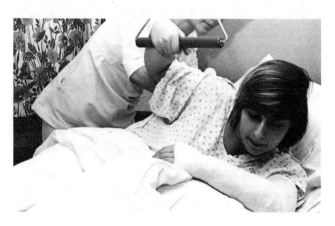

using her left hand when she normally used her right. Back and shoulder rubs several times a day relieve the aches caused by this activity and provide an opportunity for the nurse to offer encouragement.

Other Patient Activities

If the patient with a casted arm is on bed rest, she should have items placed where she can reach them when she is bathing, eating, or engaging in diversional activities. A trapeze allows her to change position when she feels like it.

Once the patient with a hanging cast is out of bed, a straight-backed chair should be used so that the cast hangs freely. It is also easier to stand up from this type of chair. If traction is not applied to the arm at night, the head of the bed must be elevated and the cast must not be permitted to rest on a pillow. If the patient has difficulty sleeping in this position, her knees may be "gatched" for comfort.

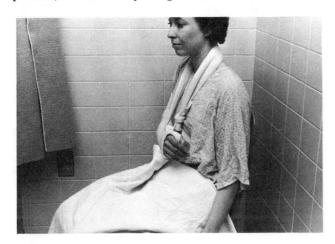

Psychological Implications

Although it is true that fracturing an arm and wearing a cast does not necessarily mean the onset of depression for every patient, it is also true that for others a tremendous adjustment must be made. Take, for example, a young mother who is right-handed and suffers a fracture of the right arm. Her mind will be crowded with worries. How will she care for her own very personal needs? How will she care for her family? What will she do when she gets home?

Pages could be written on the problems that an arm cast poses, depending on the age, sex, and occupation of the patient involved. The nurse can help the patient make a start toward resolving some of these problems by helping her to become or remain as independent as possible.

Discharge Planning

In all likelihood, a nurse will have as many questions as the patient when planning for discharge, since each patient goes home to a different set of circumstances. Since an arm cast does not usually hospitalize a person for long periods, a special effort should be made to offer suggestions at an early stage of care. Although general cast care at home is covered earlier in this chapter, a few specific observations about arm casts may be made here.

Working with an arm cast is like carrying an extra burden all day. Therefore, instructions regarding the use of the sling need to be reviewed, and the patient should be reminded that frequent rest periods for the entire body are necessary. At these times, elevation of the cast so that the fingers are at eye level will reduce swelling that occurs in the fingers and also relieve the burden of weight on the shoulders, neck, and back.

For the elderly patient who has lived alone, being discharged with a a hanging cast may mean a period of time in an extended-care facility until she regains the use of her arm. Complete data regarding her needs, personal habits, likes and dislikes, documented by the nurse and sent to the patient's destination, aid in providing continuity of care. Discussing these plans with the patient before she is discharged makes the transition from the hospital to another facility much smoother and adds to her peace of mind.

Care of the Patient in a Leg Cast

Positioning

Comfortable settling into bed of the patient with a long leg cast starts with a firm mattress, enough pillows, and an overhead bar or trapeze.

The heavier the cast, the longer it takes to dry, so more attention must be given to its position on pillows during this

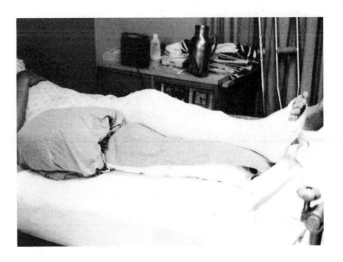

period. Pillows should be repositioned under the cast at regular intervals for 24 hours after it *feels* dry to the touch. Flat spots, meaning pressure, on the heel or posterior surface of the leg develop insidiously. The The heel of the cast should not be on the bed *at all* for the first 24 hours.

Supporting the cast so that it will remain elevated in the desired position is best accomplished by folding a pillow over and tucking it under the thigh portion of the cast and the hip joint. The hip is thus prevented from rotating the leg out and off the pillows. The same "trochanter roll" can be made by placing a folded blanket under the patient's thigh and buttock and rolling it under far enough to lift and support the pelvis. Rolling it *over* rather than *under* is not reommended, since it will unroll.

When turning the patient in a long leg cast onto his uncasted side, place a pillow between his legs to support the cast and to prevent strain on the back muscles.

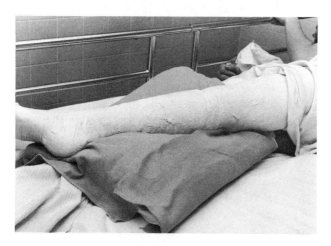

Specific points where pressure is dangerous in a casted leg are behind the knee on the popliteal artery, the upper outer part of the fibula on the peroneal nerve, the Achilles' tendon, and the heel.

Bedpan Procedure

Using a bedpan or urinal in this position may be awkward. A long leg cast that is elevated on pillows makes elimination procedures somewhat contrary to gravity. The casted leg should remain supported by pillows, however, when the patient is placed on the bedpan or is using the urinal. Otherwise, the casted leg feels as though it is dangling in space. If the cast is very long, extra care must be taken in placing and removing bedpans and urinals so that the top of the cast is not soiled. Drying the buttocks thoroughly is essential because the patient spends so much time lying on his back.

When the patient in a long leg cast seems reluctant to use a bedpan, the nurse should anticipate that he may develop problems with constipation. To help prevent this, the nurse should get an order from the physician to help this patient out of bed onto a commode or take him to the bathroom in a wheelchair. Although these procedures may be time consuming until both the patient and the nurse develop a coordinated effort, the time is well spent if the patient maintains or regains a normal elimination routine.

Very often a patient who is not enthusiastic about taking oral fluids may be motivated to do so if he knows it makes voiding and elimination easier. Fruit juices and water should be encouraged on a regular schedule. Extra milk has no value in fracture healing and may be instrumental in causing renal calculi if the patient is quite immobile.

Exercises

While patients in long leg casts are confined to bed, they should be encouraged to exercise all unaffected extremities. Routine movements in bed and self-assistance with the aid of a trapeze are usually sufficient to maintain general muscle strength. Discussing with the patient the benefits of exercises and encouraging their frequent performance helps keep the patient's mind and body occupied.

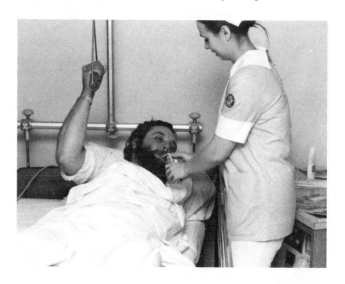

Knowing the location of the fracture becomes important in understanding the purpose of exercises. For example, fractures of the condyles of the tibia into the knee joint require a certain amount of healing before weight bearing is permitted. Since this type of fracture is often caused by a shearing force, premature weight bearing may result in impaction. Since this patient would not be allowed weight bearing on the tibia, maintenance of muscle strength by exercises may need to be emphasized more.

Psychological Considerations

For some patients, adjustment to a long leg cast involves learning to sleep in a supine position. If this is difficult, a patient may spend those long night hours quietly worrying about his convalescence or keeping his roommate awake with a radio. Back rubs, smooth bedding, and fluffed and properly placed pillows may not be enough. Sedation or pain medication are a last resort, unless the patient is very restless or uncomfortable. Perhaps the only other thing a nurse can do is allow the patient to sleep once he does, even if it means postponing early-morning routines.

Patients need moral support when progress seems slow or when the physician has given them what they consider "bad news." For example, the patient with a fracture involving a joint may be told by the physician that considerable stiffness will be present when the cast is removed and that an extensive period of regular exercise will be necessary. He may want to express his fears about a "stiff joint" and may need reassurance that he has been told the truth about eventually regaining normal motion.

A strange and endless variety of psychological problems accompany fracture injuries. A young man may be more upset about the vehicle he demolished than the leg he fractured, and he may appear uninterested in plans for his care. A 19-year-old girl, planning to be married, could be in despair over having to postpone her wedding day and all the confusion this entails. Highly sensitive or imaginative people may have guilt feelings because they are not dead, if they feel responsible for an accident that hurt or killed others. Not always willing or able to initiate a discussion of these feelings, they behave in a way that is baffling and discouraging to those around them. In spite of conscientious care, they appear irritable, demanding, or depressed. Well-meaning friends may approach such a patient with the attitude that he ought to feel "lucky to be alive." Empathy on the part of the nurse gives this patient an opportunity to air his feelings.

Assisting the Patient into a Wheelchair

The patient with a long leg cast usually is allowed to sit in a wheelchair a day before he begins crutchwalking. Two nurses should assist the patient in getting out of bed. The patient should be helped to a sitting position on the side of the bed. The wheelchair should be locked in position parallel to the bed and facing the uncasted leg. One nurse should hold the casted leg. The other nurse places her foot in front of the patient's foot and her arms around his waist or behind his shoulders as he rises to a standing position on one leg. He is then pivoted around to where he can seat himself in the wheelchair. At this time the casted leg should be elevated on the extension provided for such purposes, with a pillow

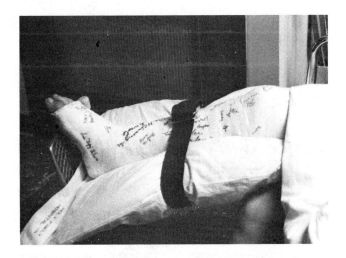

placed between the cast and extension and all three held together by a belt. For purposes of safety, the patient should have his leg secured to the extension or leg rest by a belt every time he is in the wheelchair.

Some psychological support may be necessary at this point. The patient may be discouraged because he feels so helpless and because the casted leg that was just starting to "feel better" may feel tight again, owing to the swelling that results from having it lowered.

Preparation for Ambulation and Weight Bearing

Pull-ups on the trapeze and lifting weights are exercises that can be done in bed to help strengthen arm muscles for crutchwalking. If the patient is allowed up in a wheelchair, he can do *wheelchair push-ups.* That is, he raises his hips up off the seat by pushing down with his hands on the arms of the wheelchair. The chair should be locked in position at this time.

For the lower extremities, quadriceps setting is beneficial. Straight leg raising of the unaffected leg, as well as the casted leg if possible, is also recommended and helps maintain proper hip joint motion. An added exercise includes pulling the unaffected leg into a knee-chest position.

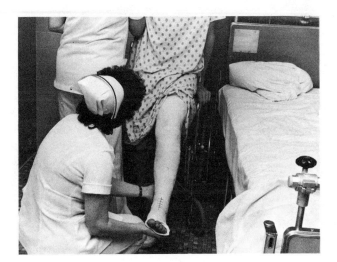

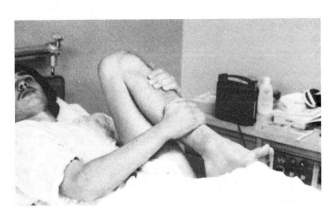

A patient who has his leg casted with the knee in extension may need a lift on the shoe on the uninvolved foot. The nurse should check with the surgeon early in the hospitalization period about the height of such a lift. The patient or his family can then be informed about what must be done in order to have the shoe ready for the patient when he is ready to use it.

Ambulating With a Walking Cast

Once a walking heel or iron is applied to the cast (p. 51) and the plaster roll used to attach it to the cast is dry, the patient is able to ambulate at will. Instead of a walking iron or heel, some surgeons prefer a cast shoe that is made of a sturdy

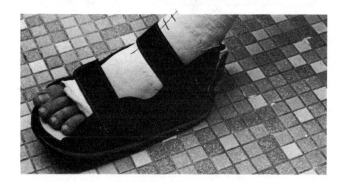

material and has a nonslip sole; it is worn over the casted foot. The strangeness of walking on such a device, the weight of the cast, and the swelling that occurs in the toes are of concern to the patient. He should be instructed to go slowly and to elevate the leg every time he sits down.

Crutchwalking

Although teaching a patient how to walk on crutches is largely the responsibility of a physical-therapy department, a nurse who does not know the basics cannot give intelligent guidance or help with independent procedures, such as taking the patient to the bathroom. Furthermore, in small hospitals therapists are not always available, so that the nurse may be required to give instruction in crutchwalking.

Crutch Fitting. Measuring a patient for crutches is ideally done in parallel bars in physical therapy. If the patient must be measured while in the supine position in bed, he should be wearing the shoes in which he will be walking. The length of a crutch is measured from a point 1 to 2 inches (2.5 – 5 cm or 2 to 3 fingers) below the axilla to a second point 6 to 10 inches (15 – 25 cm) out to the side of the bottom of the foot, about 6 to 8 inches (20 cm) from the heel. Measurement in the axilla starts next to the skin. The handpiece on the crutch should be adjusted so that there is no more than a 30-degree bend of the elbow, thus allowing for extension of the arm with minimal effort when taking a step.

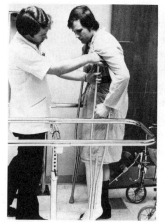
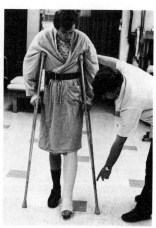

Crutch Safety. Crutches that have been used before need to be inspected for wear. The wood should not be split or slivered, and all parts must be intact. Rubber tips on the ends should not be smooth or they will slip on the floor and cause the crutches to fall away from the patient.

Initial concerns in the instruction of crutch walking deal with safety factors. The brake on the bed or wheelchair should be secured before the patient is assisted up. Both gown and robe must be checked to see that they are fastened. Many therapists recommend low-heeled oxfords as the best footwear for proper support, while some advocate gym shoes (sneakers) because they make stable contact with the floor. However, any shoe or slipper that does not have a smooth bottom may be worn.

A belt made of good strong material is needed to provide control of the patient so he will not lose his balance or put weight on the affected extremity. It should be worn by the patient whenever he is out of bed, always providing a place to "grab" him should he fall or trip.

Help the patient to a standing position on the uninvolved leg and immediately place the crutches. Check to see that they are the correct length, remembering that properly measured crutches maximize the ease of crutchwalking and

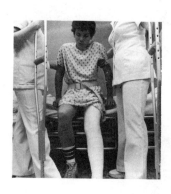
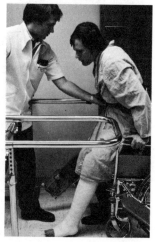

increase safety. Two people should always be present for the patient's first attempt at this procedure, in case he becomes lightheaded or dizzy.

Finally, and most important, the weightbearing status of the involved leg must be known. For example, is the patient allowed partial or full weightbearing? If a walking heel or iron is attached to the bottom of the cast, he may be allowed full weightbearing. However, orders for weightbearing for all patients in leg casts must come from the physician.

Crutch Gaits. Once the patient is safely upright, he should be allowed time to feel stable in the balanced or tripod position. His crutches should be slightly to the side and 10 inches (25 cm) in front of him.

The gait normally used by the patient in a leg cast is for non- or partial weightbearing and is called the 3-in-1 or 3-point gait. The patient moves the crutches forward, then the involved leg, taking the weight on the wrists and palms. The uninvolved leg then follows.

3-point gait

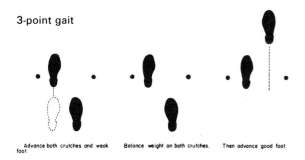

Advance both crutches and weak foot.   Balance weight on both crutches.   Then advance good foot.

Starting from the tripod position, the patient moves the casted leg forward to the crutches, then steps with the uninvolved leg, and so on. When partial weightbearing is ordered, the involved leg takes weight along with the wrists and palms. A simple rule to teach the patient is that the crutches always go with the cast.

The swing-through gait may be used for nonweightbearing ambulation, but caution is advised because it is a faster gait and requires more practice. From the tripod position, the patient pushes down on the hand grips to raise the body, always keeping the casted leg about 4 inches (10 cm) in front of the other foot, as he steps forward on the unaffected

Swing-through gait

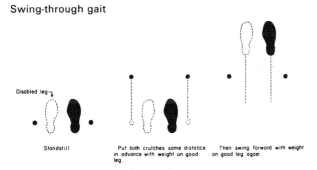

Disabled leg

Standstill   Put both crutches some distance in advance with weight on good leg.   Then swing forward with weight on good leg again.

leg. He then returns the crutches to the starting point ahead of his body.

In climbing and descending steps, the patient should be instructed always to move his crutches with his cast. Together they go first when going down stairs and last when going up. To avoid accidents caused by confusing the two, tell him, "The good leg goes up and the bad leg goes down."

Sitting and Standing. There are several ways for a patient with a cast to get in and out of a chair. The two most simple procedures are as follows. To sit down, the patient positions herself so that she stands with her back to the chair, moving her uncasted leg back until it touches the chair. She then transfers both crutches to the hand on the casted side, grasps the armrest with the other hand and sits down, pushing herself back in the chair. The crutches are placed next to the chair or against the armrest, depending on the type of chair and the convenience of the patient.

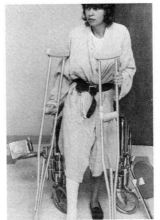 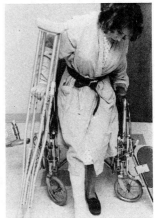

Technique for sitting

When getting up, the patient stands the crutches upright together, holds on to the crutch handgrips with the hand on the casted side, and moves her uncasted leg back so that it

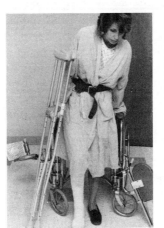 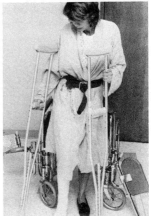

Technique for standing

touches the chair. She pushes up on the opposite armrest with the other hand and, on coming to a standing position, transfers a crutch to the uninvolved side.

Another method for sitting is to back into the chair, holding on to the sides of the crutches, working the hands down to the armrests, and then easing back on the chair seat. To get up by means of this technique, the patient positions a crutch at each side, places the palms of the hands on the armrests with fingers wrapped over the sides of the crutches, and maneuvers to the edge of the chair. She stands to an upright position with weight on the unaffected leg, and pulls the crutches up at the same time.

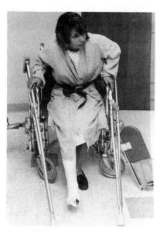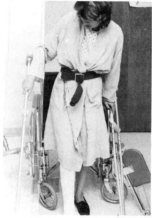

Another technique for sitting and standing

General Considerations. In crutchwalking, safety and balance are the first considerations. Following these, the patient must be taught to take steps of equal length in smooth cadence. At first, he will need reminders not to look at the floor, not to hop, and not to lift the crutches when weightbearing. He also needs to know that resting on the axillae causes compression of nerves and blood vessels.

The exposed toes or foot of the casted leg will swell and may appear cyanotic when the leg is hanging during crutchwalking. This is to be expected and the patient should be told about it beforehand. The patient should also be encouraged to wiggle toes and contract and relax leg muscles.

All instruction requires cooperation and a sharing of information with the physical therapy department at all times. Therefore the nurse should know about any problems the patient had while learning to crutchwalk and at what level of independence the patient ambulates. The nurse or other ward personnel can then supervise this activity when it is done independently. Supervision is necessary for another reason: as the patient's confidence level increases, so does the speed with which he travels on crutches.

The therapist, in turn, should know, prior to a therapy session, if the patient has just had a pain pill or has any

problem that might interfere with his learning to crutch-walk with stability.

Discharge Teaching

Talking to a person who has worn a long leg cast and maneuvered for any length of time on crutches will demonstrate to the orthopedic nurse how a sense of humor sometimes compensates, at least temporarily, for the loss of dignity present in some situations. It also provides helpful information to pass on to other patients in the same circumstances. (After all, the surface of a cast is a good place to keep track of bets and phone messages and to strike wooden matches.) And seriously, advising a patient to get a raised toilet seat if he has a small bathroom, because he may not have room to extend that casted leg, can eliminate one source of frustration. So can reminding him that he may need extra room on at least one side of his bed for getting in and out.

The nurse, as coordinator of the health team, should be the one responsible for finding out *where* the patient will walk with crutches once he is released and for consulting with physical therapy on ways to help him adapt what he is taught. What good will it do to teach a man to go up and down the stairs on crutches if he does not plan on doing it at home? Why does this happen? Maybe his steps are 2 inches

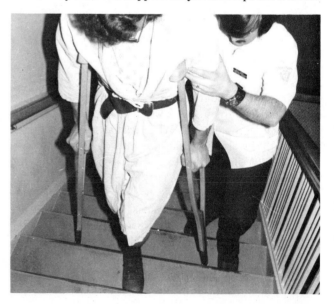

narrower than those in the hospital. So what? Perhaps it seems like nothing, but it is the sort of difference that should be discussed before discharge. All it requires on the part of a nurse is to ask the patient if stairs at home seem much like the stairs in the hospital. Another point is that it is difficult to move crutches on some kinds of carpeting. Therefore, the patient should be forewarned of this possible problem before he goes home.

On the day the patient is to be discharged, the nurse should encourage him to walk with his crutches as much as possible to gain confidence. All in all, personality has a great deal to do with how active a person is on crutches once he or she is discharged. There are those independent souls who would attempt anything, including throwing a briefcase down the steps in a school building and then kicking it all the way to class, rather than ask for help. For some, however, self-confidence and motivation come slowly, so slowly that they tend to "sit around and eat," and gain weight.

Time and rest become key words to the crutchwalker in planning activities of daily living. Advise this patient always to leave early for wherever he is going and to provide for short rest periods during the day when he can elevate the casted extremity.

Finally, remind the patient that crutches need "care" in the form of regular inspection of tips, axillary bar pads, and hand grips. They must be secure, and, as mentioned before, the tips should not be worn smooth.

Care of the Patient in a Hip Spica Cast

Patient Education

The hip spica is most commonly used in treatment of a femoral fracture following a period in traction ranging from 6 to 8 weeks.

The announcement by the doctor that "today is the day," no matter how often it was referred to earlier and how much desired, is still received with some trepidation by the patient. Remembering the pain he experienced at the beginning of his hospitalization and the length of time it took him to feel secure in traction will predispose him to fear and anxiety; these can be lessened if appropriate instruction takes place.

The procedure, like any other cast application, should be explained. The patient should be made tactfully aware of the fact that a fracture table may look like nothing he has seen before and that several people will be involved in the actual work.

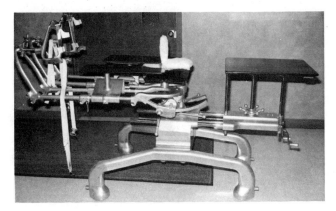

Fracture table

Reassure him that he will receive medication to help him relax and to reduce the discomfort. Then see to it that he does in fact receive the medication. Physicians appreciate being reminded ahead of time to order these medications, because they frequently schedule one or more operations on the same day and do these before applying a hip spica. If no specific medication is ordered, give the p.r.n. pain pill.

Preparing the Bed

The patient is transported from the ward to the operating room in his bed. Whoever goes to surgery to make that bed should take at least five pillows, including one small one. If the patient is put into bed in the supine position, these pillows provide support and are usually placed under the head and shoulders, the casted thigh, the lower leg, and the unaffected leg, the last one being for relief of strain on the

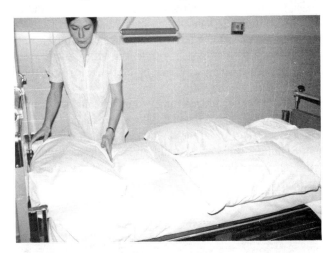

groin area. The smaller pillow is placed under the top of the cast (middle to lower back). Although the pillows may need to be rearranged once the patient is in bed, theoretically their original placement is the starting position. The rule is that the entire cast should be supported by pillows while damp.

Turning Procedure

Because turning the patient is a complicated procedure, it is wise to post written directions for the entire turning procedure near or on the head of the bed. Therefore, no matter how long it has been since the staff has handled a patient in a hip spica, there will be no confusion as to proper positioning.

Turning the patient in a damp hip spica every 2 to 3 hours requires three people, each using the palms of the hands. Remember that fingertips create dents in wet plaster.

From supine to prone position, the procedure is as follows: First, check the color, motion, temperature, and sensation of toes on the affected leg to be certain that there is no compression of nerves or blood vessels. Feel the toes, and ask the patient to flex and extend them. Next, pinch each

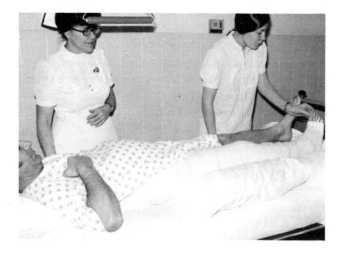

Once the patient has been moved to one side of the bed, have him place his arms over his head or at his sides. Two people go to the other side and roll the patient toward them, over his unoperated leg, by his shoulder, hip, thigh and lower leg. The patient helps by reaching for the bed rail with the hand from the affected side.

toe lightly to determine if the patient has feeling in it. Put up the bed rail on the side of the unaffected leg so that the patient can reach for it as he turns and eases himself onto his abdomen. Using the palms under the entire length of the cast, move the patient way over, on his back, to the affected side.

The pillows should be removed only while someone is supporting the cast. Note that pillows remain in essentially the same places for either position, so straightening, turning or fluffing them may be all that is required to avoid the possibility of making flat spots on the cast that would cause pressure.

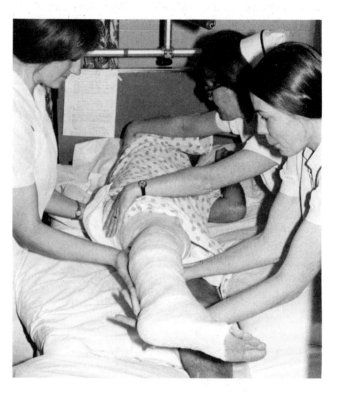

The nurse who remains on the affected side serves as a security factor since the patient is on the edge of the bed. She also helps ease his shoulder out after he is turned.

Readjust pillows as necessary to provide proper support and to keep the damp cast on a soft surface. Once the patient is turned, check for pressure on any area, make certain head and neck are comfortable and toes of both feet are hanging over the edge of pillows. The feet should be at right angles and the toes not digging into the mattress.

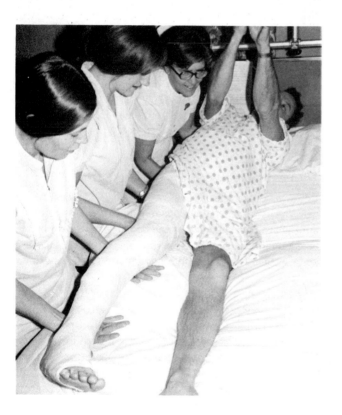

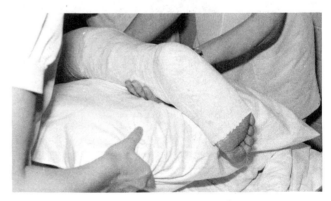

The whole procedure is far from simple. The patient in a damp hip spica is heavy. Turning him over, while on pillows, to another position on those same pillows requires a good deal of coordinated effort if it is not to feel like moving mountains.

Turning the patient onto his back involves the same steps, except he is not able to help by reaching for the bed rail.

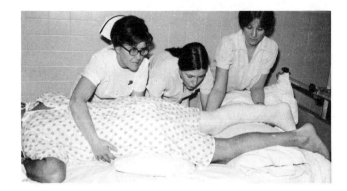

When the cast is dry, the patient should be able to turn with the help of one nurse. The patient does a major share of the work by lifting and moving to the side with the aid of a trapeze and his unaffected foot, while the nurse removes the pillows from under the casted leg. After the patient has moved to the side of the bed and grasped the bed rail, the nurse turns him over the unaffected leg and onto his abdomen.

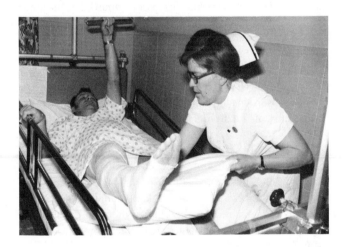

The nurse checks to see that the casted foot is hanging over the foot of the mattress and then places additional pillows for support and comfort.

When the patient is returned to a supine position, the nurse helps him move to the center of the bed and into alignment. Then the pillows can be replaced in order to raise the feet off the bed, relieve strain on the back or groin, and reduce swelling in the toes.

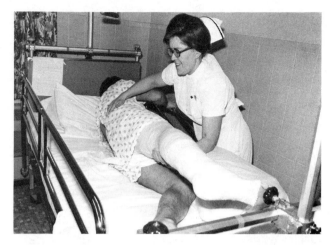

The patient should be turned every 3 hours. Most patients in hip spicas do not like lying on their abdomens; and if they are upset or uncomfortable, they should only be left in this position for 2 hours.

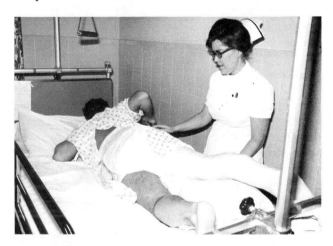

Although the turning procedure must be adapted to accommodate a bilateral hip spica or a patient of unusual size and weight, the principles remain the same. In summary, they are the following:

1. Always handle the damp cast (about 72 hours) with the palms of the hands, and support the cast on pillows.
2. Turn the patient all at once, at frequent intervals, after checking the neurovascular status of the toes.
3. If the patient is in a unilateral cast, roll him toward the unoperated side.
4. At completion of the turning procedure, check for pressure areas and make certain the call light is where the patient can reach it if pressure develops.
5. If the cast has an abduction bar, as in a bilateral hip spica or a cast that extends to the knee of the unoperated leg, this should never be used as a turning device without permission from the surgeon who applied it.

Once the cast is dry, a hip spica patient will stay on his back most of the time. If he is comfortable lying on his casted side, he should have pillows between his legs and his back and shoulders should be supported. This position is probably the least awkward one for eating meals.

Skin Care

Cast edges need to be petaled when dry. Inspect the edges, remove crumbs from underneath and around the area, and check for irritation each time the patient is turned.

Foam rubber or felt padding may be inserted, when possible, where rubbing occurs near the edge of the cast. The skin around the top edge is susceptible to sore spots where it meets a bony prominence. If the cast is high, there may be rubbing on the patient's ribs; on a low cast, the iliac crests would be affected. Refer to the section on General Care of the Patient in a Cast for more specific suggestions.

Protecting the Cast

Patients in hip spicas are helpless in matters of personal hygiene. Their casts need protection when they are on the bedpan. Once the nurse has placed a bedpan and left the room, repositioning by the patient himself is virtually impossible.

Plastic or other waterproof material should be used around the perineal edge to keep the cast from being soiled by urine or feces. This material should be inserted before a bedpan or urinal is given and removed carefully when the patient is finished. A sturdy, large plastic bag cut down the sides so it is in one piece is useful as protection and can be reused several times. Soft rubber sheeting also works well. Whatever material is used should be pliable, plentiful, and in one piece to be really moisture-proof.

Anything that is to be reused should be cleansed with soap and water and dried between applications. It is not advisable to leave the waterproof material in place, because it makes the edge airtight so that perspiration cannot evaporate.

Each time the patient finishes with the bedpan, the perineal area should be thoroughly cleansed and dried. Special attention should be given to the groin on the casted side, where movement is not possible. Fortunately, many times the surgeon leaves a large enough opening around the perineal area to avoid many problems of hygiene.

Bedpan Procedures

Fracture bedpans are the most workable for hip spica patients, because they are flat on the end that must be placed under the buttocks, which minimizes the amount of lifting required by both patient and nurse. The protective material mentioned above is inserted as much as possible while the patient is on his back. He is then turned on his unaffected side and the material is tucked in place. The fracture bedpan is placed so that the posterior lip is well up under the but-

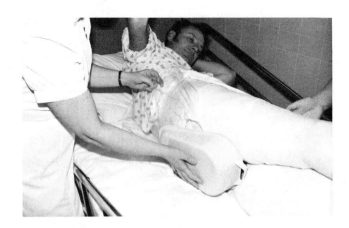

tocks. The patient is then returned to a supine position. By checking between the thighs, the nurse determines if the pan is back far enough. Both extremities and the patient's back need to be supported in a position as high as the buttocks, so that the urine does not run back into the cast.

The pan is removed in the same manner. The nurse should grasp the edge while the patient is turning, to prevent tipping and spilling.

Another, perhaps easier, method of placing the bedpan, after the patient is accustomed to his cast and moves well, is to have the patient lift himself with the trapeze. The nurse can elevate the hips with one hand and slip the pan under with the other. If the patient has a "free" leg, he can flex his knee and push up with the heel while the fracture pan is slipped into place from front to back. Ask the patient if the pan feels straight. The fracture pan is removed in the same way.

Complications

Complications due to pressure have been covered on pages 57–59. However, systemic problems may complicate the life of a patient in a hip spica, especially a high hip spica that covers part of the stomach and abdomen.

Elimination. Instruct the patient not to overeat in order to avoid pressure and cramping. Constipation is best avoided by proper diet, fluids, and education as to the importance of both. A high intake of fluids should be maintained to facilitate healing and reduce the chance of renal calculi. The supine position of the patient in a hip spica may be a contributing factor in the formation of calculi or stones. The kidney pelvises drain poorly in this position, causing minerals to settle out. Some fluids such as cranberry juice, which keeps urine acid, should be included in the diet, because more calcium precipitates out in alkaline urine.

Cast Syndrome. The nurse must be alert to the possibility of a cast syndrome characterized by complaints of nausea or vague abdominal pain and pressure. This syndrome is a dangerous complication that occurs when the superior mesenteric artery compresses the third portion of the duodenum. High intestinal obstruction results, producing prolonged nausea and vomiting. The treatment is removal of the cast and intestinal decompression by use of a nasogastric tube that is passed into the stomach and attached to a gastric-suction apparatus. The patient is allowed no oral intake until the tube is removed by order of the physician. Intravenous therapy is ordered throughout this treatment.

Exercise

The importance of exercise for all casted patients cannot be overemphasized. Again, all the unaffected extremities should be exercised, along with the toes on the affected leg. Quadriceps setting is recommended for the uninvolved thigh.

The patient should be taught to set his gluteal and abdominal muscles to maintain their strength and increase circulation. He does this by contracting the muscles, holding them in contraction, and counting to ten. This exercise should be repeated five times each hour during the day.

Footdrop and external rotation of the uncasted leg are prevented if the patient is encouraged to exercise every 3 hours during the day. Actually, a patient in a hip spica is not confined to bed very long, because the purpose of applying this cast is to shorten the period of hospitalization. Therefore, the greatest concern as far as exercise is concerned is preparation for crutchwalking. Such preparation should have begun while the patient was in traction. (See Chapter 3, section on Balanced Skeletal Traction.)

Crutchwalking

Before a patient in a hip spica begins to crutchwalk, he needs to be told that he will probably feel lightheaded, dizzy, weak, or all three, when he first gets out of bed. Patients are invariably surprised at how weak they are after a prolonged period in bed.

For this reason, the patient is taken to physical therapy for the first time on a tilt table. The therapist gradually raises him to a vertical position on this table as he adjusts to the upright position.

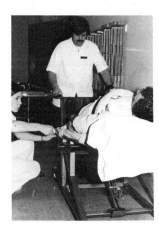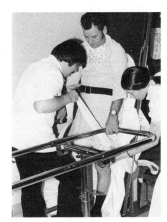

In response to the question, "How do you feel being up on crutches?" a patient was once heard to reply, "Like a lopsided mummy." As humorous as this may sound, it says a great deal about the awkwardness and limitations of the hip spica.

Because crutchwalking for this patient is a laborious process, he may spend the better part of a week learning how to ambulate before he can be discharged. First, there is the general feeling of weakness that must be overcome. The hip spica cast is heavy and clumsy, and "moving it along" while learning to bear all body weight on the opposite leg takes practice. This is done between parallel bars, initially,

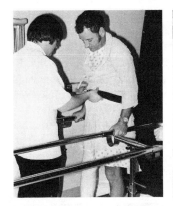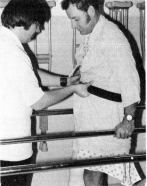

to allow the patient to achieve balance and stability. If the hip spica cast is "high," the patient may experience his greatest frustration when attempting to ease himself up and down in a reclining wheelchair.

Psychological Implications

Although it is easy for a patient to laugh at himself when learning to crutchwalk in a hip spica, the time between these efforts often brings depressing thoughts. The very young man who is anxious to be active may constantly voice discouragement and impatience. He needs reassurance that his is a normal course and that no one ever moves fast in a hip spica.

A nurse may feel at a loss for words of comfort for the patient who states he feels like "half a man." In this situation, good rapport with the family may enable a nurse to discuss this reaction with them. Together, they can decide upon ways to improve the patient's self-image by stressing the positive aspects of his progress and demonstrating love and respect in their attitudes. A wife who asks her husband's opinion on decisions made in his absence is more therapeutic than one who implies that things are going very well without him.

Discharge Teaching

One word — "clumsy" — best describes the person trying to live a halfway simple life in a hip spica cast. Managing alone after having acquired a degree of hospital dependency elicits certain responses, such as the fear of falling or frustration when trying to get to a ringing telephone. Overcoming obstacles without the aid of a physical therapist or nurse or anyone else, for certain periods of time during the day, consumes much time.

If a nurse sits down with patient and family, discusses activities the patient must perform, and tries to anticipate needs and problems, some sort of workable schedule or list of suggestions may be put together before discharge. One very important routine a patient needs to learn before discharge is how to get in and out of bed without a trapeze. The nurse should also question the patient about his bathroom. When he sits on the toilet, will he have room in front of him for his casted leg? Or will he need a commode? Tall patients need raised toilet seats.

To help overcome the fear of falling, instruct the patient that standing up and sitting down must be done slowly. In addition, inform the patient and family that scatter rugs should be removed from the floor and the furniture rearranged to provide wide pathways through the rooms.

Reclining chairs are the easiest to get in and out of when an individual is in a hip spica. Should one not be available, triangular pillows, such as those used for backrests when reading, may work if placed in the back of a chair. If possi-

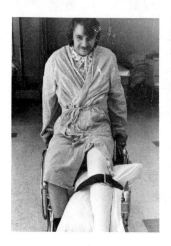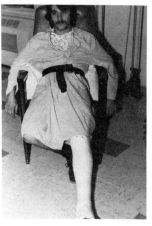

ble, strong support may be provided for the leg portion of the cast. It may be possible to rent wheelchairs with reclining backs.

Because patients with hip spicas are forced to spend a great deal of time in the supine position, all of the instruction and ideas given for cast care and turning should be written out, reviewed, and sent home with them.

Friends should be instructed to phone when other family members are home to answer the telephone, unless the patient has an extension near the chair or bed.

Looseness, as well as tightness, may become a source of irritation in a hip spica. The resourcefulness of the human mind in meeting these problems is indeed remarkable. One patient with "bony hips" found sanitary napkins to be good

sturdy padding, readily available, and economical. They can be cut in half and inserted between cast and iliac crest, with the loose end taped over the cast edge. Tightness, on the other hand, is not so easily relieved and must be called to the attention of the physician.

All other points of previously discussed cast care must be attended to, and it is a real act of charity to suggest to these patients that they call the orthopedic ward for advice and moral support when they feel it would be helpful.

Care of the Patient in a Cast Brace

Indications and Descriptions

Frequently a surgeon elects to use a cast brace in treating a midshaft or distal-shaft fracture of the femur.

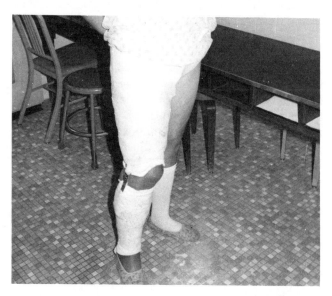

The cast brace consists of three components. Starting at the top of the leg, these components are as follows:

1. A thigh cuff made of plaster, extending as far as possible up the thigh and down to the knee joint; the cuff is applied snugly to increase the hydrodynamic compressive effect of the thigh muscles and to provide for immobilization of the fracture fragments
2. Two polycentric hinges at the knee that allow active motion of the joint and connect the thigh cuff to a short leg cast
3. A short leg cast, either a walking cast or a cylinder cast, that provides support for the thigh cuff and prevents it from slipping distally

The cast brace may be applied once proper alignment is established, the soft tissues have started to heal, and swelling is reduced. This may be anytime from 2 to 6 weeks following application of femoral skeletal traction.

Advantages and Disadvantages

The cast brace permits early weight bearing, thus shortening the period required for fracture healing. Because the brace allows for mobility of both the hip and the knee joints, the patient has a fairly normal gait when ambulating in the device. Thus his total rehabilitation period is shortened. Some patients progress to full ambulation without crutches in about 6 weeks after application of the cast brace.

Since it is not as clumsy as the hip spica, the cast brace can also have the advantage that the patient may not become as fatigued and frustrated while ambulating and getting in and out of chairs and bed.

Disadvantages are swelling in the knee and tightness around the thigh cuff edges, which may cause the patient considerable discomfort at times.

Psychological Preparation

The word *brace* often connotes "cripple." Furthermore, the patient who is going to have a cast brace applied has already undergone major trauma and endured severe pain, perhaps shock, and the treatment this entails, as well as a period in skeletal traction. It would be ideal if the nurse were present the first time the surgeon mentions the cast brace, in order to reinforce and clarify the explanation once the physician leaves. This is probably as good an example as any of why the orthopedic nurse needs to know the surgeons, their routines, and their expectations.

The patient must have a clear and simple description of what the procedure is, with the reassurance that no part of the brace will be attached to his person by any means other than a plaster cast. This is important because of the appearance of the tools that are used to attach the hinges.

Cast braces may also be applied under mild sedation, and the patient must be prepared for what he will hear and see if the procedure is to go smoothly.

The patient should be shown a photograph of the appliance. In fact, photographs of the entire procedure are an excellent teaching tool because cast braces, in contrast to other casts, are not a common sight.

Like the hip spica, the cast brace promises early ambulation and discharge from the hospital. For this reason the patient will be eager to have the procedure done. On the other hand, he has probably become relatively comfortable and accustomed to life in traction. He may be anxious and fearful that cast-brace application will mean more pain.

Physical Preparation

The nurse should know whether or not the patient is going to have his foot enclosed in the short leg cast. If so, a walking heel or cast shoe will be applied, and the shoe to be worn on the uninvolved extremity may have to be built up to match the length of the involved leg. A family member can be instructed to have this done as soon as possible so that it is ready when the patient needs it. The shoe that is selected should provide adequate support so that the patient, weak and unsteady from prolonged bed rest, will not twist his ankle when he begins ambulation.

A pain medication should be given prior to cast-brace application. The procedure is usually done in the operating room. Once more, the patient needs reassurance that although he may experience pain when traction is removed or his leg moved, the procedure itself is painless.

Care of the Wet Cast

While drying, the cast brace should be handled like any other cast. The leg needs to be repositioned on regular pillows every 3 hours, and the patient should be turned on his abdomen periodically if he can tolerate it.

Neurovascular Assessment

Checking color, motion, temperature, and sensation of the toes on the involved extremity is a priority while the patient remains in the hospital. The frequency of this routine is determined by the amount of discomfort and edema experienced by the patient.

Swelling

Once the apparatus has been applied, the nursing care is similar to that of the patient in a long leg cast, with one major difference. These patients frequently have a great deal of swelling about the knee, especially when ambulating. The affected knee may be almost double the size of the unaffected knee, causing the cast to feel tight. When this condition prevails during the hospital stay, it is difficult to convince the patient that this is normal.

Pressure

Another problem is pressure areas (more often in heavier patients), which develop around the edges of the thigh cuff. This is due partly to swelling and partly to the "total contact" of the thigh portion of the cast brace. This part of the cast is applied high and cannot be trimmed, so the groin and the fold under the buttock are especially susceptible to irritation. Cornstarch may be soothing if rubbed into these areas. The nurse must observe these areas and follow up all patient complaints of pressure with increased observation. The surgeon should be requested to check all problems due to pressure as they develop. Elevation of the leg whenever the patient is not weightbearing is the only preventive measure.

Bedpan Problems

Sitting on a bedpan or commode while wearing a cast brace often causes pinching of the skin along the top edge of the thigh cast. In addition, the extent of the cast may cause the cast to become soiled and smell if it is not covered with plastic when the patient uses the bedpan or commode.

Activity in Physical Therapy

The patient in a cast brace ambulates in physical therapy as soon as the cast dries. Because application of a cast brace is preceded by a period of at least 2 to 3 weeks in skeletal traction at bed rest, the patient's circulatory system needs time to become adjusted to the change in the patient's position. Therefore, the patient must be "weaned" from the supine position to the upright position by means of a tilt table.

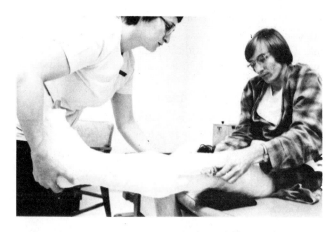

The hinges at the knee are unlocked for flexion exercises and then locked *before* the patient stands and walks. Any deviations from this routine are by physician's order. These hinges may also be unlocked when the patient is up on the commode or in a chair. The nurse must remember always to make certain they are locked before the patient stands up again. As an added precaution, they should always be checked before the patient is allowed to get out of bed.

Discharge Teaching

The patient in a cast brace is given instructions for exercising the knee joint.

The clamp is released, thus allowing flexion and extension exercising of the knee. Exercising is done either sitting

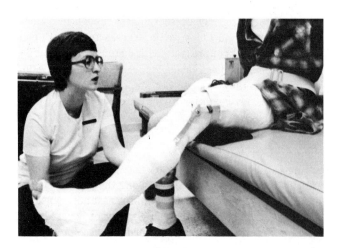

or standing, whichever is more comfortable. In a supine position, the patient flexes the knee by drawing the heel up along the surface of the bed and then extends the knee by pushing the heel down toward the end of the bed. Patients must be advised that this could cause the heel to become reddened and break down. Powder can be used on the bed. However, exercising in a sitting position is probably the best solution. If releasing the clamp is difficult, the patient should do exercises when someone else is present to be of assistance.

The patient should be told that he cannot adjust any part of the brace or trim the cast when it feels tight. This is important because swelling may occur in the knee joint as well as the toes of the affected foot for an indefinite period. The toes will also be dark in color whenever the leg is not elevated. If a patient understands that these conditions are normal, he will be less likely to become discouraged on days when it seems that he is making no progress.

Discussing safety in the home with the patient and his family is a priority in discharge planning. Safety precautions include such measures as removing scatter rugs from the floors and, whenever possible, placing some furniture where the patient can get to it safely and with the least amount of effort. In general, arrangements should be aimed at helping the patient to feel secure without "being in anyone's way."

Care When the Cast is Removed

Removing the Cast

Casts are generally removed with a vibrating saw, which is attached to a long vacuum-cleaner type hose and bag. Because the machine looks and sounds ominous, the patient needs to be reassured that the person removing the cast knows how to handle the equipment. The nurse who picks up the cast cutter and spends 10 seconds searching for the "on" button does nothing to relieve apprehension. Obviously then, the nurse should know how to use this equipment beforehand.

The blade used in the vibrating saw does not cut the patient's skin, but it will scratch the skin if it is not removed immediately after it cuts through the plaster and padding.

The nurse should demonstrate on her own skin that the saw does not cut. When giving this demonstration she should be careful not to move the saw or, indeed, it will cut.

No matter what a nurse tells the patient, he will be cut by an improperly handled cast cutter. Therefore, the saw should be held in the hand firmly, with one thumb resting on the cast to stabilize the saw as it vibrates through the plaster until the plaster "gives." Then the saw should be raised before it is advanced further. The cutting continues in this same manner.

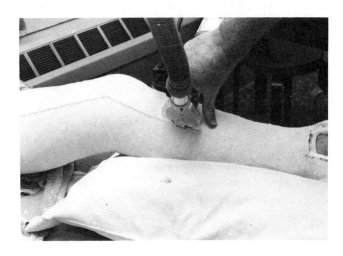

The cast edges can be separated with the cast spreader and the padding cut with a large bandage scissors.

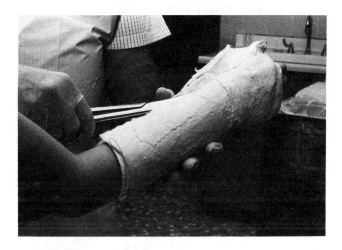

Care of the Extremity After Cast Removal

Before the cast is removed, the patient should be informed that he will have scaly, yellow, dead skin and flabby, weak muscles.

The caked exudate on the skin must not be "scrubbed" off or the skin will come off with it. Softening and removing scales with oil, or loosening them by soaking in warm water, should be a gradual process. The skin can be toned at a later date. Comfort and prevention of abrasion are the first priorities.

The limb should be moved carefully when the cast is first removed because the bone is brittle. The patient will have aches, discomfort, and joint pain he did not expect. The extremity should be supported in much the same position as it was in the cast until the patient becomes adjusted to the weakness and instability. Joints especially need maintenance.

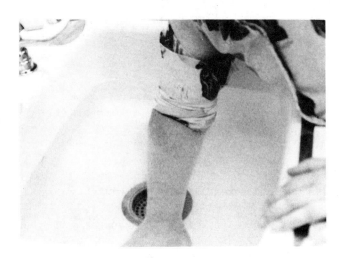

The type of support given depends on the body part casted and includes braces, splints, and elastic stockings and bandages. Pillows are also suggested support for patients who will remain in bed for a period of time. Any time the knee is involved, the patient should be cautioned against rising too quickly from a sitting position. This precaution is necessary because the quadriceps muscle group, which is essential in knee extension, will have undergone some atrophy.

Exercise

Exercise within the limits of pain and stiffness and without the use of force is the general rule. Physicians prescribe exercises according to individual needs.

For example, the patient who has had an arm cast removed needs instruction about shoulder motion, flexion and extension of the elbow, and weightlifting. If a lower extremity was involved, a program will be worked out on the basis of how much weightbearing and ambulation are allowed.

Physical-therapy departments initiate many of these exercise programs. Exercising limbs in warm water at home is often recommended.

Patient Education

Rehabilitation of a body part that has been fractured and casted is a slow process. Dependent edema in an extremity after removal of the cast is common and discouraging. Patients should be taught to elevate extremities frequently to reduce edema and to wear elastic stockings or bandages, if prescribed. These should, however, be removed at night. The patient should also be cautioned about subjecting the healed fracture to stress. Minor stresses can cause fractures in decalcified bone.

Telling a patient that careful maneuvering of a limb is necessary while he is learning to use it again may serve two purposes: it puts the proper restraint on his activities, and keeps him from becoming frustrated.

Care of the Patient Who Has Had External Fixation of a Fracture

Patient Profile

Any patient who requires external fixation of a fracture will have problems of one kind or another throughout the period of hospitalization. He presents a continuous nursing challenge. Because external fixation is used in fractures so complex that traditional methods of treatment are deemed unworkable, the patient may begin this course of treatment with a doubtful prognosis.

The typical patient is a trauma victim with a compound fracture that is often highly comminuted and accompanied by extensive soft-tissue injury, usually in the lower extremity. He may even have lost part of his bone in the accident. When his fracture is not open, he has probably undergone a period of treatment by traction and has been in pain and discomfort for a number of days.

Instruction: Patient and Family

Because the external fixator is a system of pins, rods, and clamps that defies verbal description, a nursing priority is to show both the patient and the family a picture of the apparatus before it is applied, if at all possible. However, external fixation is often done immediately after a severe injury has occurred, so that there is no time for preoperative instruction. In this case, instruction and supportive care are necessary as soon as the patient becomes aware of what has happened or a family member arrives on the scene.

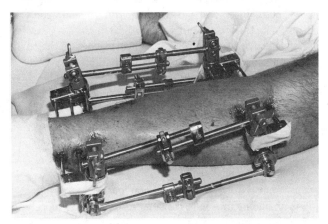

Emphasizing the positive aspects of the treatment is of psychological benefit. For instance, the patient may be told that soft-tissue healing and fracture healing can occur at the same time because the fixator is stabilizing the bone ends while allowing the treatment of open wounds. It is important to stress that pain is not a serious problem (or at least will not be any worse than it already is) once the limb has had a few days to settle down following manipulation and application of the device.

The patient needs to know that the apparatus is heavy and unwieldy, but that once it is attached to his limb, it will remain very stable until the surgeon removes it.

Position of the Limb

Postoperative elevation of the limb above the level of the heart decreases edema and allows early exercise of adjacent joints. Elevation may be accomplished by putting the leg in balanced-suspension traction or by attaching traction rope in four locations to the fixator and running these ropes up through pulleys on the overhead frame. When swelling in the limb is no longer a serious problem, the patient's leg may be elevated on pillows or by raising the foot of the bed.

The extremity should be lifted or otherwise moved by grasping the device. This may be done by the patient as well as the nurse.

Wound Care

Prevention of infection is a primary concern in the care of these patients. The extent of open wounds and soft-tissue injury, as well as surgeon preference, dictates the type of wound care that is prescribed. Irrigation may be ordered when the wounds are considered highly contaminated (*e.g.*, when the nature of the accident leaves debris buried in tissues). The main problem with irrigating a wound on an elevated extremity is that solution may run down the patient's thigh and irritate the groin, regardless of efforts to prevent it. Disposable pads must be placed under the limb and tucked and folded close to the limb to trap the fluid that escapes the suction. Fortunately, wound irrigation, when ordered, is not usually a prolonged treatment.

If dressing changes are a nursing responsibility, gloves must be worn and strict sterile technique observed. The gloves must not touch the hardware, and the dressings under the rods should be changed last. The nurse may have to use forceps, tongue blades, or applicators to maneuver the dressings into place.

Pin Sites

The type and frequency of pin-site care also varies according to surgeon preference. Typically, hydrogen peroxide or normal saline solution is used and may be followed by application of an antibiotic ointment. The use of povidone-iodine is controversial, since it is known to corrode metal. Cotton-tipped applicators, one for each pin site, are used for this procedure. Dressings may be applied, one around each pin.

While cleansing the pin sites, the nurse should be alert for signs of infection and skin tension. Serous drainage is normal. Redness, pain, and tenderness are signs that need close observation and reporting. Skin tension around the pins is a source of pain, and not only interferes with thorough cleansing, but may also result in small areas of skin necrosis. The surgeon may need to treat this condition by incising the skin around the pin.

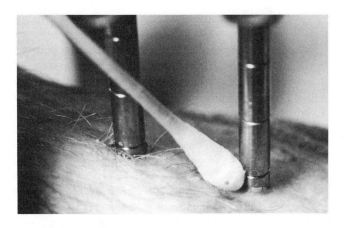

Neurovascular Assessment

The extensive soft-tissue damage and swelling make detailed neurovascular checks imperative. To increase the value of such assessments, the nurse should know if the patient has suffered injury to specific nerves or major blood vessels and what the surgeon's expectations and concerns are in regard to function of the part. Color, motion, temperature, and sensation of the toes must be recorded at 3- to 4-hour intervals in the initial phase of treatment and then as warranted by the patient's condition. Checking pedal pulses is important. When doing neurovascular checks, the nurse should ask the patient to put his foot and ankle through range of motion. Any changes or limitation of motion should be charted.

General Nursing Care

Nursing care of the patient with external fixation of a fracture is time-consuming and often frustrating for all who are involved. These patients are apprehensive every time they are confronted with a "new" nurse. Therefore, the written care plan should always reflect the "best" ways to do the procedures, as determined by both the patient and the nursing staff.

Because wound and pin-site care may require many dressings and applicators, gloves, and solutions, checking and restocking supplies in the patient's room should be a part of the regular evening or early-morning routine.

A common complaint of patients with external fixators is that "everything" gets caught on the pins. This can be avoided to a degree by using a bed cradle over the lower limbs and covering pin ends with tape, corks, or rubber tips from hypodermic needles.

Depending on his condition and ability, the patient can eventually be taught how to do his own pin-site care. The patient has the time to do a meticulous job and also benefits from the activity. He should be instructed carefully and should know the importance of avoiding shortcuts. Without causing him more anxiety, the nurse should teach the patient to report redness, a change in drainage, odors, and pain. She may do this by assessing the state of his limb with

him every day and pointing out areas that may need closer attention. When the patient is unable to reach all of his pin sites or some other injury prevents him from participating in his care, the person who will be responsible for him when he is discharged should be taught the routine.

Exercise and Ambulation

Active or passive range of motion for extremities as the patient's condition permits must be part of his care from the very beginning. Providing a pulley-weight, rope-and-handle setup on the head of the bed for arm exercises is a good idea in preparation for crutchwalking. In addition, the patient should do isometric exercises and be especially encouraged to concentrate on quadriceps setting.

Crutchwalking for these patients has its own special problems. The thought of ambulating without weight bearing, and, therefore, of actually carrying the external-fixation device around on his leg may be overwhelming for the patient. He needs reassurance that time and practice will ensure success. Initially, it will be difficult for him to achieve balance. He will be apprehensive when he finds that he has to learn to swing through the crutches without catching the ends of the pins. Furthermore, edema and discoloration of the lower limb when he is crutchwalking will be a source of discomfort and dismay.

Psychological Aspects

Physically, the patient becomes weary of the long, drawn-out period of treatment, the device itself, the immobility it demands, and perhaps the need to sleep on his back. This physical weariness affects his state of mind and often causes depression and frustration. He is ambivalent about his treatment, on the one hand being tired of it all, and on the other feeling that he can go through anything if the alternative is amputation.

Concern over his prognosis, the length and cost of hospitalization, and family and job situations adds to his worries. Consultation with a social worker may be indicated and will provide additional supportive care. The patient in an external-fixation device cannot have too many friends among the hospital staff.

Discharge Planning

The patient may go home with a cast applied around the pins if the wound is not open. Cast-care instructions will be necessary (see p. 66). All patients should have a thorough understanding of their limitations on crutches and of what the physician expects in the way of reporting and follow-up visits to the office.

A workable suggestion for adapting clothing to the condition is to slit seams on both sides of any long pants the patient will be wearing and put snaps between the pins. Inexpensive sweat pants may be comfortable in cold weather; they are loose and can easily be slipped on and off.

Discussion Questions

1. In the following three patients with fractured legs, how would the signs and symptoms differ? Compare?

   a. Comminuted fracture of the tibial plateau

   b. Compound fracture of the midshaft of the femur

   c. Transverse fracture of the distal tibia

If, on admission, the physician has only ordered a pain medication for each patient, what nursing orders would you need to write?

Consider: All three patients would have different degrees of pain, swelling, and discoloration, depending on fracture pattern and description. In (a), the patient's complaints would involve the area around the knee joint and include an inability to move or flex the knee. In (b), there would be an open wound with bleeding.

Nursing orders for all three should include the basics: ice, elevation, pedal pulses, neurovascular checks. Observations for infection would be a priority in writing orders for (b). Compression of the peroneal nerve is a potential problem for (a).

2. Make a list of questions the nurse must ask in coordinating the discharge planning for the following patients; give reasons for the questions.

   a. D. B. is a 32-year-old female and the mother of two children. She is being discharged in a cast brace. Her husband works midnight to 8:00 A.M. in a town 20 miles from home.

   b. S. L. is a 19-year-old male who plans to attend the university in his home town 1 month after discharge from the hospital in a hip spica cast. He lives with a friend in a mobile home.

Consider: (a) Before any planning can be done for D. B., the nurse must know the ages of her children and what hours of the day her husband sleeps. The neighborhood itself is an important factor. How? (b) The nurse needs to know what sort of transportation S.L. will be using to get to the university and what his relationship with his friend is in terms of how much help he can, or is willing to, provide. What are the implications for planning because the patient lives in a mobile home?

3. In each of the following situations, identify the *first* nursing intervention and give the rationale for it.

   a. A 19-year-old patient with a compound fracture of the femur has a temperature of 103° post injury and is restless.

   b. A 55-year-old female with a fractured pelvis complains of a "catch in my ribs" following 11 days of bed rest.

   c. A 19-year-old male with a fractured femur and a head injury seems slightly confused the morning after his injury.

   d. A 30-year-old patient with a supracondylar fracture of the humerus is admitted at 2:00 A.M. She has her arm splinted and is complaining of severe pain in her lower arm.

Consider: The prevention or diagnosis of complications is the nurse's responsibility in all of these. The nurse should look at the situation, mechanism of injury, time interval, and initial assessment. More interaction with the patient may be required. Why?

Bibliography

Althoff DG: External fixation of the lower extremity: Care considerations. Assessment and Fracture Management of the Lower Extremities, p 60, 1984

Arlington R: Internal fixation of the lower extremity: Care considerations. Assessment and Fracture Management of the Lower Extremities, p 65, 1984

Barden R: Use of a noninvasive electrical bone stimulator: Case study. Orthop Nurs 4(2):52, 1985

Betts-Symonds GW: Functional bracing of the femoral shaft fractures, part 8. Nurs Times 78:2127, 1982

Betts-Symonds GW: Functional bracing of the tibia and fibula, part 7. Nurs Times 78:2123, 1982

Bomalski JS: Inferior vena cava interruption in the management of pulmonary embolism. Chest 82:775, 1982

Brown R: External fixation. J Operat Room Res Inst 2:16, 1982

Brown R: Orthopedic surgery: Internal fixation. J Operat Room Res Inst 2:8, 1982

Brunner NA: Orthopedic Nursing, 4th ed. St Louis, CV Mosby, 1983

Bullas JB: Fibrinolytic therapy: Nursing implications. Crit Care Nurs 1(7):43, 1981

Burg ME: Compartment syndrome. Crit Care Q 6(1):27 1983

Callahan J: Compartment syndrome. Orthop Nurs 4(4):11, 1985

Carlson RE: The fat emboli syndrome. Med Times 107:(108) 8d–10d, (198) 15d–18d, 1979

Chaffee E, Greisheimer E: Basic Anatomy and Physiology, 3rd ed. Philadelphia, JB Lippincott, 1974

Collins DM, Weber ER: Anterior interosseous nerve avulsion. Clin Orthop 181:175, 1983

Collins P: Nursing care study: Treatment of Volkmann's ischemic contracture, pre- and postoperative care. Nurs Times 74:1038, 1978

Cooney WP: External fixation of distal radial fractures. Clin Orthop 180:44, 1983

Coping with pulmonary embolism. A guide to understanding, diagnosing, and preventing it. Nurs Life 4:35, 1984

Coppola AJ Jr, Anzel SH: Use of the Hoffmann external fixator in the treatment of femoral fractures. Clin Orthop 180:78, 1983

Crawford-Gamble P: The treatment of nonunions with electrical stimulation. Today's OR Nurse 4(11):23, 56, 1983

Cross M: Dissolving the threat of pulmonary embolism. RN 47(8):34, 1984

Crossland S, Deyerle W: Compartmental syndrome. Nursing '80, 51, 1980

Dabezies DJ, et al: Fractures of the femoral shaft treated by external fixation with the Wagner device. J Bone Joint Surg 66A:360, 1984

Dantzker DR: Alterations in gas exchange following pulmonary thromboembolism. Chest 81:495, 1982

Darkin DM: Pulmonary fat embolism: a complication of fracture. Heart Lung 5:477, 1976

Darovic G: Was this postop death preventable? RN 46(10):47, 1983

Davis P: Nursing care study: A break from the bottle. Nurs Mirror, 156(2):40, 1983

DeLee JC, Stiehl JB: Open tibia fracture with compartment syndrome. Clin Orthop 160:175, 1981

Deyerle WM, Crossland SA: Compartmental syndromes. Crit Care Update 10(8):38 1983

Digby JM, et al: A study of function after tibial cast bracing. Injury 14:432, 1983

Dossey B, et al: Pulmonary embolism: Preventing it, treating it. Nursing '81 11:26, 1981

Dossey B. Understanding pulmonary embolism. Nurs Life 4:36, 1984

Edmondson AS, Crenshaw AH (ed): Campbell's Operative Orthopaedics, 6th ed. St Louis, CV Mosby, 1980

Faoltico JB: Pulmonary embolism. Crit Care Update 8:5, 1981

Farrell J: Casts, your patients and you. A review of basic procedures, part 1. Nursing '78 (8):65, 1978

Farrell J: Casts, your patients and you. A review of arm and leg cast procedures, part 2. Nursing '78 (8):57, 1978

Farrell J: A review of hip spica procedures, part 3. Nursing '78 (8):53, 1978

Farrell J: Symposium on orthopedic nursing. Nursing care of a patient in a cast brace. Nurs Clin North Am 11:717, 1976

Farrell J: The trauma patient with multiple fractures. RN 48(6):22, 1985

Fernsebner B, et al: A vena caval filter. AORN J 39:80, 1984

Fernsebner B, et al: Home study program. AORN J 39:84, 1984

Fernandez DL: A technique for anterior wedge-shaped grafts for scaphoid nonunions with carpal instability. J Hand Surg, 9:733, 1984

Fighting fat after fracture. Emerg Med 10:221, 1978

Fitzmaurice JB, et al: Current concepts of pulmonary embolism, implications for nursing practice. Heart Lung, 3:209, 1974

Fracture repair: Conflicts and consensus, selected abstracts, part 1. Orthop Nurs 3(5):25, 1984

Fuller E: Putting a new casting material to work. Patient Care 15:129, 1981

Fuller E: Treating and preventing blood clots. Patient Care 16(20):87, 92, 97, 1982

Garland D, Chick R, Taylor J, et al: Treatment of proximal third femur fractures with pins and thigh plaster. Clin Orthop 160:86, 1981

Geary N: Late surgical decompression for compartment syndrome of the forearm. J Bone Joint Surg 66B:745, 1984

Geier KA, Hesser K: Electrical bone stimulation for treatment of nonunion. Orthop Nurs 4:41, 1985

Geier KA, Pfeffinger LL: The fully implantable direct current stimulator: Case study. Orthop Nurs 4:52, 1985

Gelberman RH, et al: Compartment syndromes of the forearm: Diagnosis and treatment. Clin Orthop 161:252, 1981

Gittman JE, et al: Fatal fat embolism after spinal fusion for scoliosis. JAMA, 249:779, 1983

Gorrell KR: A recovery. Am J Nurs 83:1672, 1983

Gosseling HR: Fat embolism syndrome: A review of the pathophysiology and physiological basis of treatment. Clin Orthop 165:68, 1982

Gosseling HR, et al: Fat embolism. J Bone Joint Surg 56A:1327, 1984.

Guenter CA, et al: Fat embolism syndrome: Changing prognosis. Chest 79:143, 1981

Hamer SS: A complication commonly overlooked: Acute pulmonary embolism. Heart Lung 11:588, 1982

Hankin FM, et al: Bleeding beneath postoperative plaster casts. Orthop Nurs 2:27, 1983

Hardy AE: The treatment of femoral fractures by cast-brace application and early amputation. A prospective review of one hundred and six patients. J Bone Joint Surg 65A:56, 1983

Hay BK, Karas CB: External fixation: Option for fractures. AORN J 34(3), 1981

Hay BK, Karas CB: A teaching plan for external fixation. AORN J 34(3), 1981

Hayden J: Compartment syndromes. Early recognition and treatment. Postgrad Med 74(1):191, 1983

Henderson OL, et al: Early casting of femoral shaft fractures in children. J Pediatr Orthop 4:16–21, 1984

Heppenstall R: Fracture Treatment and Healing. Philadelphia, WB Saunders, 1980

Hice GA, et al: The plaster-synthetic cast. J Am Podiatry Assoc 73:427, 1983

Hilt N, Cogburn S: Manual of Orthopedics. St Louis, CV Mosby, 1980

Hirsch J: Noninvasive tests for thromboembolic disease. Hosp Pract, 17:77, 1982

Hoberg A: Preventing orthopedic complications, part 2. RN 38:34, 1975

Hollinshead WH: Textbook of Anatomy, 4th ed. Philadelphia, Harper & Row, 1985

Howes DS, Kaufman JJ: Plaster splints: Techniques and indications. Am Fam Physician 30:215, Sept 1984.

Huey R: Coping with pulmonary embolism. Come quick! Something's wrong with my husband. Nurs Life 4:34, 39, 1984

Huffman MH: Acute care of the patient with a pulmonary embolism due to venous thromboemboli. Crit Care Nurse 3:70, 1983

Iwegbu CG: Preliminary results of treatment of fractures of the femur by cast-bracing using the Zaria metal hinge. Injury 15(4):250, 1984

Karlstrom G, Olerund S: External fixation of severe open tibial fractures with the Hoffmann frame. Clin Orthop 180:68, 1983

Kelly DJ: The use of fiberglass as reinforcement with plaster casts. Orthop Nurs 2(6):33, 1983

Kennedy RH, Cooper MJ: An unusually severe case of the cast syndrome. Postgrad Med J, 59:539, 1983

Kipper MS: Long term follow-up of patients with suspected pulmonary embolism. Chest 82:441, 1982

Kryschyshen P: External fixation for complicated fractures. Am J Nurs 80:256, 1980

Kushner C: A sudden complication. What's Your diagnosis? RN 44(5):123, 1981

Kushner C: A new procedure: A sudden complication. What's your diagnosis? RN 44(5):53, 1981

Kuska BM: Acute onset of compartment sydrome. JEN 8:75, 1982

Lachiewicz F: Fat embolism syndrome following bilateral total knee replacement with total condylar prosthesis: Report of two cases. Clin Orthop 160:106, 1981

Lane PL: Special care for special casts: Nursing 13(7):50, 1983

Lane PL, Lee MM: New synthetic casts: What nurses need to know. Orthop Nurs 1(6):13, 1982

Langley LL, et al: Dynamic Anatomy and Physiology, 5th ed. New York, McGraw-Hill, 1980

Larson W, Gould M: Orthopedic Nursing, 9th ed. St Louis, CV Mosby, 1979

Lenig RC: Pulmonary fat embolism. AANA J, 47:40, 1979

Levy RN, et al: Complications of Ender-pin fixation in basicervical, intertrochanteric and subtrochanteric fractures of the hip. J Bone Joint Surg 65A:66, 1983

Lippmann M, et al: Pulmonary embolism in the patient with chronic obstructive pulmonary disease. Chest 79:39, 1981

Luprin, Capt AE: Head off compartment syndrome before it's too late. RN 43:38, 1980

Marcer M, et al: Results of pulsed electromagnetic fields in ununited fractures after external skeletal fixation. Clin Orthop 190:260, 1984

Martens MA, et al: Chronic leg pain in athletes due to a recurrent compartment syndrome. Am J Sports Med, 12:148, 1984

Martin S: Fat embolism syndrome. Dimens Crit Care Nurs 2:158, 1983

Massie S: Cast-bracing of femoral shaft fractures. The method and its history, part 1. Nurs. Times 76:630, 1980

Massie S: The physics of the method, part 2. Nurs Times 76:700, 1980

Massie S: When to use this treatment, part 3. Nurs Times 76:745, 1980

Massie S: When to apply the brace: The application technique, part 4. Nurs Times 76:795, 1980

Massie S: Social benefits of the cast brace, part 5. Nurs Times 76:833, 1980

Massie S: An evaluation, part 6. Nurs Times 76:882, 1980

Matsen FA, et al: Diagnosis and management of compartmental syndrome. J Bone Joint Surg 62A:286, 1980

McCormack A, et al: The patient with pulmonary emboli. RN 47(8):40, 1984

McDermott AG, et al: Monitoring acute compartment pressures with S.T.I.C. catheter. Clin Orthop 190:192, 1984

McFarland MB: Encircling cast drainage: Is it valuable? Orthop Nurs 3:41, 1984

McFarland MB: Irrigating clotted IV lines: A potential hazard. Focus AACN, 10:45, 1983

Mercier LR: Practical Orthopedics. Chicago, Year Book Medical Publishers, 1980

Miller MC: Nursing care of the patient with external fixation therapy. Orthop Nurs 2:11, 1983

Moser KM: Diagnosis and management of pulmonary embolism. Hosp Pract 15:57, 1980

Mourad L: Nursing Care of Adults with Orthopedic Conditions. New York, John Wiley & Sons, 1980

Mullendore JW: What goes on in physical therapy. RN 45(5):54, 1982

Ng L: Position changes and their physiological consequences: Turning patients. ANS 4:13, 1982

Oh WH, et al: Fat embolism: Current concepts of pathogenesis, diagnosis and treatment. Orthop Clin North Am 9:769, 1978

Orzel JA: Proper interpretation of radioisotope lung scans. JAMA 253:40, 1985

Parkinson M: Repair of a comminuted fracture. Nurs Mirror 158(16):23, 1984

Peltier LF: Fat embolism. An appraisal of the problem. Clin Orthop 187:3, 1984

Plaster of Paris bandages: Historical perspective. Orthop Nurs, 1(6):42, 1982

Postbasic nursing procedures, 10. Plaster cast, 1. Nurs Mirror, 154(25):28, 1982

Pradka L: Use of the wick catheter for diagnosing and monitoring compartment syndrome. Orthop Nurs 4(4):17, 1985

Preventing fat embolism after fracture: A short course of corticosteroids. Emerg Med 16(5):142, 144, 1984

Pulmonary embolism. Nurs Mirror, 156(3):inside back cover, 1983

Qvarfordt P, et al: Intermuscular pressure, muscle blood flow, and skeletal muscle metabolism in chronic anterior tibial compartment syndrome. Clin Orthop 179:284, 1983

Quigley JT, et al: Compartment syndrome of the forearm and hand: A case report. Clin Orthop 161:247, 1981

Raney RB Sr, Brashear HR Jr: Shand's Handbook of Orthopaedic Surgery, 9th ed. St Louis, CV Mosby, 1978

Redheffer GM: Open fracture: Handle with care. Point View 19:9, 1982

Regan WA: Legal briefs for nurses: TX: Malpractice in cast applications; GA: neuroradiology: malpractice alleged. Regan Rep Nurs Law 22(9):3, 1982

Reichel J: Pulmonary embolism. Med Clin North Am, 61:1309, 1977

Reid H: Nursing Mirror clinical forum. Plastering in the 80s. Nurs Mirror 159(7):i, 1984

Reidel M: Long term follow-up of patients with pulmonary thromboembolism. Chest 81:151, 1982

Rockett CP: Bone stimulation: Case study. Orthop Nurs, 4:52, 1985

Rockwood CA, Green DP (eds): Fractures, 2nd ed, vols. I, II, III. Philadelphia, JB Lippincott, 1984

Rorabeck CH: The treatment of compartment syndromes of the leg. J Bone Joint Surg 66B:93, 1984

Rydholm U, et al: Intracompartmental forearm pressure during rest and exercise. Clin Orthop 175:213, 1983

Rydholm U, et al: Chronic compartmental sydrome in the tensor fasciea latae muscle. Clin Orthop 177:169, 1983

Sabiston CC Jr: Pathophysiology, diagnosis and management of pulmonary embolism. Am J Surg 138:384, 1979

Salmond S: Trauma and fractures: Meeting your patient's nutritional needs. Orthop Nurs 3(4):27, 1984

Sasahara AA, et al: Pulmonary thromboembolism. Diagnosis and treatment. JAMA, 249:2945, 1983

Searls K, et al: External fixation: General principles of patient management. Crit Care Q 6(1):45, June 1983

Shafer T: Nursing care of the patients with ARDS. Crit Care Nurse, 1:34, 1981

Shenkman B, Stechmiller J: Fat embolism syndrome: Pathophysiology and current treatment. Focus Crit Care 11(6):26, 1984

Sherman M: Thrombophylaxis with antiembolism stocking. Orthop Nurs 4(4):33, 1985

Simmons K: Angioscope "sees" chronic pulmonary emboli. JAMA 251:695, 699, 1984

Singer A: Bed rest, deep-vein thrombosis and pulmonary embolism. JAMA 250:3162, 1983

Sisk TD: External fixation. Historic review, advantages, disadvantages, complications, and indications. Clin Orthop 180:15, 1983

Smith M: Clinical forum 3: Respiratory emergencies. In care of emergency. Nurs Mirror, 154:ii, 1982

Southwick JR, Callahan DJ: A study of blood-drainage patterns on synthetic cast materials. Orthop Nurs 4:72, 1985

Spickler LL: Knee injuries of the athlete. Orthop Nurse 2(5):11, 1983

Spies WG: Radionuclide imaging in diseases of the chest, part 1. Chest 83:122, 1983

Stevenson RC: Take no chances with fat embolism. Nursing '85 15(6):58, 1985

Thomas J: Wound care, No 18. Management of compound fractures. Nurs Times 79[suppl]69, 1983

Thomas MN: Acute pulmonary embolism. Focus Crit Care 10(4):21, 1983

To clear a clogged pulmonary artery: Embolectomy for massive pulmonary embolism. Emerg Med 14(20):121, 1982

Turek SL: Orthopaedics: Principles and Their Application, 4th ed. Philadelphia, JB Lippincott, 1984

Unger KM: The causes and cures of pulmonary embolism. Emerg Med 13:21, 1981

Velazco A, Fleming LL: Open fractures of the tibia treated by the Hoffmann external fixator. Clin Orthop 180:125, 1983

Wahlstrom O: Stimulation of fracture healing with electromagnetic fields of extremely low frequency (EMF of ELF). Clin Orthop 186:293, 1984

Wang GJ, et al: Semirigid rod fixation for long-bone fracture. Clin Orthop 192:291, 1985

Wardlaw D, et al: The recovery and quadriceps function in patients treated by cast bracing. Injury 15:245, 1984

Wenger NK: Pulmonary embolism: Recognition and management. Consultant 20:85, 1980

Westaby S, Thommas J: Management of compound fractures, part 18. Nurs Times, 79(19):69, 1983

Westra B: Assessment under pressure: When your patient says "I can't breathe". Nursing 14(5):34, 1984

Williams MH: Pulmonary embolism. Emerg Med 14:84, 1982

Wittert D, Barden RM: Deep vein thrombosis, pulmonary embolism, and prophylaxis in the orthopaedic patient. Orthop Nurs, 4(4):27, 1985

Woodruff ML: Pulmonary thromboembolism: Risk factors, pathophysiology, and management. Crit Care Nurs 4(4):50, 1984

3

Care of the Patient in Traction

Ironically enough, a person who maintains a healthy, active body may be a *more* likely candidate for a traction apparatus than one who is not so active or vigorous. Such is the case of the snow sportsman who fractures a femur while skiing. The spectator fan who sits at home watching a football game on television is less likely to break any bones. But it is also true that those people whose physical status can *least* tolerate immobility may be the most susceptible to some condition that leads to the application of traction. Examples of this include the overweight person who develops back pain and the elderly person with osteoporosis who falls and fractures a humerus. The combination of either an excellently *or* a poorly functioning body and an enforced period of immobilization in traction produces a patient prone to physical and emotional frustration and the development of health problems. Since *everyone* is a potential traction patient, individualizing this kind of nursing care is an endless challenge.

Traction

Definition and Classification

Traction means that a pulling force is applied to a part of the body or an extremity while a countertraction pulls in the opposite direction. In *straight* or *running* traction, countertraction is supplied by the patient's body with the bed in one of the following positions: (1) flat, (2) tilted away from

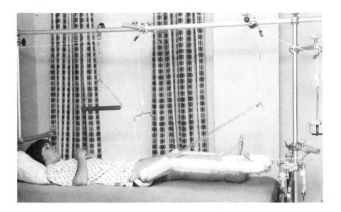

the traction pull, or (3) altered by elevating the head or knee of a Gatch bed.

In *suspension* or *balanced* traction, slings, hammocks, or splints are used to support the affected part. Although the body provides some countertraction, further countertraction is supplied by a system of balanced weights attached to an overhead frame with ropes and pulleys.

Basically, there are three classifications of traction:

1. *Skin traction* is the application of a pulling force to the skin and soft tissues. The materials used include wrapping bandages, tapes, slings, and halters. The tapes are generally of vented foam rubber or material with an adhesive backing for attachment to the skin.
2. *Skeletal traction* is traction applied directly to the skeleton with such devices as Steinmann pins. Kirschner wires, and Crutchfield tongs.
3. *Manual traction* is a pulling force exerted by use of hands. It is a temporary measure sometimes employed in handling a neck injury when a cervical-spine fracture is suspected. It is also used to apply the necessary pull to an extremity when a cast is being applied.

Purposes of Traction

1. Traction is often used in the treatment of fractured extremities to lessen muscle spasms and reduce the fracture. It provides immobilization to maintain alignment, thus promoting healing.
2. Traction is also used to correct, lessen, or prevent deformities, as in the case of the arthritic patient with flexion contractures or the child who has scoliosis and is placed in traction to help lessen the curvature of the spine before corrective surgery.
3. Immobilization by traction may be beneficial in lessening muscle spasm in back pain and in resting a diseased joint, as in tuberculosis.

Principles of Traction

Certain principles must be adhered to if traction is to be effective. Traction must comply with the following criteria:

1. Have an opposite pull or countertraction
2. Be free from any friction
3. Follow an established line of pull
4. Be continuous
5. Be applied to a patient in the supine position, in good body alignment

These five principles are so interrelated that if one principle is not applied or is interrupted, the effectiveness of the other principles will be diminished. Because the nurse uses this knowledge in the nursing care of *every* traction patient, some generalities helpful in making observations related to these principles will be discussed later.

TRACTION VARIATION: NURSING IMPLICATIONS

Physicians vary in their methods of applying traction, according to the way they have been taught, what they have practiced, and what they have found to be efficient and effective. As a result, traction application differs from region to region and from physician to physician. In addition, hospitals vary in the types of equipment they use. Footplates, types of weights, and splints are manufactured by many companies in many styles. For instance, there are other splints similar to the Thomas half-ring or full-ring splints that are mentioned in this text.

All of this means the nurse must be knowledgeable about *principles*, first of all, before she can understand the traction routines of the hospital and staff physicians. The nurse who understands the basic care of *one* patient in traction, understands the basic care of *all* patients in traction.

TRACTION EQUIPMENT

Bed Equipment

An *overhead frame* of bars should be standard equipment on all beds on an orthopedic ward. In this way, there is never a need to move a patient from bed to bed if a change in treatment requires an elaborate traction apparatus.

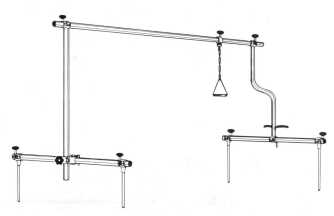

Overhead frame and trapeze constitute basic equipment for orthopedic patients. (Courtesy Zimmer Co, Warsaw, Ind)

The *trapeze* is sometimes referred to as a "patient helper." To this description should be added "nurses' helper" to describe more aptly its role in the care of orthopedic patients. Unless contraindicated by a condition in which lifting or arm movement is undesirable, the trapeze should be a standard attachment to an orthopedic bed.

A *firm mattress* is an absolute necessity for orthopedic patient care to assure efficiency of the traction and to avoid possible contracture deformities. Many companies manufacture beds with solid bottoms rather than bedsprings, thus eliminating the need for bedboards. If such beds are not available, then bedboards may be required. By one method or another, a firm foundation must be provided.

Traction Room and Cart

The amount and nature of equipment needed for traction set-ups requires a roomy storage place, plus a means of transporting the equipment to the bedside. Fracture or traction rooms, with walls covered by pegboard and hooks and large open cupboards, hold most traction components. A

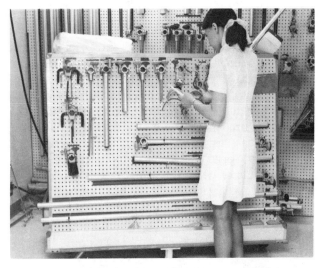

Traction room and cart. (Courtesy Zimmer Co, Warsaw, Ind)

traction cart can be stocked with the unsterile equipment necessary for applying skeletal traction, as well as such standard items as ace bandages, ropes, weights, pulleys, and weight hangers. In addition, attaching a list of supplies for procedures such as insertion of a Steinmann pin, which requires the use of an anesthetic agent, is a time-saving factor in preparing for and assisting with the procedure.

Nursing Responsibilities Prior to the Application of Traction

Assessment of the Patient's Condition

1. Data collected prior to the application of traction should include any history related to circulatory problems, such as those associated with diabetes, or to skin problems, such as allergy to tape or rubber, which may rule out the use of tapes and wrapping bandages.
2. In all patients the area to which traction is being applied should be inspected closely, especially if the patient has fallen or had any other type of accident. Open areas and bruises should be noted in the chart *before* they are covered and then covered only *after* the nurse has confirmed that the physician is aware of their presence.

3. The neurovascular status of the limb, if that is the traction site, should be checked before traction is applied, to facilitate detection of problems resulting from pain or pressure due to traction components. This means that the color, amount of motion, temperature, and sensation in the fingers or toes (CMTS) should be recorded along with the pulse.
4. Any pain in the area should be identified as to exact location, degree, and description.

Psychological Considerations and Patient Teaching

Although the patient should be instructed about the purpose of the traction and the method by which it is applied, an explanation is not too meaningful until he actually sees the equipment and experiences the procedure. The nurse should review the details of the application procedure before entering a patient's room with an armful of traction equipment. It is not very reassuring for a patient to watch a nurse unload bars, pulleys, ropes and weights, and *then* begin to get information about what is to be done with them. Because much of the equipment used in applying traction, such as ropes and pins, resembles devices that are frequently associated with torture, explanation of their use should be offered to relieve apprehension, especially if the patient has severe pain.

The patient must then be instructed as to the importance of staying in the proper position and not readjusting any part of the apparatus by himself without a lesson from the physician who applied it. He should know how much movement he is allowed, ways in which he can help himself, and, finally, the importance of reporting any pain, pressure, or discomfort that develops.

After traction is applied, the patient should be assured that someone will check on him again within an hour to see that he is adjusting to the traction and that nothing has been overlooked.

Assisting With Traction Application

Manuals that deal specifically with methods and equipment required for all types of traction should be kept near the equipment. All orthopedic surgeons have their own preferences, from splints to gauge of needle to be used for local anesthesia. If these items are listed and kept on a traction cart, even a "hurry up" preparation for the application of skeletal traction can be relatively smooth.

Because insertion of a Steinmann pin under local anesthesia is a sterile procedure and is frequently performed in the patient's room, the physician should be provided with enough assistance so that it can be done quickly and efficiently. Keeping updated lists of supplies that are needed will be helpful and will permit the nurse to assist, rather than run for missing items. The nurse should offer reassurance to the patient and answer his questions as the traction is being applied.

Knots and Weights

The method of tying a knot is unimportant. However, the *end result*—a knot that is secure—*is* important. One method of tying a knot is pictured below. Traction cord should never be reused, because it may break.

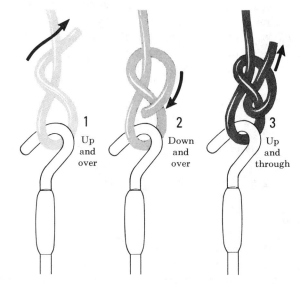

Knot-tying technique. (Courtesy Zimmer Co, Warsaw, Ind)

After the knot has been tied, the end of the rope should be brought up next to the length of rope immediately above the knot and the two wrapped together with a piece of adhesive tape. Once or twice around the ropes is sufficient. Then the free end of the tape should be folded on itself to make a tag for easy removal.

When assisting with or applying any traction to a fractured limb, be sure to hang the weights on the carriers in a slow manner to avoid a jerking, often painful movement.

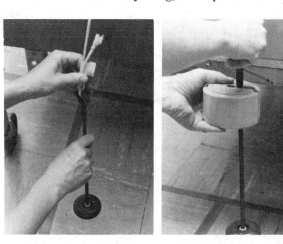

The weights should hang free, which means that they should not rest on the floor, bed, other furniture, or each other. Weights are made of metal or bags filled with sand or shot. If bag-type weights are used, they are tied directly onto the traction rope, eliminating the need for a carrier.

Nursing Assessments Relative to Principles of Traction

Knowledge of the principles underlying effective traction (p. 90) provides for a systematic check of the apparatus and the patient, since these principles are interrelated.

1. Countertraction. When patients in traction look as though they might slide into the headboard or footboard or over the side of the bed, the nurse should realize that there is a problem with countertraction. That is, the force opposing the traction pull is not adequate. This is especially true of skin traction on the leg (Buck's traction).

For ideal countertraction with Buck's traction, the foot of the bed should be elevated to allow the patient's body to provide the countertraction. However, this is not a comfortable position and the amount of weight placed on Buck's traction does not usually exceed 5 lb, so, depending on body weight, countertraction is frequently maintained just by keeping the bed flat. The patient is gradually pulled to the foot of the bed. Therefore, the nurse must check the patient's position every 3 hours and, if necessary, assist him in pulling himself up in bed. This is done by having the patient

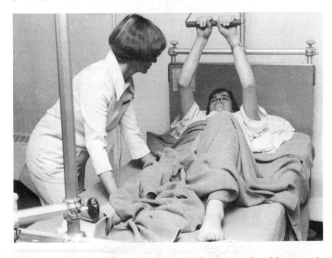

grasp the trapeze, flex the knee of the uninvolved leg, push down with his foot flat on the mattress, and move to the head of the bed while the nurse supports and helps move the involved extremity.

When countertraction is interrupted, friction may result.

2. Friction. Friction interferes with pull and is caused by traction components, bed linen, or the patient himself. All points along the traction apparatus, leading from the patient to the weights, should be checked for impingements. Some common sources of friction are (1) knots pressing against the pulleys, (2) spreaders, footplates, or splints touching the end of the bed, (3) weights caught on the bed, and (4) bed linen covering the straps or ropes. A firm mattress that does not sag is a necessity; otherwise, heels and buttocks tend to "dig in," thereby creating friction.

A potential problem is that the patient's movements may cause a weight to catch under the end of the bed. An excellent way to prevent this from happening is to tape an old x-ray film to the foot of the bed behind the weight. When the patient moves, the weight slides over the x-ray film.

Friction-free traction is troublesome in terms of keeping the patient adequately covered and the linen on the bed, since bedding cannot be tucked in over straps or ropes. Therefore, linen must be arranged around straps and ropes to cover the patient's extremities. When it is not possible to see the apparatus because part of it is covered by bedclothes, it is difficult to check the line of pull.

3. Line of Pull. Although the line of pull should always be checked in all traction patients, it is most important in the reduction of fractures, in which the physician has aligned

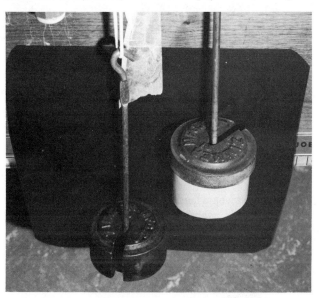

the distal fragment with the proximal fragment in the type of traction he or she considers most beneficial. The line of pull must never be interfered with by changing the position of a pulley and extension bar to remove them from a point of friction. For example, the restlessness of a young man in skeletal traction may cause one rope to shift next to another many times during a day, but this is basically a positioning problem, and either he or the sling should be moved, not his line of traction pull. A patient's position should be checked regularly to see that his body is resting in line with the traction pull.

4. Continuousness. Parallel to the principle of maintaining the line of pull is the one that states that traction should be continuous. If this were not true, there would be no point in having the pulling force in a fixed line, since releasing weights would disturb it. All orthopedic personnel are aware that patients in pelvic or cervical traction for reducing muscle spasms are allowed out of their traction for varying periods of time. However, this requires a physician's order and should be accompanied by some sort of assessment of patient reaction to the release of traction. Also, if traction is to be continuous, the tapes should not be slipping from their points of attachment, and all pulleys should be operating normally.

5. Positioning. The patient should be positioned in good body alignment on a firm mattress. This entails a good deal more than having him flat on his back and perpendicular to the ends of the bed. With the limb in proper alignment, the remainder of the body should be positioned comfortably,

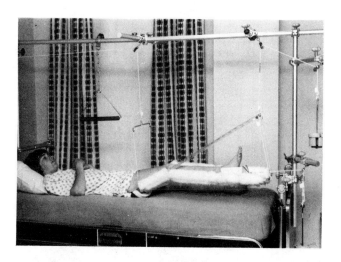

with support given where needed to shoulders, head, or leg to relieve muscle strain. The head of the bed is only elevated when it provides countertraction and as ordered by the physician. However, with all these precautions, it is not necessary to restrict movement.

General Nursing Care to Prevent Complications

Complications resulting from immobility must be considered in caring for the bedridden traction patient. Age, general condition, and limitations caused by specific types of traction are factors in the development of certain problems. Keeping this in mind, the nurse should be able to anticipate needs and plan nursing care that aids in the prevention of complications.

Skin Care

Beginning with careful and comprehensive inspection, skin care is of utmost importance in the care of every traction patient, because body movement is limited so that traction can be continuous. It is important to record any observable skin problems in the nursing care plan if such problems exist. Assisting the patient in bathing provides an opportunity for daily inspection.

Back and buttocks should be rubbed at least three times a day to increase circulation. However, for the patient who spends most of his time in the supine position, back care is necessary every 3 to 4 hours during the day. When dryness is the problem, a lotion may be used. When dryness is desirable and the skin is not irritated, alcohol may be used. Only powder that does not cake is desirable for long-term use. Aerosol powder sprays with protectants and drying agents such as cornstarch, zinc oxide, purified talc, and magnesium stearate are preferable.

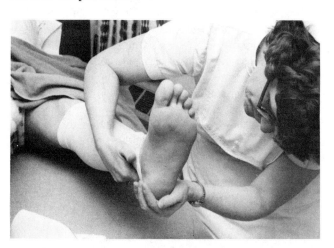

Skin must be inspected as well as rubbed. Heels may still develop pressure sores, even when they are rubbed regularly. Looking at them is the only way to evaluate whether or not the care given is adequate. A rubber glove filled with water and placed under a problem heel is an excellent preventive measure. However, the glove should be covered with

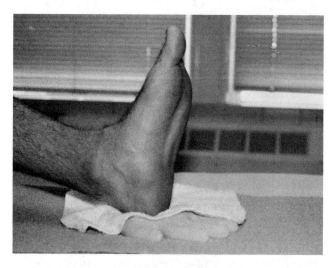

a washcloth, or the nurse will be exchanging one problem for another. The air-tight situation of skin against rubber may cause perspiration and a burning sensation in the heel.

With a trapeze, the patient can lift himself for some aspects of skin care and inspection. He may also do so at will

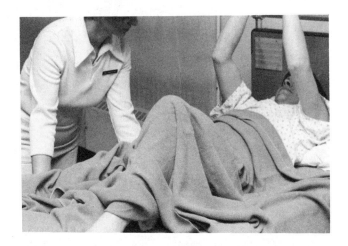

in order to relieve pressure on his buttocks and improve circulation. Instructing the patient in proper use of a trapeze is also part of nursing care. He should attempt to pull himself straight up rather than twist the body. He should also be shown how to place his unaffected foot flat on the bed and push with the foot (not the heel) when raising himself with the trapeze.

General Pressure Points

All bony prominences, back, buttocks, heels, and even the ears, are potential pressure points. Although body parts in traction may be the least mobile, it is frequently other extremities or parts that suffer from pressure while the nurse concentrates solely on traction care.

Take the example of a girl who weighs 110 pounds and has 20 pounds of weight on a Steinmann pin in her tibia. She may need to pull herself up to the top of the bed quite frequently. Unfortunately, she may tend to push herself up with her elbows rather than to use the trapeze. Consequently, she could develop raw spots on her elbows. Suppose she also has one injured hand. That elbow probably rests on the bed more than is healthy for the ulnar nerve. Tingling or numbness in her ring and little fingers from pressure on that nerve would be one of her complaints. It is fairly common for bedridden patients to develop an ulnar-nerve problem, and this aspect of observation, aimed at prevention, must be included in a nursing care plan. The patient should be en-

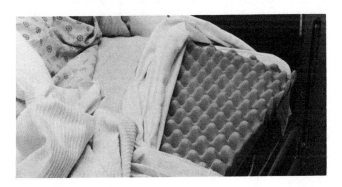

couraged to change arm positions frequently to prevent the elbows from resting continuously on the bed. In addition, the elbows should be rubbed with lotion at the same time that other skin care is given. Furthermore, any patient who is in traction for a long time requires an alternating-pressure mattress or a convoluted bedpad made of foam rubber.

Pressure Sores

Pressure sores, or decubitus ulcers, need not and should not occur in traction patients at all. Reddened areas will develop on occasion, no matter how conscientious the orthopedic nurse has been in changing position, attending to skin care, or keeping a bed dry. There are always those patients who tend to slip back into the same bed position no matter how often they are turned, or how they are "propped," when such methods are permitted. Some people have sensitive skin that breaks down overnight. However, the nurse who is scrupulous in making observations recognizes reddened areas on her patient as danger spots and plans nursing care accordingly. This may involve rubbing the reddened area or checking the position of the patient every hour until redness diminishes or disappears.

Exercise

Exercise increases circulation and maintains muscle tone and must be stressed as part of daily patient care. Movement of all unaffected limbs should be encouraged and range of motion explained to a patient. Using the trapeze is an excellent way to keep arms and shoulders exercised when they are not the body parts in traction.

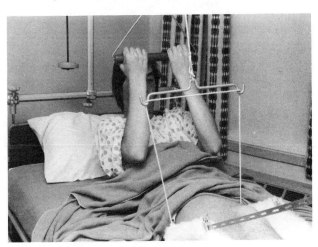

Muscle weakness and contractures occur from disuse. Exercises of all unaffected extremities should be regular so that muscles do not atrophy. Patients tend to guard joints near a fracture, and the nurse must explain and promote range-of-motion exercises, when possible, to prevent contractures.

Initially, the patient in skeletal traction with a fractured femur is most reluctant to move the foot on the affected leg.

Yet active or passive exercising of that foot prevents contracture of the Achilles tendon much better than use of a foot support.

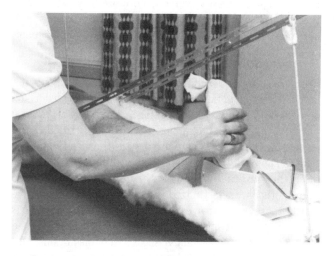

Every orthopedic nursing text would do well to emphasize that the quadriceps muscle begins to atrophy in about 1 week if not used. Patients confined to bed, especially when their legs are immobile to any extent, must be taught quadriceps-setting exercises if they are to ambulate with stability and strength once they are out of bed. For the long-term, immobilized traction patient, an active exercise program including progressive resistive exercises and bedside exercise set-ups may be appropriate. Consulting the physician about a physical-therapy referral for these instructions may assist the patient both physically and emotionally.

Proper positioning and body alignment are also important, as already noted. Keeping a patient warm enough helps keep him in proper position. A nurse may waste a lot of time trying to prevent an elderly patient in traction from attempting to "curl up" in bed, if that patient is cold. When the placement of traction apparatus makes tucking bed

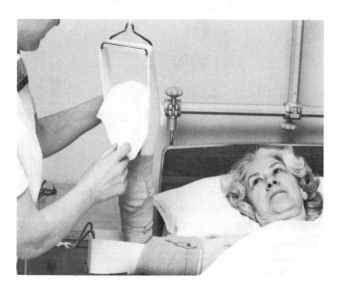

linen around fingers and toes impossible, some covering such as stockinette or a washcloth may be feasible.

The temperature of the patient's room is a factor in promoting comfort. A busy evening nurse who is wearing a sweater may overlook the possibility that the room is too cool for an immobile patient. Whether or not he is warm enough is a judgment the patient should make and a question the nurse should remember to ask.

Digestive Disorders

The slowing down of cell metabolism due to decrease in activity manifests itself in digestive disorders, mainly anorexia and constipation. The problems can be dealt with, first of all, by taking into consideration the eating habits and diets of the individual patient.

The elderly patient with dentures may or may not require a softer diet. Some people with dentures can and do eat "anything," whereas others have difficulty chewing meat that is not chopped or very tender. An added consideration is the fact that the elderly patient requires less food normally than a younger patient. Inquiring extensively into likes and dislikes in food and perhaps providing small feedings with nourishment at bedtime could be a partial solution to nutritional problems.

Once a younger patient becomes comfortable enough in traction to move as much as he is allowed, anorexia is only a problem if he does not like hospital food. If enough efforts are made to satisfy his food tastes, he may even gain weight, especially if he is bored.

Narcotics prescribed for pain relief and lack of adequate privacy when using the bedpan contribute to constipation in a traction patient. These may be unavoidable factors. However, proper nutrition and fluids reduce the incidence of constipation.

Patterns of bowel elimination differ in individuals and are usually of most concern to the older person. All the best nursing intentions in the world will not solve the problem of constipation for this patient as quickly as his own ideas of what he finds effective in the way of foods that maintain regularity or the type of laxative he is used to taking.

Voiding and Urinary Problems

The prevention of urinary problems—cystitis, retention, and renal calculi—is to a great extent a nursing responsibility. Fluid intake must be supervised to ensure that it is adequate and that it includes some juices, such as cranberry juice, which will keep the urine acid. Urinary output should be noted as to amounts and concentration, particularly when the limitations imposed by traction, such as arm or cervical traction, discourage drinking.

Whenever adequate perineal care is difficult to do or give, the chance of cystitis is increased. In many types of traction, therefore, where the pelvis or legs are immobile, prevention of this condition is a priority of nursing care. In an effort to avoid this complication, fluids should be encouraged every 3 hours. The patient should be instructed to report any burning sensation or difficulty when voiding.

A fracture bedpan is best suited for the traction patient because it is easier for the nurse to place and more comfortable for the patient to sit on. The flat lip slips under the lower back and therefore does not place a strain on the lumbar spine or necessitate much lifting on the part of patient or

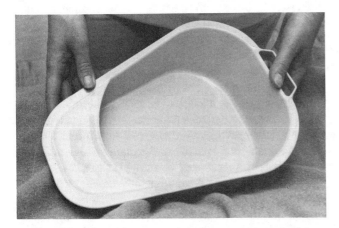

nurse. Because a patient is more likely to void normally when seated comfortably on a bedpan, the fracture pan reduces the possibility of urinary problems.

Hypostatic Pneumonia

Inactive patients need to be taught the importance of deep breathing and coughing to prevent the collection of secretions in the lungs and the occurrence of hypostatic pneumonia. Again, the elderly patient who is immobilized in Buck's extension or arm traction is most prone to this hazard. The nurse should assess respiratory status daily by questioning the patient about the presence or absence of a productive cough and pain or difficulty on inspiration or expiration. Most important, the nurse should listen to the lungs with a stethoscope.

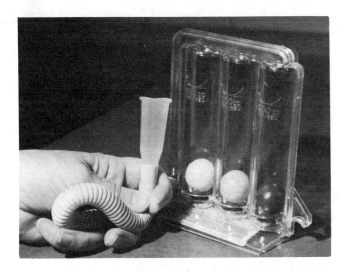

Intermittent positive-pressure breathing (IPPB) treatments or an apparatus the patient can use independently, such as an incentive spirometer that operates on an inhalation principle, may be ordered when coughing and deep breathing do not seem effective in keeping lungs clear. As the patient inhales, the balls rise in their columns. The goal is to maintain all three balls at the tops of the columns for as many seconds as possible. Although the design and structure of incentive spirometers varies, the principle remains the same.

Thrombophlebitis

Measures to prevent *thrombophlebitis*, or inflammation of a vein with clot formation, are extremely important. Not only is this complication painful in itself; it carries with it the possibility of fatal pulmonary embolism. As a prophylactic measure, leg movement needs to be encouraged. When leg movement is restricted, pressure from pillows and knee gatches is to be avoided or relieved by changes in position. Observation for reddened areas or pain in the calf should be regular and such signs must be reported when noted.

Elastic stockings are also used in an effort to prevent venous stasis and are ordered fairly routinely for patients who spend any length of time in bed. Although elastic stockings come in different styles, they have one thing in common. They are generally hard to put on, especially over a painful extremity. One very successful method of application is to turn the stocking inside out except for the part that covers the toe. Place the end of the stocking over the toes

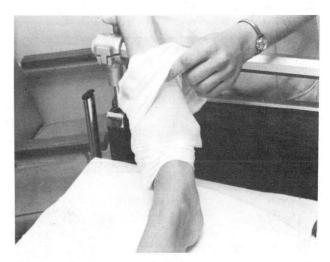

and work the stocking over the foot. It is then fairly simple to pull it up over the leg.

Osteoporosis

There is no way the nurse can prevent *osteoporosis*, or demineralization of bones due to lack of stress. However, encouraging the patient confined to bed to exercise may be helpful. The elderly patient and the postmenopausal woman are susceptible to osteoporosis even *before* becoming bedridden. Therefore, careful positioning and planned exercise become even more important in their care. The nurse should understand that bones that are not being stressed by exercise become fragile and can fracture with little or no trauma.

Psychological Considerations

When the initial shock of injury has subsided, traction patients often suffer from periods of panic and frustration and tend to cry easily. Because they are still in an acute phase, it is easy to assess such behavior as pain related. However, other explanations should be explored. For example, a farmer may have injured himself at the beginning or height of his harvest season and at this time may have no idea about who will carry on in his absence. Every effort must be made to put this kind of patient in touch with someone who can reassure him that "things are being looked after."

Disorientation and boredom frequently cause more nursing problems than the physiologic effects of immobility. Perhaps this is because the manifestations of both are different for each patient, and so the solutions need to be individualized.

Knowing what day it is and what is happening in the world and having some familiar objects in the environment will contribute to mental and emotional health. For example, the patient who is accustomed to an active life in the business world may be lost if someone forgets to bring a daily newspaper. Obviously, patients with prominently displayed pictures of their children need to talk about them. More examples of providing diversion, maintaining orientation, and taking into consideration the unique needs of patients are given in specific care sections.

Maintaining a Therapeutic Environment

Keeping a traction patient physically and mentally comfortable requires common sense as well as nursing skill. Creativity is also helpful.

Only by investigation will the nurse know if complaints about the apparatus are real or imagined. Therefore, they should never be ignored. The care and maintenance of both

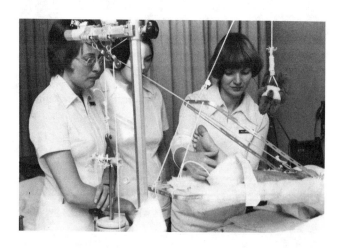

patient and traction is better seen than said. One of the most effective ways to teach personnel and the patient about the possible sources of complaints is to show them the potential cause of the trouble. The nurse should take team members who are responsible for the care of a traction patient into that patient's room and point out the various sources of friction on the traction apparatus and areas where pressure is likely to develop. The patient can be included in these discussions. Remember, there are always some patients who think they are not supposed to complain. These are the ones who experience pain under wrapping bandages and never mention it.

Creativity in orthopedic nursing is often born of sheer frustration. For instance, a patient in skeletal traction with exercise equipment added to his bed frame often has as many as five different ropes that can get tangled together. Using wide-tipped felt markers to make each rope a different color enables *anyone* to tell at a glance which rope goes where, thereby saving time when the traction is checked.

A doctor may decide that immobilization in Buck's traction is the wisest course of treatment for a terminal-cancer patient who has pathologic fractures of the pelvis and femur. However, if in daily assessment and observation the nurse learns that the patient can be encouraged in self-help even slightly, balanced skin traction for the affected leg may be suggested to the physician, since this type of apparatus allows more movement. Once applied, it provides ease in handling the patient when care is given and prevents skin breakdown by allowing greater mobility and a more comfortable position for the leg.

At this point, it would be good to stress that nurses should not be timid about making what they consider to be practical suggestions to the attending physician. As specialized areas of nursing such as orthopedics receive more attention and recognition, the decision-making responsibilities of the nurse also increase. The ability, for example, to assess the individual needs of a traction patient and to suggest ways of meeting them based on knowledge of this type of treatment is appreciated by orthopedic surgeons, who are able to see their patients only for minutes each day. The end result of such comprehensive care is certainly appreciated by both patient and family.

Getting an adequate amount of rest at one time can be a problem for traction patients. Sleeping may be difficult, and some patients never sleep longer than several hours at a time. When traction patients do wake up at night, they should know that this is a good opportunity for the nurse to check their apparatus, rub their back, and straighten the bed. On the other hand, in the early phase of hospitalization a traction patient needs to be awakened frequently during the night for care and observation. The result may be a patient who is irritable from interrupted sleep or loss of sleep. Sometimes this type of patient does not want to eat breakfast; he would rather just sleep.

In conclusion, a traction patient quite often feels

"trapped." He needs to know that all these things (such as coloring of ropes) are being done for him, not because he is "that much work," or "that sick," but because he is "that important."

Skin Traction: Features and General Care

Indications for Use

Skin traction is applied to the skin and soft tissues in instances in which a light or temporary pull is desired or the traction force need not be continuous. Most types of skin traction may be applied or readjusted by the nurse as well as the physician.

Advantages and Disadvantages

The main advantage of skin traction is that no device is introduced into the skeleton. Thus, a possible source of infection is eliminated. However, because the traction is applied to the skin, the amount of force that can be exerted is limited to what the skin can tolerate. The tapes, wrapping bandages, slings, halters, and belts that are commonly used are potential sources of skin irritation and pressure problems. As previously noted, skin traction is often contraindicated in patients who have skin problems arising from poor circulation, diabetes, dermatitis, varicose ulcers, or an injury to the skin and soft tissues.

Implications for Care

Conscientious observation by the nurse is necessary to prevent skin problems or neurovascular problems in these patients. To make intelligent observations the nurse must also be familiar with the correct method of applying tapes, wrapping bandages, and other "soft goods," and must have an awareness of when they can and cannot be reapplied.

Skeletal Traction: Features and General Care

Indications and Site for Skeletal Traction

In skeletal traction a Steinmann pin, Kirschner wire, Crutchfield tong, or similar device is inserted into the bone, enabling direct longitudinal pull to be applied directly to it. When wires or pins are used, the traction force itself is applied to a traction bow (spreader, stirrups, or calipers), which is attached to the wire or pin. These attachments can withstand the stress of 15 to 40 lb of weight for extended periods and are therefore an effective means of providing traction when a strong, steady force is required. Examples include fractures of the femur below the trochanters, in which the strong muscle pull on the proximal fragment of the fracture complicates maintenance of alignment, and

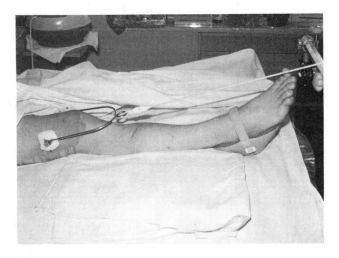

fractures of the cervical spine, in which stability is of prime importance. Displaced fractures of the pelvis are at times treated with skeletal traction.

Sites most commonly used for skeletal traction on the extremities are the distal end of the femur, the proximal end of the tibia, the calcaneus, and the proximal ulna. Skeletal traction of the toe or finger is also employed, although rarely. Tongs are used in the skull for traction and immobilization of cervical-spine fractures.

Insertion of the Device

Since insertion of a pin, wire, or tong is a surgical procedure, aseptic technique must be used in the interest of preventing infection. Osteomyelitis (bone infection) may be a serious complication of skeletal traction. Skin preparation prior to the procedure varies, but one suggested method includes a scrub with a germicidal solution such as povidone-iodine (Betadine), followed by cleansing with alcohol and the application of merthiolate.

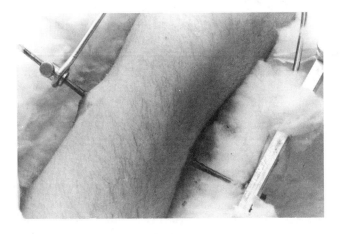

Special Care

Following the procedure, some physicians place gauze dressings around the pin area and direct that the dressing not be removed, for fear that frequent changes and excessive wound care may lead to infection. Others feel that daily wound care is necessary to remove accumulated drainage which, if not removed, could clog the pin tract and create a medium for bacterial growth. Hydrogen peroxide is frequently used in pin-site care, followed by an antibiotic ointment.

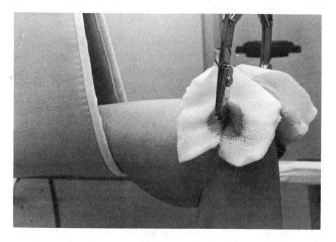

Some physicians request that the pin area not be covered but be kept clean; still others cover the pin area with collodion and specify that it should not be touched. Whatever the situation, it is imperative that the physician's orders be followed in this regard. If the physician does not order pin care, do not do it!

Whatever the physician's instructions, the nurse can and *must* inspect the area around the wire, pin, or tongs for redness, swelling, and drainage. Since these findings may indicate infection they should be recorded and reported promptly.

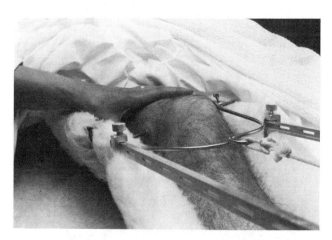

The nurse should also observe the general condition of the suspension device to see that it is intact. If the sharp ends of the wire extend beyond the U loop, cork covering or adhesive should be placed over the protruding edges so that they will not scratch the patient or those giving care, or snag on the sheets and bed linen. If wires or pins appear to have loosened or slipped, the physician should be notified imme-

diately, because the pin or wire can easily cut into the soft tissue, causing injury and creating the danger of infection. The patient is usually the first one to notice this and will become alarmed. He should be told that this will not affect healing.

Care of the Patient in Cervical-Halter Traction

Definition and Indications for Use

Traction may be applied to the cervical spine by means of a head halter. It is most commonly used for relief of neck pain, neck strain, or "whiplash" and in cases in which subluxations or minor fractures are suspected. Cervical-halter traction is rarely used for prolonged periods because it is skin traction and, as in other forms of skin traction, continuous use causes skin irritation. Therefore, it is not desirable for severe injuries or major cervical-spine fractures when release of traction is liable to cause injury to the spinal cord.

Application of Cervical-Halter Traction

The nurse often applies cervical-halter traction except in instances of cervical fracture or when the diagnosis has not been definitely established. The standard components of cervical-halter traction include some type of head halter, a spreader bar, weight carrier, weights, and traction cord. The *kinds* of clamps, bars, and pulleys used vary with the type of equipment in use at a particular hospital. The amount of equipment used may depend on the kind of bed to which the traction is going to be attached and on whether or not the head of the bed will be elevated, as indicated by the physician's orders.

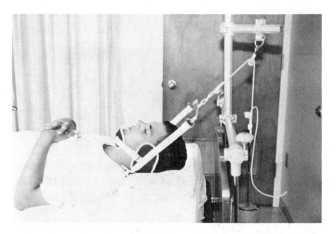

When the patient is to remain flat, it is often simpler and requires less equipment to turn the bed around and attach the traction apparatus to the foot of the bed. There are types of cervical-traction devices available that are designed to attach the unit to the upper end of the backrest of the bed. Such devices allow the backrest to be elevated or lowered without altering the traction forces. However, orthopedic beds are now being manufactured with solid supports for the mattress rather than a frame with bedsprings. This change in bed design may make it impossible to use some clamp attachments for cervical traction.

The nurse with adequate knowledge of the five basic principles that make traction effective should be able to adapt whatever equipment is at hand when cervical traction is prescribed for her patient.

The basic procedure for applying cervical-halter traction is as follows:

1. Make sure that the patient is comfortable, with body in good alignment, shoulders level and relaxed, and back flattened against the bed.
2. Make sure that the patient is down far enough in bed to allow room for the spreader bar and rope.
3. Attach the bars and pulleys to the frame.
4. Make sure that the spreader bar is wide enough so that when the halter is attached it will not press against the sides of the head or pinch the patient's ears.
5. Tie traction cord to the spreader bar, thread it through the pulley, and then tie it to the weight carrier.
6. Attach the weight carrier and then the weight.
7. Apply the head halter to the patient.
8. Make sure that the chin piece is on the chin, not the throat, and that the ears are free.
9. Make sure that the patient is comfortable in the halter before slipping the spreader through the ropes or rings on the head halter.

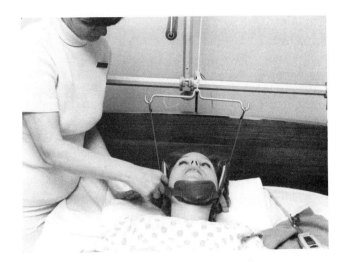

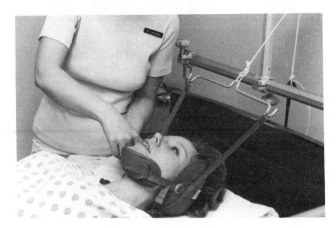

Adverse effects of improperly applied cervical traction (*i.e.*, an unequal pull on either side of the head or a force that is on the chin or ears rather than the occiput), may not be felt for several hours, since the greatest weight used is usually 5 lb. These effects include increased neck or head pain, pressure on the ears, or discomfort along the chin or jawline. Before leaving the patient, the nurse should make another inspection to make certain that the chin piece is centered correctly, the lateral straps appear even and away from the ears, and the posterior strap is on the occiput.

Pressure Points

Fortunately, most patients in cervical-halter traction are permitted to be out of traction for short periods. This helps prevent pressure sores on the areas that must be inspected regularly—the occiput, chin, ears, and mandible. Keeping the chin dry, perhaps with the use of rubbing alcohol or cornstarch, is imperative unless the patient is suffering from some skin inflammation such as severe acne. If the patient does suffer from acne, the skin may require more frequent observation. The physician may need to be consulted and special ointment or medication ordered. If rubbing on the ears is a problem, using a wider spreader bar may be the solution.

Men in cervical traction should use their time out of traction to shave, since stubble may cause prickling or itching when a chin piece rests securely against it. A full beard may inspire the owner to shave completely, since besides causing prickling, a beard is very conveniently located to catch dribbles of food and fluid!

Placing material in the chin piece only adds to the pressure. If the patient's chin is especially susceptible to irritation, it is best to ask the physician if the patient may pull the chin piece down for a few seconds at frequent intervals.

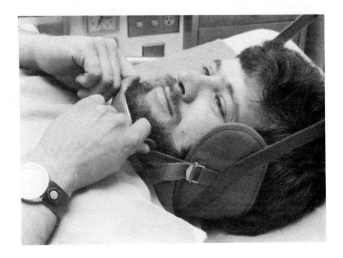

Problems Due to Position

An immobile head and fairly immobile jaw create many problems for a patient. Eating, chewing, and drinking may cause crumbs and drops of fluid to fall on the face and consequently the chin pad. A napkin and other protective material tucked over the pad may minimize this problem. Swallowing may also be difficult. A soft diet may be indicated along with careful observation of food and fluid intake.

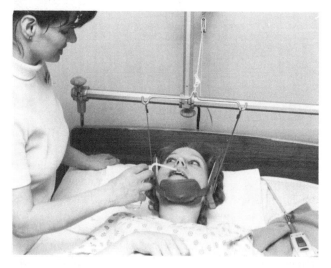

Leave a straw in a glass only partially filled with water and remember to keep it readily accessible to the patient. Visual perception may be impaired because of restricted head movement, and some patients complain that they have trouble judging how far an object is from their reach.

Even talking may be difficult for these patients because it can put strain on the jaw and throat muscles. To help relieve boredom, prism glasses may be used to enable the patient who is flat in bed to watch television or read.

Changing Bed Linen

Common sense dictates that for patients in cervical traction who are not seriously injured, it is less uncomfortable to remove the traction for the minute or two required to

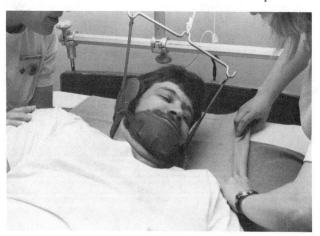

change bottom bed linen than it is to push sheets or towels under the patient's head and neck. However, if this is not possible, the drawsheet is usually the only bottom linen that is changed daily. For this patient it is also a good idea to place plastic under the head and shoulders and cover it with a towel, which is more easily changed than a bottom sheet. Care must be taken to use only plastic sheeting that can be tucked in so that it will not wrinkle. The patient in a cervical halter can be logrolled about 45 degrees if his shoulders are supported, and if the rope is threaded through a hanging pulley. As the patient is turned, the apparatus turns with him.

Skin Care

The patient can also bathe when out of traction. Good back rubs are essential every 3 hours during the day. The patient's elbows and heels should also be examined at these intervals and lotion rubs given when indicated.

General Observations

The patient should be observed for any reaction to temporary release of traction. Any increase or decrease in neck discomfort, numbness, tingling, or pain in arms and hands should be recorded. Patients quite often become adept at getting in and out of their own halters and should be taught to inform the nurse each time they do this. This ensures

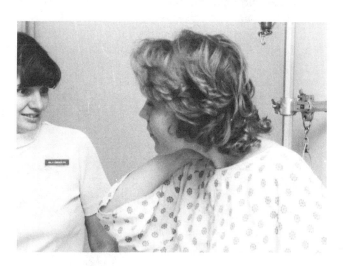

proper application of the apparatus and provides an opportunity for assessment of symptoms. The ears, chin, and occipital areas can be inspected closely for signs of irritation.

Psychological Considerations

The physical discomfort experienced by patients in cervical-halter traction may have a demoralizing effect. A woman with undiagnosed neck pain may have a headache from her tiresome position in the cervical traction, may worry over her house, or may be annoyed by the bright ceiling lights in her eyes. If the condition requiring traction is a recurring type caused by an old injury, the patient may often feel discouraged.

Although a lot of physical care may not be required for these patients, the nurse who comes to the bedside to visit and who establishes eye contact in doing so reduces the patient's sense of isolation and allows for expression of feelings.

The physician may order a head-halter traction setup to be used in the home after the patient is discharged. The traction is a vertical pull on the occiput provided by a pulley-and-rope system running vertically from the head halter to a door bracket. The halter and traction apparatus is worn

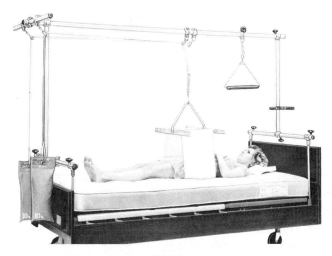

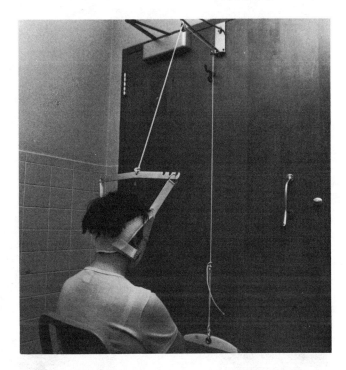

while sitting on a chair under the bracket. The amount of weight varies but is generally more than the amount used in the hospital, because the patient is not in an acute phase of neck pain. The patient is introduced to the apparatus while still in the hospital.

Care of The Patient in a Pelvic Sling

Description and Indications for Use

The pelvic sling, used for some types of pelvic injuries, is made of canvas and is attached both to a spreader and to a spring that supports the patient's pelvis off the bed. Metal rods or wooden bars are inserted at each of the side ends of the sling, with the ends of each rod protruding enough to be placed into slots on the spreader. The physician decides where the rods are placed according to whether or not he

Pelvic sling. (Courtesy Zimmer Co, Warsaw, Ind)

desires a compression force to be applied. The position of these rods should never be changed by anyone except the physician.

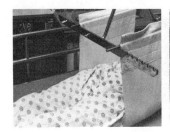 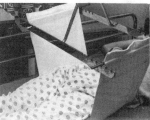

Traction is accomplished by attaching the spreader to a spring, which takes up the slack and is further attached to a rope drawn up through a pulley on the overhead frame. The rope is threaded through another pulley on the frame at the head or foot of the bed, and weight is attached. The construction of spreaders for pelvic slings varies somewhat and may employ the use of two ropes and separate weights. Compression of the pelvis occurs as the side ends of the sling are drawn toward each other over the patient, and the rods are placed as described above.

The use of the pelvic sling for fractures of the pelvis is somewhat controversial. Theoretically, it should provide compression for innominate bones that are laterally displaced. Although it is an effective compression force when in place, it is so difficult for a patient to use a bedpan while in a pelvic sling that it may need to be released or moved for the procedure. Consequently, the compression force is temporarily lost.

Care Plan Based on Two Considerations

The nursing care plan of the patient who has sustained a pelvic fracture and is in a pelvic sling is based on two considerations. The first is the knowledge that any patient with this type of fracture needs to be observed for injury to pelvic or abdominal organs. Especially important are observations for adequate urinary output, hematuria, rectal bleeding, abdominal pain, spasm, rigidity, or distention, plus symptoms of shock from internal bleeding.

The second consideration relates to exactly how much movement the patient is allowed according to physician's orders and whether or not the sling can be released or moved.

Back Care

Knowing the limitations of both patient and sling, the nurse can decide how to give back care. If the sling must remain in place, the back should be massaged by working the hands between the patient's body and the sling. The entire back should be rubbed every 3 hours. The sacral area needs careful massage, because the patient is so flat. Total inspection may be impossible, so careful attention must be given to complaints or irritation or pressure.

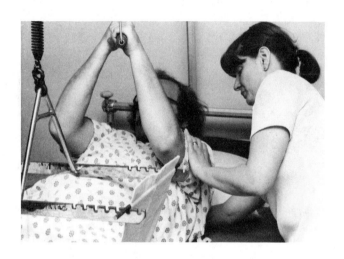

Some sources suggest the use of a pad in the sling to prevent wrinkles. If a pad is placed, it should be large enough so that the patient is not lying on the "edges," which then become an added source of skin irritation.

Elimination and Hygiene

Protection of the sling against soiling by urine or feces is a major problem. The edge should be covered by plastic or a disposable pad when the bedpan is placed.

If the pelvic sling has been applied to compress the pelvis to any extent, it is all but impossible to place a fracture bedpan. For this procedure the sling usually needs to be released. If the sling is immobilizing the patient with minimal compression, it may be released or slid slightly toward the patient's head. Moving the sling or placing a bedpan with the sling in place also depends on the patient's condition and how much sliding and handling he can tolerate. For a woman a female urinal may be more workable for voiding than a bedpan. If both prove too awkward, the physician usually orders an indwelling catheter.

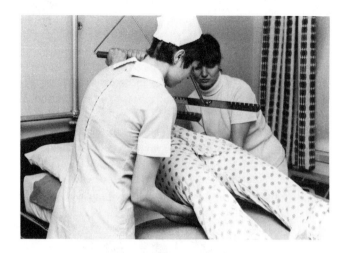

Obviously, the less movement the patient is allowed, the harder it is to maintain a clean, dry perineum. Each time the bedpan is used, perineal cleansing with warm water and a mild soap is suggested. The area should then be dried with a soft towel, followed by application of a protectant powder.

Exercising and Foot Support

The legs of a patient in a pelvic sling need exercise to prevent venous stasis and muscle weakness. Unless the patient has a real problem keeping the feet active, a footboard is unnecessary. Whenever a footboard is omitted from nursing-care plans, the nurse must make a special effort to assist the patient with foot exercises. For the patient, exercising is more valuable than foot support. Elastic stockings may be ordered as an aid to increased circulation.

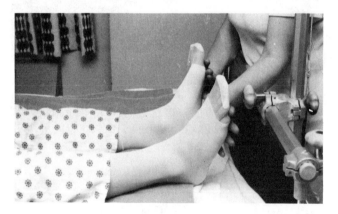

Although pillows may lessen muscle strain by enabling leg position to be changed, a physician's order should be obtained before pillows are placed under the legs and feet of a patient in a pelvic sling. Prolonged flexion of the knee and pressure on the popliteal space must be avoided. The pillows should not be placed under the sling.

Typical Problems

Nursing approaches to some typical problems of the patient in a pelvic sling are presented in the chart below.

THE PATIENT IN PELVIC-SLING TRACTION: PROBLEM SOLVING (NURSING PROCESS)

Patient Situation: L.W. is 46. He has a pelvic fracture and has been in pelvic-sling traction for 14 days. His wife visits twice daily. This patient is undemanding, pleasant, and rarely complains of anything unless he is questioned. The following complaints and problems were identified at a 7:00 A.M. shift report.

Problem/Complaint	Assessment Data	Intervention	Evaluation
1. Pruritus: buttocks and right groin.	1. Right groin reddened. Buttocks area: what is visible is covered with spotty rash. Sling is damp from perspiration.	1. Change sling. Increase back care to q 2 hr while awake. Use alcohol. Keep groin dry and apply cornstarch q 4 hr while awake.	1. No increase in rash. Decreased pruritus in 48 hr.
2. Muscle pain: left leg.	2. Homans' sign negative. Calf not inflamed. States his legs ache when not exercised.	2. Remind patient to exercise legs with each nursing routine.	2. Decreased muscle pain left leg 48 hr.
3. Wants to "help" when being lifted by pushing up with his feet.	3. "Forgets" he should not be lifting.	3. Instruct patient that lifting takes him out of sling and alters traction force. May be reason his sling shifts (see 4).	3. Allows himself to be lifted without helping.
4. Sling "feels like it's moving up around my waist."	4. Sling edge at waist. May need to be adjusted closer to body.	4. When changing sling, move bars one notch toward patient's body, since this will not alter compression force.	4. No further complaints of sling slipping.
5. Had an emesis shortly after 11:00 P.M., following glass of grape juice.	5. Denies gastric distress at present or any history of GI problems. Temp. 98.8. Stress?	5. Check daily for complaints of gastric distress (see 6).	5. No further signs of gastric distress (see 6).
6. States he did not sleep well but appeared to be sleeping when checked during night.	6. Takes a sleeping pill that usually works, is upset. Doctor told him he would be in traction 4 more weeks. States he was told that a week ago. Says his father had "trouble" with a hip pin, and "Doctors don't know everything." Denies this kept him awake, but it is a possibility.	6. Reassure patient that 6 weeks is average for this type of treatment. Spend some time with him and encourage him to verbalize feelings and ask questions. Tell him that he is allowed to complain and that internalizing negative feelings may be causing him anxiety and problems such as restlessness and gastric distress. He should be told that restlessness may affect the alignment of his traction and aggravate skin irritation already present. Include patient's wife in this discussion.	6. Sleeping better. Decreased signs of anxiety.

Psychological Considerations

The patient in a pelvic sling may have some apprehension about the state of his pelvis. When observations are made for damage to pelvic organs, he may become quite concerned, especially if he has not been informed as to the reasons why a nurse is so interested in the condition of his abdomen and his urinary output. An alert patient notices how carefully his sling is moved or released and how gently he is handled. Without daily reassurance and emotional support, he may even wonder how stable his pelvis will be when it is healed. Prism glasses help him do things that keep his mind occupied.

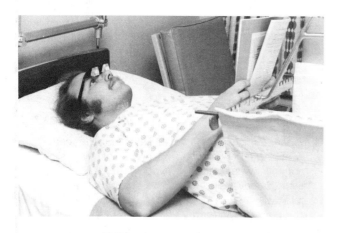

Care of The Patient in a Pelvic Belt

Use and Therapeutic Value

Any discussion by orthopedic personnel of back pain and the use of pelvic traction usually brings forth a variety of opinions concerning this affliction and its treatment. This is understandable because the complaints of "back" patients are variable and the condition often is chronic. The patient may find traction comfortable one day and uncomfortable the next. Furthermore, over a period of a couple of years, the nurse may see the patient admitted three or four times for treatment.

Physicians are generally skeptical about the therapeutic effects of pelvic traction, except that it does provide a degree of immobilization and gives the patient a sense of being treated. As long as some relief from pain is obtained and the patient feels better emotionally as well as physically, pelvic-belt traction will be used in the treatment of low back pain.

Applying Pelvic-Belt Traction

Probably the most common type of traction applied by nurses is the pelvic belt, because it is used primarily in the conservative management of back pain. Pelvic belts that are

made of canvas and lined with flannel are no longer in common use. However, a nurse may encounter one from time to time. These belts are darted to fit the contours of the body, marked with a size, and chosen for the patient based on measurements of the patient's waist and hips. They are secured snugly over the iliac crests and fastened with straps and buckles. However, these belts are reusable and tend to shrink when laundered. The nurse who uses this type of belt should bear this in mind and perhaps choose one that is marked a size larger than the patient's measurements would require.

The more commonly used belts are adjustable and disposable and are secured in place by surfaces that adhere to each other, thereby ensuring a proper fit. These belts come in several sizes, or one universal size, depending on the manufacturer. They are applied directly onto the skin over

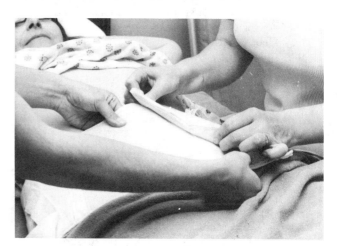

the iliac crests and secured by crossing the ends over each other and down slightly over the abdomen. Once the correct fit is determined, the excess at the ends of the belt may be cut off. The belt should not be applied like an abdominal binder or it will be loose at the upper edge.

On all pelvic belts there are straps that attach to ropes and weights to exert a downward pull on the lower back. On canvas belts, these straps are sewn on, making them nonadjustable. On disposable belts, the straps have a self-adhering side that sticks to the belt in the desired position. There are two possible ways of placing the straps. The straps may be attached so that the patient is lying on them, making the pull of the traction downward and upward on the lower back. Or, as is frequently done, they may be attached at the sides of the belt, parallel to each other as well as to the patient's thighs, in which case the pull on the lower back is strictly downward. The height of the pulleys through which the ropes are run also helps provide the direction of traction pull.

After the straps are attached and adjusted to the same lengths, a traction rope is tied to each. The ropes are threaded through pulleys that are secured, one on each side,

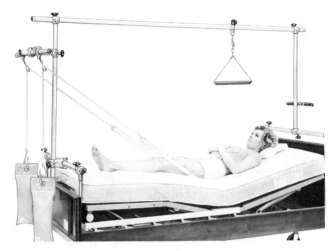

Pelvic belt traction. (Courtesy Zimmer Co, Warsaw, Ind)

to a crossbar that is clamped in a horizontal position to the vertical bar at the foot end of the bed. These ropes are tied to weight carriers and weight is applied equally to each side, to a total of 14 to 20 lb, as prescribed. Bed position is head and knee gatch elevated into a modified jackknife or Williams' position.

Another method of attaching ropes and weights to the belt is to use a spreader bar attached to the ends of the pelvic straps, with one traction cord attached in the middle of the bar. This cord runs through a pulley that is clamped to a bar attached to the vertical or upright bar at the foot of the bed.

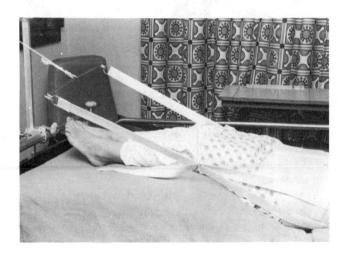

A drawback in this method is the tendency of the spreader bar and rope to shift and rest against the upright bar of the basic frame when the patient moves. Also, it is more difficult to keep bed linen over the patient's legs with this type of attachment of weight.

An initial check after the traction has been on 1 to 2 hours readily indicates if it has been applied correctly. If not, the belt will be slipping or the patient may complain of an uneven pull as the result of unequal strap lengths.

Initially the patient may complain of more back pain while adjusting to the traction. At this point a prescribed pain medication and TLC (tender loving care) may be the best solution. Since the purpose of pelvic traction is to exert pull on the lower back, thus flattening the lumbar curve, placing a pillow under the lumbar spine is not recommended.

Importance of Reporting Symptoms

When chronic back pain is undiagnosed or the patient is experiencing his first episode of back discomfort, an accurate and complete description of symptoms is most important. The nurse must question the patient about the presence of any urinary problems and elicit a clear description of the pain and its exact location. This aids in ruling out kidney problems or involvement of the autonomic nervous system.

Pressure Points and Skin Care

The areas over the iliac crests are subject to rubbing or pressure from the belt and should be inspected at intervals. Special padding over the crests of thin patients helps relieve

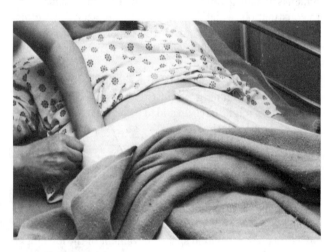

pressure. The elbows become reddened as the patient shifts about in bed. The buttocks are quite stationary and need rubbing, along with the entire back, three or four times a day. Lotion may be used where skin care is indicated.

Routine Nursing Care

Rarely does a patient in pelvic traction have to remain at complete bed rest. Physicians generally agree that it is just as uncomfortable to sit on a bedpan as it is to get out of bed and walk to the bathroom. It is also easier and more comfortable for the patient if the bottom bed linen is changed while he is up going to the bathroom, rather than while he is in bed. However, if the patient is not allowed out of bed, he should be encouraged to use a trapeze to lift himself as a fracture bedpan is being placed. If it is absolutely necessary,

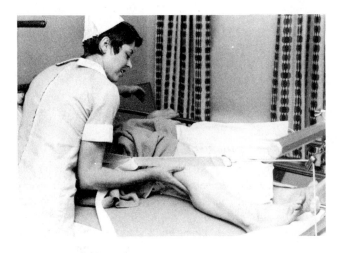

the patient may be logrolled onto the bedpan with a pillow between his legs.

Solving Elimination Problems

One problem for patients in pelvic-belt traction is constipation. The combination of an Empirin and codeine compound, which is usually given for pain, and relative immobility leads to constipation, which in turn adds to low back discomfort. Thus, the nurse should teach the importance of drinking fluids and eating a balanced diet with more roughage and fruit to alleviate this problem.

Sometimes these patients are slightly overweight to begin with. Teaching good nutrition as an aid to relieving constipation might have an added beneficial effect if weight loss can be encouraged.

Exercises and Positioning

Encouraging the patient to move his extremities and to put his feet through range-of-motion exercises while he is in bed will help him maintain muscle strength and promote circulation. When the knee gatch is elevated, thereby putting pressure on the popliteal space, movement of the lower legs

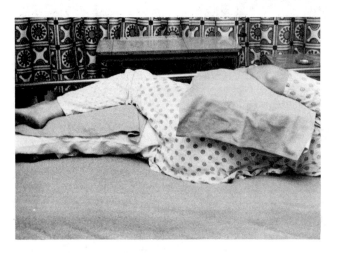

and feet is especially important in the prevention of venous stasis.

One position that is correct and that provides relief from traction is lying on the side with hips and knees bent, with pillows placed under the head and upper arm and between the knees.

The nurse can aid the physician in the evaluation of back pain by talking to and observing the patient both in and out of traction.

Specific Problems

Keeping the traction applied properly, according to principles, is frustrating to the nurse and patient. Feet and legs are hard to keep covered when bedclothes must be off the straps. The newer disposable belts may be cut and altered to fit most people. However, getting in and out of one at intervals, as is usually allowed, wearing it over nightclothes, and enduring the pull of 14 to 20 lb, all are factors that cause problems in keeping the belt in place. When the patient is removing the belt, it is wise to assist by holding on to the weights to relieve the traction pull and to prevent the weights from falling to the floor.

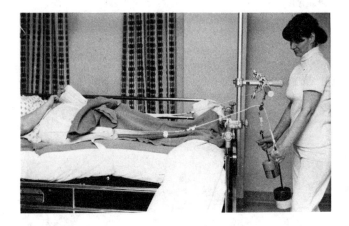

Heating pads, when ordered for back and thigh in conjunction with traction, need careful observation so they do not cause burns.

The position of the bed, with head and knees elevated, along with the traction components, makes it difficult to keep the linen free from wrinkles, which can be frustrating to both nurse and patient.

Psychological Considerations

Chronic back pain is discouraging both to the person who has it and to those involved in treatment. A truck driver or laborer who strained his back while on the job and undergoes periodic hospitalization because of back trouble may have guilt feelings if the pain is not severe. Very likely he also has periods of depression, particularly if he is employed by a company that does not want him back unless he is "cured." So he may have persistent questions about his treatment, his physician, and the possibility of surgery and permanent disability. Much of what he has a need to know, no one can tell him with absolute certainty. Often the most therapeutic thing a nurse can do for a patient in pelvic traction is demonstrate an acceptance of his feelings and a willingness to listen.

Care of The Patient in Buck's Extension

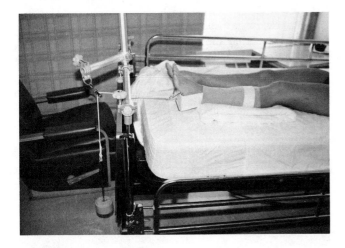

Description and Indication for Use

Buck's extension, also known as unilateral or bilateral leg traction, is a form of skin traction in which a pulling force is exerted on the affected part by means of running traction. No balanced support is provided by a splint or a sling. Buck's traction can be applied only for short periods and is limited to traction weights of less than 10 lb, so it is usually a temporary form of treatment.

Buck's extension is unilaterally applied after reduction of a dislocated hip and for immobilization of (1) a hip fracture prior to surgery, (2) a leg in abduction following total hip replacement, (3) a locked knee, and (4) a fracture of the femur. However, in most femoral fractures in adults, Buck's traction is not suitable, because it cannot maintain the traction weight necessary to reduce the fracture and cannot be used for the length of time necessary for healing. However, it may be used as a temporary measure before surgical reduction.

Applying Buck's Extension

Buck's extension is frequently applied by the nurse. Assistance is needed in this procedure in order to tape and wrap the leg efficiently.

Shaving the extremity may be necessary if adhesive tape is used. Care should be taken to avoid scratches: an electric shaver or clippers are recommended because a razor is more

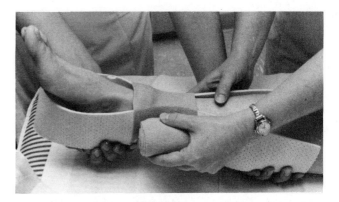

likely to cause small lacerations and abrasions of the skin, which could lead to skin breakdown once the tapes are applied.

Regular adhesive tape and moleskin, to which some people are allergic, are generally being replaced by two other varieties of tape. One is made of a spongy material with a gummed surface on one side that enables it to adhere to the skin. It allows perspiration to evaporate and is nonirritating to the skin. The other kind of tape is sponge rubber without the sticky surface; it adheres to the skin by means of suction created by the sponge.

The tape should be attached in one strip, down the inner aspect of the leg, then left loosely unattached around the foot, and attached once more up the outer aspect of the leg. The portion of the tape that is unattached and extends around the foot should extend from about 1 inch above the medial malleolus to 1 inch above the lateral malleolus, and should be prepared so that neither side will stick. This is accomplished by placing a piece of tape over the sticky side. There must be enough slack in the tape around the foot to allow for attachment of a spreader, block, and footplate.

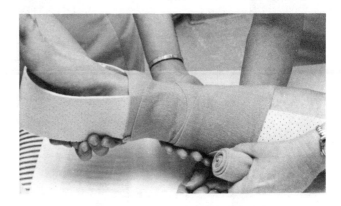

The reason for preventing the tape from sticking to the area above the malleoli is to allow room for the tape to slip, after weight is applied, without the tape covering the malleoli in the process. The skin over these bony prominences will break down rapidly if subjected to the stress of traction

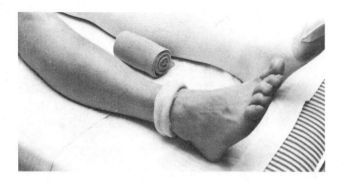

tape. An effective method of keeping tape off the malleoli is to slip a doughnut made of stockinette over the foot to a point just above the malleoli, before applying the tape.

The tapes extend from the malleoli to either the thighs or just below the knee. When tape is to extend onto the thigh, the knee should be in slight flexion as tape is being applied to prevent hyperextension of the knee joint. If applied on a leg for which surgery is anticipated, as in the case of a fractured hip, the tape should probably stop below the knee to avoid irritating the skin at the surgical site. Tape should never cover the patella or the popliteal area, to avoid skin breakdown and compression of blood vessels. Furthermore, traction should never extend over the fracture site, for if it does, the pull will not be entirely over the distal fragment where it belongs. Actually, since Buck's extension is most often a temporary measure for immobilization, application to a level below the knee is sufficient.

The only advantage in applying tapes over the thigh is to provide a greater surface area to withstand the stress of weight. This may be desirable if more than 5 lb of weight is ordered or if the traction is to remain on the leg for any length of time.

Another way of using more surface area is to apply several adhesive-type tapes from a level below the knee. They

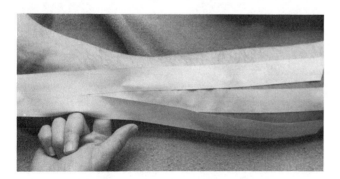

should converge at the foot spreader and thus take the stress of more weight over a period of time.

Traction tapes should never be applied so that they encircle the limb. Any slipping of such tapes would constrict circulation. The method of applying tapes obliquely around the leg in a "criss-cross" fashion is not recommended.

Should such tapes slip, they would take along any areas of skin left exposed by the criss-cross pattern.

Since creases in the tape may cause pressure areas on the skin, the tape should be applied without wrinkles. This is difficult unless the nurse has someone to hold the leg and assist with smoothing and pressing the tape into place. Notching the tape at intervals makes it more adaptable to the contours of the extremity, but is only manageable if it can be done beforehand. This makes it applicable to tape with a backing that peels off for application. Plain sponge rubber tape is simply held in place by one nurse or assistant as elastic bandages are applied.

If the traction is to be on for longer than 2 or 3 days, sheet wadding should be applied over adhesive tapes to provide added protection for bony prominences. When the sponge rubber tape is used, the leg should be wrapped with sheet wadding prior to application of the tape. This helps prevent the tape from slipping, thereby reducing irritation of the skin.

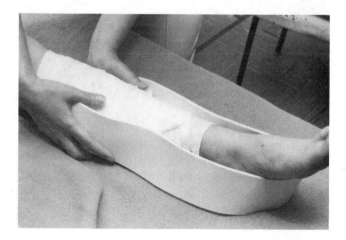

Once the traction tape is in place, elastic bandages are applied, starting above the ankle and avoiding the achilles tendon, which can become extremely irritated if covered.

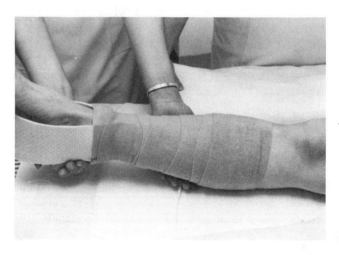

Care must be taken not to wrap too snugly over the upper 3 inches of the fibula, where the peroneal nerve lies close to the surface and is easily compressed by the bone. A diagonal or modified figure-eight method of applying a bandage, which excludes the foot and ankle, gives a more even distribution of pressure and remains in place longer. Bandages should be secured with clips or safety pins.

Next, the spreader is attached. The important point to remember in choosing a spreader or block, which is to be attached below the foot, is that it needs to be wide enough so the tapes are kept off the sides of the foot, but not so wide that the tape will be pulled off the leg. Some hospitals use

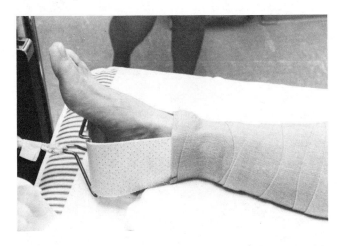

footplates rather than spreading attachments. Likewise, in some areas, foam rubber boot-type splints with self-adhering straps substitute for tapes, bandages, and footpieces. They come equipped with an attachment for the rope.

The rope is tied to whatever footpiece or spreader is being used and then is threaded through a pulley over the foot of the bed and attached to a weight carrier. Weight is slipped on the carrier *slowly* and in the prescribed amount. The weight should be positioned high enough from the floor so that if the patient slips down in bed, the weight will not come to rest on the floor. At the same time, the weights

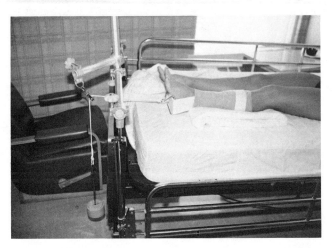

should not be so high that the knot comes to rest against the pulley when the patient changes positions. Nor should any change in the patient's position cause the weight to rest on the bed frame. It goes without saying that the rope should be in good condition. As previously stated, the knots must be secure to avoid any possibility of sudden release resulting in painful jarring.

The bed may be placed in a flat position or the foot may be elevated on shock blocks.

After the traction has been applied and checked for mechanical efficiency, it should be rechecked in 1 hour to determine if either the tape or wrapping bandage is causing skin irritation or compression of nerves and blood vessels.

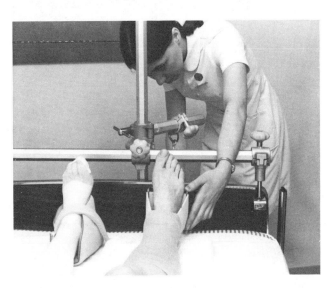

Skin and Pressure Problems

Whatever type of material is used for skin traction, it is ultimately attached to the weight and puts tension on the tissues. As a result, the skin under it may become irritated and break down. Recognition of *early* signs of this condition is imperative in the prevention of severe maceration of the skin.

The following sections on problems and nursing observations associated with tapes and wrapping bandages are applicable to any kind of traction in which the patient's leg is wrapped.

Tape Irritation

Irritation from tape may come from many sources. When adhesive tapes slip because of the stress of weight, they pull the skin off with them. Skin irritation may also result from perspiration under sponge rubber tapes, even though the tapes are vented to enable evaporation. When the patient who has a leg in skin traction complains of soreness or burning, and the elastic wrapping bandage appears properly applied, the tape is probably the offender. The nurse should run a hand over the tapes gently to locate the af-

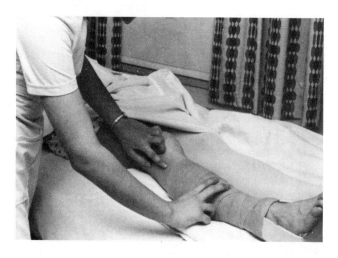

fected area. The physician should be notified as soon as possible, and the nurse should remove and reapply the wrapping and tape unless she has specific orders otherwise.

Patients may need to be *questioned* about discomfort in areas where tape has been applied. A nurse who does not become suspicious of developing problems until she detects drainage or an odor through a wrapping bandage, when none is to be expected, has waited too long.

Problems Caused by Wrapping Bandages

Wrapping bandages, used on extremities to secure the traction tapes, need to be checked so that they are not too tight over the pressure points. This should be done four to fives times daily from early morning until bedtime. A wrapping bandage needs to be removed and reapplied at least once in an 8-hour shift, and more often if it slips. The physician who does not want this to happen should be asked for specific alternatives. While rewrapping is being done, manual traction on the limb is necessary. A tight bandage on a leg may cause pain or numbness due to *general* nerve and blood vessel compression. Tight wrapping is to be avoided especially over the proximal end of the fibula, where the superfi-

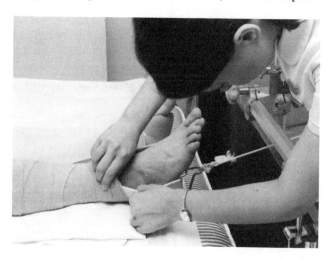

cial peroneal nerve lies close to the bone. A patient whose peroneal nerve is in trouble will complain of pain or tingling on the anterior surface of the leg and dorsum of the foot. Difficulty in extending the toes or a tendency of the foot toward inversion is also an indicator of pressure on the nerve. The patient should be able to feel each toe as it is pinched slightly. Remember that the real problem with footdrop in orthopedic patients comes from pressure on the peroneal nerve (once it has been proven intact after injury or surgery) due to inadequate attention by the nurse, and not from lack of foot support.

Sandbags along the affected leg to maintain alignment are not recommended unless specifically ordered. They are another source of pressure, especially in the area of the peroneal nerve.

Numbness and coldness of the toes or dorsum of the foot may be signs that the circulation has been impaired signifi-

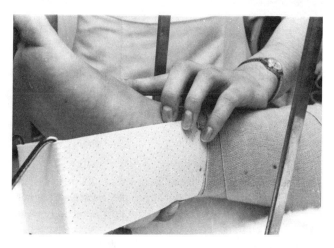

cantly. Often swelling occurs in the toes along with these other signs. Check for a pedal pulse when observing vascular status.

Another source of trouble is a wrapping that slips, either loosening the traction or acting as a constricting band on the extremity. The skin over the tibia is especially subject to breakdown from this sort of pressure because it is so close to the bone. Likewise, the *edges* of wrapping bandages can cause pressure and erosion in specific areas.

The edges of wrapping bandages on the leg rest on the popliteal space, causing pressure on blood vessels and soft tissues. The hamstring tendons at the back of the knee and the Achilles tendon at the heel are spots to check regularly. The skin over these tendons breaks down rapidly from pressure. The soft tissues on the top of the foot are also subject to irritation from bandage edges.

The foot in traction must not be allowed to slip down against the spreader plate. This interferes with the effectiveness of the traction by causing friction. Indentations or pressure on the sole of the foot may result in skin breakdown.

Preventing sore heels is a priority. They are best kept off the bed by a folded bath blanket under the calf. A bath blanket is firm and provides even support. However, it is important to place the blanket so it does not put pressure on the popliteal space or the Achilles tendon. If heel protectors are used, they should not be a replacement for rubbing and inspection. Rather they should serve to remind the nurse

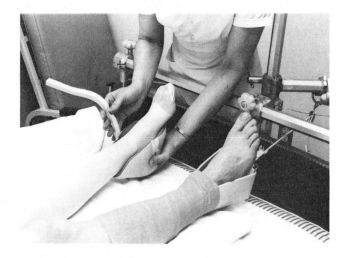

that the heels are there and need attention. Protectors only alter, they do not eliminate, the type of pressure on the heels. Heels blister or become red from pressure in several hours.

The traction splint, or "boot," used in place of the conventional elastic bandage and tapes for Buck's or leg traction, is comfortable for the patient and a timesaver for the nurse. The boot is made of convoluted foam rubber with straps that adhere to each other and a place of attachment for a rope on the bottom.

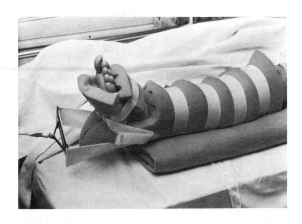

Meticulous attention must be given to the leg and foot in a traction splint, because foam rubber causes perspiration. The boot should be removed every 8 hours and the entire lower leg, especially the heel, should be inspected carefully and the necessary skin care given. Straps must be tight

enough to secure the splint but not so tight that they cause pressure.

An orthopedic nurse, obviously, must constantly be aware that there is more to complaints of a painful arm or leg in traction than the original problem requiring the traction.

Back Care

One of the disadvantages of Buck's extension is that the patient is forced to lie flat on his back. Therefore, back care, including the buttocks, should be given every 3 hours. These patients generally are able to use a trapeze to lift the top half of the body off the bed. If they are unable to do this, they may be turned 45 degrees to either side, with a pillow between the legs.

Bedmaking

If the patient is able to use the trapeze and assist with the unaffected leg, changing bed linen will be easier if started from top to bottom. As shown here, two people loosen a soiled bottom sheet at the top as the patient lifts shoulders and upper back. At the same time they start to put the clean

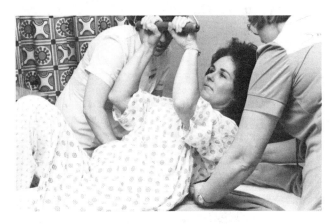

sheet in place. Then the buttock or buttocks are lifted by the patient for that part of the change. If the patient is unable to lift both buttocks, the sheets can be pulled under the raised side and then one nurse can lift on the other as the sheets are pulled down.

To remove the sheets from under the legs, the patient can raise the unaffected leg and a nurse may support the affected leg just enough to work the sheets down the length of the leg. Two nurses lifting the leg a little at a time may be required until the patient has adjusted to traction and feels secure.

Fortunately, since the period of time spent in Buck's traction is usually 24 to 72 hours, the drawsheet is the only bottom linen that will require changing. This is done efficiently by turning the patient from side to side, 45 degrees, with a pillow between his legs to maintain the line of pull in the affected leg.

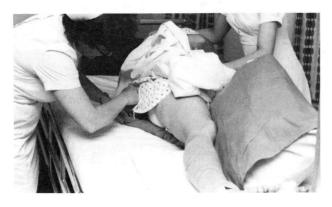

For the very immobile patient in Buck's extension, several people may be required to change the bottom linen. The procedure then involves turning the patient from to side to side, as when changing a drawsheet. Remember that wrinkles cause skin irritation and should be avoided.

Maintaining alignment of the involved leg as the patient is being turned is not a problem with a "hanging" pulley. The pulley and the rope shift slightly as the patient turns.

Bathing

Bathing the patient in Buck's extension is a problem only if the patient is confused or otherwise uncooperative, as may be true in the case of an elderly patient with a hip fracture. Otherwise, the patient should be encouraged to do as much self-care as possible, because it is a form of arm exercise. However, bathing while lying flat is awkward, and a nurse should be at the bedside to assist the patient as necessary. It is important to remember that any turning during the bathing procedure must be done with a pillow between the patient's legs.

Bedpan Procedure

When the patient in Buck's traction is in severe pain from a hip fracture or is exceptionally heavy, two people may be required to place and remove the fracture bedpan. The patient flexes the unaffected hip and leg and pushes with the foot on the mattress, using the trapeze to raise as much of the body as possible. One nurse places an arm under the shoulder and leg or hip on the affected side for added support. The other nurse slides the fracture pan in or out of place. At first, this is not as easy as it seems, because the patient will be apprehensive and tense. In the care of any traction patient who is in pain, trust and cooperation may be won by the confident manner in which the nurse does procedures.

The patient in Buck's extension who is weak, uncooperative, or stiff (as may be the case of a patient with a fractured hip) can be turned toward the affected side by one nurse while another pushes down on the mattress under the buttocks and works the pan into place. In removing the pan, care must be taken to dry and cleanse the perineum thoroughly.

Exercise and Immobility

The extent of an exercise program for a patient in Buck's traction depends on how long he will be in traction.

Since Buck's traction is usually temporary, the daily routines of turning for back care and bedpans may be sufficient along with encouraging foot movement. Deep breathing and coughing are beneficial and, for the convenience of both nurse and patient, should be done on the same schedule as back care.

Again, the length of time in traction is a factor in how susceptible the patient is to problems of immobility. Age and general condition contribute to this susceptibility, and all three factors determine the kind of preventive measures that should be taken.

Care of The Patient in Russell's Traction

Definition and Indications for Use

Russell's traction, like Buck's, is a type of skin traction that is applied to the leg. The difference is that Russell's traction makes use of a sling under the knee, with suspension of the

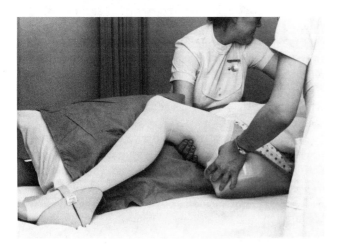

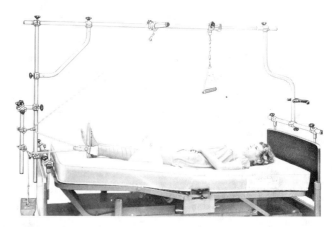

Russell's traction. (Courtesy Zimmer Co, Warsaw, Ind)

limb in traction. If a heavy traction force is desired, a skeletal pin through the calcaneus or distal tibia and fibula may be used.

Although Russell's traction is indicated for the same conditions as Buck's extension, most frequently it is used in the treatment of femoral-shaft fractures in the adolescent and fractures of the tibial plateau in adults.

Principles of Use

The pull in Russell's traction is exerted both vertically on the sling and horizontally on the footplate by one cord that is run through four pulleys and attached to one weight. Owing to the pulley arrangement, the pull on the foot is twice that of the weight applied. The resulting pull, as shown by the parallel-of-force diagram, should be in line with the femoral shaft. The position of the overhead pulley and the sling may vary according to the direction of pull that is desired. The pulley on the overhead bar, carrying the rope as it comes from the sling, is referred to as the first pulley. The position of the second pulley may vary and may be placed higher than or almost directly in line with the pulley that is attached to the footplate. Some physicians do not use a footplate with a pulley and instead run the rope through a spreader plate at the foot. These variations are often due to the type of bed and equipment available, as well as to the physician's preference. The *important* aspect of application is that the *resultant* pull is exerted in the correct line.

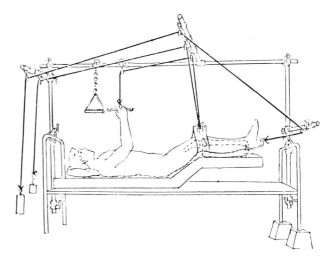

Split Russell's traction. (Schmeisser: A Clinical Manual of Orthopedic Traction Techniques. Philadelphia, WB Saunders)

The flexion in the knee depends on the angle that the physician wishes to maintain in treating the condition. A physician may order pillows placed under the knee and lower leg to aid in maintaining proper knee flexion and in keeping the heel off the mattress. Countertraction is established by elevating the foot of the bed or the knee gatch. The position of the patient is flat in bed unless otherwise ordered.

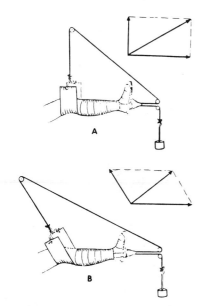

Pulley arrangement and line of pull in Russell's traction. (Schmeisser: A Clinical Manual of Orthopedic Traction Techniques. Philadelphia, WB Saunders)

Sometimes the weights on the knee and the foot are applied by using separate cords, running them through pulleys on the overhead bar and over the head of the bed, and attaching them to separate weights. This arrangement is called *split Russell's.*

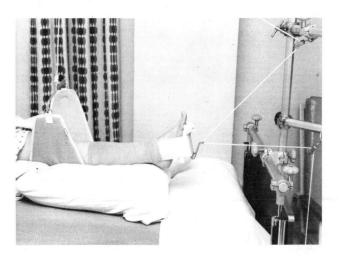

Advantages and Disadvantages

The advantage of Russell's traction is that the suspension weights usually allow movement of the body without disturbing the line of traction on the affected limb.

As with other types of skin traction, the effectiveness of Russell's traction is limited by the amount of stress the skin can tolerate.

Traction Observations

In addition to general traction observations as discussed on pages 93–94 there are certain points about Russell's traction that should be stressed. Because there are variations in the application of Russell's traction, the nurse should be aware of how the apparatus "looked" when it was originally applied. She must know the degree of angle that has been established between the affected thigh and the bed and make frequent observations to see that it is being maintained.

Foot support is usually provided by the use of a footplate. This should be checked for position as often as other traction checks are done, preferably every 3 hours.

Movement of The Patient and Nursing Routines

Although turning from the waist down is not permissible, the patient may lift, sit up, and move quite well. When nursing care is given, assistance is provided by lifting the patient's body and not his affected leg. The fracture bedpan may be placed from the unaffected side as the patient pulls up with the trapeze, flexes his unaffected knee, and pushes down against the mattress with his foot.

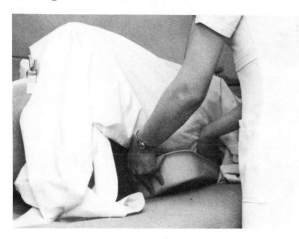

Changing the bottom sheet is not a problem when the leg is off the bed and is most efficiently done from top to bottom in the same manner as for the patient in Buck's traction (p. 113). When pillows are used to support the leg, care must be be taken to replace them immediately and in the same position after the sheet has been changed. If the involved extremity is resting on the bed, the bottom half of the sheet must be carefully worked down under the entire leg by pushing down on the mattress with one hand and pulling the sheet down with the other. The back and buttocks should be rubbed with lotion every 3 hours during the day and evening.

Keeping the lower extremities covered without covering the ropes may be a futile task because patients in Russell's traction are usually young and active. A towel over the lower part of the leg in suspension may be a partial solution.

Potential Pressure Points

An alternating-pressure mattress or convoluted bedpad is desirable as an extra precaution against skin breakdown over bony prominences.

Since the sling can cause pressure areas to develop in the popliteal space if it becomes wrinkled, the patient should be questioned frequently about how the sling "feels" under his knee. The combination of pressure on the blood vessels in the popliteal space and immobility may cause thrombophlebitis. Although some sources advocate placing a piece of felt

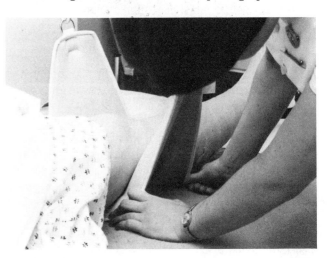

to pad the sling, the edge of the felt may cause a dent in the skin and, thus, defeat its purpose. The skin at the edges of the sling needs to be inspected and rubbed with alcohol or cornstarch if it becomes reddened. When a sling causes a patient obvious discomfort, the physician should be informed.

Because the footplate can also be a source of irritation, the sole of the foot should be inspected for reddened areas. When a foot spreader is used the nurse must check to see that the foot is not pressing against the spreader. Placing a folded washcloth between the sole of the foot and the foot spreader provides some foot support and prevents the foot from resting directly on the metal.

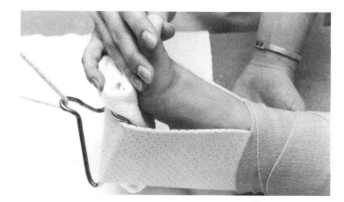

Tension stress on the skin may cause breakdown under the bandages and tape. A wrapping bandage that is too snug is also a source of problems. (See Buck's traction, p. 112)

If pillows are placed under any part of the affected leg for support, they must not be allowed to cause pressure areas.

The heel should be off the mattress. A folded bath blanket under the calf of the leg accomplishes this end if a pillow has not been ordered. The heel on the unaffected limb may become reddened as the patient uses it to push himself up in bed. Good nursing care includes regular observation of both heels along with lotion rubs. The patient's elbows should also be checked for redness.

Exercises

Preparation for eventual crutchwalking should begin as soon as the patient is adjusted to the traction apparatus. Arm workouts on the trapeze and routine movements of the unaffected leg should be stressed. The foot of the affected leg should be exercised. Besides maintaining muscle strength, exercise improves circulation and helps prevent venous stasis.

Psychological Considerations

A patient in Russell's traction might worry less about length of convalescence if the nurse keeps him informed about his progress. For instance, when the physician tells him his x-ray films "look good," the nurse should take the time later to ask the patient if he has any questions. There is always the possibility that he feels the physician tells this to everybody, and positive reinforcement by the nurse at this point may go a long way toward lifting his spirits.

The Bohler-Braun Splint

Description and Advantages

The Bohler-Braun splint is still used in the treatment of fractures of the femur, or as limb support in the case of multiple injuries. This splint is a frame that rests on the bed and elevates the lower limb. The knee joint should meet the beginning of the inclined plane, and the entire leg should be supported. This splint may be used with either skin or skeletal traction and maintains leg position more easily than Buck's traction.

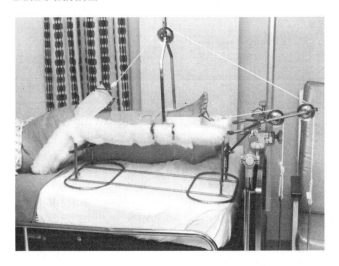

Implications for Nursing Care

Much of the nursing care of the patient with a Bohler-Braun splint involves observations for problems due to the leg wrapping (pp. 111–112) and pressure points. The prox-

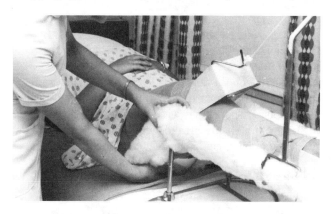

imal arm of the frame may make contact with the perineum or groin. These areas must be inspected every 3 hours for skin irritation. Cornstarch is soothing and may be applied if irritation occurs.

Patients can usually be turned toward the splint when back care is given or the drawsheet changed.

Changing bottom bed linen presents no difficulty if that linen was originally applied in the following manner. One sheet is placed from the proximal end of the splint to the top of the bed with the excess tucked under the mattress. Another sheet is folded and placed under the entire splint. In this way the sheet under the patient can be changed as necessary, and the one under the splint can be left in place.

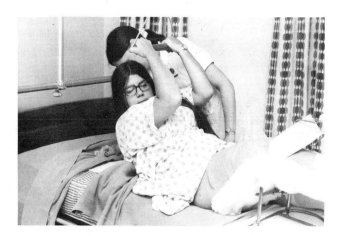

The Thomas Leg Splint and Pearson Attachment

Use and Description

The Thomas leg splint, either full-ring or half-ring, with a Pearson attachment, is one of the most popular splints for suspension of the lower limb in the treatment of femoral fractures.

A Thomas splint consists of a large ring or half-ring connecting two rods that are placed on either side of the limb and are linked by a cross bar at the distal end. When the splint is in place, the ring encircles the thigh (or half the thigh if a half-ring is used). Modified Thomas splints consisting of a posterior half-ring splint with a flat ring covered by a disposable padding are also common.

Some authorities recommend a half-ring splint with an anterior orientation, claiming that since the patient does not have to "sit" on the ring he is less susceptible to pressure problems in the groin. However, the posterior half-ring is very popular. The truth is, either splint will cause pressure in the groin and skin breakdown if countertraction is improper or nursing care is inadequate.

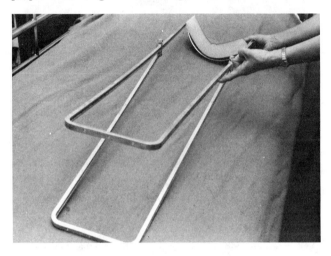

Slings are attached to the splint rods and act to support the upper leg. These slings must hold firmly in place and not slide or stretch when in use. Nor must they allow wrinkles to form that can place uneven pressure on the skin and lead to skin breakdown. Foam-rubber pads or slings made of material similar to sheepskin often replace cloth or canvas slings

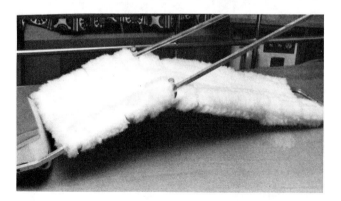

for use with this splint. These materials do not wrinkle and they provide more comfortable support for the limb. The thickness of the padding eliminates pressure from "thin" sling edges.

A Pearson attachment supports the lower leg off the bed in the same manner as the Thomas splint supports the upper

leg. It allows the knee to be flexed and the lower leg to be moved, if the surgeon orders, for purposes of knee-joint exercise. The ends of the rods in a Pearson attachment are fastened to the Thomas splint at the knee, with clamping devices that allow the attachment to move independently of the splint.

The height to which the distal end of the splint is elevated is at the discretion of the physician who applied it. The lower leg usually lies in the Pearson attachment in a neutral position and parallel to the mattress.

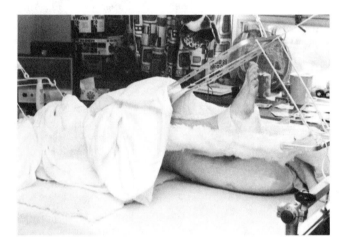

Advantages

There are several advantages to the sort of suspension this splint and attachment provide. The limb itself can be lifted easily by its owner. Circulation in the leg is better. As part of a traction apparatus, the splint contributes to more freedom of the whole patient, which means less chance for pressure areas to develop.

The Thomas leg splint with the Pearson attachment is commonly used in the application of balanced traction (skin or skeletal) for suspension of the lower extremity.

Care of The Patient in Balanced-Suspension Traction

Definition

In balanced traction there are two related systems in operation. One is the traction system; the second is the balanced suspension of the lower limb. When the Thomas splint is used, the lower limb rests or "floats" in the Pearson attachment. The traction force is exerted by skeletal traction or skin traction.

Description and Set-Up

Equipment and method of applying the "balance" in balanced traction vary, but the end result is a distribution of weights through pulleys that provide countertraction, as well as suspension of the lower limb. In looking at a patient in balanced traction, the nurse will observe that a spreader

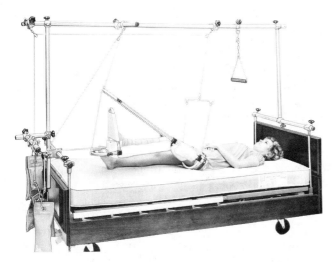

Balanced skin traction. (Courtesy Zimmer Co, Warsaw, Ind)

bar is attached to the proximal end of the splint by a rope that runs through pulleys on the overhead frame and over the head or foot of the bed. A rope is tied from the distal end of the Pearson attachment to the distal end of the Thomas leg splint and taken up through pulleys on both the overhead frame and the bars on the foot of the bed.

There are surgeons who prefer suspending the Thomas splint and Pearson attachment by using one continuous rope, two overhead pulleys, and a single weight in the center. This is called the *flying W*. One of the advantages in this suspension is that it aids in keeping the ring from

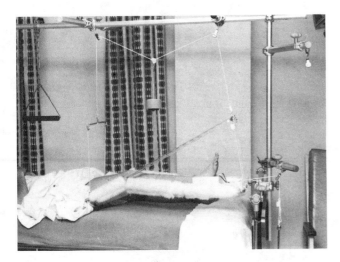

causing pressure in the groin. A disadvantage is the fact that a weight hangs over the patient's extemity. Surgeons who use this form of traction are careful to tape the weight securely to the rope.

BALANCED SKIN TRACTION

Description and Use

In balanced skin traction, the pulling force is applied to the leg as in Buck's extension, and a Thomas splint with Pear-

son attachment is added. A distribution of weights through pulleys exerts the traction force, helps provide countertraction, and also suspends the lower limb.

Balanced skin traction has limited use. It may be applied when a light force is sufficient on a fractured femur, as for example, in a pathologic fracture. It is commonly used for immobilization and abduction of the affected leg in a patient who has had a cup arthroplasty. Again, this method of traction is only applicable in this case because a light force is all that is required.

Advantages and Disadvantages

The complications due to immobility are more easily prevented with this kind of traction then with Buck's traction. The patient is more comfortable because he can move himself about freely in bed. However, the nurse must be watchful for signs of skin breakdown under the wrapping bandages (p. 112).

BALANCED SKELETAL TRACTION

Description and Use

Generally, when balanced skeletal traction is applied to a lower extremity, the device used for skeletal attachment is a Steinmann pin or Kirschner wire. The point of insertion of the pin or wire is most often the distal femur or proximal tibia, depending on location of the fracture and the surgeon's preference.

The Thomas splint with the Pearson attachment and the suspension system are applied by one of the previously described methods.

Most of the countertraction is provided by body weight with the patient flat in bed. Some sources advocate positioning the half-ring of the splint against the ischial tuberosity for countertraction. However, in this situation the splint must be pulled away from the perineum frequently, because it tends to dig in, causing skin irritation.

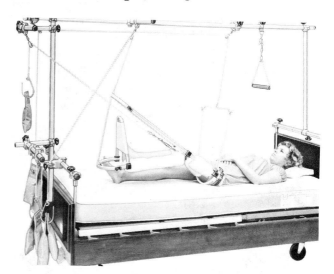

Balanced skeletal traction. (Courtesy Zimmer Co, Warsaw, Ind)

Fractures in the distal two-thirds of the shaft of the femur are commonly treated (at least until callus formation has taken place) with this type of traction.

Checking the Extremity in Traction

A thorough inspection from groin to toes of the extremity in traction is essential every 3 hours from early morning until bedtime.

The groin, adductor muscle, and ischial area must be observed closely for signs of pressure from the ring. Padding should not be "shoved" between a leather ring and the skin, because it will wrinkle. Nor should any padding that is part of a half-ring be removed. Pressure points along the leg include the heel, the Achilles tendon, and popliteal space where the proximal end of the Pearson attachment corresponds with the knee joint.

The sling and metal parts of the splint should not be allowed to put pressure on the peroneal nerve. This could

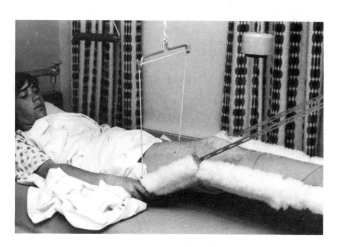

occur if the Thomas splint and Pearson attachment tip gradually to one side, as often happens with very active patients. It is not unusual for a surgeon to teach a patient such as this to "shift" the splint into place while grasping it on both sides of the ring. Actually this is the best way to restore proper

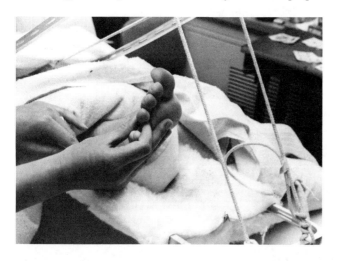

positioning, because the patient tends to be more careful in handling his leg than the nurse. Another sign that the splint has tipped is when one rope is resting against another.

A tendency of the foot towards inversion and difficulty in extending the toes are indicators of peroneal-nerve trouble. The patient should be asked to move his foot and extend his toes fully each time the extremity is checked.

Skin Care

The more bathing these patients can do independently, the better, because it provides some exercise. The leg in traction needs careful, but not daily, bathing. The sling on the splint and Pearson attachment must be kept dry, so how much and how often the leg is bathed is a nursing judgment.

As a daily procedure, rubbing alcohol may be applied, not massaged, into the entire leg including the heel, except for

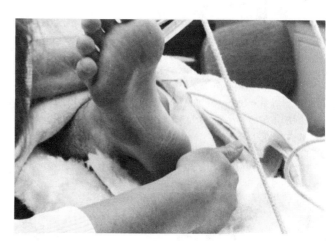

the area very close to the pin. For some patients, lotion may be better if the skin is dry. This phase of skin care provides an excellent opportunity for the nurse to observe the pin and surrounding area for any signs of inflammation or loosening.

The foot and toes on the affected leg need daily cleansing and massage with lotion. Alcohol swabs keep the areas between the toes dry. Elbows should be rubbed with lotion if

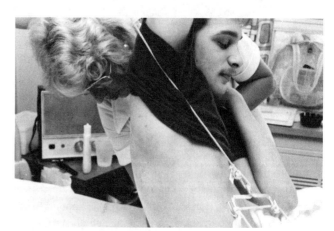

they are raw from being used by the patient to change position.

For back care, the patient lifts himself with the trapeze and turns slightly toward the splint. Nurses must remember that special attention should be given to the sacral area, because this is usually the first spot on the back to become reddened when a patient is on bed rest.

Buttocks can be washed, dried, and rubbed with the help of another nurse. This nurse helps the patient lift his hips as he pulls on the trapeze, flexes the unaffected hip and knee, and pushes his foot on the mattress.

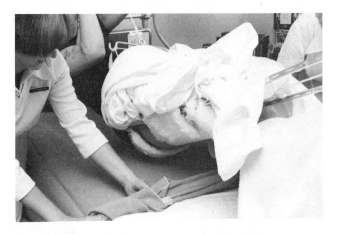

Bedmaking

The bottom sheet is more efficiently changed from top to bottom by two nurses. The patient lifts the top half of his body by means of the trapeze while the sheet is brought down as far as the buttocks. One nurse helps him lift his buttocks in the same manner as for skin care. The sheet can then be pulled down under the legs.

Bedpan Procedure

Placing and removing the bedpan is done easily, with the patient doing the lifting while the fracture pan is slid in and out. When the patient is first placed in traction, the bedpan

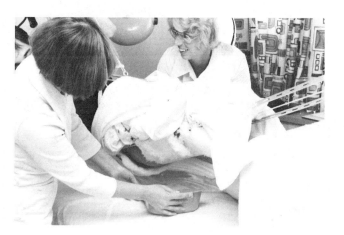

should be placed from the unaffected side. But once the patient is comfortable and no longer apprehensive about the traction apparatus, the bedpan may be placed from either side. Care should be taken that the ring does not become soiled when the bedpan is used.

Complications

The early complications the nurse must watch for in these patients are fat embolism, plus gas gangrene, tetanus, and infection if the fracture was compound in nature. Pulmonary embolism is always a possibility, especially in the older patient. These complications are discussed in Chapter 2.

Immobility problems, *for the most part*, are not as likely to develop in these patients as in those in Buck's extension. Balanced skeletal traction allows the patient great freedom to move about in bed, so supervising food and fluid intake, encouraging exercise programs, giving good skin care, and establishing good elimination habits will probably suffice in preventing complications due to immobility. However, boredom *is* often a problem.

Boredom

Once the patient is adjusted and somewhat comfortable, he will have periods of boredom and restlessness. He may be silent and depressed some days, and on others he may be boisterous or "pesty." It is important for the nurse to understand that this is normal behavior. Keeping this type of patient from being bored means being flexible in scheduling routines and even tolerating clutter around his bedside unit when friends bring things for him "do do."

Typical Problems

Nursing approaches to some typical problems of the patient in balanced skeletal traction are presented in the accompanying chart.

Psychological Considerations

How the patient responds to and cooperates during his care depends on several things. First of all, the level of patient apprehension and restlessness is often high, since many of these patients are very young males who have been in automobile accidents and are hospitalized for the first time in their lives. To this is added the trauma of having had a pin inserted, whether under local or general anesthesia. Finally, the patient probably has bruises and soreness on other parts of his body which are manifested when the nurse attempts to move him.

Obviously, the patient will be apprehensive about everything that is done for him until he has had a few days to adjust to hospitalization. He also needs to know what is happening around him and to him, and why. He can be told that his pain will continue to decrease, and if the nurse is careful not to bump into the weights and apparatus while working with him, he will believe it.

THE PATIENT IN BALANCED SKELETAL TRACTION: PROBLEM SOLVING (NURSING PROCESS)

Patient Situation: D.M. was in an automobile accident 3 weeks ago and has been in balanced skeletal traction with a fractured left femur ever since. She also has a healing fracture of the left tibia. Her left eye, cheek, and neck still show evidence of contusions, and she often jokes about her "shiner." She and her husband have no children, and he visits every evening. She is a talkative, pleasant patient. Although she claims to be a "nervous type," her complaints are always realistic. At 8:00 P.M., the following complaints and problems were identified.

Problem/Complaint	Assessment Data	Intervention	Evaluation
1. Had refused supper because she was "not hungry."	1. Denies any gastric distress. States supper "looked good." Too tired to eat. Does appear pale and lethargic.	1. States she is getting enough sleep. Ask physician about recheck on Hgb. and Hct.	1. "Too tired" will not be reason for refusing meals.
2. Agitated because she has problems with constipation even though she is on a stool softener.	2. Had an enema today. Drinks prune juice with breakfast. Taking all the fluids she can "hold." Does not take pain medications. Wants more bran in diet.	2. Change or increase stool softener? Laxative daily? Ask dietician to see patient regarding more bran in diet.	2. Patient verbalizes satisfaction with bowel elimination pattern in 2-3 days.
3. Ropes "hurt" thigh.	3. Traction ropes from half-ring to spreader bar above thigh are causing skin irritation on lateral aspects of thigh.	3. Change spreader bar to a wider one (because to add padding may add pressure to irritation). Talk to patient about traction in general to identify any other possible sources of irritation.	3. No further complaints of skin irritation from ropes.

An accident that put a patient in femoral skeletal traction may have killed or injured someone else. This fact carries many psychological implications, which vary depending on the patient and the circumstances. The nurse must bear this in mind when establishing rapport with such a patient.

Preparation for Ambulation

Because the patient with a fractured femur in balanced skeletal traction faces a long convalescence, the sooner he can begin a prescribed program of exercise, the better. Arm-strengthening exercises that are helpful in preparing the patient for crutch-walking include squeezing a hand grip, lifting weight that is strapped on the arm, or lifting dumbbells. A system of pulleys, weights, ropes, and handles may be added to the head of the bed for active arm and shoulder exercise.

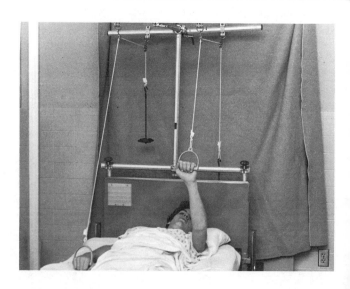

4. "Pressure" in chest.

4. Auscultate lungs. Normal sounds. No complaints of respiratory distress. Patient suggests "nerves" could be cause.

4. Continue to auscultate lungs q shift. Increase stirrups. Ask patient to report any symptoms of respiratory distress immediately (see 5).

4. No further complaints of pressure in chest (see 5). Any sign or symptom of respiratory distress will be identified immediately.

5. Feels "weepy." Is upset with care.

5. When asked to talk about care, states, "I'm not a crabby person, and I'm not hard to please. I'll do whatever you want, but I wish everyone would make up their minds and quit changing things around." Looks like she is going to cry. Has been having her bath at different times each A.M. Today she was in the middle of it at noon, and the doctor "always comes at noon and today was no exception." Had her enema in late afternoon and understood she was having it earlier. Squeezes nurse's hand while she is talking about all of this. She needs more TLC!

5. Review her plan of care with her and schedule daily bath for 10:00 A.M. Make note on plan to inform her ahead of time of all new orders and pending routines, such as enemas, x-ray films, so she can prepare for them psychologically. Review current diversional activities with her and evaluate whether or not changes are necessary. Touch her or hold her hands when talking to her about any plans or concerns. Assure her that no concern is trivial if it is causing her anxiety.

5. Patient will verbalize satisfaction with scheduled care tomorrow. She will be "happier" in 24 hours.

Range-of-motion exercises for the three uninvolved extremities are recommended, and quadriceps setting of the uninvolved leg is essential.

The patient will be more receptive to exercising, especially the foot of the affected leg, if he has been handled gently and skillfully by nursing personnel. He will also be more receptive if he has been taught the importance of maintaining muscle strength in order to walk with crutches.

Preparation for Spica Cast

There is an excellent chance that this type of patient, after 6 to 8 weeks in skeletal traction and the formation of sufficient callus at the fracture site, will leave the hospital in a hip spica cast. For this procedure the patient is transported to the surgical department in his bed. Because moving these patients requires extremely careful handling, they must be

relaxed and cooperative. The amount of medication prescribed prior to the procedure is influenced by the patient's emotional status and the amount of discomfort he is having.

The pin is removed as a sterile procedure after the skin around it has been scrubbed with a preparation such as Betadine, cleansed with alcohol, and covered with merthiolate. One end of the pin is cut off close to the skin and the pin is removed from the other side.

As soon as the physician discusses the casting procedure with the patient, the nurse must begin the necessary cast-care teaching (see Chapter 2). Discharge planning should start, however, as soon as the patient appears to have accepted the length of his confinement in traction. When casting and ambulation are in sight, the nurse and discharge planner must coordinate teaching and planning for patient and family.

Care of The Patient in Sidearm or Overhead (90–90) Traction

Definitions and Indications for Use

Fractures of the humerus with or without involvement of the shoulder and clavicle may be indications for traction on the arm. Whether this is skin or skeletal, overhead or sidearm, depends on the location of the fracture and associated injuries, as well as physician's preference.

Sidearm Traction

Sidearm traction is used when alignment of the fracture fragments is effectively maintained with the arm in this position. Skin traction may be indicated in treating a fracture of the humerus if there is damage to tissues around the elbow, where a pin would have to be inserted for skeletal traction. Overhead (90–90) skeletal traction is sometimes used when the proximal fragment of a fractured humerus is adducted and flexed.

For sidearm traction the pulleys are attached to a basic frame that clamps to the bed frame under the mattress. This allows the position of the headrest to be changed without disrupting the traction. If the frame that is available cannot be attached in this manner, the bed must remain flat.

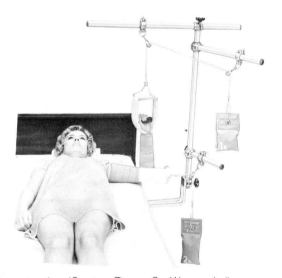

Sidearm traction. (Courtesy Zimmer Co, Warsaw, Ind)

In sidearm traction the forearm is flexed and extended 90 degrees from, and in the same plane as, the upper part of the body. It is maintained in this position by some form of traction tapes that extend upward from the forearm and attach to a spreader and pulley-weight setup. A suspended handle within this apparatus allows the patient to flex his fingers and exercise his hand.

The traction pull is outward. It is achieved by two adhesive straps extending from the upper arm to a spreader on the side, or by a skeletal pin near the elbow, which is attached to a hoop. Either arrangement is attached to a traction cord and a pulley-weight setup. The same tape material

as is used for Buck's traction (p. 109) may also be used for arm traction, and all tapes are secured in place by wrapping bandages.

Sidearm traction requires that a countertraction be provided. One way to achieve this is to place shock blocks under the head and foot of the bed on the side of the affected arm so that the pull of the patient's weight provides the necessary counteraction. However, this may result in the patient's sliding too far to the side of the bed opposite the traction. An effective way of providing countertraction for

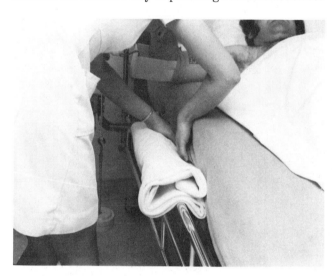

the patient in sidearm traction is to place a folded blanket under the mattress near the traction frame.

One reason some physicians prefer overhead to sidearm traction is that the vertical force in overhead traction eliminates the need for countertraction. With the traction pulling upward on the arm, the weight of the patient's body, in the supine position, is the countertraction.

Overhead Traction

In overhead or 90–90 traction the elbow is flexed to 90 degrees and the arm is at right angles to the body, over the upper chest. The vertical traction force on the upper arm is

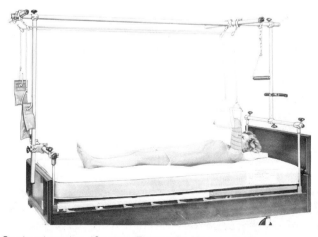

Overhead traction. (Courtesy Zimmer Co, Warsaw, Ind)

applied in the same manner as for sidearm traction. The pulley-weight setups are on the overhead bar and at either the foot end or head end of the bed. The forearm rests in a sling that is attached to ropes and weight in the same manner. When skeletal traction is the treatment of choice, the traction tapes and sling may be replaced by a long arm cast applied over the Steinmann pin, with the pin attached to a hoop and rope. A rope is also tied around the forearm portion of the cast for the purpose of suspension.

Special Observation and Care

Nursing care and observations are similar for overhead and sidearm traction.

Inspection and care of the arm of patients in sidearm or overhead traction starts at the shoulder. Muscle stiffness from maintaining one position requires a gentle massage if the area has been involved in the injury and is bruised. Swelling of the shoulder, elbow, or hand is to be noted, and relieved, if caused by tight bandages. The nurse must loosen tight bandages and allow the bandage to retract slightly before fastening it in place.

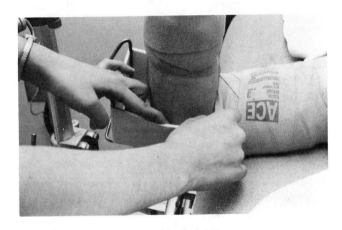

Because circulatory impairment can be a critical problem, the presence of a radial pulse must be noted at least four times within each 24-hour period, more frequently if the patient's fingernails do not blanch well. Cyanosis or

pallor of the hand and fingers, as well as numbness, is an indication of circulatory difficulty. Pinching the fingernail and noting the speed with which color returns to the nail is a good test of circulation. Delayed return should be reported to the physician immediately. The patient should be requested to extend the fingers *fully* as part of checking the circulation. Pain in doing so may be due to a developing compartments syndrome (pp. 57–59). Failure to act promptly when circulatory impairment is evident could result in serious ischemia.

Tingling or pain in the hand can be a sign of pressure on a nerve and should be attended to quickly. Each finger should be pinched or pricked slightly to determine sensation. Neurovascular checks, or the assessment of color, motion, temperature, and sensation (CMTS) should be done every 3 hours.

Fingers that have good color, sensation, and motion may be cold from elevation and immobility. Some light covering is indicated.

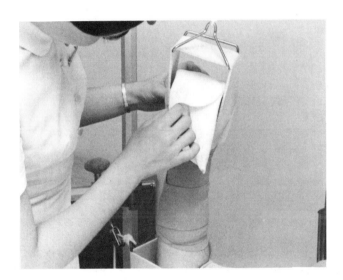

The areas that may become irritated from the edges of wrapping bandages are the soft tissues near the shoulder, the anterior surface of the elbow joint, and the palm at the

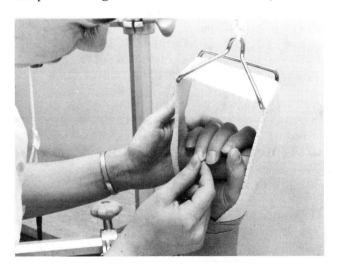

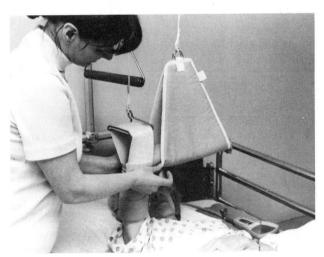

wrist. When the patient complains of pain under the wrapping the nurse should run her hand gently over the wrapping bandages to localize the area of pain and thus determine whether or not the patient is having skin breakdown under the traction tapes. Sling edges in overhead traction may be irritating and should be checked and adjusted as necessary.

General Nursing Care

The patient in overhead traction cannot turn the upper half of one side of the body; therefore, care of the upper back and shoulder on the affected side is awkward, and inspection of the area is almost impossible. Discomfort in this area is most pronounced, and skin care should be given every 3 hours to avoid breakdown. Lotion should be used sparingly to avoid stickiness. Alcohol rubs are better. Discomfort may also develop around the bony prominences of the wrist. Gentle rubbing here is beneficial.

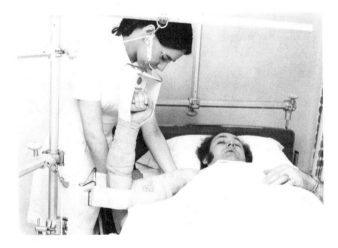

Because the patient is on his back, the linen must be kept dry and wrinkle free to reduce the chance of skin irritation. Soilage of linen under the shoulders is unlikely; the bottom sheet should not be changed because the traction force could be disrupted. The area under the shoulder could be covered by towels, but these only provide a source of more wrinkles. Wide drawsheets should be used, with the top edge at the level of the patient's axillae.

Thromboembolic stockings may be ordered to reduce the risk of thrombophlebitis, although range of motion of all three unaffected extremities must be encouraged frequently during the day.

Psychological Considerations

The older patient in arm traction is rendered quite helpless in caring for herself and needs encouragement in self-care, especially if she has severe pain in the fracture area. An elderly woman may find it very tiring to comb her hair and brush her teeth while lying flat on her back. If she is normally right-handed and is forced to carry out these activities with her left hand because her dominant hand is immobi-

lized, her fatigue may be even greater. In addition, her appetite may be restricted severly by the fact that she is immobile and has only one arm with which to eat.

Scheduling self-help activities when she feels able to do them herself aids in creating a feeling of independence and self-worth. Prism glasses for reading and watching television are helpful if the patient's eyesight permits.

A community resource for the nurse to investigate is the local library. These institutions often have special racks for holding books that may be placed across the patient on the bed. A "talking book" service may also be available.

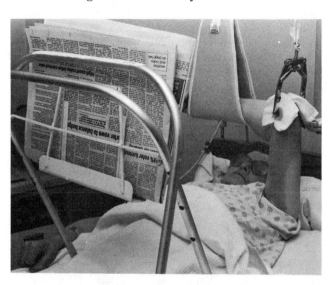

An older patient who is severely restricted in activity will derive psychological comfort from knowing that those who are caring for her are involved from the outset in plans for her rehabilitation program before she leaves the hospital. Older people have an intense need to know what will happen to them when they become dependent. The average patient benefits most from knowing as soon as possible what the plans are for continued treatment. That is: (1) How long will traction be maintained? (2) What form of immobility will be necessary after traction is removed? (3) What kind of exercise will be needed to regain use of shoulder and arm? The only person who can give this information is the physician, because length and type of treatment are dependent on the location and the nature of the injury. However, the nurse should recognize the anxiety that stems from such concerns and encourage the patient to ask questions of the physician as they arise.

Care of The Patient in Crutchfield Tongs

Description and Indication for Use

Skeletal traction for the reduction of fractures and dislocations of the cervical spine is often provided by Crutchfield tongs, placed in the top of the skull by a surgeon to a depth of about 1/2 inch. Prior to insertion the area is shaved and prepared for a sterile procedure. Although there are other kinds of tongs for cervical traction, all are similar to Crutchfield tongs and are designed to accomplish the same goal.

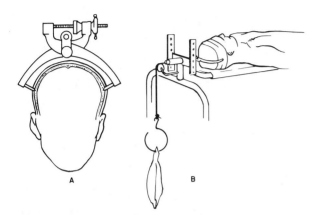

Crutchfield tongs. (Smith and Germain: Care of the Adult Patient. Philadelphia, Lippincott)

Tongs are designed so that the physician may tighten them once they are in place to maintain the neck in extension or hyperextension. Sterile gauze dressings are usually placed around the points of insertion. As much as 30 pounds of weight may be applied. The initial weight is applied gradually and may be increased slowly.

The type of bed used (regular or turning frame) depends on the extent of neurological symptoms and the physician's preference. The head of the bed may be elevated slightly by order of the physician.

Patient, Family, and Staff Education

Needless to say, the insertion of Crutchfield tongs may be an extremely traumatic experience for patient and family. To begin with, cervical injuries often cause panic for the patient and family because of the possibility of paralysis. Furthermore, it is emotionally traumatic for many patients to have their heads shaved.

Adequate explanations of treatment and positive reinforcement at intervals are helpful in gaining patient cooperation and in reassuring both patient and family.

Besides knowing what the traction is all about, the patient and his family should know that the traction cannot be adjusted, nor the weights bumped or removed. They should be aware that the bed must stay in the same position. If possible, the bed should be locked in that position.

Staff education is also extremely important. Perhaps nothing is as frightening to a patient with Crutchfield tongs as a fearful or timid expression on the face of the staff member who answers his call light. Crutchfield tongs are not all that common on orthopedic wards, and a review of the nursing care and problems involved is necessary with each patient.

Initial Assessment

A complete nursing assessment must be done before the tongs are inserted or subsequent assessments will be of little value. The nurse should record complaints, degree and location of pain, numbness, weakness, and loss of motion. The status of bowel and bladder functioning is also important to note. Records of vital signs and level of consciousness are imperative if even a slight head injury was incurred. All of the details the patient can remember about how he was injured need to be part of a nursing history.

Daily Nursing Observations

Any symptoms indicating motor sensory changes must be reported and recorded. Vital signs are monitored as warranted by the patient's condition. Loss of muscle strength, respiratory distress, and projectile vomiting are danger signals, because they indicate damage to the cervical spine. The physician needs to know about them immediately.

Generally speaking, the patient with Crutchfield tongs and neurological involvement is on a neurological ward or in an intensive-care unit for evaluation. However, the orthopedic nurse should be aware that if the above signs and symptoms develop in any patient with Crutchfield tongs, they could indicate spinal-cord injury.

Nursing Care

Bathing, bedmaking, and bedpan procedures require planning, but since this type of traction is very stable, these procedures present few problems when the personnel understand what is to be done. Placing a fracture bedpan, changing bottom linen, and giving skin care to the back and buttocks may be done when the patient is logrolled.

The patient can usually be logrolled 45 degrees to either side with a pillow between the legs. If desired, a pillow may be placed in front of the patient's chest during the turning procedure, for support of the arm and shoulder. To maintain alignment the entire patient should be logrolled with head, shoulders, and pelvis turned simultaneously. The cervical spine must not be flexed. When turning the patient, the nurse must be alert to any sign of respiratory distress. If cyanosis or dyspnea should occur the patient must be returned to a position that relieves the respiratory distress, and the physician should be notified promptly.

Patients with tongs are frequently placed on CircOlectric beds or Stryker frames. General care of the traction patient as described in an earlier section is applicable to the patient in Crutchfield tongs.

Special Considerations and Problems

Physicians should specify the type of tong care they prefer. Quite frequently, daily cleansing with hydrogen peroxide of the skin around the point of tong insertion is ordered. This is necessary with Crutchfield tongs because exudate is usually present. Bleeding around the tongs is not to be expected and should be reported to the doctor immediately.

Since the back of the head is prone to pressure sores, sheepskins or small pillows may be ordered for under the head. However, they should never be placed without an order. Shaving and giving a shampoo require a specific order by the physician.

Initially, getting accustomed to eating with Crutchfield tongs in the skull is a problem for a patient because of the fixed position in bed. Soft food may be ordered until the patient is confident he will be able to chew and swallow. Prism glasses enable him to watch television.

Patients are usually fearful that the tongs will fall out. Although this could happen, it is rare, and the patient should know it. If the tongs do fall out, the physician should be notified, and manual traction or a cervical halter should be applied to the head in the interim.

Range-of-motion exercises of the extremities are necessary and whether they are active or passive depends on the patient's condition.

Prevention of immobility problems is a priority, because these patients may be on bed rest for a period of weeks or months. General suggestions for nursing care and observations may be found on pages 94–98.

Psychological Considerations

Patients with Crutchfield tongs need much moral support. Many of them are young people, males especially, who have been in accidents. The fear of paralysis may persist for a long time, no matter what the physician tells them.

Depression that comes with the feeling that they are "out of it" is hard to overcome. After all, they *are* "out of it," and rehabilitation may be a long process.

When the tongs are removed, some form of hyperextension neck brace may be applied that will be worn for several weeks or months. Such a patient does not need to be told that he is "lucky" he is not paralyzed. This does not alter the fact that in many ways, unknown to the nurse, his life-style may be seriously disrupted.

Discussion Questions

1. What thoughts and feelings about body image might affect the behavior of the following two patients in femoral skeletal traction, and how?

    a. Snowmobile accident. A 24-year-old male. No insurance. Works for a construction company. Two girlfriends. "Top" bowler.

    b. Automobile accident. A 65-year-old female, widow of the former mayor. Active and outspoken in civic affairs. Only child, a daughter, lives out of town. Drives a car. Social-security income. Medicare.

Consider: What combinations of factors suggest the personality of each? Compare with people you know.

2. Prepare a care plan for the following patient. R.S. is a 72-year-old woman with a comminuted fracture of the right proximal humerus. Her shoulder is bruised and painful. Sidearm skin traction with 5 lb of weight has been applied. This patient weighs about 170 lb and is 5'2" tall. She smokes a package of cigarettes a day. She has one son who is a Catholic priest. Her husband is living and well.

Consider: What care will her traction require? Think about the nursing implications of her smoking and her weight. Discuss the importance of her relationship with her son and husband.

3. What are the potential problems in the following situation, and what nursing actions will be necessary to prevent or lessen them?

D.E. is a 20-year-old male who is 5'11" tall and weighs 240 lb. He is admitted to the hospital following a motorcycle accident in which he suffered a highly comminuted fracture of his right femur with marked displacement. In addition to this, he has blisters on his anterior and lateral right thigh, probably from gasoline, and multiple abrasions on both lower legs. He has no other apparent injuries and was not drinking before the accident. His right leg was placed in 25 lb of balanced skeletal traction, with the pin through his tibia.

Consider: What kind of fracture symptoms will this patient have? The blisters and abrasions will contribute to his symptoms. What are all the possible sources of leg pain? What is a potential complication of the open areas on his legs? The combination of his weight and traction will produce some problems. How comfortable will he be in the Thomas splint?

Bibliography

Boos ML: A program of home traction for congenital dislocation of the hip. Orthop Nurs 1(2):11, March–April 1982

Briscol S: Fractured femur. Nurs Mirror 156(26):50, June 29, 1983

Brown S: Skeletal traction for supracondylar fractures of humerus. ONAJ, 4:9, January 1977

Brunner N: Orthopedic Nursing, 4th ed. St. Louis, CV Mosby, 1983

Carini E, Owens G: Neurological and Neurosurgical Nursing. St. Louis, CV Mosby, 1974

Cassels CJ: Fundamentals of long bone traction, Part I. Crit Care Update 10(3):36, March 1983

Cassels CJ: Fundamentals of long bone traction, Part II. Crit Care Update 10(4):26, April 1983

Cassels CJ: Fundamentals of long bone traction, Part III. Crit Care Update 10(5):38, May 1983

Celeste et al: Identifying a standard for pin site care using the quality assurance approach. Orthop Nurs 3(4):17, July–Aug 1984

The do's and don'ts of traction care. Nurs 74, 4:35, November 1974

Fairbrother C: One nurse's bright idea. Nurs Times 78(1):59, January 6-12, 1982

Gates SJ: Helping your patient on bed rest cope with perceptual/sensory deprivation. Orthop Nurs 3(2):35, Mar–Apr 1984

Hilt N, Cogburn S: Manual of Orthopedics. St. Louis, CV Mosby, 1980

Iveson-Iveson J: Orthopaedic traction: You're pulling my leg. Nursing Mirror 53:44, Oct. 7, 1981

Larson W, Gould M: Orthopedic Nursing, 9th ed. St. Louis, CV Mosby, 1978

Mourad L: Nursing Care of Adults with Orthopedic Conditions. New York, John Wiley & Sons, 1980

Nursing care of the patient in traction (programmed instruction). AJN, October 1979

Silverstein P: The Hare traction splint. Ambulance J 9:23, Jan–Feb 1981

Smith C: Nursing the patient in traction. Nurs Times 80(16):36, Apr 18-24, 1984

Sproles K: Nursing care of skeletal pins: A closer look. Orthop Nurs (4)1:11, Jan–Feb 1985

The Traction Handbook. Warsaw, Ind, Zimmer Co, 1975

4

Care of Patients With Specific Spinal Conditions

Two fears are common among patients with back problems. One is the prospect of chronic pain with restricted mobility if the condition is left untreated or is treated unsuccessfully. The other is the fear that spinal surgery may cause paralysis. Although many patients do not verbalize these fears, they may be manifested in apprehension, tension, or depression. A nurse should recognize this fact when giving these patients instructions about their care and should encourage them to ask questions. Positive reinforcement and clarification of the physician's explanations is also important.

Care of the Patient With a Herniated Intervertebral Disk

An intervertebral disk is located between two vertebral bodies, and is composed of two cartilage plates that are separated by a gelatinous center or nucleus pulposus. A thick ring of fibrous tissue extends from both plates, forming a protective covering around the nucleus pulposus. This tissue, the annulus fibrosus, also extends into and is attached to the anterior and posterior longitudinal ligaments and the vertebral bodies themselves. the function of the disk is that of shock absorber for the spine.

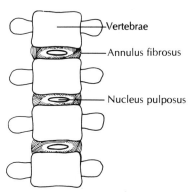

Portion of vertebral column showing vertebrae, annulus fibrosus, and nucleus pulposus (Adapted from Hoppenfeld: Scoliosis, Philadelphia, Lippincott)

CAUSE OF HERNIATION

The posterior ligament is normally weak, and the attachment to it is loose. When part of the nucleus pulposus herniates or seeps through this ligament into the spinal canal, it is called a *herniated, ruptured,* or *slipped disk.* Herniation of the nucleus pulposus may occur suddenly, as a result of (1) lifting an object from a stooped position, (2) suffering direct injury to the back, or (3) twisting the back in a sudden motion. Gradual degenerative changes in the disk, common to all cartilage, may cause it to rupture following a minor injury or for no apparent reason at all.

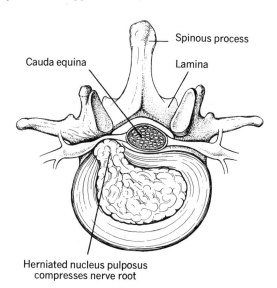

Ruptured vertebral disk (Chaffee and Greisheimer: Basic Physiology and Anatomy. Lippincott)

Most ruptured disks occur in the lumbar and lumbosacral regions of the back. The compression of spinal nerve roots caused by this condition produces the symptoms that necessitate treatment.

SIGNS AND SYMPTOMS

Usually the first symptoms of a ruptured lumbar disk are severe low back pain and muscle spasm that is aggravated by sneezing, coughing, and bending. The patient is most comfortable lying down. The pain eventually radiates into a leg and foot, and the patient may list toward the unaffected side. Pain of a cramping nature in the back of the leg and thigh is often present. Numbness and paresthesia may occur in the involved dermatome (the area of skin innervated by the compressed spinal nerve root). For example, sensory loss of the S1 nerve root, as depicted in the following figure, is due to compression at the L5 interspace.

The back appears "flat" in the lumbar region. Weakness and atrophy of the leg muscles and loss of reflexes are later signs of the herniated disk.

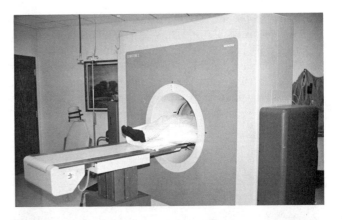

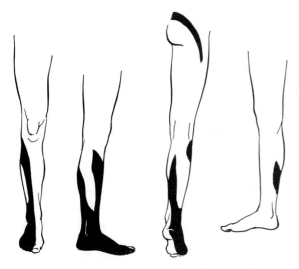

Sensory loss from pressure on the S1 nerve root (Turek: Orthopaedics. Philadelphia, Lippincott, 1977)

DIAGNOSIS

A history of the circumstances prior to onset of pain and the signs and symptoms aid in the initial diagnosis. Sciatic pain on straight leg-raising, (flexing the hip with the leg extended) is a positive test. The patient with a herniated disk also offers resistance or pain to having the knee extended when both hip and knee are at 90 degrees of flexion (Kernig's sign). Loss of the ankle reflex or knee jerk is a sign of spinal nerve-root compression.

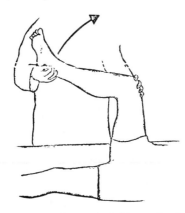

Testing for Kernig's sign. (Bates: A Guide to Physical Examination. Philadelphia, Lippincott)

X-ray films are valuable in detecting degenerative changes or an old ruptured disk. In these cases, the x-ray film will show a narrowing of the disk space. Two diagnostic tests are commonly performed. Computerized scanning (known as "computed tomography, CT scan, or "Cat" scan) of the lumbosacral spine may reveal the defect. In this noninvasive test the radiation source and detectors rotate around the patient, imaging specific points which can be seen on a monitor and processed on film.

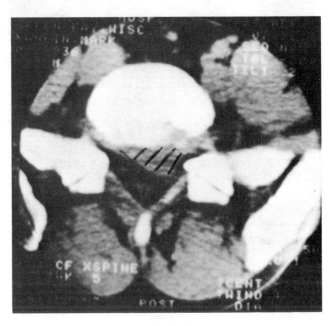

The myelogram is another diagnostic test and may be done in conjunction with a scan. A radiopaque substance, usually water soluble, is injected into the dural space, and the path of the dye through the lumbar canal is followed by

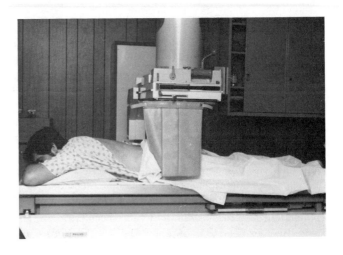

the fluoroscope. Where there is a ruptured fragment, a filling defect is visible, and films are taken for further study.

Since most contrast media contain iodine, the nurse must be alert for allergies the patient might have to substances (such as salt-water shellfish) that contain iodine. When a patient has such an allergy, the radiology department must be notified.

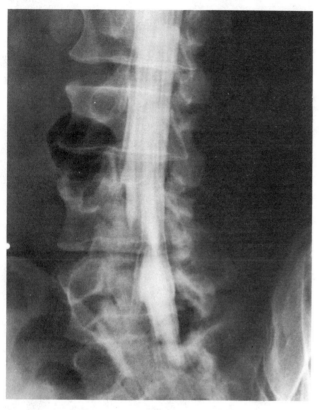

Metrizamide (Amipaque) myelogram.

The Myelogram: Nursing Implications

Patient instruction for computerized scanning can be simple. The patient should be told that the scanning is done while he is lying on a table, with the machine taking X-rays around him rather than just in front or in back. However, most people are apprehensive at the prospect of a spinal puncture, and patients need psychological preparation for myelograms. The surgeon will explain the procedure and the necessity for doing it, but it is the nurse's responsibility to follow this instruction with any needed clarification and to give emotional support.

Instruction given before the myelogram is aided by the use of a teaching tool such as a photograph album with pictures and captions related to the herniated disk, the myelogram procedure, and post-myelgram care. A word of caution about photographs and explanations: the patient does not need to see a photograph or read about anything he will not actually see because this may cause needless apprehension. He does need to know about the spinal puncture and

the fact that a local anesthetic will be injected into the tissue. However, a photograph showing the various needles that will be used is unnecessary, because he will not see them. Drugs that lower the seizure threshold (except in the case of epileptics) are withheld for 48 hours prior to the myelogram. Food and fluids may also be withheld for 4 to 6 hours before the procedure is done.

A premedication should be ordered for the patient by the physician to promote relaxation and assure cooperation. The patient who is relatively comfortable prior to the myelogram as a result of being properly instructed and premedicated will experience little discomfort during the procedure. Post-myelogram care and observations for the patient having water-soluble myelography generally include the following. The patient will return to his room with the head of the stretcher elevated to prevent the contrast medium from entering the cranial cavity. The head of the bed should remain elevated 15 to 30 degrees for 8 hours. Patient activity following that period of time is variable. Vital signs and neurologic status must be checked immediately after the myelogram and at regular intervals for 24 hours. Fluids are encouraged and diet is ordered as tolerated. The first voiding is measured. Although nausea and vomiting may occur, the patient should not be given phenothiazines for 48 hours. A padded tongue blade, to be used in case of seizure activity, may be taped to the head of the bed if hospital policy permits, and the patient is informed of its purpose. Analgesics are ordered for headaches.

METHODS OF TREATING THE HERNIATED DISK

Three basic methods may be used for treating a herniated disk: conservative management, laminectomy, and chemonucleolysis.

CONSERVATIVE MANAGEMENT

Most physicians prefer to treat the patient with a herniated disk by conservative measures for several weeks at least, unless there are signs of severe cord compression such as loss of motor or bladder function. The objective of this treatment is to relieve the pain by reducing the compression force of normal weightbearing activities on the involved disk. The regimen consists of prolonged bed rest, usually in pelvic belt traction, physical therapy in the form of deep heat, specific exercises, and intermittent pelvic traction. Ice massage may be indicated in cases of acute muscle spasm. Narcotics may be necessary for relief of pain during the acute phase, and muscle relaxants are commonly given.

Transcutaneous electrical nerve stimulation (TENS), may be ordered in the conservative management of back pain. The TENS device consists of a battery-operated pulse generator and a pair of cables with electrodes. The electrodes are normally applied to the skin overlying the painful

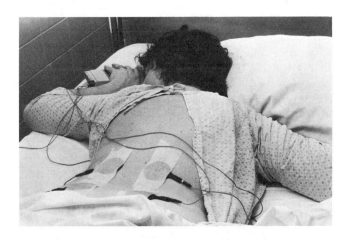

area or the nerves supplying the painful site. The sensation produced by electrical stimulation is similar to tingling and theoretically masks the pain. The physician or physical therapist places the electrodes and initiates the treatment. The patient is taught how to handle the unit and produce stimulation when pain is present and requires relief. The nurse assumes responsibility for supervision of this treatment. TENS may also be ordered for relief of postoperative pain as an adjunct to narcotics.

Positioning

If the patient is in severe pain and greatly incapacitated (some of these patients can barely move or bend), bed rest in continuous pelvic traction is ordered until the patient feels more comfortable. During this period the greatest comfort is most frequently achieved with the head of the bed elevated 30 to 45 degrees, and the knee gatch elevated to flatten the lumbosacral curve. This is known as Williams' position, modified Williams' position, or modified jackknife position, according to the reference used.

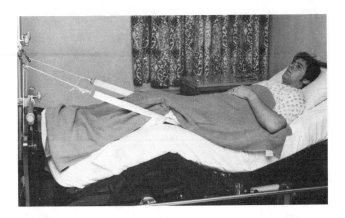

The therapeutic benefits of pelvic traction in Williams' position for a herniated disk are questionable. However, this does keep the patient at bed rest and in good body alignment, thereby decreasing muscle spasm.

While in traction, the patients movements are limited. He should not use a trapeze (and cannot if he is in severe pain or spasms) without a physician's order.

The patient should be instructed not to turn sideways in the traction and to keep his lower back immobile. When he is in acute pain there is not much likelihood that he will move around anyway.

Turning Procedure

A fracture bedpan or a child's bedpan will be easier for the patient to use, because both are smaller and flatter than the standard bedpan. If the patient can use a trapeze, he will not need to lift his buttocks very much to have either of these bedpans placed. If he must be turned, a pillow should be placed between his knees to prevent his back from twisting. He can grasp the bed rail with the hand on the side to which he will be turned, and with the nurse supporting buttock and shoulder to ease him over, he can readily grasp the bed rail with his opposite hand as he turns. The same turning procedure may be used for giving skin care. (See pp. 107 for care of the patient in pelvic traction.)

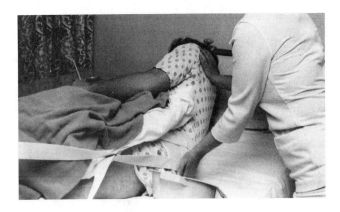

Anticipating the patient's needs and checking with him every hour for the first day or until he becomes moderately comfortable is better than trying to keep everything in his reach all of the time. The call light, however, should be in reach at all times.

Physical Therapy

When the patient is given bathroom privileges, the physician also may begin the physical therapy program. The purpose of deep heat, massage, and the Hubbard tank is to decrease muscle spasm and promote relaxation. Pain medication or muscle relaxants should be given to the patient before he goes to physical therapy. Exercises are prescribed based on the physician's philosophy of what "works" for a protruding disk, those exercises that decrease pressure on the nerve root and relieve symptoms, and those that strengthen the back and abdominal muscles. The patient's general condition, including strength and weight, are taken into consideration.

After several sessions with the patient, the physical therapist will often suggest those exercises or modalities which he believes will be most beneficial. Some exercises are designed to promote total joint mobility and strengthen the back.

The exercise program may include extension exercise such as:

1. Stomach-lying

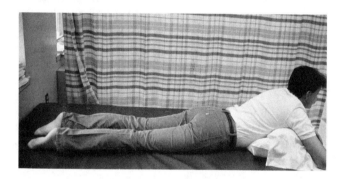

2. Prone pushups

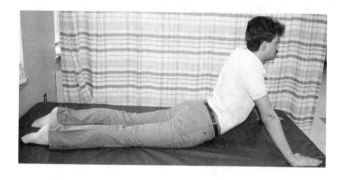

3. Upper trunk extension

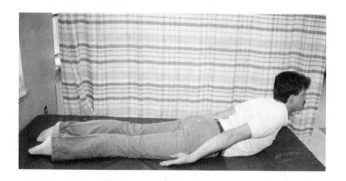

All exercises are performed according to the patient's tolerance. The therapist will "do nothing to increase symptoms."

Flexion exercises include:

1. Semi-situps. The patient lies on his back on the physical therapy table with his knees and hips flexed. (A mattress is placed on the table for comfort.) He can either clasp his hands behind his head or extend them toward his knees. He is then told to bring himself up to a "curl" position, as if he were reaching to touch his knees with either his hands or

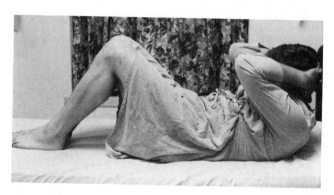

elbows. He does this without moving his legs or feet. He holds the position for a count of 5 or 10 as tolerated and then lowers himself back down to his original position.

2. Pelvic tilt. The patient is in the same position, on his back with knees and hips flexed. The therapist places his hand under the lumbar region, requesting the patient to tighten his abdominal muscles to flatten the lumbar region of the back, thus touching the therapist's hand.

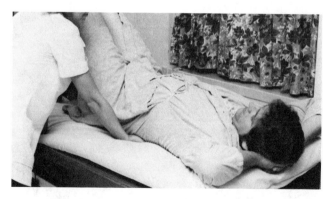

3. Knee–chest. The patient is asked to maintain a pelvic tilt, while bringing one or both knees up to his chest, holding for a count of 5 to 20, then relaxing.

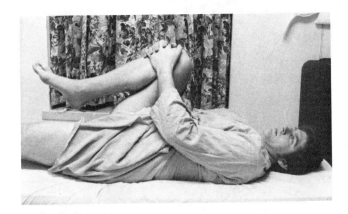

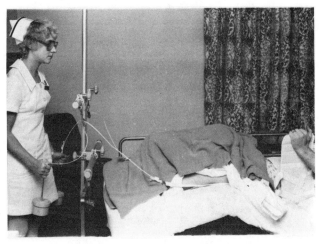

Intermittent pelvic traction in physical therapy may also be prescribed. The patient lies on a table and is fastened into a thoracic belt that is attached to the end of the table. A pelvic belt is also applied, with the straps of the belt positioned under the lumbar spine. The patient's legs rest on a stool so that his hips and knees are slightly flexed. The straps are attached to a spreader bar, and this is attached to the traction machine. The traction force is exerted gradually and ranges form 30 to 90 pounds, depending on the patient's tolerance, the physician's prescription, and the capacity of the machine to exert force without pulling the

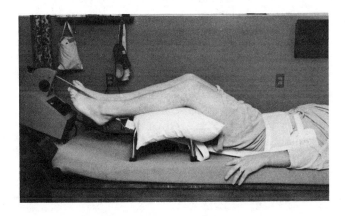

belts apart. A session of intermittent traction therapy is about 20 minutes in length. The position of the patient in this traction setup may be changed to promote comfort. He may have his legs in a neutral position or he may lie prone. Hot packs may be ordered and applied before, during, or after treatment.

Removing Traction

The patient should not remove his traction without proper instructions, so that the weights will not crash to the floor when the belt is unfastened and slides toward the foot of the bed. It is preferable for the nurse to remove the belt or hold the weights while the patient loosens the belt. When the

patient is mobile enough to hop in and out of the traction, or to adjust the components at will, he probably does not need it at all.

Avoiding Problems of Immobility

If the patient must remain on strict bed rest for longer than a couple of days, measures must be taken to prevent problems of immobility. Thromboembolic stockings may be ordered. Deep breathing, coughing, or some form of mechanical respiratory support such as the incentive spirometer (p. 97), quadriceps setting, and exercises of the extremities as tolerated should be added to the nursing care plan. Encouraging fluids is essential to help prevent renal calculi and constipation. Constipation is one of the most common physiological problems in patients with low back pain. Because this problem may increase back pain, it should be anticipated, and preventive measures should be a part of the initial care plan. Besides having an increased fluid intake, the patient should be given a stool softener or laxative as required if he is taking narcotics. A well-balanced diet is also important.

Post-Traction Regimen

Once the patient has become comfortable and the physician has determined that ambulation is permissible, a back support may be ordered. Typically, the back support device is similar to a corset, with a number of rigid stays and an adjustable fastening system, either belts and buckles or self-adhering ends. Patients should be instructed in exercises for strengthening the lower back and in the importance of maintaining good body mechanics at all times.

How successful the conservative treatment of the herniated disk is depends a great deal on how the patient cooperates with those who are involved in the treatment and how well he follows instructions when he gets home. The extent of disk disease and the condition of the fibrous tissue and ligaments surrounding the intervertebral disks are also factors in the success or failure of conservative management.

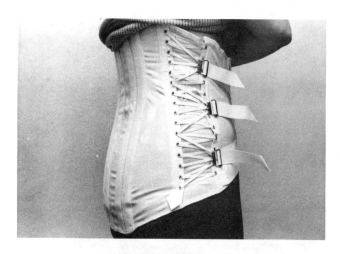

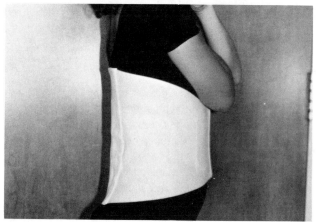

Post-traction corsets for patient undergoing conservative treatment for herniated disk.

LAMINECTOMY

If conservative treatment of the ruptured disk has proven ineffective, a laminectomy may be done. This surgical procedure involves removal of parts of one or more vertebral laminae along with the protruding disk (nucleus pulposus).

Preoperative Assessment of Condition

When a patient is admitted to the hospital for a laminectomy, the nurse must do a thorough assessment of his signs and symptoms in order to have baseline information for postoperative comparisons. The patient should be asked to describe exactly where and what his pain or paresthesias are. Pain and numbness associated with a herniated disk usually radiate to the lower extremity. The nurse must record the data in the patient's own descriptive terms. The neurovascular status and range of motion of both lower extremities should be checked, compared, and recorded. Gait and posture when standing or walking are also noted. A patient with a herniated disk often favors the affected side.

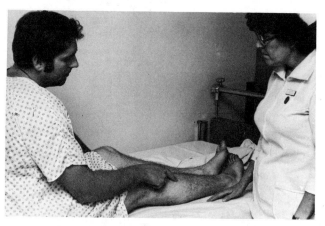

Preoperative Teaching and Psychological Consideratons

People with back and leg pain and other symptoms that accompany a "slipped" disk have generally undergone a long period, or intermittent periods, of conservative treatment before deciding to have surgery. Because of chronic pain and discomfort, they have lost time in working hours and have been limited in many of their activities. The decisions to undergo a laminectomy is accompanied by feelings of relief, mixed with anxiety about the outcome. How these feelings and reactions affect nursing care and patient convalescence depends greatly on patient teaching.

Initial preoperative instruction should focus on alleviating fears about spinal surgery. Often this requires a review of what has already been discussed between surgeon and patient, especially in regard to postoperative pain. The patient should be told that whatever numbness or pain he has had in his leg or legs before surgery will remain with him a while. He will be easier to care for postoperatively if he expects to experience "pins and needles" or a feeling of weakness in his legs that makes it difficult, for a couple of days, to believe that he can move them.

All postoperative routines that the patient will be required to submit to, or participate in, should be explained to him and the family member who will be at his bedside. A wife is likely to be alarmed at the frequency with which her

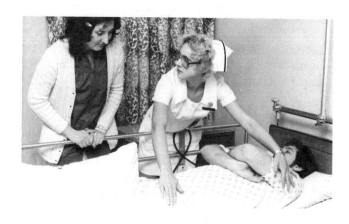

husband's vital signs are checked if she does not know this routine. More undesirable still, she may attempt to help him turn the minute he is recovered enough to ask if he can do so. Preoperatively, both should be taught the importance of the patient being turned without twisting his body—that is, that he should be logrolled all in "one piece."

The preoperative intramuscular injection should be given in the unaffected buttock, or in the deltoid muscle if both buttocks are subject to pain from the herniated disk.

Vital Signs

Once the patient has returned to his room, his vital signs should be monitored closely until stable, and then as often as is deemed necessary for the first 24 hours.

Positioning and Logrolling

The bed of a laminectomy patient should have a solid bottom or be equipped with boards under the mattress. Postoperatively, the nurse must know how soon the patient may be turned and how frequently. Usually laminectomy patients are turned every 3 hours immediately after surgery, according to the following procedure.

First, all pillows are removed. When the patient is conscious he may be instructed to cross his arms across his chest. If two nurses work together, beginning on the same side of the bed, they place their hands under the patient's shoulders, back, buttocks, and legs and pull him slightly to one side of the bed. One nurse can then go to the other side

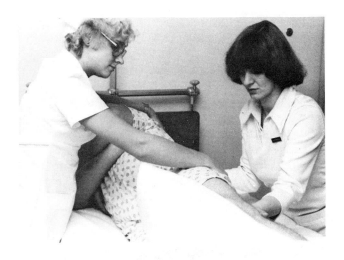

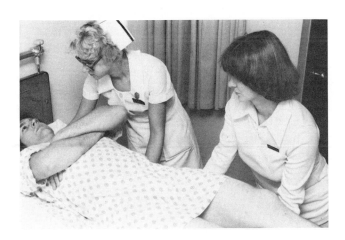

of the bed. A pillow is placed between the patient's knees, and he is instructed to keep his arms crossed over his chest and to roll to one side. One nurse assists him in rolling by supporting his back and buttocks as he turns away from her. The nurse on the other side of the bed places her hands where additional support is needed as the patient turns toward her. She then helps him maintain this position while

the other nurse places pillows for support. The pillow under the patient's head is replaced. Two pillows may be needed to support his back and buttocks. One should remain between his knees while he is on his side, and one can be placed in front of his chest to support his arm (see next photo).

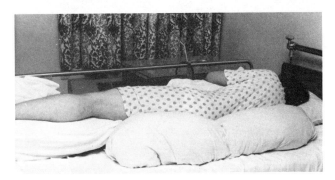

Many hospitals advocate the use of the turn sheet, sometimes called the *"laminectomy sheet."* This is a double-thickness drawsheet that is placed on the bed before the patient returns from the operating room. The side ends are not tucked under the mattress. The purpose of the sheet is for lifting or pulling the patient to the side of the bed and turning him. The ends of the sheet are rolled as close as possible to the sides of the patient's body. One nurse on each side of the bed holds on to the rolled-up portion of the sheet as the patient is lifted and turned. However, it is just as

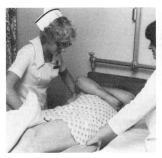

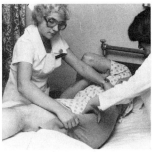

expedient (since two nurses are needed for either procedure) and just as comfortable if the patient is turned without a sheet. Furthermore, if he is to be propped on his side, the rolled sheet under that side will have to be pulled out and may wrinkle. It then takes added time to straighten it out.

Whatever method of turning is used, perfect alignment of the body should be maintained in all positions. The head of the bed is elevated as the surgeon permits. Back rubs are also given when the patient is repositioned.

Once a laminectomy patient is able to turn and move about in bed without assistance, the nurse must remind him not to "bunch" pillows up under his knees when he is lying on his back, because this promotes venous stasis in his lower legs.

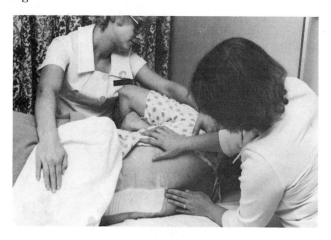

Dressing

The dressing should be checked for drainage when the patient is repositioned. It is not common for oozing to occur through the dressing after a laminectomy. Any oozing should be reported with specific description of type and amount.

The "Stir Up" Routine

To "stir up" a postoperative patient means what it suggests: to get the patient moving. Aside from having the patient move his arms and legs to increase circulation, en-

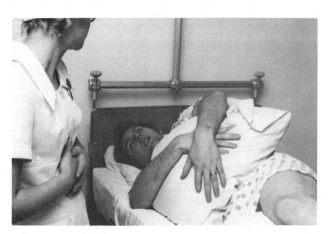

courage him to breathe deeply and to cough. In the past, nurses were taught to be cautious about encouraging these patients to cough, for fear of putting stress on the incisional area and causing undue discomfort. However, the average laminectomy patient coughs very gently, with his back pressed firmly against the mattress or a pillow held against his chest for restraining or splinting purposes. Because most patients are out of bed within 24 hours, such measures as intermittent positive-pressure breathing (IPPB) or the incentive spirometer are not necessary.

The patient who has had a laminectomy should be "stirred up" every 3 hours until he begins to ambulate; after this it is still a good idea to remind him about deep breathing and coughing. There are patients who do not expand their lungs adequately, for fear it will create a "pulling" sensation in the incisional area.

Checking the Extremities

The neurovascular status of the legs is observed by noting the color, motion, temperature, and sensation (CMTS) of the toes, as well as the patient's ability to move the entire extremity. Here again, it is important for the nurse to be

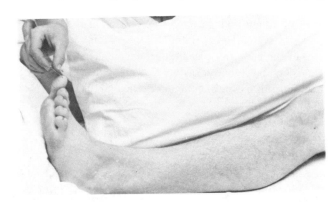

aware of any numbness or pain that was present in the extremity before surgery, in order to make an accurate postoperative assessment. The nurse must be certain that the patient is differentiating between "coldness" and "numbness."

Use of Analgesics

The amount of pain varies with each patient. Some patients experience pain or discomfort and muscle spasms for most

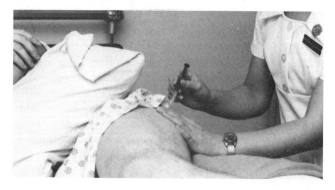

of the time they are in the hospital. Some, in comparison with their preoperative states, become comfortable fairly soon.

Postoperative discomfort is intensified by apprehension about movement, which makes clear the importance of adequate preoperative instruction.

The nurse must remember to evaluate the patient's need for pain medication every 4 hours. Many times, the patient is so accustomed to low back pain that he waits too long to request medication. Then, when it is given, it provides little relief. It is a fact that some people, especially young men, do not like "needles" and that they suffer in silence rather than ask for medication.

Usually after 48 hours, oral medication may be substituted for intramuscular injections. Throat lozenges are beneficial for those patients who complain of sore throats for a day or so because of the use of the endotracheal tube in the recovery room.

Bedmaking

The patient must be logrolled when the bottom linen is changed. The bed is made on one side first, with both soiled and clean linen rolled to the middle of the bed and pushed as far as possible under the patient. The patient has to roll back over this ridge of linen. Therefore, it should not be left directly under his incisional area, so that the move to the other side of the bed will be less uncomfortable.

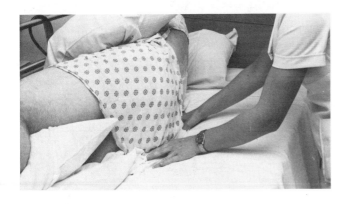

Temperature

Temperature should be taken every 4 hours for 48 hours; some surgeons continue this order for 7 to 10 days. An elevation of temperature is to be expected for about 72 hours postoperatively. To what degree it should be allowed to rise before the nurse makes a telephone call to the doctor should be determined well before 3 A.M. on the first postoperative day. It is permissible to rely on nursing judgment when the surgeon is not specific. However, many of them are specific in this matter, and the nurse eliminates problems by obtaining this information ahead of time.

When aspirin is given to reduce body temperature, the patient may perspire. If allowed to remain on damp linen he may become chilled. Thus, bed sheet and hospital gown should be changed when needed.

Diet and Fluids

Intravenous fluids are not routinely administered to patients who have had laminectomies. Oral fluids are encouraged as soon as they are tolerated, and adequate intake may help the patient to void without the need for catheterization.

Diet is also increased as the patient desires. As he begins to eat, the nurse should stress the importance of well-balanced meals in preventing constipation.

The laminectomy patient has to eat lying on his side until he can sit on a straight chair. His body should be well

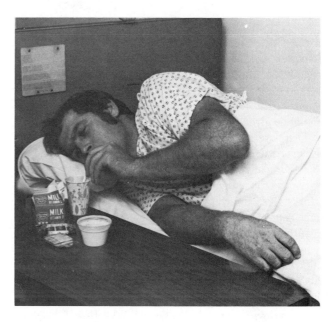

supported with pillows. The tray table should be close to the bed and as close to the height of the bed as possible. The nurse should be certain that the patient can reach all the food on his tray and should provide him with straws for fluids. The patient should be assured that he may have as much time as he needs to eat the meal.

Voiding

Pain and position often create problems in voiding. The patient may require catheterization or even an indwelling catheter if difficulty persists. However, getting the laminectomy patient out of bed to void is preferable to catheterization. The decision on whether the patient is able to get out of bed to void is usually considered a matter of nursing judgment. The male patient may be assisted to a standing position at the bedside, and the female patient can be helped to a bedside commode. Shock to the sympathetic nervous system causes a temporary loss of bladder tone; for this reason it is advisable to measure and record urinary output for 24 to 48 hours postoperatively.

When the laminectomy patient does use a bedpan, being logrolled onto a fracture bedpan is the most comfortable procedure.

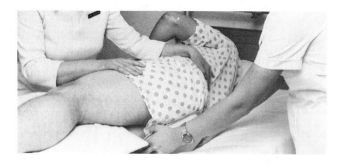

Dangling

Some surgeons allow laminectomy patients to dangle in the evening on the day of surgery. Dangling should be explained to the patient at the same time that the nurse announces that he will "dangle soon." A pain medication should be given 30 minutes prior to this procedure.

There are at least two efficient ways of getting a laminectomy patient onto the side of the bed for the first time. The objective of any method of mobilizing a laminectomy patient is to move the patient without twisting either his back or a nurse's. This is facilitated by allowing the patient to have some control over his own movements.

If the head of the bed is to be elevated before the patient is helped up, he should be positioned so that he bends in the same place as the mattress without twisting his body. With the bed elevated, his buttocks should rest on the flat half of the mattress, just past the point where the mattress bends. Usually, the patient can help himself up with a trapeze.

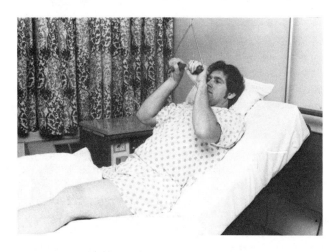

As the patient brings himself around to a sitting position on the side of the bed, with a pillow between his legs, one nurse helps him move his legs while a second nurse stands by to support his shoulders.

If the patient gets up from a flat bed, he should be turned on his side as close to the edge of the bed as safety permits, with his hips and knees slightly flexed and a pillow between his legs. Then he can help himself by pushing up with one or both hands as one nurse supports his shoulders and the other brings his legs over the edge of the bed.

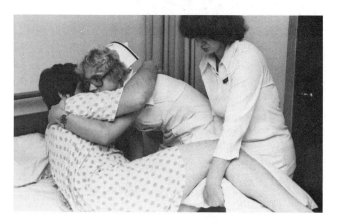

Not infrequently, the surgeon prefers to assist the patient personally in sitting up for the first time.

As the patient sits at the edge of the bed, his shoulders and back should remain supported as he is encouraged to

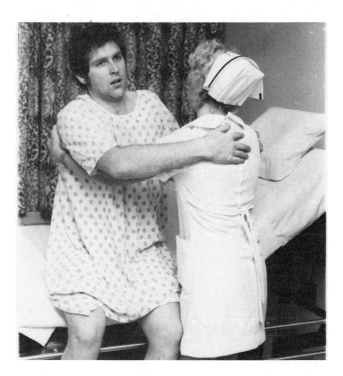

take some deep breaths. Then he is asked to "paddle" his feet. Not only does this increase his circulation, but it takes his mind off his discomfort and dizziness.

When the patient is lowered back into bed, the procedure is done in reverse, except that the head of the bed should then be elevated for comfort.

For a summary of priorities in the preoperative and postoperative care of the laminectomy patient, see the accompanying chart.

THE LAMINECTOMY PATIENT

Priorities in Preoperative Assessment

Significant Admission Data

L. S. is a 35-year-old male.
Ht.: 5'11"   *Wt.:* 190 lb.
T.: 97.8   *P.:* 60   *R.:* 16   *B.P.:* 115/80

Reason for Admission

He is admitted to the floor in a wheelchair and accompanied by a business associate. He states that he is to have a myelogram and "surgery on his back."

History of Present Condition

Injured his back 12 years ago while pouring concrete. Has been in hospital three times for conservative treatment. For the last 2 to 3 months, he has had increasingly severe pain, very little in back, mostly in left hip region radiating down to the back of his thigh with a constant aching pain in his calf. States he has numbness in his left lower extremity when he walks.

Orthopedic Assessment

Appears to have marked spasm of back muscles. Cannot lie with left leg straight. Barely able to do left straight leg-raising. Straight leg-raising on right is painful, with pain referred to left lower extremity. Color, motion, temperature, sensation (CMTS) of both feet comparable. Toes warm, move, and can feel pinch. Bilateral pedal pulses present and same. Achilles-tendon reflex absent on left side. Can feel pin pricks on both extremities. Cannot walk more than ten steps without increased pain. Favors left side when he walks. See history for complaints of pain.

General Health Status

Good. T & A when 10 years old. On no medications. Denies allergies. Does have "smoker's cough." Significant family history: father is obese with bilateral osteoarthritis in knees.

Personal Profile

L. S. smokes one pack of cigarettes daily. States he drinks about three martinis every day. Has no hearing or vision problems. Showers daily. Eats "everything." Retires late. Does not like to get up early but does because of his job.

Mental/Emotional State

Alert, cooperative, oriented. Restless and has occasional twitching of face muscles. Slight tremors of hands noted. States he has "had it" with treatment and hopes he can have surgery and "be done with it."

Social History

Is a salesman. Sells office equipment. States job is "high pressure." He travels a lot. Has just been separated from his wife. Has two daughters, ages 13 and 15.

Additional Assessment

Nurse should assess patient knowledge concerning the myelogram and laminectomy. This will be helpful in planning initial supportive care and correlating preoperative instruction with that of the surgeon.

Priorities in Postoperative Management

GOALS

Patient Goals

1. To be relieved of signs and symptoms of herniated disk.

2. To be discharged with a clear understanding of the alterations necessary in his life-style to prevent recurrence of back problems.

Nursing Goals

1. Prevent complications due to
   a. Surgery
   b. Limited mobility
2. Deliver supportive care to promote patient's psychologic comfort.
3. Assess patient's health education needs and provide instruction p.r.n.

(continued)

THE LAMINECTOMY PATIENT (*Continued*)

EARLY POSTOPERATIVE PERIOD

Routine Postoperative Care

1. Vital signs q 30 min until stable, then q 1 hr × 4, then qid for 48 hr
2. Check dressing.
3. CMTS both feet and compare.
4. "Stir ups"*
5. Back care
6. Heel care
7. Logroll with pillow between legs.
8. Check for abdominal distention.

q 4 hr for 48 hr and then decrease or discontinue as nursing judgment dictates

9. Elastic hose. Remove q shift for skin care.
10. Measure voidings × 3.
11. May stand at bedside (with help) to void

11. May require surgeon's order; often a nursing decision.

12. Catheterize p.r.n.
13. Food and fluids as tolerated
14. Analgesic and sedative

12–14. Require surgeon's order and specifics vary.

15. Additional measures to promote lung expansion

15. Nurse should suggest such measures when routine stir ups do not seem to be adequate.

PRIORITIES — ONGOING CARE

1st Postoperative Day — 3 P.M. Report

Implications for P.M. Assessment and Intervention

1. Slept most of A.M. until noon. Restless when awake.

1. Do HS routines as late as possible. If patient is awake at 11 P.M., evaluate if this is a good time to encourage him to verbalize feelings and establish rapport. Observe for tremors. (See admission data, m/e state.)

2. Has been medicated for pain only twice since surgery. States back feels "better" than before operation.

2. Check q 4 hr to see whether he needs pain medication.

3. Walks in room with assistance of one person.

3. Instruct not to walk alone. Remind him he should lie down or walk, not sit. Observe posture.

4. Is being allowed to smoke (per physician order) when someone is with him.

4. Ask his daughter to tell nurse when she leaves. (Patient might forget he cannot smoke alone.) Continue stir ups q 3 hr while awake.

5. Asking about laxative but does not feel constipated. Is voiding in good amounts.

5. Discuss stool softeners, laxative with patient. How is his appetite? Encourage fluids. Check preference.

6. T. 100.2 P. 88 R. 16 B.P. 134/82. Asked about his B.P. and is surprised it is higher than usual. Told he should take pain medication if uncomfortable, because this will help him to relax and keep B.P. down.

6. Reinforce day instruction about B.P.

7. Youngest daughter is here at present. They seem to get along very well. Mr. S. is cooperative and pleasant but seems a bit hyperactive.

7. See 1.

* "Stir up" patient by encouraging deep breathing, coughing, and a movement of extremities

THE LAMINECTOMY PATIENT (*Continued*)

FURTHER CONSIDERATIONS IN INDIVIDUALIZING NURSING CARE

1. Patient should be evaluated periodically to see if any additional respiratory support measure is necessary because he is a heavy smoker.
2. Because of what is known about patient's father, he should be instructed regarding relationship between obesity, exercise, and knee problems.
3. Discharge planning will have to focus on fact that patient sits for long periods of time behind the wheel in his car and may have to handle office equipment.
4. Patient is intelligent and realizes that the stress of his job may cause physical problems. Perhaps discuss signs and symptoms of stress, importance of regular checkups.

Getting the Patient Up

Getting out of bed to stand and walk is the next milestone and may be done as early as 24 hours postoperatively. The

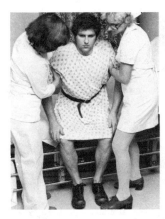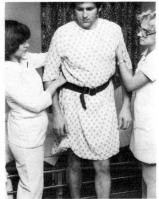

patient is brought to a sitting position on the edge of the bed by the same maneuver used to position him for dangling.

Generally, it is better to have two people available to help the patient take those first few faltering steps. A belt around the patient's waist is a good security measure while he is still walking with assistance. Once the patient is able to ambulate, he is advised to walk, rather than merely to stand. Standing leaves the lumbar spine without support, thus putting stress on the operative area. Walking causes this stress to be intermittent rather than continuous. When the patient becomes tired, he should lie down.

Sitting on a straight firm chair to eat meals is preferable to sitting on the edge of the bed, because a chair provides support for the back.

Convalescing

As the patient becomes stronger, there are ways he can make his convalescence more comfortable. The nurse should advise him to stand and walk as straight as possible.

This is slower and more painful at the start, but he will gradually be able to do so without great fatigue. Limping or hunching his shoulders may be more comfortable at first but will eventually cause him more fatigue. There may be times when the patient feels unusually tired or as if he is making no progress. If he is assured that this is natural, he may feel better.

Preparation for Discharge

When the patient is beginning to think and ask questions about what he will be allowed to do at home, the nurse should encourage him to make a list of his concerns. Then, when the physician gives him instructions, he will have a point of reference for deciding whether or not all of his questions are answered. One thing a nurse can tell him is that he should not undertake any exercise or activity that is not permitted. The patient should be informed by the surgeon of the limitations that have been placed on his daily activities and to what extent they are permanent.

Laminectomy patients are often concerned about how soon they may be allowed to resume sexual activity after they are discharged from the hospital. Sometimes they are reluctant to introduce the subject when receiving discharge instructions from the surgeon, and the surgeon does not always provide guidelines. Therefore, it is a nursing responsibility to remind the patient to ask questions about sexual activity if this is a matter of concern to him.

Patients who have had laminectomies do not normally require braces or corsets postoperatively. However, they should have a clear understanding of prescribed exercises and the importance of proper body mechanics and good posture. The basic objectives of postoperative instruction for the laminectomy patient are to strengthen the back and abdominal muscles and maintain the normal mobility of the spine. A combination of flexion and extension exercises (p. 134) may be ordered.

Good posture and proper body mechanics will prevent back strain, develop strong muscles, increase circulation, and allow room for internal organs to function normally. Key points include the following:

1. Avoid stretching (bowing out) of the lower back in any position or activity. Maintain normal curves.

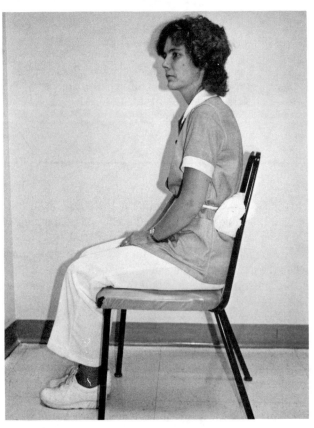

2. Rest your feet alternately when standing.
3. Lift heavy objects close to your body and maintain normal curve.

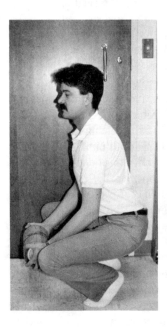
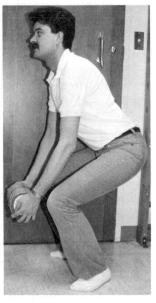

4. Get enough rest.

In addition, the patient should be taught to stop any activity that causes pain and advised to avoid becoming overweight.

Postlaminectomy patients are often troubled by the thought of recurring back problems, especially if they know someone who has had such an experience. The only reassurance the nurse can offer is that backs, like people, are all different, and that following the advice of the physician may help make the difference.

CHEMONUCLEOLYSIS

The removal of herniated disk tissue by means of the enzyme chymopapain may be indicated for some patients. Chymopapain, which is derived from the papaya plant, acts as a meat-tenderizing enzyme, dissolving the projecting disk material. The procedure is performed under fluoroscopy in the operating room or radiology department. General or local anesthesia may be used. The patient is positioned on his side with support for his spine, and his knees

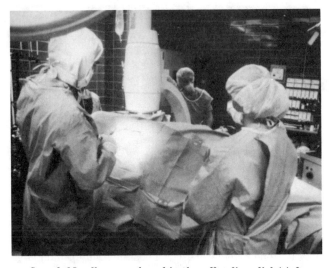

are flexed. Needles are placed in the offending disk(s) from a posterolateral approach, to avoid damaging the nerve roots. A discogram is done by injecting radiopaque dye into

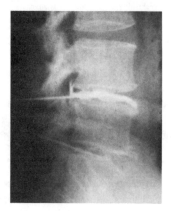

the disk. The pathology is diagnosed by the way in which the dye is distributed. A very small amount of the chymopapain is injected through the same needle to test for allergic reaction, or anaphylactic shock. About 15 to 20 minutes later the entire amount, 1 cc to 2 cc, is injected to hydrolyze the involved disk material.

Preparing the Patient for the Procedure

Psychological preparation for chemonucleolysis is of the utmost importance, because the patient is aware that this treatment is "different" from surgery and that it may not be successful. The best way to accomplish this is to establish rapport with the patient and family as soon as possible and begin instruction.

When the patient is admitted to the unit, the nurse, in collecting data and making observations, can assess the patient's emotional state and physical condition. Asking questions about pain and limitation of motion is only a part of the interview. Noting how the patient moves in getting up and down and whether he needs help to do so gives the nurse some indication of how he may do these things in the early stages of recovery. Family reactions to the patient's limitations may be clues to how supportive they are and how much support they need from the orthopedic nurse.

Patient history in regard to allergies, previous surgery, and medical treatment is very important. Chemonucleolysis is contraindicated in patients who are allergic to meat tenderizers, chymopapain, or radiopaque dyes. Individual surgeons also have their own criteria, and the nurse must be aware of these.

Specific literature for patient education is most helpful because it can be shared with family members.

The nurse should plan on spending enough time with this patient preoperatively so that the patient goes to surgery fully aware of what will happen every step of the way.

The preoperative medication should not be given in the affected hip, to avoid any masking of disk symptoms after the procedure has been performed.

Postoperative Care

The patient who undergoes chemonucleolysis will remain on bed rest for 24 to 48 hours, depending on the surgeon. The total length of time in the hospital averages 3 days. How quickly the patient resumes normal activities of daily living depends on how strenuous these activities are.

On the operative day, bed rest is maintained in whatever position is comfortable for the patient. Several pillows

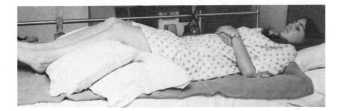

placed under the knees, with the backrest flat, have proven to be comfortable for most patients. When the patient's knees are flexed over pillows, the nurse must remember to encourage frequent leg movement to avoid pressure on the popliteal space.

Turning is done with the pillow between the legs. Side positioning includes leaving the pillow in place. The patient may require assistance in turning for 24 hours.

Placing a fracture bedpan is accomplished by placing a pillow between the patient's legs, turning the patient to the side and then back on the pan. If voiding proves to be difficult, a Foley catheter may need to be inserted.

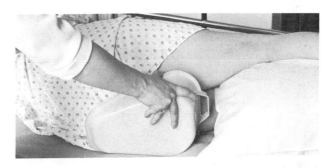

Deep breathing and movement of arms and legs are encouraged on a regular schedule to promote circulation.

The patient should be kept comfortable with analgesics (again, injections are not given in the affected buttock), and the nurse should assume a positive attitude so that the patient does not anticipate a great deal of discomfort. Spasms of the back muscles occur in some patients and heating pads may be used to aid in relaxation.

Food and fluids are given as tolerated. Usually intravenous fluids that were started in surgery are discontinued by the end of the operative day.

Progression of Activity

Getting out of bed does not need to be an ordeal. The backrest is elevated according to patient comfort. The patient is then instructed to flex her knees and use the trapeze to come to a sitting position on the edge of the bed. As the

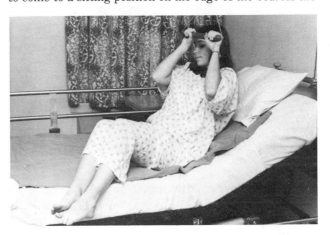

patient first sits at the edge of the bed and then steps down, it will be more comfortable if most of the weight rests on the hands, rather than on the buttocks. The bed should be high enough so that the patient does not have to bend forward to get off the edge and can slide back on the edge with minimal

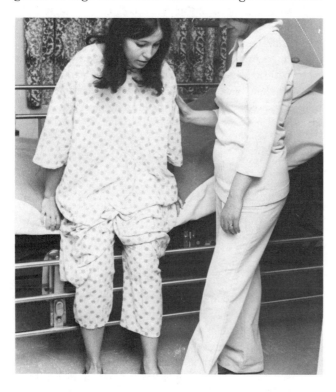

effort. The patient is allowed as much ambulation as can be tolerated.

Any procedure that requires the patient to be standing should be modified if possible, to rest the affected side. For example, when brushing her teeth, the patient might rest the affected foot on a footstool.

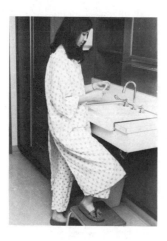

All activity depends on the patient's individual tolerance. Patients who have painful spasms may be given muscle relaxants and deep heat or ice massage.

Discharge Planning

Special exercises for the back are written out and should be started only after the physician has determined that the patient is ready for them. These may include the exercises described on p. 134.

The instructions for the postlaminectomy patient regarding posture and body mechanics (p. 144) are also appropriate for the patient who has undergone a chemonucleolysis.

Many times the physician suggests swimming as an appropriate activity following discharge, because the buoyancy of water permits exercise without placing strain on the back muscles.

Audiovisual aids, reinforcing what the patient has been taught about proper exercise and positioning, are excellent for use in discharge planning.

Care of the Patient With a Spinal Fusion

Spinal Fusion Procedures

In spinal fusion, an ankylosis is created surgically between two or more vertebrae. The most common procedure is the posterolateral fusion.

In this procedure, bone is laid down onto the transverse processes and may or may not include the facet joints. There are probably two reasons why this procedure is preferred. Many patients who undergo spinal fusion have had previous back surgery, and the parts of the vertebrae that were involved do not usually include the transverse processes and facets. Therefore, the bone of the bed for the fusion graft is still normal. The second reason is that, following spinal fusion, the disks immediately superior to the fused area may rupture because they become subject to more trauma; a posterolateral fusion allows a surgeon to remove a protruding disk without going through the fusion site.

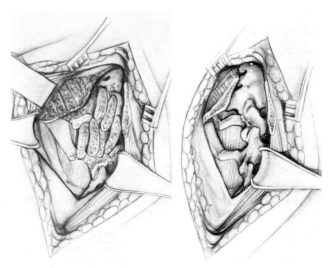

The lateral bed for this fusion extends from the tip of the transverse process to its base and from the superior facet along the pars interarticularis to the inferior facet. The size of the lateral graft site, the total amount of bone covered, and the blood supply have been cited by some sources as the reasons why this particular spinal fusion has good results.

Probably a more significant reason is that the posterolateral fusion site is near the center or axis of motion of the vertebra. This decreases the chance that there will be motion at the fusion site, which would result in a *pseudoarthrosis*, or "false joint."

The ilium is usually preferred as a source of bone graft because it is composed of cancellous bone. Also, a graft from the ilium can be taken through the same incision that is made for fusion in the lumbar region.

Indications for Spinal Fusion

A spinal fusion is done to eliminate motion in a section of the spine and to relieve pain. The conditions that warrant this procedure include the following:

1. Degenerative disk disease at a single level
2. Spondylolisthesis, or the forward slipping of one vertebra on another
3. Active tuberculosis of the spine
4. Selected fracture
4. Scoliosis
6. Failure of other methods of treatment to relieve chronic back pain sufficiently

In treatment of these particular conditions, many surgeons consider spinal fusion to be the last resort because of the risk of recurrent problems or the development of pseudoarthrosis at the fusion site.

Aftertreatment

How to treat a patient who has had a spinal fusion, in terms of activity and external back support, is a matter of opinion. Although this treatment depends somewhat on the type of fusion and the pathological condition, it is generally a matter of surgeon's preference.

The incidence of pseudoarthrosis seems to be the same no matter how early patients begin ambulating. Although 5 days of bed rest is not uncommon, a spinal fusion patient may be out of bed in 48 hours and ambulating independently in 5 days.

External support is provided by casts, orthoplast jackets, or braces.

Preoperative Care and Instruction

Generally, preoperative teaching about postoperative routines is the same for a patient scheduled for spinal fusion as for one undergoing a laminectomy.

Besides becoming acquainted with hospital routines and learning what is expected of him and what he can expect from others, the patient should be informed that some pain or discomfort in the hip, due to removal of bone from the iliac crest for grafting, is to be expected.

A number of the patient's questions will center on his fear of spinal surgery and whether or not his mobility will be

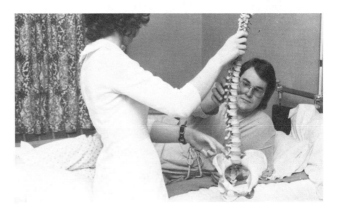

limited because of the fusion. The nurse must reinforce the surgeon's explanation, allow the patient to express his concerns, and help him achieve a comfortable state of mind.

Before the operation, the patient may be fitted for some type of back brace, or orthosis, which he will have to wear postoperatively when out of bed. He is discharged with this brace; how long it must be worn is a decision that is made by the surgeon for each individual patient.

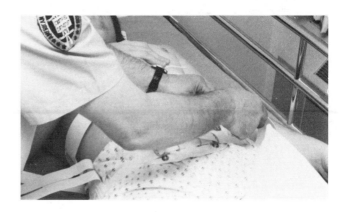

Postoperative Transfer

In some hospitals it is routine to take the patient's bed to surgery. However, if he has to be transferred to bed on the orthopedic unit, at least four people are necessary to assist with the procedure. There must be enough "hands" to hold the ends of the stretcher sheet along the side of the patient's

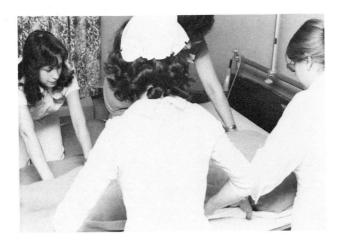

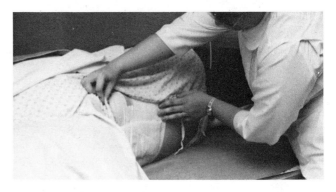

body so that his back does not sag during transfer. The postoperative bed must have a solid bottom or bedboards to provide good back support.

Vital Signs

Spinal fusion operations take longer than laminectomies and involve more blood loss. Thus, in the immediate postoperative period, the patient may appear pale, with a lower blood pressure, increased pulse rate, and other signs of the shock state. Vital signs need to be checked frequently until they are stable and then every 3 hours for 24 hours.

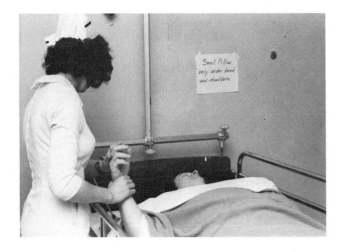

Dressing and Drainage

Slight oozing of blood from the incision for about the first 24 hours is not uncommon in these patients, and the dressing may need to be reinforced. The dressing must be checked at least every 3 hours for 24 to 48 hours, or longer if the patient exhibits signs of shock. Leakage of cerebrospinal fluid is always a possiblility; therefore, if the dressing is "wet" (not with urine), it should be reported to the surgeon. Because

the incision is over the lumbar spine, it may become contaminated with urine. When this happens, the dressing should be changed. Some surgeons use a wound drainage system which remains in the incision for 24 to 48 hours. These need be emptied only when they appear full or decompressed, unless other orders are given. The nurse should be aware of what the surgeon considers "too much" drainage in order to report concerns. The apparatus should be placed so that the tubing is free of kinks and the container is not under any part of the patient's body.

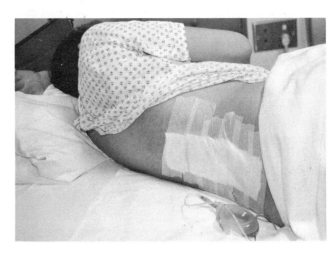

Positioning and Turning

Surgeons, even in the same hospital, differ in orders about the postoperative position of the bed and the patient. Therefore, the nurse should make certain that written orders are clear and complete on this point. If the patient is to be kept flat or immobile for a specific length of time, a sign should be placed on the head of the bed or on the overhead frame. Whether or not a flat pillow is permitted under head, neck, and shoulders should also be spelled out.

The nurse must know if the patient is to be positioned on his back, side, or abdomen, and how far he may be turned on his side. The important point is to keep the body in good alignment and the spine from twisting.

Regardless of what a nurse has been taught about placing pillows, not all patients are comfortable in the same position. For instance, some people are never comfortable on their backs or abdomen for very long and will move their own pillows around to promote comfort if left too long in one position. Much placing and replacing of pillows may be required . The implication here is that positioning the patient and placing the call light within his reach does not mean he is "set" for 3 hours. Frequent observation constitutes good nursing practice.

Supporting the entire length of the legs on flat pillows may be beneficial in relieving strain on the lower back, but the nurse must check every hour to make certain that the

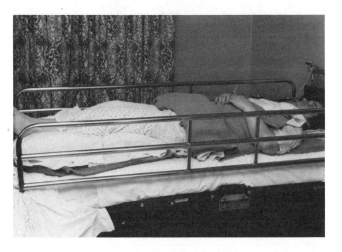

patient has not maneuvered the pillows so that his knees are in flexion. Although the patient may consider this an even more comfortable position, it is not advisable, because the folded pillow under the knee puts pressure on the popliteal space.

When the patient is positioned on his side he should be lying with his spine straight and his hips pulled slightly back to maintain balance. The upper leg should be flexed and a pillow should be placed between the legs. Placing a pillow crosswise so that one end supports his upper arm while the other end rests against his chest will also provide a resting place for his lower arm.

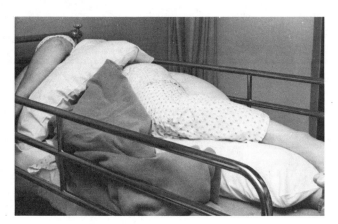

If the physician permits, the patient should be logrolled every 3 hours. The procedure for logrolling the patient with a spinal fusion is the same as for a laminectomy patient (p. 137). A turning sheet may be used but is not required.

At all times, turning and positioning the patient requires extreme caution. Twisting of the spine is detrimental to healing in the graft site and may be the cause of pseudoarthrosis.

Pain and Analgesics

The amount of pain and spasm experienced following spinal fusion varies considerably from patient to patient and is partly related to the symptoms the patient had preoperatively. Spinal-cord edema and irritation of nerves during surgery are also responsible for postoperative discomfort. Medication should be offered to the patient every 3 to 4 hours for the first 48 hours.

Often the patient complains of as much pain in the donor site as in the operative site. If the bone graft is taken from the tibia, the nurse must take into consideration the fact that leg movement will be painful. It is important for nurse and patient to realize that symptoms that were present preoperatively in terms of pain and spasm may persist for a period of time after surgery. Proper positioning in good body alignment helps keep the patient comfortable.

Other Nursing Considerations

In general, nursing care and observations relative to functioning of body systems and neurovascular status of extremities are comparable to those outlined for the patient who has had a laminectomy (pp. 138–140).

Several aspects of care, however, require special comment. These are as follows:

1. Bedpan Procedure. The patient with a spinal fusion should have his back and legs supported while he is on the bedpan, so that his entire body is as level as possible.

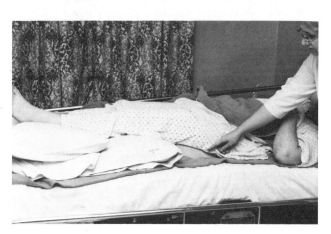

2. Skin Care. The skin of the patient who must remain in any one position for a prolonged period is susceptible to reddened areas over bony prominences. Frequent massage is indicated, along with visual inspection, if possible.

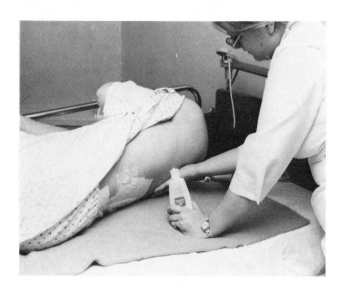

When the Patient Remains on Bed Rest

Conscientious nursing management, including attention to the everyday habits and routines of the patient such as having bowel movements, drinking fluids, and eating properly, will help to prevent constipation and urinary problems. In the patient who must be on prolonged bed rest, these are major concerns.

In daily assessment of pain or muscle spasms in a patient immobilized for this length of time, the nurse should bear in mind that thrombophlebitis is a possible and serious complication. Elastic stockings are a preventive measure. The use of respiratory support systems, such as IPPB treatments or the incentive spirometer, may be required if deep breathing and coughing do not keep the lungs clear.

No matter how long he is bedridden, or how comfortable he has become, this patient must still be handled gently and turned without twisting his body. Proper support with pillows should always be given to his entire back when he is on his side, and a pillow should remain between his legs.

A change of position and back care should be scheduled at least four times a day.

A consultation with the surgeon should precede any exercise of the legs other than moving the lower legs with the hips and knees flexed. Exercises that place strain on the lower back (straight leg-raising) are contraindicated. Range of motion for the feet and ankles (rather than a footboard), as well as range of motion for the upper extremities, should be done at least five times daily. A bed cradle may be used to keep bedding off the feet.

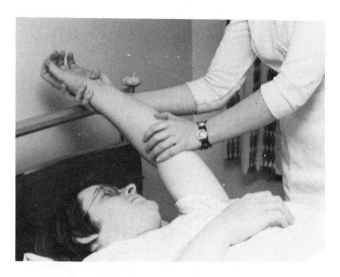

Boredom could be a major problem. Flexibility in scheduling nursing routines may make it possible for the patient to watch television programs of his choice, read, or have visitors when he is in the mood.

Dangling

Having the patient sit on the edge of the bed and dangle his feet within 24 to 48 hours after surgery is often routine.

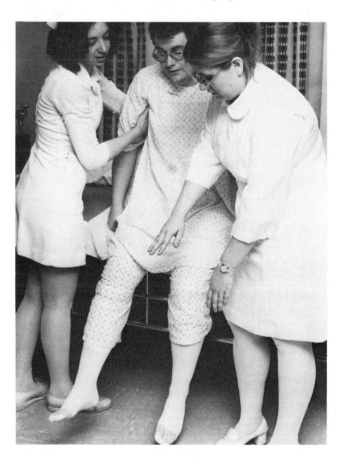

With a spinal fusion patient, as with a laminectomy patient, the surgeon may wish to do this procedure himself the first time it is done. When the responsibility is placed on her, the nurse must take care that the patient's body is not twisted. The steps in getting the patient to a sitting position, as described under care of the laminectomy patient, should be followed (p. 140).

The Orthosis or Brace

The purpose of postoperative bracing in a patient who has had a spinal fusion is to splint the spine. Usually the brace is not applied until shortly *before the patient is allowed out of bed*. A certified orthotist applies the apparatus for the first

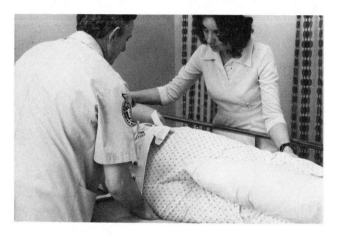

time, and in doing so, instructs the nurse. To apply the brace, the patient must be logrolled to his side and the brace applied from the back.

Although many types of braces are used for lumbar support, basically they all fit the patient in the same way. The brace must be applied so that the upper part of the buttocks is held snugly. Yet it should not be so low that it impinges on the groin when the patient is sitting. Dorsal uprights, com-

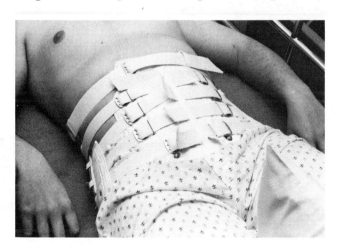

monly made of stainless steel, fit on either side of the spine, close enough to lie between the scapulae but not pressing on the vertebral prominences.

Once the brace is in place, the patient is rolled back and any pressure points are relieved. The abdominal support must be laced more snugly at the lower end than near the top.

After the sutures are removed, some sort of lightweight knit material similar to stockinette, such as an undershirt, may be worn under the orthosis to make it more comfortable.

The brace will be worn until solid bony union occurs at the fusion site as indicated by x-ray. How long this takes varies from patient to patient.

Ambulation and Activity

Two or three days after surgery, the patient may be allowed to stand at the bedside and take a few steps in the room. When he gets up for the first time, he will be lightheaded and weak and will, therefore, need physical and emotional support. This means at least two people must be present throughout the procedure. The patient must also be relaxed if he is to be cooperative.

Often the surgeon prefers to bring the patient slowly from a supine to a standing position, especially if he has been on prolonged bed rest. In this case, the tilt table is the best method for getting the patient out of bed. The patient's

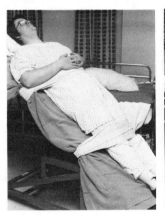 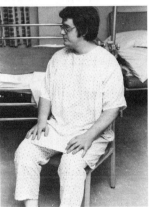

head must be elevated slowly and he must be observed for dizziness and nausea.

When the patient is permitted to sit up in a chair, he must be provided with one that is straightbacked and allows him to place his feet flat on the floor.

In fusions for which a brace is not used postoperatively, the patient must be taught not to flex the lower back. In all probability such a patient will be apprehensive, and nothing could induce him to move his lower back anyway. Nevertheless, the instruction should be given. The patient who has a brace should never get up without it.

All patients should wear slippers with nonskid soles; stockings and shoes that provide good foot support are indicated as soon as the patient is able to ambulate for any length of time.

The amount of ambulation and activity allowed the patient who has had a spinal fusion varies according to the procedure performed and the protocol of the surgeon.

The earliest that independent ambulation is allowed is about the fifth postoperative day.

The Body Cast

Postoperatively, a patient may be placed in a body cast, which he must wear for several months. The cast may be made of plaster or a synthetic material and is applied to the patient after the sutures have been removed and the patient is ready to ambulate. Until the patient regains strength and becomes accustomed to lying in bed and turning over in a body cast, he will require help and instruction.

When the patient in a body cast is being turned from his back to his abdomen, he must first be moved over to the edge of the bed. Two nurses, one on each side of the bed, can then logroll him onto his abdomen. He is instructed to put his arms above his head and remain rigid while being turned. A pillow is placed between his legs, and support is given to his shoulders and buttocks, as well as to the cast. Once on his abdomen, he will need to be moved back to the center of the bed. His legs should be placed on a pillow with his feet hanging over the edge of it, so his toes do not dig into the mattress.

Lying on the abdomen may be awkward at first, but it is beneficial to circulation and relieves pressure on the back, legs, and heels. The ease with which a patient adjusts to this position depends on how efficiently he is turned, how comfortably he is positioned, and whether or not the nurse has explained why it is necessary.

As with a brace, the body cast is worn until x-ray films demonstrate solid bony union at the fusion site. Cast finishing, maintenance, and general care after discharge are discussed in Chapter 2.

Discharge Planning for the Spinal-Fusion Patient

Exactly what kind of assistance and how much planning are needed depend on the patient's general condition and the surgeon's instruction about activity. It is helpful if a nurse is with the surgeon when this instruction is given. This enables her to answer questions from the patient and the family as they arise. Having the patient go over the modification of activity as explained by the surgeon and the rules for posture and exercise will help determine how well the patient understands their importance. How soon the patient resumes normal activities depends to a large extent on his preoperative diagnosis.

Independent teaching by the nurse is appropriate in the realm of safety measures. Patients who have had spinal fusions should be cautioned against doing activities "in a hurry." For example, walking too fast does not always permit a patient to watch where he is going, and turning his ankle when stepping off a curb or walking on uneven surfaces would jar his spine and perhaps even cause him to make a twisting movement. Safety also includes avoiding fatigue.

Care of the Patient With Scoliosis

Definition

Scoliosis is a lateral curvature of the spine. It is described as a *C-shaped* or *S-shaped* curve according to the deviation of the spinal column that occurs. The "C-curve" is called a

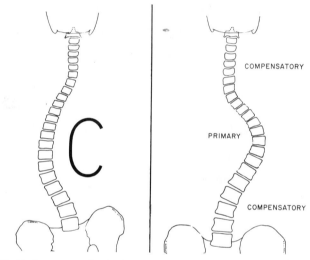

(*Left*) C-curve scoliosis. (*Right*) S-curved scoliosis (Hoppenfeld: Scoliosis, Philadelphia, Lippincott)

simple or total curve. In an "S-curve", or compound curve, there is a primary and secondary, or compensatory, curve.

Spinal deformity in scoliosis may be thoracic, lumbar, or thoracolumbar. Curvatures of the thoracic spine are usually right-sided, as are thoracolumbar curvatures. Curvatures of the lumbar spine are usually left-sided.

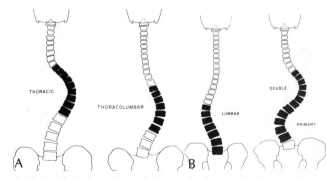

(A) Right-sided thoracic and thoracolumbar scoliosis curvature. (B) Left-sided lumbar curvature (Hoppenfeld: Scoliosis, Philadelphia, Lippincott)

Functional Scoliosis

Functional or postural scoliosis means that there is no fixed deformity of the spinal column.

Poor posture due to muscle weakness is a common cause of the appearance of a lateral curve. In this instance, exercises and the formation of new postural habits cause the scoliosis to disappear.

A leg-length discrepancy also causes functional scoliosis, because the righting reflex of the spine attempts to place the occiput over the sacrum as the individual stands erect. Elevating one shoe or equalizing leg length corrects the condition.

Structural Scoliosis

In structural scoliosis there is deformity of the vertebral bodies, causing lateral curvature of the spine to develop. As

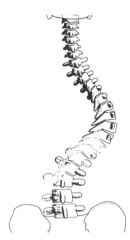

Vertebral rotation in scoliosis (Hoppenfeld: Scoliosis. Philadelphia, Lippincott)

deviation increases, the vertebral bodies tend to rotate toward the convexity of the curve, and one vertebra turns upon another in the longitudinal axis.

Types of Structural Scoliosis

Congenital Scoliosis. Congenital scoliosis is usually related to an anomaly of the vertebral body.

1. The most common anomaly is the hemivertebra, or half of a vertebra, which acts as a wedge between two normal vertebrae. (See following figure, left.) This congenital anomaly is characterized by an incomplete development of one side of a vertebra. More than one vertebra may be involved.
2. Congenital bars of bone that act as staples and keep the vertebra or vertebrae from growing on one side turn them into wedged vertebrae. (See following figure, right.) The vertebrae on the concave side of the curve are under greater compression forces, which causes wedging.

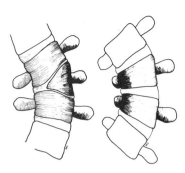

(*Left*) Hemivertebra. (*Right*) Wedged vertebrae. (Hoppenfeld: Scoliosis. Philadelphia, Lippincott)

Musculoskeletal Scoliosis. Musculoskeletal scoliosis occurs when muscles pull on the spine in an imbalanced way. Poliomyelitis, although rare now, is an example of paralysis due to disease, which is one cause of this type of scoliosis. Muscle imbalance on either side of the spine does not permit the spine to grow normally.

Idiopathic Scoliosis. Idiopathic scoliosis means that the pathology is unknown. It is the most common type of scoliosis and falls into three classifications: infantile, idiopathic, juvenile idiopathic, and adolescent idiopathic.

Infantile idiopathic scoliosis almost always occurs in boys and consists of left thoracic and right lumbar curves. When it does occur in girls, the curvature is right thoracic and left lumbar. Frequently, these curves straighten out by age 3 or 4. If they progress 20 degrees, they must be braced. Juvenile idiopathic scoliosis appears in both boys and girls, usually between ages 2 to 5. The type of curve varies and almost always responds to nonoperative treatment such as bracing and exercises. Adolescent idiopathic scoliosis predominantly affects girls and does not disappear spontaneously. The curvature occurs during the rapid growth that begins at about 10 years of age.

Idiopathic scoliosis, particularly in the preadolescent or adolescent periods, is the condition that will be under discussion in later sections. This form of scoliosis is the one most commonly encountered by the orthopedic nurse in the hospital setting.

Miscellaneous Causes. Other, rare, causes of structural scoliosis are tumors of the ribs or spinal cord, lung diseases such as empyema, metabolic bone disease, and hysteria, to mention a few.

Clinical Findings

As lateral curvature of the spine occurs and compensatory curves develop to maintain body balance, the deformity may not be evident unless one is looking for it. Diagnosis may be delayed by the fact that scoliosis rarely presents subjective symptoms until the deformity is well established. These subjective symptoms include fatigue, dyspnea, and backache. The modesty of the teenager, that is, a reluctance to have her parents "look" at her, is another contributing factor in delayed diagnosis. Many parents notice "something wrong" when a hemline is uneven or slack legs are different lengths.

When examined, the patient should be standing with feet together. A tape measure (plumb line) is then dropped from

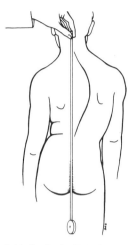

Plumb line. (Hoppenfield: Scoliosis. Philadelphia, Lippincott)

the occiput. The amount of lateral deviation of the spine should be noted. If the plumb line passes through the gluteal fold, the spine is usually considered balanced or compensated.

When the patient's back is exposed and examined, a discrepancy in shoulder height, elbow level, and the height of the iliac crests is found, plus infolding of one loin and flattening of the other.

Asymmetry of the paraspinal muscles may be noted. The muscles on the convex side of a curve are rounded out, and those on the concave side are flattened.

On the convex side of the curve, the shoulder is higher and the ribs protrude backward. In scoliosis of the lumbar spine, the patient commonly has a more prominent hip and a hollow waistline on the concave side of the curve. In relation to the pelvis, the thorax deviates laterally.

The range of motion of the spine in all directions is helpful in evaluating the rigidity of a curve. When the patient bends forward to a right angle at the hips, protrusions of the rib cage, shoulder blade, and iliac crest may sometimes be noted, depending on the shape, direction, and severity of the curve.

X-rays taken with the patient bending as far as possible laterally, first to one side and then the other, demonstrate the primary curve. This curve is the one that is least flexible and therefore least correctable. Other x-rays may be taken with the patient supine, shoulders and pelvis kept flat on the table, and the trunk bent laterally in each direction to the point of discomfort.

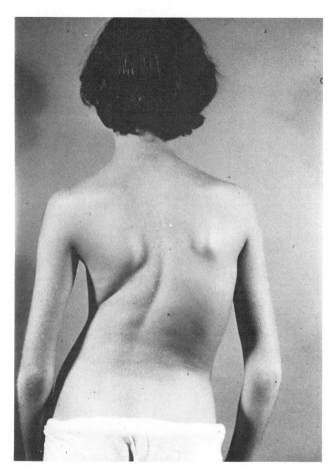

(O'Connor BJ: Scoliosis: Classification and diagnosis in pediatric orthopedics. ONAJ 3:84, Mar 1976)

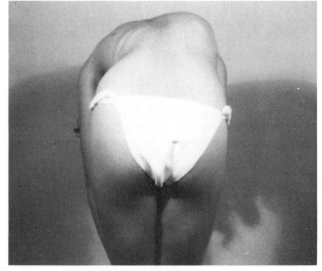

(O'Connor BJ: Scoliosis: Classification and diagnosis in pediatric orthopedics. ONAJ 3:84, Mar 1976)

In any instance of scoliosis, a standing x-ray confirms the diagnosis and allows the degree of the curve to be measured and any associated deformity identified. Photographs

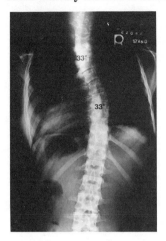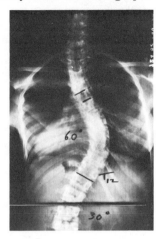

X-ray films showing *(Left)* scoliosis curve of 33 degrees (O'Connor: ONAJ 3:84, Mar 1976), and *(Right)* curve of 60 degrees (Courtesy Zimmer Co. Warsaw, Ind)

of the patient are taken and used following treatment for as a "before and after" comparison of body asymmetry.

Considerations on Treatment

Angle of the Curve. Variables that are considered in deciding on the course of treatment include age of onset and size and pattern of the curve. The younger the child is when the curve is observed, the greater the chance of deformity, because the curve progresses during growth periods. When the main curve is in the thoracic spine, progression to deformity is more likely.

The angle of the curve is determined by the Cobb method of measurement, as indicated in the following example.

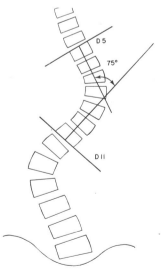

Measurement of spinal curve (Turek: Orthopaedics Philadelphia, Lippincott, 1977)

1. The top vertebra in the curve (D5) is the first of the upper vertebrae whose top or superior surface tilts toward the concave side of the curve being measured.
2. The bottom vertebra in the curve (D11) is the lowest vertebra whose bottom or inferior surface tilts toward the concave side of the curve.
3. Perpendicular lines are drawn from the superior surface of the top vertebra and the inferior surface of the bottom vertebra of the curve. The angle formed by the intersecting perpendiculars is the angle of the curve.

Emotional Factors. Any treatment requires an extended period of time with frequent evaluations of progress. Close cooperation between physician, child, and parents is essential if treatment is to be successful. Therefore, the attitudes of the parents and the emotional status of the child must always be considered in the presentation of facts and plans. *Trust* is the key word and is established through rapport and teaching.

NONSURGICAL TREATMENT

Exercise

A child with a curve of less than 20 degrees is given a program of exercise to follow and is instructed by the physician to return in 3 months for a follow up x-ray. Exercise programs are designed to strengthen the torso muscles and keep the curve from progressing. A typical set of instructions for exercise is as follows:

1. **Pelvic Tilt.** Lie on your back with your knees flexed or bent. Push the lower part of the back down against the floor or exercise table, keeping the abdomen pulled in and buttocks slightly raised. Hold this position for a count of 5 and then relax. Repeat the exercise 10 times.

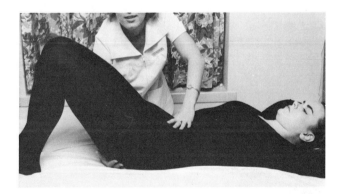

2. **Situp Pelvic Tilt.** While lying on your back with knees bent, tilt the pelvis and come to a half-sitting position. Hold this for a count of 5 and then slowly lower the body to the

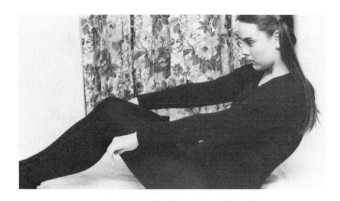

floor or table and release tilt. Repeat 10 times. If the situp is difficult with the knees bent, begin with the knees straight, until abdominal muscles become stronger.

3. Hyperextension. While lying on your stomach, tilt the pelvis by tightening the abdominal muscles. Bring shoulders back with head up. Have someone exert pressure between shoulder blades. hold for a count of 5. Relax. Repeat 10 times.

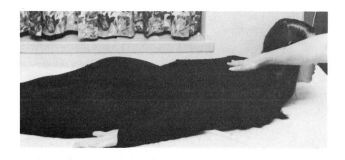

4. Pushups. While lying on your stomach, tilt the pelvis by tightening the abdominal muscles and then do a pushup. *Keep the body straight,* and lower slowly, nose touching the floor or table first. Release tilt. Repeat exercise 10 times.

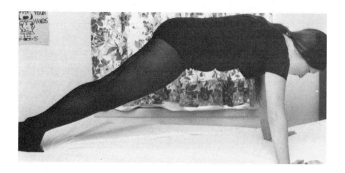

5. Wall Exercise. Stand against the wall, with the heels 4 inches away from the wall. Tilt the pelvis by pushing the

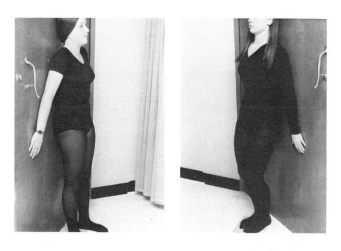

lower back against the wall. Then try to walk maintaining the tilt *Always try to walk* with the pelvis tilted.

6. Breathing Exercises. The child with a thoracic curve must be taught to spend time each day concentrating on deep breathing to promote adequate lung expansion.

ORTHOTIC TREATMENT

The child whose curve progresses 3 to 4 degrees in three months on an exercise program, in other words, fom 20 to 24 degrees, is commonly placed in a brace. The purpose of the brace is to balance the curves in the back and to halt progression. It does not reverse the scoliosis.

Scoliosis orthoses fall into one of two categories: cervico-thoraco-lumbo-sacral orthoses (CTLSO) and thoraco-lumbo-sacral orthoses (TLSO). The CTSLO is an orthosis that includes a neck ring, as in the Milwaukee brace. A TLSO is an orthosis that does not encompass the neck region, as in the various low-profile orthoses. A Milwaukee brace (CTLSO) is utilized for curves in which the apex of the curve is above T8. A low profile brace (TLSO) is utilized for curves in which the apex is below T8.

The Milwaukee brace consists of a pelvic girdle that fits snugly and holds three uprights with a neck ring. The posterior uprights are made of steel and are placed on either side of the spine. The anterior upright is made of aluminum to allow x-rays to be taken. All three uprights support the throat mold and occiput pads, which are adjusted so that the patient's head is just above the supports and distracts the spine. A lateral holding pad is attached to the uprights below the apex of the major curve to apply medial pressure.

The low profile braces consist of a one-piece shell made from plastic and fit snugly to stabilize the pelvis. The linings are generally of soft foam. The lumbar lordosis is markedly reduced. Pads to provide lateral corrective forces are built into the brace. TLSOs, are called "low-profile orthoses because they do not have a metallic superstructure.

The posterior opening of the orthosis is the width of one vertebra, which allows the lumbar pad to push on the transverse processes of the vertebral column so as to derotate the spine. This type of orthosis is more cosmetically acceptable to the patient.

The Milwaukee brace metal superstructure is adjustable so that it can "grow" with the patient. The pelvic sections of the Milwaukee and the low-profile braces must be refabricated to accommodate growth. Scoliosis orthosis (braces) must be worn until bone growth is completed. The average wearing time is 34 months, with the range between 1 and 8 years, depending on the patient's age when treatment is begun. The patient and family should know how the brace is supposed to fit and understand the importance of visiting the orthopedic surgeon and the orthotist for regular adjustments and follow-up x-ray films. Appointments are necessary about every 3 months.

Initially, the patient may only be allowed to remove the brace for bathing. This means spending 23 hours a day in that brace, and for a child or teenager, this may create emotional stress, requiring a great deal of support from family and friends.

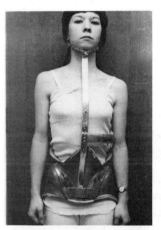
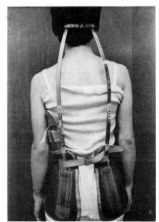

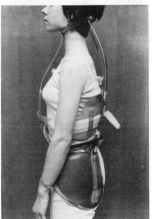

The Milwaukee brace as seen from *front*, *back*, and *side*.

Special exercises are a part of the therapy, and they should be taught before the brace is applied. The basis of all the exercises is the pelvic tilt. Two types of exercises are indicated for the scoliosis patient in the braces. The first group deals with strengthening the abdominal muscles, whose activity is automatically restricted by the brace itself. The exercises for the scoliosis patient described on pages 155 and 156 can be modified for the patient in a brace.

Skin care is very important to prevent skin breakdown. The skin under the brace needs to be toughened, especially where the brace presses the hardest. To protect the skin, the patient must bathe daily and apply rubbing alcohol to all parts of the skin that the brace covers, especially the areas where the skin is pink. The alcohol, in addition to the friction between the hand and the body, toughens the skin. Under the brace the patient must always wear a 100% cotton undershirt or T-shirt, without side seams, to absorb perspiration and prevent heat rashes. Creams, lotions, or powder are contraindicated because they soften the skin. Good skin care also requires that the brace be washed each day with alcohol and water.

The second set of exercises is designed to diminish to major curve and rib deformities. There are two routines. The first consists of tilting the pelvis and then taking a deep breath to round out the back posteriorly against the thoracic pad. The second exercise is done by tilting the pelvis and holding the tilt while shifting the torso toward the concavity of the major curve.

Patients are usually encouraged to increase rather than decrease their participation in all activities at home and at school, with the exception of strenuous gymnastics and contact sports.

Weaning from a brace depends on skeletal maturity and how well correction of the curve is maintained when the brace is removed. Skeletal maturity usually occurs in a girl at approximately 18 years of age. For a boy it may occur closer to 20. Before a child is allowed to spend any length of time out of the brace, the brace should be removed for several hours and an x-ray film taken to determine the

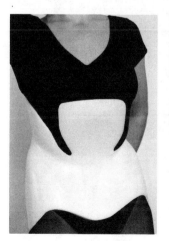
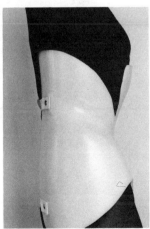

A thoraco-lumbo-sacral (TLSO) low-profile brace as seen from *front* and *side*.

stability of correction. The time out of the brace is gradually increased as stability improves.

The greatest stimulus to exercising is knowing that maintaining and improving muscle tone may result in longer periods out of the brace once weaning is begun.

The scoliosis brace is usually worn at night for a year or two following skeletal maturity.

While misery may love company, by the same token, any communication that a physician or nurse can establish between adolescents in scoliosis orthoses may prove supportive and helpful to both.

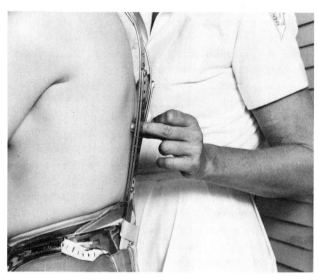

(Blount WP, Moe JH: The Milwaukee Brace. Baltimore, Williams & Wilkins, 1973. Photos courtesy ONAJ)

Halo Traction

The *halo* is a metal traction device that is attached by four pins, under anesthesia, to the outer table of the skull to immobilize the head and neck. It is used in the treatment of

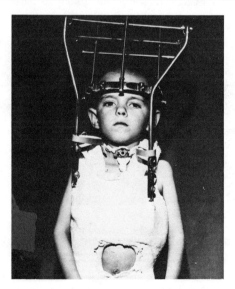

Halo traction. (From Perry J: The halo in spinal abnormalities. Orthop Clin North Am 3(1):68, 1972)

paralytic scoliosis when the cervical and thoracic spine are involved. A body cast or Milwaukee brace may be attached to the halo. The molding of the cast or brace over the pelvic portion of the body provides the countertraction. An advantage of the brace is that it does not further restrict chest expansion in a patient who may already have decreased respiratory function. However, the brace does not provide rigid spinal immobilization as does the body cast. Both forms of traction allow the patients to be ambulatory

Halo Distal Skeletal Fixation

Skeletal traction for a distal pull may be applied by use of a pelvic hoop, similar to the halo, or by inserting pins through the distal femurs or proximal tibias. The pelvic hoop is desirable for the management of severe thoracic and spinal malalignments and permits the patient to ambulate while maintaining fairly rigid spinal traction and immobilization.

Traction of the lower extremities is usually used prior to spinal fusion, and the patient is confined to bed for a period of 3 to 4 weeks. During this time, weights are gradually added to the traction apparatus. Nursing care of this type of patient is intensive owing to the prolonged period of bed rest and the fact that the patient may have a limited respiratory capacity. The appearance of the traction apparatus and the adjustment of weights may cause the patient apprehension; therefore, supportive care is a priority. A specially designed wheelchair for attachment of this type of traction may be used instead of placing the patient on bed rest.

INSERTION OF THE HARRINGTON ROD AND SPINAL FUSION

The patient with a curve of 45 degrees becomes a candidate for surgery, even if she has stopped growing. This is true because after skeletal maturity, a lateral curve continues to progress at the rate of about 1 degree a year.

Basic Principles and Procedures

Insertion of the Harrington rod after spinal fusion reduces the curve that is already present by means of a distraction rod on the concave side and a compression rod on the convex side. Alterations in this spinal instrumentation system to increase its strength, improve stability, or decrease the period of postoperative bracing are being made continually, but the basic principle of mechanical correction and spinal fusion remains the same.

Fusion of the spine is corrective and prevents progression of the scoliosis. In the area to be fused, the spinous processes and the facet joints are excised, and the lamellar surfaces are decorticated. Chips of bone from the spinous processes and the iliac crest are packed in this area, and then bone strips are laid down to linearize the fusion. The fusion of vertebrae is thus accomplished by a continuous mass of bone. The Harrington rod actually serves two pur-

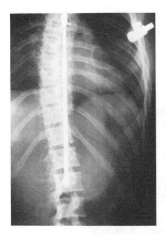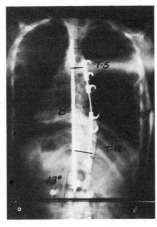

(Left) Harrington rod in place following spinal fusion. *(Right)* Harrington rod and compression rod. (Right photo courtesy Zimmer Co, Warsaw, Ind)

poses. It jacks up and straightens the spine. It also acts as an internal splint, allowing the fusion that has been done to go on to a solid union.

Psychological Considerations

Very often the patient who is scheduled for insertion of a Harrington rod is a teenager whose scoliosis was discovered accidentally on a routine physical examination, such as prior to going to camp. With the establishment of state programs for screening scoliosis in the public schools, more cases are being detected in the early stages. But in the meantime those adolescents who suddenly learn they have a serious curvature of the spine experience a number of shocks before that of surgery.

The orthopedic surgeon who first shows the diagnostic x-ray film to parent and child will be faced with reactions from disbelief to panic. Most probably, the patient was a referral from a family doctor or a screening clinic, and the relationship between the orthopedic surgeon and the patient and her parents is a new one. The patient and her family are very likely overwhelmed at the prospect of this surgery and

the alterations in life-style that will be necessary for the patient and the whole family.

Along with other feelings, the patient may experience a sense of being suddenly set apart from her friends, different and alone. This is exactly what most teenagers do *not* want. The orthopedic nurse must have insight into some of the anxieties and problems to which this type of patient is prone and must be aware that when the patient is admitted to the hospital, she has already undergone emotional trauma. Although her basic needs are the same as those of any other teenager, her individual feelings and fears and how they are handled may determine her behavior pattern while she is hospitalized.

Preoperative Risser Cast

In preparation for Harrington-rod insertion, it is routine for many surgeons to admit the patient to the hospital 2 weeks before surgery for application of a Risser corrective cast. In this type of body cast, the corrective forces are applied by head and pelvic distraction and lateral pressure, just before and during the application of the cast. Over a 2-week period, the body cast stretches the ligamentous structure and muscles on each side of the spine to allow more correction. The cast is applied, allowed to dry, and the patient is discharged until the day before surgery.

In order to prepare the patient properly for the application of a Risser cast, the orthopedic nurse should be acquainted with the procedure. Although the surgeon and his assistants explain the process while applying the cast, the patient should have some previous knowledge of what to expect; otherwise, the sight of the Risser table alone would cause her much apprehension. Sometimes preoperative medication is ordered.

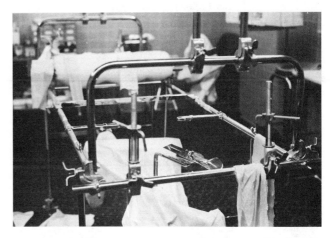

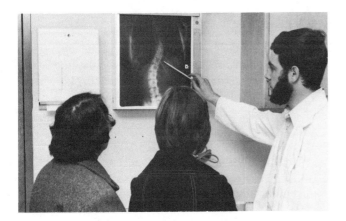

The cast is applied on what is called a Risser table, which is actually a large frame, not unlike a "torture rack" in appearance. The patient needs to know immediately that she will be completely supported by the frame and held in place by straps, and that there will be several assistants

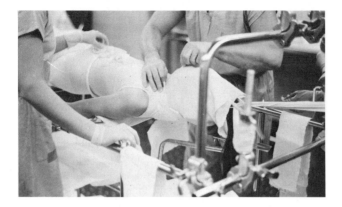

working with the doctor. She should know that she will be encased in stockinette, with only her limbs exposed. Her face will be covered a good deal of the time, to protect it from

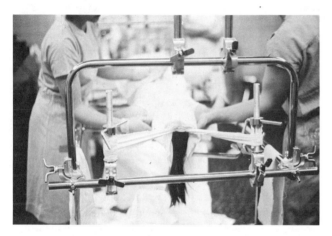

the plaster. Her neck will be stretched slightly by tightening the straps that secure her head at one end of the table. Muslin straps over her hips will provide the means to stretch the other end of her body. This stretching is done to reduce the curve and is not painful. The patient should be informed that an additional strap may be used to apply pressure on her chest. This is the Cotrel strap.

The cast will be applied by at least two pairs of hands and will be heavy and cold at first. It will gradually become hotter and then lighter as it dries and is cut away in places. The patient may be less fearful if she knows that casts are routinely trimmed with a scalpel and saw. She should also

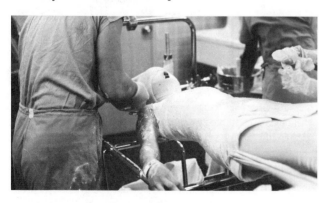

be told that she does not need to watch and, in fact, should close her eyes to keep them from being irritated by plaster dust.

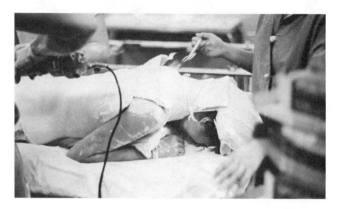

The finished product has a high collar and a large opening over the patient's stomach; it extends just far enough over hips and abdomen to provide support without digging into her thighs and buttocks when she sits down.

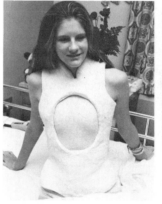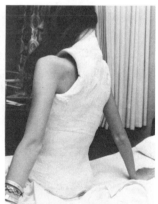

Nursing Responsibilities. During the 24 to 48 hours when the patient is waiting for the cast to dry, she must have her position changed every 3 hours. Her body and the cast must be supported by pillows during the drying process. If a synthetic cast has been applied, the drying process is quickly completed.

Petaling the cast should not be necessary, unless rough edges develop, because the stockinette is brought tightly over the edge and secured by plaster strips after the cast is applied. The edges should be inspected regularly to be certain that no pressure spots are present, and the skin directly under all edges should be kept dry. Plastic may be placed over the bottom edges of the cast when the patient uses a bedpan.

Patient Instruction. The patient and her family are instructed in the importance of keeping the cast dry, preventing skin breakdown, and reporting any persistent discomfort to the physician.

Preoperative Care for Harrington Rod Insertion

Admission to the orthopedic ward is not a new experience for the adolescent who arrives to have a Harrington rod inserted. She spent at least 48 hours there as a patient when

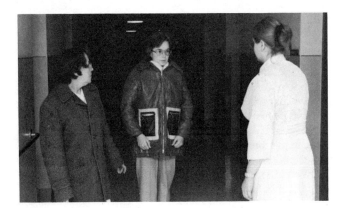

the Risser cast was applied 2 weeks earlier. Some of the staff look familiar. The nurse who greets her as if everyone has been "waiting" for her to come back will increase her feeling of security. She needs this emotional support, because she will be in the hospital for about 2 weeks and during much of the time she will be completely dependent on others for everything. Some guidelines for establishing rapport with the patient are presented in the chart on pages 161–162.

All of the postoperative routines are explained the day before surgery. The nurse should spend time with the patient and family to allow expression of feelings and to clarify anything about this hospitalization that they may have difficulty understanding.

Specific preoperative preparation of the patient may involve several things. Frequently, surgeons will order an in-

dwelling catheter to be inserted preoperatively. The cast is bivalved and removed. Occasionally a surgeon will request that the bottom half of the cast go to surgery with the patient. In this case it should be lightly lined with clean padding. The patient will return from surgery positioned in the bottom half of the cast and will remain in it while on bed rest to keep her back straight.

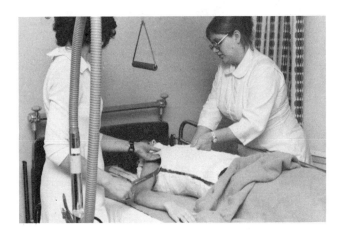

The bottom sheet of the bed is applied over an alternating pressure mattress or convoluted bedpad. Bedboards should automatically be in place.

Immediate Postoperative Care and Observations

The surgical procedure is a lengthy one, and the blood loss is considerable. Therefore, it is necessary to take and record vital signs every 15 minutes until stable, and then according to routine.

Coughing and deep breathing should be initiated as soon as possible and are especially important because of the change in the size of the chest cavity. Signs of respiratory

---

THE HARRINGTON-ROD PATIENT: ESTABLISHING RAPPORT IN THE PREOPERATIVE PERIOD

Patient Situation: Lynn, a 14-year-old, well-developed female, 5'5" tall, weighing about 125 lb. enters the hospital for insertion of a Harrington rod. She has two older sisters, ages 16 and 17, and two younger brothers, ages 8 and 6. Both sisters have had Harrington rods inserted. Lynn is in Jr. High, active in volleyball and in girls' chorus.

Considerations in Mental/Emotional/Social Assessment	Possible Approaches in Communication	Data Collection	Implications for Supportive Care
How does her physical development at age 14 affect her self-image and activities?	"You're tall enough to be a good volleyball player" or, "Nice thing about being tall, you stand in the back row on the stage!"	More eager to talk about volleyball than chorus. Is taller than all her girlfriends. Seems self-conscious?	Make note on the Kardex emphasizing that Lynn seems self-conscious about size and not to comment on her size for her age.

(Continued)

THE HARRINGTON-ROD PATIENT:
ESTABLISHING RAPPORT IN THE PREOPERATIVE PERIOD (*Continued*)

Considerations in Mental/Emotional/Social Assessment	Possible Approaches in Communication	Data Collection	Implications for Supportive Care
What problems did her sisters have following surgery?	"This operation must have been frightening for your oldest sister and a different experience for your whole family."	Whole family was nervous about oldest sister's surgery. However, the only problem she had (at 15) was that she didn't want her boyfriend to see her in a cast. Evidently she endured much teasing because of this attitude. The second sister (surgery at 14) did not have a boyfriend and did not have any unexpected problems. Lynn has no special boyfriend. Both sisters got tired of being in bed and were apprehensive about application of the postoperative cast.	Recognize that patient expects to be bored while on bed rest, and plan accordingly. Have patient explain exactly what she knows about sisters' experience with postoperative cast application and instruct, clarify, and reassure as necessary.
Does she resemble her sisters physically?	"You and your sisters are close enough in age to share a lot, maybe even clothes."	Gets along "better" with both sisters now that they have part-time jobs. They do not share clothes with each other but they both share with her.	Talk to sisters to learn more about Lynn—little things she may be reluctant to mention but that may be helpful.
How significant is her place in the family (third girl and youngest child for 6 years before birth of first boy)?	"All those years without a boy in the family— someone must have been the tomboy."	None of the three girls were tomboys. Discussed the tomboy role and father–daughter relations. Father travels a lot. Not too involved with activities of any of the children except to fish with the boys. This does not seem to bother Lynn.	Mother will probably be source of needed information and most frequent visitor.
What are her relationships with her brothers, sisters, parents?	"Your mother has built-in babysitters for your brothers."	Little brothers are a "pain." Does a lot of babysitting with them. Also does most of housework, because mother works outside of home. Seems proud of ability to do housework but "hates" fact that "it never lasts."	Make a special effort to involve Lynn in decision making about her care, and acknowledge the fact that she is a capable and responsible young person. Also note that she may not always express her anxieties and may minimize her discomfort.

embarrassment should be reported to the surgeon, because a lung may have been punctured during the surgical procedure. The dressings should be checked frequently at first.

The patient should be turned, by two nurses, only as far as is necessary to visualize the dressing. Slight oozing of bloody drainage is normal in the very early postoperative period.

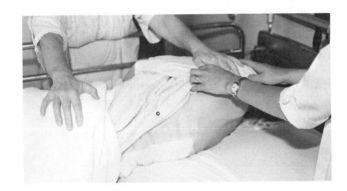

Paralysis is a dreaded complication of any spinal surgery. The neurovascular status of *all* extremities should be observed and recorded immediately and at 3-hour intervals for at least 24 hours. Thereafter, the motion and sensation of the extremities may be observed and recorded several times each day.

Intravenous antibiotics may be administered if the procedure was especially long and difficult. The insertion of a Harrington rod usually requires more time in an older adolescent. This is true because the bones of an 18-year-old, for example, are more rigid than those of a 13-year-old.

Positioning

Although surgeons vary in their orders regarding position, it is customary to keep the bed flat and allow the patient a folded bath blanket under the head.

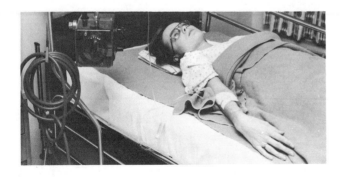

Logrolling 20 to 30 degrees on either side is usually permitted to give back care or place the bedpan. Extreme care must always be taken when logrolling the patient to

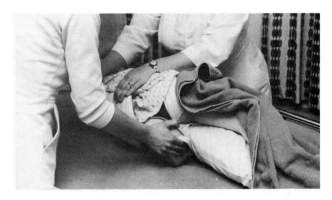

avoid twisting her body. A logrolling procedure has been described under laminectomies (pp. 137–138).

Pain and Discomfort

The amount of pain experienced by Harrington-rod patients is not great, considering the extent of surgery. Movement always produces pain, but generally speaking, narcotics every 4 hours for the first 24 hours keep the patient comfortable. After that, the intervals between pain medication are gradually lengthened. Muscle spasms are infrequent, but pain in the graft site on the iliac crest is a factor.

Abdominal Distention and Intake

Paralytic ileus is common following insertion of Harrington rods. For this reason oral intake is prohibited until function is reestablished. The patient must be able to expel flatus.

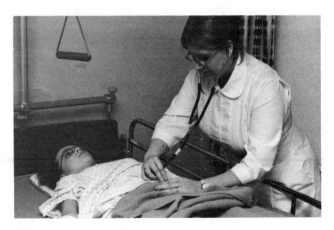

Intravenous fluids are ordered for an average of 3 to 4 days. When oral intake is allowed, it is administered sparingly at first in the form of ice chips only. Fluids and diet progress slowly and with careful observation of the patient's condition.

During the time that the patient is on bed rest, some abdominal distention may be present. If this condition causes undue discomfort, the surgeon may allow a moderate degree of knee flexion. Distention is sometimes one of

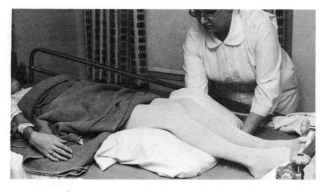

the main problems encountered in caring for a patient following insertion of a Harrington rod. A rectal tube should be inserted for periods of 20 to 30 minutes when the patient complains of flatulence.

Constipation should be avoided. Rectal suppositories may be ordered for insertion once or twice daily to stimulate the bowel.

Urinary Output

The indwelling catheter simplifies the recording of urinary output, which tends to be decreased in the early postoperative period. When the nurse observes that the patient is excreting small amounts of concentrated urine, the surgeon should be notified. With an increase in the rate of intravenous flow, the condition is gradually corrected.

Daily Observations and Care

Priorities in the postoperative assessment and care of the Harrington-rod patient are indicated in the accompanying chart. Good skin care is necessary, and the buttocks and back need special attention. Because the patient is restricted in how far she can be turned, rubs must be given on both sides, as far under as possible. Heel protectors, if used, should be removed three times a day, and the heels exposed, inspected, and rubbed.

THE HARRINGTON-ROD PATIENT: PRIORITIES IN POSTOPERATIVE ASSESSMENT AND CARE

Second Postoperative Day

7:00 A.M. Shift Report	*8:00 A.M. Assessment*	*Data Collected*	*Nursing Implications*
P.R., a 16-year-old patient who had a Harrington rod 2 days ago, did not have a particularly good night. Checked her at 6 A.M. She is still having periods of nausea and retching. Her abdomen is soft and flat, and she has faint bowel sounds in LUQ. She gets medication for nausea, but it only lasts several hours.	Check exactly when nausea is occurring. After pain medication? Auscultate abdomen. Is IPPB causing nausea? Does turning make her nauseous?	No specific time; same findings	Question possibility of IV antibiotics causing nausea, or is patient getting "flu?"
Complains of some discomfort in lower back, not incisional area.	Menstrual period due? Is pillow properly placed under knees? How often is this done? Does it seem to relieve strain on back muscles?	Period "may be due." Is irregular. Pillow under knees "does not help much." She becomes restless easily.	Increase back care, especially rubs in lumbosacral region q 2 hr.
She has a slight cough that she has had since surgery. Lungs are clear, and stir ups are nonproductive.	Auscultate lungs. Discuss cough with patient. Is she a smoker?	Admits to being a smoker. "Don't tell my mother!"	Order throat lozenges.

(Continued)

THE HARRINGTON-ROD PATIENT: PRIORITIES IN POSTOPERATIVE ASSESSMENT AND CARE (*Continued*)

Second Postoperative Day

7:00 A.M. Shift Report	8:00 A.M. Assessment	Data Collected	Nursing Implications
Toes sometimes feel "numb," but she can feel touch, has motion, and toes are warm. Pedal pulses are strong. Logrolls with assistance of one.	Check elastic hose for fit. Are they constricting around her thigh or wrinkling behind her knees? Are toes cold?	Hose seem snug but are not rolling down. Toes feel warm. She states they often feel cold.	Encourage range of motion for ankles and toes frequently. Remove hose q 6 hr for ½ hr. Keep feet and legs warm.
T. 100 P.100 R. 20 Intake: 100 ml IV Output: 510 ml dark amber urine	Check color of urine; has patient any burning or discomfort around catheter?	Urine same as reported. Negative for symptoms.	Question possibility of increasing IV rate.
Dressing dry and intact.			
Last pain medication 5:45 A.M.	Evaluate effect of pain medication and time desired.	Satisfactory. Would prefer it "just before bath."	Give IM pain medication 15 min before bath.

Short or long elastic stockings are ordered and should be removed daily when the bath is given.

Footboards are unnecessary because the patient should be exercising her feet. The nurse must encourage as much movement of limbs as the surgeon will allow. Any activity

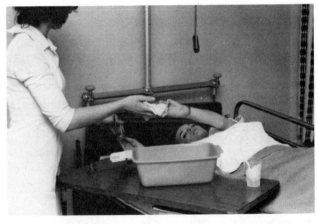

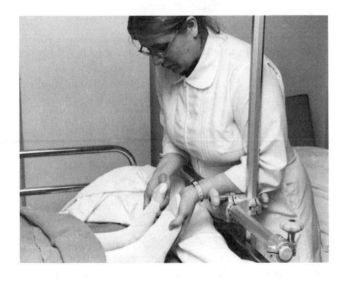

the patient can perform with her hands, such as bathing her own face and arms, involves range of motion and helps maintain muscle strength. Nurses often neglect to explain to the patient that the purpose of bathing herself is to provide her with exercise, not to relieve the nurse of her work. Quadriceps-setting exercises are equally beneficial.

Body temperature in excess of 102° for 2 or 3 days postoperatively is not unusual but should be reported and recorded. Continued inspection of the dressing at regular intervals is necessary to note any signs of drainage that would indicate developing wound infection.

Intermittent positive-pressure breathing treatments or the incentive spirometer are needed if the patient shows signs of respiratory congestion.

Psychological Aspects of Care

The moods of teenagers who have undergone this surgery may vary from day to day. Much of the time, when they are comfortable, they behave like any other individual of the same age. Understandably, though, they often have periods of depression or times when they appear withdrawn. Many of them tend to regress to a certain degree and exhibit childish behavior. It is not surprising if a 15-year-old girl decides that she cannot sleep without the presence of three stuffed animals in her bed.

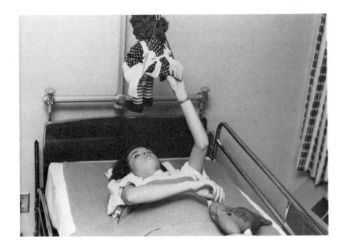

A major part of orthopedic nursing is concerned with supportive communication as patients cope with the concepts of an altered body image, long-term rehabilitation programs, and adjustments in life-styles. In the care of young patients following Harrington-Rod insertion, the importance of such communication cannot be overemphasized. To communicate therapeutically with them, the nurse must realize that their family situations are all as unique as their individual personalities. For example, the home life of one 13-year-old girl my be such that she will brood over who is doing her share of the housework. Another frets because tomorrow's weather forecast may prevent her mother from visiting her on her birthday.

Whatever her mental preoccupation, diversion should be provided when the patient is comfortable enough to become bored. Prism glasses make it possible to watch television and read.

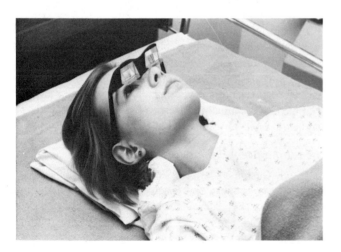

Rehabilitation Program

Sutures are usually removed after 10 to 14 days and a new Risser cast is applied. Current practice in the rehabilitation of patients with Harrington rods involves getting them out of bed when the new cast is dry. The rationale for this is that loading the spine helps to lay down more new bone. The first few times the patient gets up, a tilt table is used. Weakness, dizziness, and sometimes nausea are present when the patient becomes upright, and she is left on the tilt table until she feels able to stand. However, these patients are naturally eager to "get going" and respond positively to a smiling, encouraging therapist and supportive nurse.

The physical-therapy department assumes responsibility for the patient as she begins to stand and take steps. She is discharged when this goal is reached, probably after 2 or 3 days.

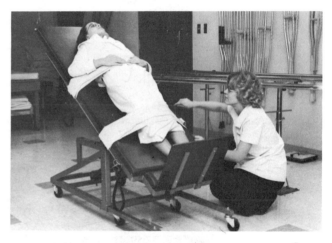

At the time of discharge, general cast-care instructions should be given, in writing, along with information about the importance of increasing daily activities at a slow rate, getting plenty of rest and eating a balanced diet. A typical set of written instructions that should go home with these patients appears below.

Every orthopedic nurse should make a home visit to a Harrington-rod patient. This provides insights for a nurse that are useful in teaching and planning for the next patient. For instance, the nurse learns what type of clothes look and wear best over a cast. The individuality of the teenage patient is demonstrated by the "tricks" she devises to keep herself mobile and independent. For example, one teenager learned that if she tied one end of a rope to the corner of the bed frame under the boxspring at the foot end of her bed and kept the rope on the floor next to her bed, she could reach down and pick it up and use it to pull herself up and out of bed.

It is helpful to both parents and child if they have the name and phone number of another Harrington-rod patient. The sharing of information can be invaluable in reducing frustration and maintaining a positive, health self-image.

SOME GENERAL INSTRUCTIONS FOR HOME CAST CARE FOR THE PATIENT WITH A HARRINGTON ROD

1. Make sure that the bed you sleep in has a firm mattress or bedboards.
2. Skin care is necessary around the edges of your cast. Rub the skin daily with lotion. Use alcohol for rubbing under the cast edges, because it will dry and leave no sticky feeling. Cornstarch in small quantities may be used under the cast edges that have the most contact with your skin.
3. When washing, use a damp washcloth that is not dripping, in order to avoid getting the cast wet.
4. Should the cast become wet, use a hairdryer to aid drying.*
5. Tape the edges of the cast if they begin to irritate the skin.
6. Do not wash the cast if it becomes soiled. Use a *small* amount of shoe polish to cover large soiled areas. A small amount of cleanser on a lightly dampened cloth will remove smaller soil spots.*
7. Use plastic around the edges of the cast when sitting on the toilet for bowel movements, if there is the slightest chance that the lower edge of the cast may become soiled. You may need a plastic covering during menstrual periods also.
8. Do not use knitting needles, hangers, or any other sharp pointed objects for scratching under the cast. Rough terrycloth may work, as may a belt (not the buckle end) slipped under the cast edge.
9. Report *any* pain, burning, pressure, loss of feeling, unusual feeling, or cast odor to the physician immediately.

* If your cast is synthetic, your doctor will tell you how wet you can get. Your cast can be dried off with a towel, and if you get the cast wet inside, use a hairdryer on "cool" to dry it. You can wash the cast off it if becomes soiled.

Cast Removal and a Brace

Total cast time varies with the individual surgeon. The patient may have a cast change in 3 months and remain in the cast for another 3 months before she goes into a thoracolumbar support. Or she may go into the support when the

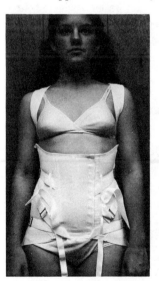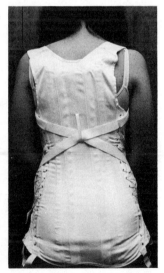

first postoperative cast is removed at 3 months. Some surgeons prefer longer periods of time in a cast and no back support when the last cast is removed; others use a brace once the final cast is off.

The cast is removed in the physician's office. The patient is forewarned that she may experience some weakness when the cast is first removed.

A thoracolumbar support is fitted and applied by an orthotist. This support stabilizes a long area of the spine and extends over the buttocks and shoulders. The orthotists shapes the metal stays to the contours of the patient's body. The thoracolumbar support is worn for 3 to 6 months and is removed only at night.

Dwyer Instrumentation

THE PROCEDURE

Dwyer instrumentation, also known as the Dwyer spinal technique or simply the Dwyer procedure, is another operation for the correction of scoliosis or lordosis. This procedure is used for severe lumbar and thoracolumbar curves, usually of paralytic origin, and employs an anterolateral approach to the convex side of the spinal column. The pleural cavity may be entered, depending on the curve that requires correction.

Intervertebral disks are removed. A staple is impacted over the first vertebral body that is to be instrumented, and a screw with a cannulated head is inserted into that vertebral body. Next, a cable is started through the head of the screw. The process is repeated down the length of the vertebrae that are to be included. Bone chips from a resected rib are placed between the vertebral bodies. Tension is then applied to the cables to shorten the distance between screws. The cable is locked by means of a button positioned next to the last screw head and is collared to prevent unraveling. Finally, the remainder of the cable is cut off.

Preoperative Preparation

Preparation of the patient's spine depends on the rigidity of the curve and include the previously mentioned procedures of traction or casting. Pulmonary function studies are mandatory to evaluate the risks to the patient who has impaired function and to provide guidelines for appropriate postoperative pulmonary support.

Postoperative Management

If the pleural cavity is entered, a chest tube is inserted and connected to closed water-seal drainage. The tube remains in place for about 72 hours, or until the lungs are reexpanded on x-ray and pleural drainage is less than 30 ml in 24 hours. A nasogastric tube may also be inserted and gastric suction maintained for 24 to 48 hours to keep the area around the operative site "quiet."

Postoperative management of the patient who has had Dwyer instrumentation is otherwise the same as that of a patient who has a Harrington rod.

Complications

The possibility of damaging the spinal cord, aorta, or vena cava is always present during Dwyer instrumentation. Atelectasis is an early postoperative complication because these patients tend to hypoventilate. The importance of close nursing observation and vigorous intermittent positive-pressure ventilation cannot be over emphasized. Other possible complications are fracture of the vertebral bodies, deep wound infection, and failure of the screw-and-cable system.

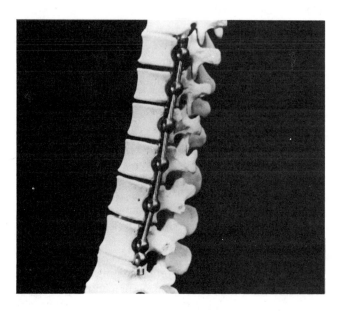

Segmental Spinal Instrumentation

The Luque method of segmental internal splinting of a scoliotic spine, along with a posterior spinal fusion, is a more recent development in this field. A disadvantage of this procedure is that the patient must be under general anesthesia for a prolonged period. The advantage of the technique is that it allows postoperative mobility without casting. The principles of nursing care are similar to those for the patient with a Harrington rod.

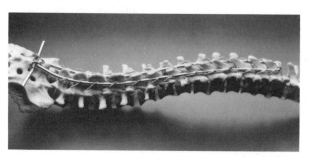

Luque segmental spinal instrumentation. (Courtesy Zimmer Co, Warsaw, Ind.)

Care of the Patient With a Stable Vertebral Fracture Without Cord Involvement

The orthopedic nurse cares for many patients who fall out of trees or off ladders, are stressed by seat belts in automobile accidents, or suffer other direct and indirect blows to the back. Any of these patients may enter the hospital with a diagnosis of vertebral fracture. Further investigation defines the fracture as "stable."

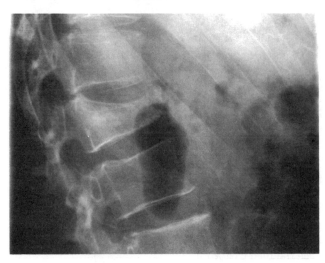

Compression fracture of L1, lateral view.

Definition

A stable vertebral fracture is one that is not expected to change its position. There is little or no ligament disruption. compression fractures of the vertebral bodies and fractures of the spinous or transverse processes are included in this classification.

All of these patients enter with complaints of pain and may have some paresthesias in the upper or lower extremities. The back of such a patient lacks the angles and swelling normally associated with fracture, and because there are many possible vertebral fracture locations, the pathology may be difficult to visualize. In initiating care for these patients the nurse must base many of her orders for care and observation on patient history.

Patients with osteoporosis or bone disease may sustain vertebral fractures as a result of minimal trauma or normal stresses. The following discussion on history is more pertinent to the patient who has had an accident.

Nursing Assessment

History of injury is important in doing thorough assessments. For example: A 69-year-old man falls backward off a three-wheeled vehicle. Why? Did he hit another object, "black out," or experience any other symptoms related to balance and coordination, such as dizziness? The possibility of another problem contributing to the fall must be considered.

The patient with vertebral fracture usually gives an account of a sudden violent episode of trauma followed by severe back pain that increases if he moves. He should be asked to describe his actions and reactions immediately after the injury. Did he lose consciousness? Exactly how did he feel? Did he try to stand up or walk? When did this happen and how soon did he get help, and what kind? Maybe someone tried to sit him up and he became dizzy and had to lie down. What "hurt"?

The entire trunk should be inspected first, with observations appropriate to the mechanism of trauma. For example,

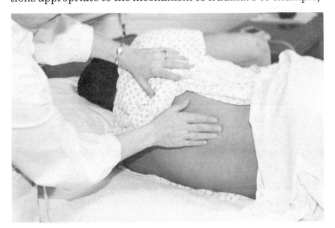

if he fell on a gravel road, the back of his head and hair should be carefully examined for evidence of gravel, dirt, laceration, and bleeding. The patient will need to logroll on his side so that his back can be examined for swelling, ecchymoses, open wounds, and tender areas. The spinous processes should be palpated.

The appropriate extremities must be evaluated and compared. The chest, abdomen, and pelvis should also be examined, with careful attention to the areas of impact and patient complaints (see Chapter 1). A neurological assessment is imperative for a neck injury or if the patient lost consciousness after the accident or had neurological symptoms prior to the trauma. A cerebrovascular accident may have preceded the fall in an elderly patient.

THE PATIENT WITH A CERVICAL FRACTURE

This type of patient is usually ambulatory if there are no accompanying prohibitive injuries. The nursing care depends on the mobility allowed by treatment. The management of the patient in cervical halter traction is described in Chapter 3. Range-of-motion exercises and heat may be prescribed. The patient may be fitted with some type of cervical collar and discharged when comfortable in it.

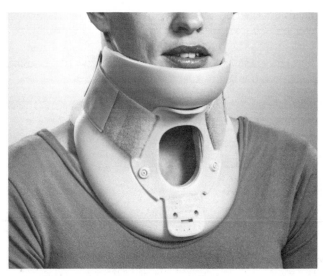

Philadelphia collar. (Courtesy Zimmer Co, Warsaw, Ind)

NURSING CARE OF THE PATIENT WITH A THORACOLUMBAR FRACTURE

A convoluted bedpad or alternating pressure mattress should be placed on the bed as soon as the nurse knows the patient is coming. Measures to prevent problems associated with immobility are paramount while the patient is on bed rest. The duration of bed rest varies according to the patient's condition. Neurovascular status and vital signs will be checked on a regular basis while the patient is on bed rest.

Nursing routines include frequent skin care measures with special attention to the heels and coccyx, encouraging deep breathing and coughing and movement of extremities, and position changes. If the patient is a smoker, respiratory support measures may be indicated. Elastic hose should be ordered. The patient will need to be logrolled and instructed in this procedure because the supine position will be uncomfortable and he will try to turn himself.

Paralytic ileus is almost a certainty. The condition occurs in about 24 hours and may last 3 days. For this reason nourishment may be restricted to clear liquids at the outset of hospitalization.

The abdomen should be checked routinely for distention, and distention should be promptly reported to the physician. As paralytic ileus develops, the patient needs nasogastric suction and intravenous fluids.

The color and amount of urine voided by the patient should be monitored if kidney contusions are suspected. Voiding may be difficult if the patient must remain flat, and an indwelling catheter may be indicated.

The physician's intention when prescribing "bed rest" must be clear from the beginning. May the patient have the head of the bed elevated (and how far) for meals? How much can he turn? When the head of the bed is elevated, the patient must be positioned with his back straight and his hips where the mattress "cracks." In other words, he must bend with the bed to keep his spine in neutral alignment.

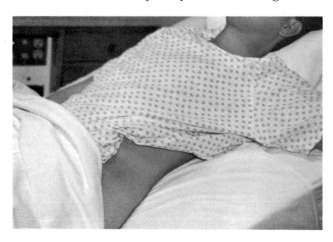

Constipation should be prevented. The nurse needs an order for stool softeners and laxatives or enemas in the initial plan. Fluids should be given as allowed by the state of the ileus.

The lungs need regular auscultation, and the nurse should watch for signs of respiratory distress and possible pulmonary embolism (p. 49). Calf tenderness is also a constant concern.

Activity

After 2 to 5 days of bed rest the patient may begin ambulating in the physical therapy department with help. If a longer period of bed rest is necessary, the tilt table may be employed the first couple of times the patient goes to the physical therapy department. The nurse should assist the patient in getting out of bed in the same manner in which she helps a laminectomy patient.

An orthosis will be ordered and fitted while the patient is still in the hospital.

Discharge Planning

When the patient is tolerating ambulation, the brace, food, and fluids, and when he is comfortable on oral analgesics, he is discharged. Instructions for restriction of activity are highly individual and are based on the fracture and the patient's general condition and lifestyle.

Discussion Questions

1. What nursing actions must be taken in the following situations?
  a. A patient who is scheduled to have a lumbar myelogram at 1:30 P.M. complains at 12:30 P.M. that she is nauseated and has developed tingling and numbness in her fingers.
  b. The nurse receives the following report on a laminectomy patient 7 hours postoperatively. Patient is restless, has just been logrolled, and will not stay on his side; he says he cannot stay on his back.
  c. An 18-year old girl is in surgery having insertion of a Harrington rod. The mother expresses concern that her daughter has been "gone more than 4 hours."
  d. Nine days postoperatively. A Harrington-rod patient refuses supper, stating that she "feels okay" but is not hungry.
  Consider:
  a. What are some common manifestations of anxiety? What has been the patient's activity up to this time? Does she have any other physical problems?
  b. What are the causes of restlessness at this time? What is normal behavior for a new laminectomy patient?
  c. Does the girl's age have any significance?
  d. After 9 days, what are the problems of immobility? What is significant about the fact that this *is* 9 days after the operation?

2. Identify the steps in reassessment based on the following data:
  a. Harrington-rod patient has 3 plus occult blood in her preoperative-urine specimen.
  b. A laminectomy patient admitted the night before his

surgery has an elevated cholesterol on his early morning screening panel.

c. A Harrington-rod patient complains of a prickly feeling in her feet on the first postoperative morning.

d. Four days postoperatively, a laminectomy patient has a temperature of 100.6°.

e. Two days after admission, an elderly patient with a compression fracture of L-4 complains: "it's hard for me to breathe."

Consider:

a. How significant are single abnormal laboratory reports? The patient's age and sex?

b. What other laboratory test results need to be looked at? Of what importance is the time element, that is, time admitted and time of test?

c. When and how is the patient being positioned?

d. What is normal for a postlaminectomy patient in terms of body temperature? What systems require assessment?

e. What complication is most common in this type of patient?

Bibliography

Agre K, et al: Anaphylaxis from chymopapain. JAMA 251(15):1953, 1984

Allard JL, Dibble SL: Scoliosis surgery: A look at Luque rods. Am J Nurs 84(5):609, 1984

Allard JL, Northrop WA: Nursing care: Segmental spinal instrumentation . . . Luque rod instrumentation. AORN J 38(1):45, 1983

Anderson FJ: Self-concept and coping in adolescents with a physical disability. Issues Ment Health Nurs 4(4):257, 1982

Apfelbach H: Technique for chemonucleolysis. Today's OR Nurs 6(1):20, 1984

Barton CR, et al: Anaphylactic reaction to chymopapain injection: A review and anesthesia considerations. AANA J 52(3):280, 1984

Battit GE: Anaphylaxis associated with chymopapain injections. JAMA 253(7):977, 1985

Berman AT, et al: The effects of epidural injection of local anesthetics and corticosteroids on patients with lumbosciatic pain. Clin Orthrop 188:144, 1984

Bernstein IL: Adverse effects of chemonucleolysis. JAMA 250 (9):1167, 1983

Bowen C: Spotlight on children. Scoliosis—a care study. Nurs Times 80(26):65, 1984

Branson KA: Patient management following amipaque myelography. Orthop Nurs 1(6):38, 1982

Bruce J: Nursing Mirror clinical forum. Treatment for scoliosis. Nurs Mirror 158 (3):ii, 1984

Brunner NA: Orthopedic Nursing, 4th ed. St. Louis, CV Mosby, 1983

Bryant SA: Crossing over. J Pract Nurs 33(4):34, 1983

Burton CV: Conservative management of low back pain. Postgrad Med 70(5):168, 1981

Carini E, Owens G: Neurological and Neurosurgical Nursing. St. Louis, CV Mosby, 1974

Carruthers CC: Surgical treatment after chemonucleolysis failure. Clin Orthop 165:172, 1982

Chaffee E, Lytle I: Basic Physiology and Anatomy, 4th ed. Philadelphia, JB Lippincott, 1980

Ciba. Symposia on Scoliosis. 24 (1), 1972. Summit, NJ, Ciba Pharmaceutical.

Connolly, JF: The thoracic and lumbar spine . . . fracture pitfalls. Emerg Med 15(1):183, 1983

Cooper S: Low back pain caused by rupturing of the nucleus pulposus. ONAJ 2:224, 1975

Crenshaw AH (ed): Campbell's Operative Orthopaedics, 6th ed. St. Louis, CV Mosby, 1980

Cyriax J, Cyriax P: Illustrated Manual of Orthopaedic Medicine. London, Butterworth, 1983

Davis SE, Lewis SA: Managing scoliosis: Fashions for the body and mind. MCN 9(3):186, 1984

Devoti AL: Lumbar laminectomy: Diagnosis to discharge. J Neurosurg Nurs 15(3):140, 1983

Dionne KE: The no-strain approach to back-breaking work. RN 48(1):45, 1985

Drug bulletin: Chymodiactin R (chymopapain). Orthop Nurs, 2(2):27, 1983

Dunn HK, et al: Fixation of Dwyer screws for the treatment of scoliosis. A postmortem study. J Bone Joint Surg (Am) 59(1):54, 1977

Dunwoody CJ, Pais MB: Scoliosis. Nursing (Horsham) (Can Ed) 13(9):24, 1983

Edgar MA, et al: Pre-operative correction in adolescent idiopathic scoliosis. J. Bone Joint Surg (Br) 64(5):530, 1982

Ejeskar A: Surgery versus chemonucleolysis for herniated lumbar discs. A prospective study with random assignment. Clin Orthop 174:236, 1983

Erwin WD, et al: The postoperative management of scoliosis patients treated with Harrington instrumentation and fusion. J. Bone Joint Surg 58:479, 1976

Farrell J: Caring for the laminectomy patient. Nurs 78 8(5):65, 1978

Farrell NA: Cast syndrome. Orthop Nurs 4(4):61, 1985

Ferguson RL, Allen BL, Jr: A mechanic classification of thoracolumbar spine fractures. Clin Orthop 189:77, 1984

Flanders A, et al: Osteotomy of the fusion mass in scoliosis. J Bone Joint Surg (Am) 64(9):1307, 1982

Floman Y, et al: Osteotomy of the fusion mass in scoliosis. J Bone Joint Surg (Am) 64(9):1307, 1982

Folkard PM: The halo pelvic traction operation. S Afr Nurs J 40:21, 1973

From the editor: Issues related to the distribution of chymopapain. Ortho Nurs 2(2):8, 1983

Fuss M: Disk therapy without surgery. Today's OR Nurs, 6(1):18, 1984

Gainer JV, Nugent GR: Herniated lumbar disc. Am Fam Phys 10:127, 1974

Goldberg C, et al: A retrospective study of Cotrel dynamic spinal traction in the conservative management of scoliosis. Ir Med J 74(12):363, 1981

Goldsmith MJ: Chymopapain—injection an often fruitless endeavor? JAMA 251(1):13, 1984

Grammer LC, et al: Chymopapain allergy: Case reports and identification of patients at risk for chymopapain anaphylaxis. Clin Orthop 188:139, 1984

Gunby P: Chymopapain: Tropical tree to surgical suite. JAMA 249 (9):1120, 1983

Gurnham RB: Adolescent compliance with spinal brace wear. Orthop Nurs 2(6):13, 1983

Halladay J: Update on scoliosis. Can Nurs 81(8):44, 1984

Hancox V: Cotrel traction for patients with scoliosis. Physiotherapy 67(3):71, 1981

Hausman DL: Percutaneous lateral discectomy: Another approach for the treatment of a herniated nucleus pulposus. Orthop Nurs 3(6):9, 1984

Hayne C: Counting the cost of sickness. Nurs Times, 80(33):50, 1984

Hejna WF: Chemonucleolysis of herniated lumbar discs. Am Fam Phys 27(5):97, 1983

Henning JH, et al: Preparation for the Luque procedure: patient education booklet. Orthop Nurs 3(5):50, 1984

Herriotts KF: Anaphylaxis and chemonucleolysis: A case report and treatment summary. AANA J 52(3):296, 1984

Hilt N, Cogburn S: Manual of Orthopedics. St. Louis, CV Mosby, 1980

Hollinshead WH: Textbook of Anatomy, 3rd ed. Hagerstown, Md., Harper & Row, 1974

Holmes P: Back pain, part 3. Shops that bend over backwards. Nurs Times 81(3):29, 1985

Holt EP, Jr: Chemonucleolysis. Clin Orthop, 154:296, 1981

Hoppenfeld S: Scoliosis. Philadelphia, JB Lippincott, 1967

Hsu LC: Dwyer instrumentation in the treatment of adolescent idiopathic scoliosis. J Bone Surg (Br) 64(5):536, 1982

Hutsan L: Laminectomy. Nurs Mirror 146:18, 1978

Jackson C: Nursing care study: Scoliosis. Nurs Times 78(14):567, 1982

Jacobs DM, et al: Anaphylactic reactions following intradiscal injection of chymopapain under local anesthesia. J Bone Joint Surg Am 66(5):806, 1984

Javid JM, et al: Safety and efficacy of chymopapain (Chymodiactin) in herniated nucleus pulposus with sciatica. JAMA 248(18):2489, 1983

Jonasson-Rajala E: Boston thoracic brace in the treatment of idiopathic scoliosis: Initial correction. Clin Orthop 183:37, 1984

Kahanovitz N, et al: The part-time Milwaukee brace treatment of juvenile idiopathic scoliosis: Long-term follow-up. Clin Orthop 167:145, 1982

Keene JS, et al: The Wisconsin Compression System. Spine 7(1):83, 1982

Konings JG, et al: The effects of chemonucleolysis as demonstrated by computerized tomography. J Bone Surg (Br) 66(3):417, 1984

Kumano K, Tsuyama N: Pulmonary function before and after surgical correction of scoliosis. J Bone Joint Surg (Am) 64(2)242, 1982

Lande RE: Luque rod instrumentation. AORN J 38(1):35, 1983

Langley LL, et al: Dynamic Anatomy and Physiology, 5th ed. New York, Mc Graw-Hill, 1980

Larson C, Gould M: Orthopedic Nursing, 9th ed. St. Louis, CV Mosby, 1978

Legislative review: Chymopapain. Orthop Nurs 2(2):33, 1983

Lichter RL, et al: Treatment of chronic low-back pain. A community-based comprehensive return-to-work physical rehabilitation program. Clin Orthop 190:115, 1984

Lonstein JE, Carlson JM: The prediction of curve progression in untreated idiopathic scoliosis during growth. J Bone Joint Surg (Am) 66(7):1061, 1984

Luque ER: Segmental spinal instrumentation for correction of scoliosis. Clin Orthop, 163:192, 1982

Macek C: Electrical stimulation of muscles replaces braces for scoliosis. JAMA 247(8):1097, 1982

Macnab I: Backache. Baltimore, Williams & Wilkins, 1977.

Maida MJ: Chemonucleolysis: A new approach for patients with herniated lumbar disc diseases. J. Neurosurg Nurs 15 (3):144, 1983

McCarthy RE: Coping with low back pain through behavioral change. Orthop Nurs 3(3):30, 1984

Mercier LR: Practical Orthopedics. Chicago, Year Book Medical Publishers, 1980

Mims BC: Back surgery: Helping your patient get through it. RN, 48:26, 1985

Moe JH, et al: Harrington instrumentation without fusion plus external orthotic support for the treatment of difficult curvature problems in young children. Clin Orthop 185:35, 1984

Moss V: Chemonucleolysis: Enzyme eases back pain. AORN J 38(6):965, 1983

Musolf J: Chemonucleolysis: A new approach for patients with herniated intervertebral disks. Am J Nurs 882, 1983

Pelino T: Chymopapain: Alternative to laminectomy for herniated lumbar discs. Orthop Nurs 2(2):14, 1983

Powell, GM: Evaluation of low back pain. Occup Health Nurs 32(5):266, 1984

Raney RB, Brashear HR: Shand's Handbook of Orthopaedic Surgery, 9th ed. St. Louis, CV Mosby, 1978

Roberts RS, et al: Use of a bivalved polypropylene orthosis in the post-operative management of idiopathic scoliosis. Clin Orthop 185:25, 1984

Rodgers S: Back pain, part 1. Shouldering the load. Nurs Times 81(3):24, 1985

Romankiewicz N: Treatment of ruptured intervertebral disc by chemonucleolysis with chymopapain. J Pract Nurs 33(9):7, 1983

Schafer MF: Dwyer instrumentation of the spine. Orthop Clin North Am 9(1):115, 1978

Scoliosis terminology. Orthop Nurs 1(5):38, 1982

Self Rx . . . exercise. Kans Nurs 59(2):6, 1984

Simmons JW, et al: Update and review of chemonucleolysis. Clin Orthop 183:51, 1984

Smith D: Nursing your lower back, part 1. Nurs Success Today 1(2):36, 1984

Smith D: Nursing your lower back, part 2. Nurs Success Today 1(3):30, 1984

Smith WS, et al: Chymopapain injection. JAMA, 251(19):2515, 1984

Speck G: Chymopapain in intradiscal therapy. J Bone Joint Surg (Am), 66(5):808, 1984

Spelman MR: Back pain: How health education affects patient compliance with treatment Occup Health Nurs 32(12):649, 1984

Stewart JR: Thorne RP: Complications of metrizamide (Amipaque) myelography. Orthop Nurs 4(4):53, 1985

Swaffield J: Back pain, part 2. Out of court, out of mind. Nurs Times 81(3):247, 1985

Thomas PC: Nursing care of patients undergoing posterior spinal fusion with segmental (Luque) spinal instrumentation. Orthop Nurs 2(3):13, 1983

Thomassen PF: Helping your scoliosis patient walk tall. RN 47(2):34, 1984

Tompkins JS, Brown MD: Dissolving a lifetime of lower back pain with chemonucleolysis. Nursing 85 15(7):47, 1985

Turek SL: Orthopaedics: Principles and Their Application, 3rd ed. Philadelphia, JB Lippincott, 1977

Urbanski P, O'Donnell J: Chymopapain: A New therapeutic agent. Infusion 7:75, 1983

Vandenburgh VJ: Nursing care study: Plain sailing. Correcting curvature of the spine. Nurs Times 77(18):770, 1981

Vercauteren ME, DeGroote WF: A mobile: Halo. Spine 5(3):297, 1980

Watkins P: Straightening up. Nurs Times 81(8):40, Feb. 20, 1985

Watkins RG: Surgical approaches to the spine. New York, Springer, 1983

Weinstein SL, Ponseti IV: Curve progression in idiopathic scoliosis. J Bone Joint Surg (Am) 65(4):447, 1983

Weitz EM: Paraplegia following chymopapain injection: A case report. J Bone Joint Surg (Am) 66(7):1131, 1984

Wells R: Lumbar laminectomy and/or fusions. ONAJ 1:33, 1974

Wiltse LL, et al: Surgery for intervertebral disk disease of the lumbar spine. Clin Ortho 129:22, 1977

Winter RB: Combined Dwyer and Harrington instrumentation and fusion in the treatment of selected patients with painful adult idiopathic scoliosis. Spine 3(2):135, 1978

Yamada K, et al: Etiology of idiopathic scoliosis. Clin Orthop 184:50, 1984

Your back and how to care for it . . . posture. Kans Nurs 59(1):6, 1984

5

Care of the Patient With a Hip Fracture and Internal Fixation

The vascular supply to the head of the femur comes mainly from a series of arteries that enter at the junction of the head and neck. Fractures may tear the blood vessels and disrupt the blood supply. This fact becomes important in the treatment and healing of fractures of the neck of the femur and will be discussed under fracture types. Of equal importance is the fact that the amount of blood supplied by the metaphyseal arteries and through the ligamentum teres (which attaches the head of the femur to the acetabulum) is minimal.

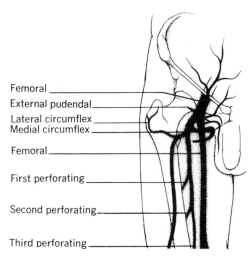

Femoral

External pudendal

Lateral circumflex
Medial circumflex

Femoral

First perforating

Second perforating

Third perforating

(Chaffee and Greisheimer: Basic Physiology and Anatomy, 3rd ed. Philadelphia, Lippincott, 1974)

Since it is the elderly person who is most prone to this sort of injury, the incidence of hip fractures will increase as the older population increases. Basic knowledge of the specific nursing needs of the geriatric patient and an understanding of the value systems of older people are as necessary to the orthopedic nurse as an orthopedic theory base. Even with the best preparation and intentions, caring for these patients, who are for the most part fragile and in some instances senile, continues to be the supreme challenge in orthopedic nursing.

Anatomy of the Hip

The part of the anatomy involved in fractures of the hip is the upper part of the femur. The head of the femur, covered by a layer of cartilage, fits into the cup or acetabulum on the side of the pelvis, forming a ball-and-socket joint. The head is followed by a short femoral neck, at the distal end of which are located the greater and lesser trochanters.

Muscles that move the hip tend to displace fracture fragments. They are therefore responsible for some of the clinical features and complications of the fractured hip. The abductor muscles, or the gluteus medius and minimus, in-

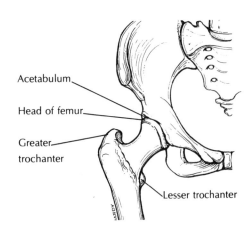

Acetabulum

Head of femur

Greater trochanter

Lesser trochanter

(From Chaffee and Greisheimer: Basic Physiology and Anatomy, 3rd ed. Philadelphia, Lippincott, 1974)

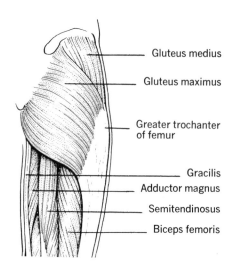

Gluteus medius

Gluteus maximus

Greater trochanter of femur

Gracilis
Adductor magnus
Semitendinosus
Biceps femoris

(Chaffee and Greisheimer: Basic Physiology and Anatomy, 3rd ed. Philadelphia, Lippincott, 1974)

sert on the greater trochanter. The gluteus maximus, which rotates the femur outward, inserts on the gluteal tuberosity. The iliopsoas muscle is attached to the lesser trochanter and acts as a hip flexor. Apart from this function, its actions are a matter of conjecture.

In fractures in which the fragments have been separated, one or a combination of these pulls may cause the distal fragment to pull upward and rotate outward, so that the fractured extremity is lying on its lateral side. It also appears shorter than the extremity that is not fractured.

Types of Hip Fractures

Fractures of the hip are intracapsular or extracapsular, depending on whether or not they are located within the joint capsule, which extends along the neck of the femur.

Hip fractures may occur along the femoral neck or in the intertrochanteric or subtrochanteric regions.

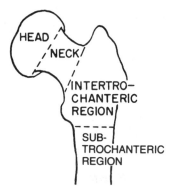

(Smith and Germain: Care of the Adult Patient, 4th ed. Philadelphia, Lippincott)

Femoral-neck fractures are called subcapital, transcervical, or basilar neck fractures, taking their names from anatomic locations. Such fractures, when displaced, cause serious disruption of the blood supply to the head of the femur. This, in turn, may result in avascular necrosis of the femoral head. Femoral-neck fractures are not usually associated with major trauma. Osteoporosis is considered partially responsible, along with minor injury or stress. Consequently, patients with these fractures may have few initial symptoms and are not always seen by a physician for prompt attention.

If immediate diagnosis and treatment are possible, these fractures are reduced by internal fixation with a hip pin (or nail). When 2 or 3 days have elapsed since the probable time of fracture, or when the femoral head is grossly misplaced or comminuted, avascular necrosis is a prime consideration. Under these circumstances, many surgeons customarily insert a femoral prosthesis rather than a pin. (See p. 176.)

The *impacted fracture* is one in which the neck of the femur is driven up into the head, more or less reducing itself. These fractures, therefore, are often treated as if they are in the postoperative stage. In other words, the patient whose x-ray shows an impacted fracture is allowed the activity of one who has just had internal fixation.

Intertrochanteric fracture lines run between the greater and lesser trochanters and are classified as extracapsular. They are usually the result of a fall or similar injury. Although they occur through cancellous bone and do heal if properly immobilized, surgical fixation by pinning is the treatment of choice. This is because of the long period of immobilization required for nonoperative union, plus the fact that, even with traction, the leg may be somewhat shortened.

Subtrochanteric fractures, just below the trochanters, are generally the result of severe direct trauma. Likewise, they are reduced by surgical fixation to permit early ambulation.

Methods of Reduction

Traction

Buck's extension traction (see Chapter 3) may be used to immobilize and, hopefully, promote healing in an intertrochanteric or femoral neck fracture in a patient who is too debilitated to undergo surgery. Most of the time, however, traction is used as a temporary measure until an operative procedure can be performed.

In the case of a subtrochanteric fracture, the flexion pull of the iliopsoas muscle makes 90-90-90 traction effective in

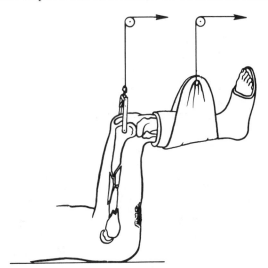

90–90–90 traction is especially applicable to fractures of the subtrochanteric area with associated wounds of the groin and buttock. Traction through the femoral condyles is most efficient, and it is not associated with stiffness at the knee. Suspension of the leg in plaster casts is optional. (Rockwood and Green: Fractures. Philadelphia, Lippincott, 1975)

aligning the distal fragment with the proximal fragment. (See figure p. 175.)

The primary reason for delaying surgery at all is the patient's general condition. Many surgeons feel that the sooner operative fixation is done the better, not only for healing purposes, but also because it is more humane than keeping the patient so completely helpless for a longer period than is necessary.

Internal Fixation

Since the success of the Smith-Peterson nail, many devices in the form of pins, nails, or screws have been designed and manufactured for the purpose of repairing a fractured hip. There are triflanged nails with or without side plates, sliding screws and nails, and multiple pins. The effectiveness of any individual device is probably most dependent on the surgeon's skill at using it.

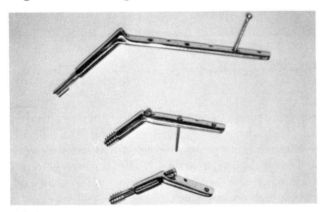

In the operating room, under anesthesia, the femoral neck is reduced by means of the fracture table (p. 75). The patient's feet are attached to stirrups, and the leg section of the table is adjusted to pull the fracture ends into alignment. If an x-ray film or fluoroscopy (continuous throughout the procedure) confirms satisfactory reduction, the surgeon proceeds with the pinning.

From the outer aspect of the hip a small guide wire is drilled or driven across the fracture line. A small reamer is used to produce a hole in the bone extending from below the greater trochanter, up the neck, across the fracture line, and deep into the head. This hole is made to accommodate the threaded pin that is placed in the head of the femur.

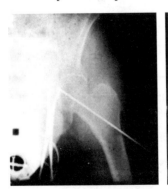
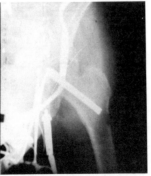

Next, a larger hole is reamed below the trochanter to accommodate the plate that anchors the pin. After the pin is properly seated, the plate is slipped over the pin and attached to the outer side of the femur by means of screws that are driven through the holes in the plate into the shaft of the femur. This anchors the plate securely. The final step

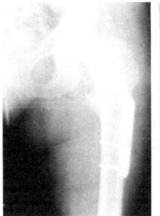
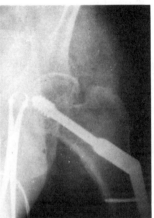

in the procedure is the application of a compression force to the fracture line by means of a small bolt that is inserted up through the plate, engaging the pin. Drawing the pin and plate together creates a high level of compression across the fracture line.

The Hip or Femoral Prosthesis

Insertion of a prosthesis is the treatment of choice in subcapital fractures, in which avascular (aseptic) necrosis is likely to occur. Two hip or femoral prostheses are pictured here.

The special nursing considerations for the patient with a femoral prosthesis are discussed at the end of this chapter, pages 193–196.

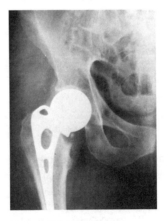
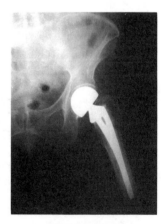

Austin-Moore prosthesis.

Bi-polar prosthesis includes acetabular cup, which reduces friction.

Major Complications Following Hip Surgery

Nonunion

Hip fractures that fail to unite are rare. When they occur, they may be treated by bone grafting across the fracture site. A very successful method of promoting union of the fragments is to place the fracture line in a more horizontal plane by means of a subtrochanteric osteotomy and then to establish fixation by a compression screw.

Avascular (Aseptic) Necrosis

Failure of a subcapital fracture to unite results in avascular necrosis of the head of the femur. This condition is manifested by the presence of pain in the area months, or even years, after the fracture has been treated. It is diagnosed by demonstration of collapse of the femoral head on x-ray film. The head of the femur is then replaced by a prosthesis as shown above.

Infection

A superficial wound infection may progress to a deep infection, resulting in osteomyelitis or septic arthritis. These conditions are very serious and may involve long, complicated treatment.

It is imperative, therefore, that good nursing care be provided, to help prevent infection and other complications. In fact, it might be said that the prognosis of the elderly patient with a hip pinning is greatly dependent on the quality of nursing care he or she receives.

Initial Nursing Assessment of the Patient With a Fractured Hip

Appearance on Admission

A typical patient with a fractured hip is an elderly woman admitted to the orthopedic unit by ambulance stretcher. She will appear pale, helpless, and in severe pain. Frequently,

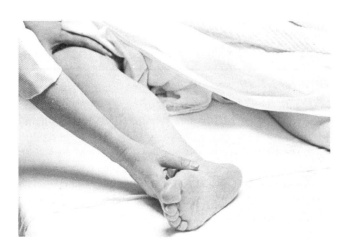

the only information the nurse has at this point is that the patient "broke her hip." The classic sign of a fractured hip is the appearance of the leg — it may be slightly shorter and in a position of lateral rotation. Ecchymosis, contusions, and swelling may also be present in the hip area.

The patient usually complains of severe pain in the hip and the leg and wards off attempts by anyone to touch that part of her body. She is not able to move the affected leg at all and may be extremely fearful that someone else will try to do so.

Transfer to Bed

When being transferred from stretcher to bed, the patient may manifest apprehension by becoming rigid and uncooperative. For this reason, as many as four people may be required to transfer the patient from the stretcher to the bed. Her hands should be placed on her abdomen and the stretcher moved directly next to the bed. The bed should be raised or lowered to correspond, if possible, with the height of the stretcher. Two people on the opposite side of the bed roll the edge of the sheet that is under the patient as close to her body as possible. The two people at the side of the

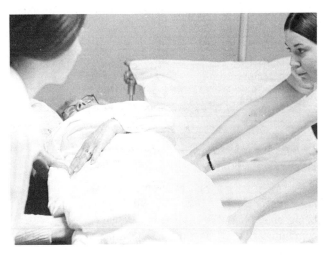

stretcher do the same. The top bed linen should be folded well over the foot of the bed. At the count of three, all four persons lift slightly and move the patient onto the mattress. It is desirable to place a convoluted bedpad on the bed before transferring the patient.

Communication

When attempting to communicate with the patient, the nurse may find her to be slightly confused, disoriented, or emotionally upset from the shock of trauma. No matter what her level of understanding at the time, she needs reassurance that she will be handled carefully.

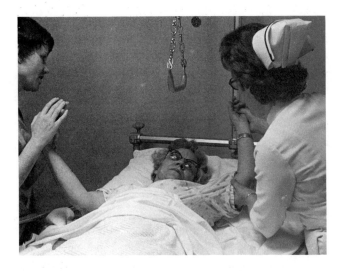

If the patient is unable to provide details about her injury and disability, the nurse may make pertinent observations as the patient's clothing is being removed and she is being settled into bed. In making these observations, the nurse should ask herself the following questions:

1. What is her speech like, if she is able to answer questions?
2. Can the patient move one or both arms? Maybe her arms were injured when she fell, if she fell. Perhaps she has had a previous stroke or suffered one that caused her to fall.
3. Does she appear to have chest pain or difficulty breathing?
4. Are there bruises anywhere on the patient's body?
5. Is she able to move the uninjured leg without difficulty?

Collecting and Sharing Data With the Family

One of the greatest frustrations in providing adequate nursing care for the elderly patient with a fractured hip is not being able to identify her needs because of problems with communication. Conferring as soon as possible with a family member or someone closely associated with the patient is extremely helpful. For example, the family may provide important information by indicating that the patient had been alert and able to feed herself before the injury. Therefore, if in the first few hours after admission the patient proves to be confused, incontinent, perhaps even noisy and uncooperative, then this behavior may clearly be related to her present mishap.

Such behavior will, of course, make nursing care, observations, and assessment of pain more difficult. It is important to realize this if the nurse is to be effective in helping the orthopedic surgeon with a preoperative evaluation. As part of the evaluation, the surgeon needs to know if this patient was bedridden or in a wheelchair before she was

admitted to the hospital. The decision to operate may be influenced by this piece of information. Therefore, the family should be asked specifically about the patient's status in this regard.

Having the family indicate the likes and dislikes of the patient in relation to food and fluids is helpful in maintaining her nutrition. All too frequently, these patients cannot or will not give out this information. They just simply do not eat or else they eat and drink very little, thus exasperating everyone who tries to feed them.

Every new face that appears, added to the strange surroundings and unfamiliar routines of admission, increases this patient's disorientation. Because of this, settling her comfortably into bed may prove to be a slow process.

At the same time, relatives of the patient will be distressed and perplexed to find her becoming increasingly confused, disoriented, and helpless, if she was fairly alert and self-sufficient 24 hours earlier. An effective method of communicating with the family and friends of the patient with a fractured hip is through a printed pamphlet explaining what to expect and pointing out how they, the visitors, can be helpful. This material can be presented, explained, and then left near the patient's bedside. An example of the contents of a pamphlet that has proven to be useful can be found on page 179.

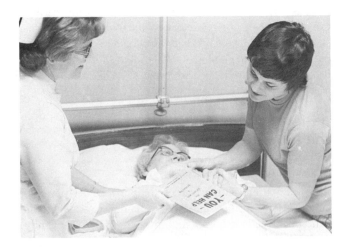

Preoperative Management and Nursing Care

General Health Assessment

Although it is current practice to repair a fractured hip surgically without delay, some preoperative evaluation and preparation is necessary. The objective of the surgeon is to have the patient in the best physical condition possible to reduce the surgical risk.

When the patient has been admitted, many orthopedic surgeons routinely order an electrocardiogram, chest x-ray film, and serum electrolytes, as well as routine laboratory

---

YOU CAN HELP THE PATIENT WITH A BROKEN HIP*

If the patient is elderly, he or she may become confused at times because of the shock of the injury and suddenly finding him/herself in strange surroundings.

These patients are sometimes afraid that they will remain bedridden for a very long time or become totally disabled. In the past, this was often true and it is likely they remember this happening to someone else. With newer, better surgical procedures it is now possible to get these patients up and about quite soon. Remembering this will help you, the patient, and the staff. Keep the following facts in mind:

1. The nurses and floor personnel will be turning the patient often and encouraging deep breathing and coughing. Although these procedures may cause discomfort, they are not harmful and will produce a faster recovery.
2. The patient will be encouraged and often assisted in exercising the unaffected leg and both arms by the nursing or physical-therapy staff. This will help maintain muscle strength necessary for when the patient gets out of bed. In this, encouragement from you will be helpful. Usually these patients are out of bed in a wheelchair in 1 to 3 days.
3. Shortly thereafter, he/she will be going to physical therapy and gradually using a walker or crutches. Here again, you can help by offering encouragement and moral support. Not all patients with a hip injury are allowed to bear weight on the operated leg. In fact, they may not be allowed to bear full weight on that leg for several months or longer.
4. AT ALL TIMES, unless there is a special reason, the patient should be encouraged to drink fluids, such as water, milk, and juices. This will promote healing and general well-being.
5. AS SOON AS POSSIBLE, you should begin thinking about where the patient will be going when he/she leaves the hospital. Will it be home? Will it be your home or the home of another relative? Or will it be a nursing home? What financial adjustments or help will the patient need?

* Pamphlet excerpt courtesy of Bellin Memorial Hospital, Green Bay, Wisconsin

---

studies done on both blood and urine. If the patient has a history of other health problems, such as diabetes, hypertension or a cardiac condition, either the patient's family physician or an internist may be called in for consultation and to prescribe treatment.

Nursing Assessment

Nursing assessment has two objectives.

1. The nurse should be familiar with the patient's present physical and mental condition in order to make accurate judgments about postoperative status. For instance, auscultation of the lungs before surgery is the basis for determining early in the postoperative course whether any congestion is developing.
2. Knowledge of the patient's general health history is necessary in planning independent nursing care.

Besides the specific problems associated with aging, such as poor nutritional status, poor skin condition, and osteoporosis, and the dangers from complications, the patient may have other chronic health problems. Some of the more common ones include heart and vessel disease, diabetes, and gastrointestinal disturbances, such as diverticulosis. These factors need to be considered in the surgeon's evaluation and influence nursing care and observations greatly. For example, maintaining effective traction is a problem in a patient whose cardiac condition requires the head of the bed to be elevated, and meticulous skin care

becomes even more important if the patient has diabetes or circulatory disturbances. This is especially true for the leg in traction.

Immobilization of the Fracture

Buck's traction is often ordered preoperatively to decrease muscle spasm and to immobilize the leg in order to prevent further damage to the soft tissue around the ends of the

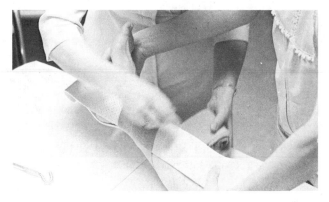

bone fragments. Because no dramatic change in alignment of fragments is expected from this procedure, the nurse usually applies the traction. Alignment of the leg should not be attempted. If the neurovascular status of the foot is satisfactory, there is no need to attempt to align the leg. The nurse should wrap the leg in the position that seems natural to the patient at this point. Some stiffness of the leg, espe-

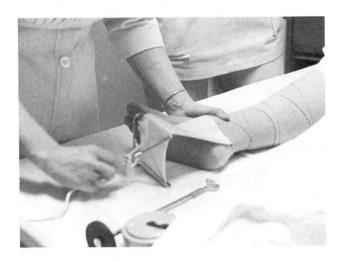

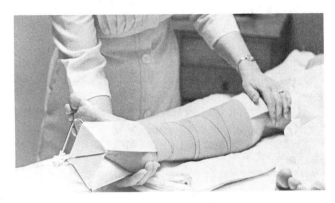

cially the knee, is to be expected in an elderly patient. The knee joint may be more comfortable if supported by a small pillow. A folded blanket under the calf keeps the heel off the bed.

2. Part of the tibia, or shin bone, is thinly covered with skin and subcutaneous tissue, so care must be taken not to cut off the circulation in this area. Too much pressure would cause breakdown of the skin.
3. The traction tape around the footplate, the footplate itself, and the ropes must not be resting on the bed.
4. Knots should be secure, not resting against the pulleys.
5. Weights should hang free.
6. The heel should clear the bed.

To help maintain the alignment of the leg, a trochanter roll is preferable to sandbags. A leg resting against a hard

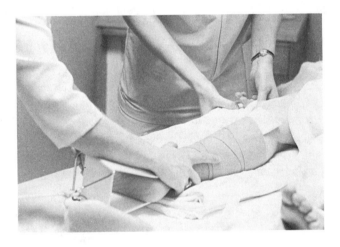

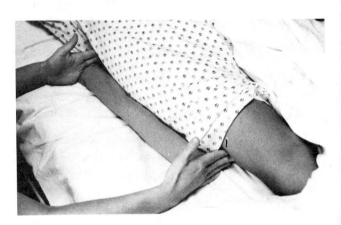

The details of Buck's traction with regard to application and nursing care are discussed in Chapter 3. However, the specific observations are worth repeating. These checkpoints must be observed every time nursing care is given:

1. Elastic bandages or traction boots should be checked to see that they are neither too loose nor too tight. If they are too loose, the apparatus may slip down, cutting into the flesh of the foot and causing pressure on the dorsalis pedis artery with resulting ischemia. If bandages slip down to the heel, there could be soreness and injury to the Achilles tendon. Tight bandaging may compress the peroneal nerve on the outer aspect of the calf just below the knee, causing paralysis of the foot.

sandbag perspires, predisposing the skin to irritation. More important, sandbags may put pressure on the peroneal nerve. When placing the trochanter roll, make sure that it is well under the patient's buttocks and extends from the iliac crest to the midthigh.

Skin Care

With the patient in a state of immobility, even for a matter of 24 to 48 hours, good skin care to promote circulation is essential. If an alternating pressure mattress or convoluted foam-rubber bedpad is not available, a sheepskin pad is indicated. The elderly patient has delicate skin, and areas

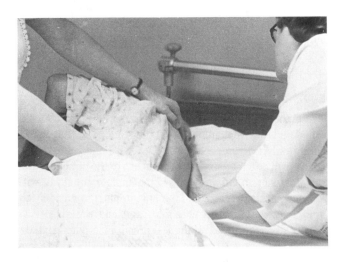

over bony prominences, especially the sacrum and heels, become reddened from pressure in a few short hours. Heel protectors are useful but must be removed every 3 hours for heel care; which consists of observation and massage. General circulation should be stimulated by giving the patient a backrub at least every 3 hours and turning her as indicated in the following paragraphs.

Turning the Patient

It is essential to turn the patient from side to side. In fact, a thorough backrub cannot be given unless she is turned.

Turning 45 degrees in either direction, even with the assistance of two nurses who are both gentle and encouraging, can still be a difficult and painful procedure for the older person with a hip fracture. Turning should be done with a pillow placed between the patient's legs and two nurses assisting, one on each side of the bed. (See Chap. 3, pp. 113–114 for details on turning.)

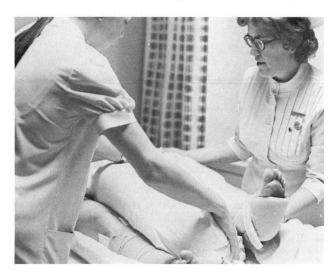

The amount of stiffness that is normal in old age, compounded by arthritic pains, adds to the patient's general

discomfort. Most nurses learn early in their careers that it often takes every communication skill they were taught to convince an 80-year-old patient that she will not fall out of bed when she turns—if falling out of bed was how she injured herself in the first place.

Because of apprehension about turning, the patient should be encouraged to cough and deep breathe before the turning procedure. This routine helps prevent hypostatic pneumonia and bronchial congestion.

Exercise

When the patient is able to assist by using the trapeze to lift the top half of her body off the bed, it not only makes skin care easier but also provides her with some arm exercise. Good circulation and muscle tone is maintained by having the patient move her uninvolved extremities at regular intervals.

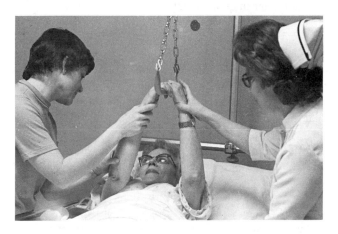

Nutrition

Keeping the patient adequately hydrated and nourished is difficult when she must be flat in bed, is in pain, and is perhaps slightly disoriented. Sincere nursing efforts should be made to provide oral nourishment.

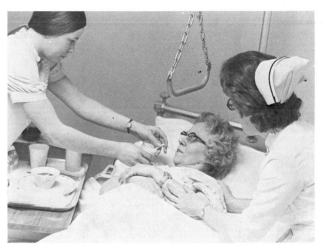

The fact that many elderly patients have false teeth affects the type of food they can eat. However, this varies from patient to patient and may depend on other health problems that necessitate special diets. In addition, older people usually have decreased appetites. Their eating habits often depend a great deal on general well-being. Elimination patterns are a common determinant of what they eat.

To promote fluid intake, liquids of the patient's preference should be offered frequently. Many elderly people are adamant about the kind of juice they drink and may only like warm milk. Although their tastes differ from that of the younger patient, their attitude does not. It is interesting to note that younger people are seen as having "likes and dislikes," whereas older people are generally considered "set in their ways."

If the patient cannot or will not feed herself, as is often the case, the nurse must assist her. Feeding the patient or assisting her in eating and drinking is often time-consuming, since older people usually eat more slowly. But promoting adequate intake may be a factor in maintaining electrolyte balance and mental orientation.

An accurate record of oral intake and output indicates whether the patient is taking enough fluids and aids the physician in determining if intravenous fluids are necessary.

Urinary Problems

Intake and output records are also important in detecting urinary difficulties. The shock and fright experienced by the elderly patient with a hip fracture often cause urinary incontinence. On the other hand, urinary retention and overflow may be a problem because of inability or reluctance to use a bedpan. The fracture bedpan should be placed under the patient at 3-hour intervals if she is confused or otherwise unable to request it. Hopefully, she can use the trapeze to lift herself. If not, she should be turned onto the pan.

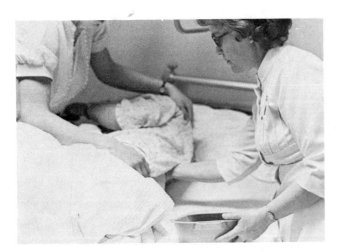

Inducing normal voiding is desirable to avoid the possibility of infection from an indwelling catheter. Nurses are well aware that when a patient is confused or restless, the catheter is the first thing he or she attempts to remove.

Elimination Problems

The orthopedic nurse should approach the patient who is scheduled for a hip pinning from the standpoint that constipation is likely to develop after surgery, and that when it does it will be a major source of concern to the patient. There is a tendency in old age toward incomplete emptying with one defecation, which could result in impaction. In addition, intestinal motion decreases with age and the supportive intestinal structures weaken. Forced inactivity and decreased food and fluid intake preoperatively add to any elimination problems the patient may already have. Narcotics and sedatives help cause or increase constipation. Bowel elimination in older persons is apt to be a concern to them normally, as they realize that physiological changes and inactivity slow them down. They also have the *time* to worry about changes in bowel habits.

In an attempt to avoid this problem, the nurse should find out when the patient last had a bowel movement and what constitutes normal defecation habits for that patient. A laxative or enema may need to be given. It may be wise to request the physician to order stool softeners. Gas-forming foods should be avoided and fluids encouraged. Forcing fluids also reduces the chance of urinary infections and kidney stones.

Psychological Considerations

Nurses often tend to categorize the elderly much more readily than they do other patients. Indeed, a great deal of the time the 80-year-old lady with a fractured hip is stubborn, "childish," and noisy. How much of this is due to arteriosclerosis and impairment of hearing and sight is difficult to evaluate. How does the nurse determine the amount of pain a patient is having if that patient cries *most* of the time? There are no easy solutions to the problems encountered in nursing the aged patient with a fractured hip.

But taking into consideration the following factors may be helpful in lessening the frustration of caring for these patients in the preoperative period. Most older women remember when going to the hospital with a fractured hip meant dying or being crippled, because they had friends and relatives to whom this has happened. Added to the shock and pain of her own fracture is the strangeness of surroundings, routines, and many new faces. The motives of those who are caring for her are baffling to a partially confused patient, when their actions seem to make her more uncomfortable. Gentleness and constant reassurance by the nurse are often ineffective. Still, just as often they are the only solution.

Three suggestions for promoting the cooperation and emotional comfort of the elderly patient are as follows.

1. To keep the patient from becoming confused, schedule treatments and routines that involve personnel from other departments so that only one person at a time is trying to explain his or her actions or intentions. Along with this, personnel should remember to introduce themselves each time they come in contact with the patient. It is not unusual for an elderly, slightly confused patient to believe that all of the people in white coats who visit daily are physicians, even though some are, for example, respiratory therapists. The patient who is concerned about finances may become more anxious if she believes she is being cared for by several physicians.

2. All personnel should be specific about what they are doing and what is required of the patient, every time that action or interaction takes place.

3. When dealing with the elderly patient who has had a hip pinning, it is important to avoid extremes in sensory input. For instance, any time more than one person is required to do a procedure, conversation should be kept a minimum. The television should not be on while the nurse is instructing or talking to the patient. In general, "one person talking at a time" is all that should be happening.

It is the path of least resistance to replace "tender loving care" with sedation and restraints to keep the patient quiet and to prevent her from trying to get out of bed or traction, or from pulling on her Foley catheter. Yet sedation and narcotics produce or add to many of the problems just mentioned and, along with restraints, they often serve to increase agitation and restlessness. While analgesics and sedatives are indicated, very often kindness, tolerance, patience, and a sense of humor accomplish what a sleeping pill cannot, both pre- and postoperatively.

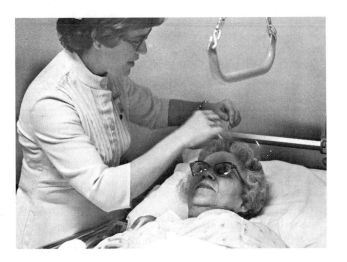

In this youth-oriented culture, the attitudes acquired toward aging tend to cause some nurses to shun the elderly patient. The nurse needs to understand her own feelings before she can accept and care for the older individual. The little old lady with a fractured hip may neither feel nor think of herself as old. She may have lived alone for years and be normally shy, independent, and unwilling to complain about a wet bed, should she have an "accident." It is a mistake to assume that old women are deaf or that they like being called "Grandma."

The nurse who understands these aspects of the care of the elderly patient with a hip fracture will find it possible to give more effective nursing care and eliminate undue frustration, while coping with the inevitable.

Postoperative Nursing Care

Vital Signs

Immediate postoperative care involves the routines of checking vital signs until stable, encouraging the patient in

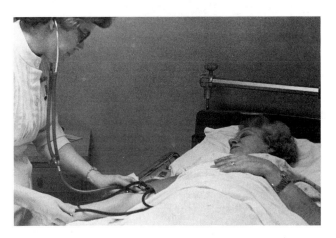

deep breathing and coughing, checking dressings, and changing the patient's position every 3 hours. If an icebag has been ordered for the incisional area, it must be checked regularly and changed when necessary.

Fluid Therapy

Intravenous fluids should be infused at a rate of approximately 100 ml per hour to prevent circulatory overload, and are generally discontinued after 1 liter unless the patient is dehydrated. Therefore, the emphasis in early postsurgical care is on giving oral fluids when tolerated. Encouraging fluids is as important postoperatively as preoperatively. Many elderly people do not take enough fluids when they are healthy and take even less when they are ill. Offering small amounts of juice, milk, or water at frequent intervals may be the most successful approach.

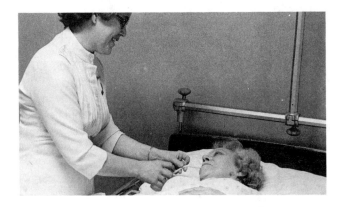

Medications

Antibiotics should be given as prescribed with observation of side-effects. Pain medications should be administered judiciously, bearing in mind the adverse effects they may have on the elderly. The nurse should check with the surgeon before restarting any medications the patient has been taking for a chronic condition.

Turning

Early activity for the patient involves coughing, deep breathing, and being turned from side to side at 3-hour intervals. The first time the patient is turned, two nurses should assist, with a third person in attendance in anticipation of resistance. Remember that, besides having pain in the operative area, the patient is stiff and apprehensive. For the same reasons, these patients are not very comfortable for very long on either side. They should be turned 45 degrees in each direction for necessary care and observations and then be allowed to remain supine with the affected leg in a neutral position.

A pillow should be placed between the patient's legs before she is turned, in order to help maintain good body

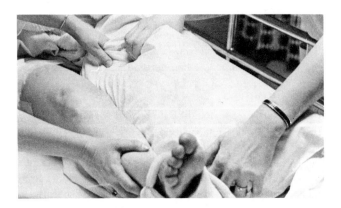

alignment and prevent twisting movement or adduction of the involved extremity. The pillow also prevents strain from being placed on the fracture or surgical area.

To turn the patient, two nurses should face one another on opposite sides of the bed. The bed rail is raised on the side toward which the patient is being turned, and the nurse on that side assists by placing one hand on the patient's shoulder and one on the hip (below the dressing, if that is the operated side.) The other nurse supports the lumbar

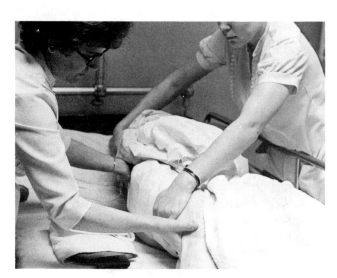

region and the calf of the uppermost leg as the patient turns. When the patient has the bed rail in hand, the nurse on that side can support her long enough for the other nurse to straighten and inspect the drawsheet quickly and to rub the exposed part of the patient's back. The same procedure is then repeated to turn the patient in the opposite direction.

Communication

The nursing goals involved in planning and caring for the patient with a hip pinning include (1) assisting the patient in returning to normal function, if possible, and (2) preventing the complications arising from relative inactivity and helplessness.

Achieving either aim demands an awareness of the obstacles that arise in communicating with the elderly. Attention span is diminished, as is memory, because of the aging process. The nurse may have to establish rapport all over again, *every day*, if the patient is very forgetful. Additional health problems may create further difficulties. A workable approach to building confidence is not always easy to find when the patient is hard of hearing, has cataracts, or is somewhat senile.

However, there *are* elderly patients who are quite alert, usually good-natured, and mostly trusting. Perhaps the best place to start with these patients is to ask them what they would like to be called. This gesture immediately shows respect for the patient as an individual and encourages her to have confidence in the nurse's ability.

Maintaining Nutrition

Although older people have the same fluid and nutritional needs as younger patients, their energy output may be less. For this reason, the caloric requirement is also less and may be reduced by decreasing proportionately the amount of fat and carbohydrates in the diet. Eating habits and feeding problems have been discussed in the section on preoperative care and are applicable here.

Because the geriatric patient usually needs encouragement to eat and drink, she is subject to electrolyte imbalance. Her system will not tolerate the problems that develop from this disturbance as well as that of a younger person would. Careful observation of what she eats and a record of fluid intake and output are essential. It is important to remember that mental confusion in these patients may be the result of such imbalance, rather than senility.

Avoiding Complications

Preventing Pressure Sores

There are always unavoidable exceptions to every rule. But *in general*, a hip-pinning patient who developes pressure sores (decubitus ulcers) is the victim of inadequate nursing care.

All of the previous information on turning the patient and using heel protectors, alternating-pressure mattresses, and sheepskins should prevent pressure sores. The only way a nurse can evaluate the effectiveness of any of these measures is by conscientious observation, every hour if necessary.

Bathing and caring for the patient's skin are easier after the hip has been pinned and the danger of causing further injury has passed. The elderly tend to have dry skin, so complete daily baths may be contraindicated. However, lotions or baby oil should be used freely. The perineum and buttocks need frequent, careful cleansing, especially after bedpan procedures. Powders containing drying agents are beneficial in soothing reddened groins. Caring for the skin of the elderly is much like caring for the skin of a baby.

A clean, dry bed is as important in fighting pressure sores as a clean, dry patient.

Avoiding Contractures

Keeping the patient in good body alignment and encouraging and assisting her in exercises are the best ways to prevent contractures. Flexion deformities of the hip and knee may develop in the inactive patient. A "dropfoot" deformity due to contracture of the Achilles tendon will occur if the foot is not exercised. Because exercise is more effective than a footboard, range of motion of the foot and ankle should be done every 3 hours.

Attending to *comfort* while maintaining proper body alignment may help discourage the well-meaning visitor who wants to place a pillow under the patient's knees to make her "feel better.' The older patient will remain in good body alignment more readily if she is warm enough. The nurse must remember that even though *she* is wearing a sweater and the thermostat is set at 75°F, the *patient* may still be cold.

An older patient who has undergone a hip pinning should not be left to do exercises independently. The patient will need assistance, supervision, instruction, and support. As soon as she is able, she should be taught to grasp the trapeze and lift herself off the bed, in an attempt to maintain muscle strength in her arms. This will prepare her for using a

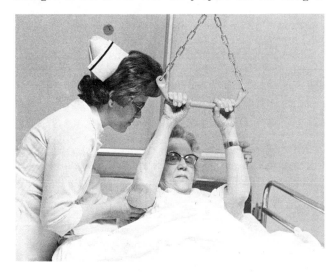

walker or crutches when she becomes ambulatory. Isometric exercises for the gluteal, quadriceps, and abdominal muscles are also helpful. The nurse may encourage movement of all parts of the body as well as rhythmic breathing.

All of this is more complicated than it seems. Elderly patients often need repeated instructions and much moral support to be motivated. They tire easily and experience weakness and stiffness in many areas of the body. Therefore, although it is simple enough for a nurse to realize what would be beneficial to her elderly patient with a hip pinning, it is not always possible to have activities go as planned. This is true in all aspects of her nursing care but is especially noticeable when the patient is exercising in preparation for ambulation. Sometimes perserverance is needed just to gain the patient's attention and cooperation before any physical activity can begin.

Two or three days postoperatively, the surgeon may prescribe muscle-strengthening exercises to be done in the physical therapy department or at the bedside. These consist of working the arms and shoulders with the use of pulleys and lifting sandbag weights with the unaffected foot.

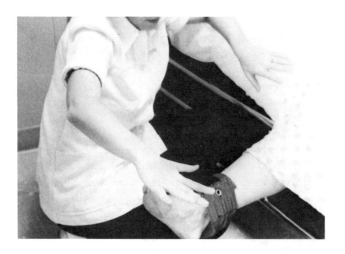

Preventing Pneumonia

Inactivity, decreased lung expansion, and poor circulation make the elderly patient a likely candidate for pneumonia.

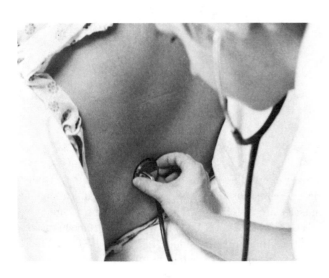

Symptoms of pneumonia are not as dramatically evident in the elderly patient as they are in a younger patient. Therefore, regular auscultation of the lungs aids the nurse in detecting the development of bronchial congestion.

When deep breathing and coughing fail to keep the lungs clear, some assistance, such as intermittent positive-pressure breathing (IPPB), may be required. Elevating the head of the bed assists the patient in coughing. An added precaution is to see that the patient does not become chilled.

Preventing Pulmonary Embolism

One of the leading causes of death in elderly patients who have undergone major surgery on the lower extremities is pulmonary embolism. The signs and symptons of this complication may resemble postoperative pneumonia, and the degree of chest pain and dyspnea depends on the location and size of the embolus. Pulmonary embolism is often "silent," emphasizing the need for close nursing observation of patients with hip surgery. Special attention should be given to changes in respirations or chest sounds (p. 49).

The treatment of pulmonary embolism is basically two-fold: (1) anticoagulation to prevent the formation of further emboli and (2) symptomatic.

Preventing Thrombophlebitis

Encouraging leg movement and assisting the patient in changing her position help prevent thrombophlebitis. Elastic stockings are usually ordered for the patient who has had hip surgery and are a preventive measure against venous stasis, which is a causative factor in thrombophlebitis. How-

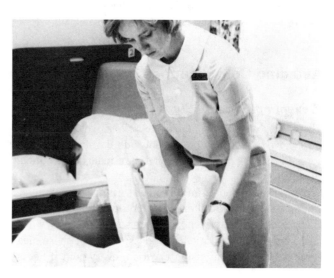

ever, the nurse should be aware that the dependent edema present in the fractured extremity may compress nerves and blood vessels more when the patient is wearing elastic stockings. Color, motion, temperature, and sensation (CMTS) of the toes, and pedal pulses, should be checked routinely. The stocking should be removed twice a day to observe the condition of the leg and foot, especially the heel.

Some surgeons prescribe prophylactic anticoagulation for the patient with a fractured hip. In this case, the nurse must observe the incisional area for evidence of bleeding. Increased swelling, hardness, and ecchymosis in the area may indicate the development of a hematoma.

Preventing Urinary Infection

Incontinence, frequent micturition, inadequate fluid intake, and catheters are contributing factors in the development of urinary infection.

Getting the patient up on a bedside commode, offering the bedpan at frequent intervals, and keeping the bed dry are standard nursing measures to prevent urinary complications.

Catheters present their own problems. When they are inserted, removed, and reinserted, for various reasons, it is almost impossible to avoid irritation of the perineum.

Urging fluids and making diligent efforts to keep the patient's perineum clean and dry are still the best suggestions for preventing urinary-tract infections.

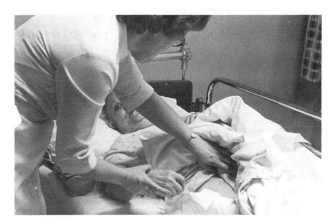

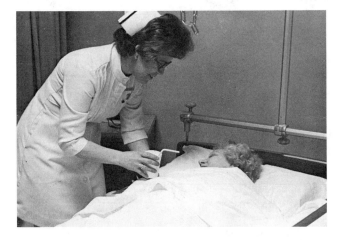

Avoiding Constipation

If concern over constipation were a stimulus for the bowel, the elderly patient would not be plagued with this problem. Those patients who take numerous laxatives or administer their own enemas at home present the nursing staff with problems when they become relatively helpless.

Conservative measures such as prunes or prune juice and vigilant attention to the diet and fluid intake have merit. If stool softeners were prescribed before surgery, they should be continued postoperatively. They aid in lessening constipation and fecal impactions. Laxatives and enemas are almost invariably indicated to some degree.

Bedpan Procedure. To promote elimination, the fracture bedpan should be used, because it slides under the patient with more ease than a regular bedpan. Turning the patient onto the bedpan may be easier postoperatively than having her lift herself with the aid of the trapeze. Much of this is dependent on her orientation, how fearful she is of hurting herself, and how much strength she has.

Preventing Superficial Wound Infections

Strictly speaking, this complication is not the result of inactivity or helplessness. However, because the elderly patient with hip pinning is not always able to express her needs, she may attempt to "help" herself by eliminating sources of discomfort, usually the dressing. It is not uncommon for the patient to pick at the tape, dressing, and finally, the incision. Wound infection may occur after she has done this several times. To avoid this kind of problem, inspection of the dressing should be routine at least twice on each shift.

Avoiding Psychological Problems

The days, and more specifically the nights, that follow the immediate postoperative period test the ingenuity and perhaps the patience of the orthopedic nurse. A commitment to providing TLC is never outdated in nursing and is the best guideline of all in nursing the elderly patient with a hip pinning.

Settling the patient for the night involves much more than positioning her in correct alignment with the proper support of pillows and checking whether or not the siderails are up. The combination of her age and limited mobility, along with thoughts of a long period of convalescence, will produce in this patient a pessimistic outlook. The natural tendency for all people who are ill is to worry more at night. While her night nurse is wondering why she won't sleep following "good" nursing care and a sedative, the patient may be plagued and depressed over such things as how her husband who has cataracts is managing for himself; how he *would* manage if she died, since he hasn't cooked a meal for himself in 60 years; how their finances have been affected by her hospitalization and what assistance is available from other sources; whether or not she will be crippled for the rest of her life; and whether or not she can possibly do all the things the hospital staff requires of her to help herself recover.

In the still unfamiliar environment, she has feelings of loneliness and insecurity. Her bedtime ritual, composed of habits of a lifetime, has been severely altered. She may not only be unable to sleep without her old shawl, but unable to make anyone understand that she would like it brought from home. Although the hospital hot chocolate is not as tasty as hers, it would be more pleasant to drink if some words of comfort were offered with it.

Aside from dealing with these psychological problems, the nurse should learn to identify problems concerning pain or general discomfort. Is the patient having incisional pain or gas pains? Or is the pain somewhere else in her body? Palpate her abdomen or listen to her lungs if either seems appropriate. When is she just restless because of apprehension? In the long run, taking the time on a busy night to put an elderly lady with a hip pinning to bed properly will save time.

Many older people do not require much sleep at night; many older people do not sleep *well* at night. The lifestyle and background of the elderly patient will reveal information that will be helpful in deciding what to do about those who do not seem hopelessly confused and yet attempt to get up over siderails or continually cause commotion. Perhaps the patient had a night job for 50 years or was accustomed to getting up at 3:30 A.M. to do farm chores. The male patient who saw combat in a war may not know much in the way of a "good night's sleep" ever, because of dreams of combat experiences. The patient who cannot or will not sleep at night should be allowed to sit in a wheelchair, perhaps near the nurses' station. This may avoid a nursing exercise in futility.

A preoperative care plan and a summary of considerations in postoperative care planning are presented in the chart below.

THE PATIENT WITH A FRACTURED HIP

PREOPERATIVE CARE PLANNING

Significant Admission Data

Name: Mrs. T. *Age:* 74
Ht. 5'3" *Wt. 160#*
T. 98 *P.* 88 reg *R.* 22 *B.P.* 160/100

Personal Profile:

Hearing slightly impaired. Broke glasses in fall. Has dentures. No problem eating. Eats all but fatty foods. Showers daily. Requires mild laxative occasionally. Retires by 10:00 P.M.. Early riser.

History of Present Condition:

Fell on way home from store this A.M. Admitted per ambulance to emergency room, accompanied by eldest son. Pain in left hip and leg. Slight swelling in thigh with moderate bruise in lateral thigh. Unable to more leg by herself. No other injuries or limitations of motion. (X-ray film from ER shows intertrochanteric fracture of left hip.)

General Health Status:

Good. Hospitalized with miscarriage 30 years ago and surgery for ruptured appendix 3 years ago. Takes antacid p.r.n. for hiatal hernia diagnosed 6 mo ago. Sleeps with two pillows. On no meds for high B.P. States she "never had it before."

Mental/Emotional State:

Is alert, oriented, talkative. Seems distressed at thought of having to use bedpan. Cooperative.

Social History:

Seems to relate well to son. They laugh together. Has been living alone and keeping house in two-story home. Is a widow with six married sons, three of whom live in town. No religious affiliation.

Surgeon's Orders

1. Bucks traction—left leg 5#
2. NPO past midnight
3. Prepare for OR
4. Type and crossmatch for 2 U blood
5. Preop medication per anesthesiologist
6. Demerol 75 mg IM q 3-4 hr p.r.n.
7. Light diet
8. Antacid p.r.n. preoperatively*

Nursing Orders

1. Check traction q 6 hr.
2. Convoluted bedpad
3. Turn patient with pillow between legs ⎫
4. Back and heel care   ⎬ q 3 hr
5. Cough and deep breathe   ⎭
6. CMTS and pedal pulse
7. Speak slowly, clearly, close to patient (hard of hearing)
8. Keep call light near hand
9. Bed rails up at all times
10. Two pillows under head and shoulders
11. B.P. 6 P.M. and 6 A.M.
12. Help with supper and offer fluids (her glasses are broken)
13. Preoperative teaching
14. Encourage fluids until midnight
15. Offer bedpan with other routines

Additional Nursing Responsibilities

Because Mrs. T. has been an active individual and is alert and cooperative, she should have her preoperative teaching done as soon as possible to reduce or prevent anxiety. The nurse should communicate with family members who visit during the evening to identify and fulfill their learning needs regarding their mother's treatment and care.

* This kind of order is easily forgotten, especially if this is the first time the surgeon has had contact with the patient. The nurse should be alert for such situations.

THE PATIENT WITH A FRACTURED HIP *(Continued)*

POSTOPERATIVE CARE PLANNING

NURSING GOALS

1. Promote healing of hip fracture.
2. Assist in restoring the patient to maximal functioning.
3. Prevent complications associated with
   a. The surgical procedure
   b. Immobility
4. Assist patient in maintenance or improvement of present health status.
5. Provide individualized nursing care to meet the patient's total needs.

I. NURSING CARE: INTERNAL FIXATION

A. 24-48 Hour Care

1. Check vital signs frequently until stable.
2. Check dressing and reinforce p.r.n.
3. Icebag to incisional area
4. Turn with pillow between legs.
5. CMTS and pedal pulses of operated leg. Compare frequently with other leg.

B. Ongoing Care

1. Continue to position and turn with pillow.
2. Continue CMTS and pedal pulses bid.
3. Do not flex hips 90 degrees when transferring from bed to chair.
4. Pivot on unaffected leg.
5. No weight bearing on affected leg.
6. Check incision for signs of infection.
7. Evaluate all complaints of pain in left lower extremity.
8. Evaluate effects of pain medications and administer as required.

II. PREVENTION OF PROBLEMS DUE TO IMMOBILITY

A. Respiratory Distress

1. Encourage "stir ups."
2. Auscultate lungs.
3. Evaluate and report any need for additional respiratory support.

B. Gastrointestinal Irregularities

1. Encourage proper nutrition.
2. Assist when eating meals (while eyeglasses gone).
3. Laxative of choice p.r.n.
4. Assess to determine need for stool softener.
5. Up on commode with help.
6. Allow patient time and provide privacy while she is on commode

C. Urinary Problems

1. Check voiding as to amount and color.
2. Encourage fluids.

D. Skin Breakdown

1. Back and heel care
2. Keep skin dry and clean.
3. Change patient's position frequently.

E. Contractures

1. ROM unaffected extremities.
2. Maintain body alignment.
3. Keep temperature of room comfortable.

F. Thrombophlebitis (Pulmonary Embolism)

1. Elastic hose
2. Encourage movement of feet.
3. See I B-7.
4. Observe for any signs of respiratory distress.
5. Be alert to subtle signs of pulmonary embolism: "catch" in chest muscles, diaphoresis, pallor, rapid pulse.

G. Boredom

1. Establish rapport.
2. Provide patient with diversional activities she enjoys.
3. See IV D.

III. PRESENT HEALTH STATUS

A. Hiatal Hernia

1. Elevate head of bed 45 degrees at all times unless patient requests otherwise.
2. Evaluate knowledge of treatment of condition and provide necessary instruction.
3. Report signs of gastric distress (if unrelieved by antacids) to physician.

B. Elevated Blood Pressure

1. Monitor blood pressure bid.
2. Discuss possibility of further medical treatment with physician.
3. Identify patient learning needs regarding relationship between diet, weight, and high blood pressure and provide instruction.

(continued)

THE PATIENT WITH A FRACTURED HIP *(Continued)*

POSTOPERATIVE CARE PLANNING

IV. INDIVIDUALIZING PATIENT CARE

A. Sensory Loss

1. Evaluate extent of visual impairment (while eyeglasses are being repaired).
2. Evaluate hearing loss and plan care and instruction accordingly.

B. Personal Habits

1. Check if she prefers bath before or after P.T.
2. Settle for sleep before 10:00 P.M.

C. Rehabilitation

1. Involve patient and sons in discharge planning as soon as feasible.
2. Read P.T. notes daily and validate with patient. Offer encouragement.*

D. Diversion

1. In view of her cheery disposition and willingness to converse with others, she will probably have, and enjoy having, many visitors. Is evidently close to sons, and their visits may be the best times of her day.
2. Talk to patient about her family.

* Mrs. T. has been so active and independent that, if anything, she may minimize her problems with, or concerns about ambulating. She is anxious for recovery.

Progression of Activity

Getting the Patient Up

It is frequently possible for a patient who has undergone a hip pinning to be out of bed within 24 hours of surgery. Getting the elderly patient out of bed as soon as possible helps prevent the problem of immobility.

The first time a patient is assisted out of bed, it is imperative that enough people be present to ensure a smooth, safe transfer from bed to chair. Mishaps and discomforts in transfer are long remembered, no matter what else the patient may forget!

If available, an orderly, male nurse, or male physical therapist should be asked to assist. Such male assistance provides psychological as well as physical aid, because men are traditionally considered to be the "lifters."

Two people may be required to help the patient to a sitting position on the side of the bed. If she can help pull herself up with the trapeze, she should be encouraged to do

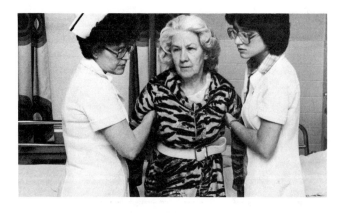

so. A wheelchair with removable arms is recommended the first time the patient is gotten out of bed. The chair should be placed parallel to the bed and locked into position. Whether it faces the foot end or head end of the bed depends on who is doing the lifting and which direction seems the "easiest" to take. When the chair is slightly lower than the bed and when the arms of the chair are removed, it is possible to move the patient with a minimum of upward lifting.

The patient should be lifted from behind the shoulders and under the axillae, with another person helping to place her in a geriatric chair or a wheelchair. If the patient is obese, a Hoyer lift may be needed to move her.

Certain precautions should be kept in mind when the patient is up in a chair. A belt should always be used to secure the patient in the chair if she is to be up for more than a few minutes. Also, the patient *should never be left unattended the first time she is out of bed.* A geriatric chair, if available, is excellent because it comes equipped with a tray, which, when attached in front of the patient, serves as an added safety measure to prevent her from slipping.

Pivoting

The question of when the patient is ready to pivot into the chair is usually a matter of nursing judgment. If possible, the nurse should have assistance, preferably from a physical therapist, when the patient is learning to tolerate this maneuver. The entire procedure of getting the patient up and helping her pivot into a chair for the first time must be done efficiently. This calms her fears of falling or hurting herself when she moves, thus making subsequent preparation for ambulation less difficult.

Reassurance will have to be given again in the following areas:

1. Weakness and the pain of muscle spasm will go away eventually.
2. The stiffness in her joints will lessen as activity increases.
3. Getting her out of bed will be done slowly and carefully.

There are times when all of this has to be explained over some loud "ow–ow-ing" or other noises that indicate that no matter how carefully the nurse is proceeding, the patient is still apprehensive. She may remain so until seated comfortably in a geriatric chair or wheelchair. Even when it appears that her instructions and efforts are not being comprehended, the nurse must keep repeating and explaining in the hope that her patient is listening and understanding some of what is happening. *Establishing rapport is a continuous process.*

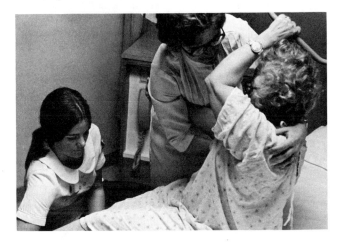

The patient should be swivelled to a sitting position in bed. The chair should be placed parallel to the bed facing the uninvolved extremity and locked into position. The patient should be allowed to sit on the edge of the bed, with support, for a few minutes until she feels steady. At this time, the nurse should encourage her to take deep breaths, sit erect, and contract her abdominal and gluteal muscles. Then the patient is helped to a standing position.

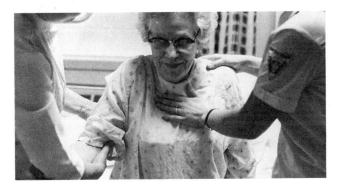

There are several methods of doing this, and the one that is chosen will depend on the preference of the nurse doing the lifting. The nurse may lift the patient by placing her

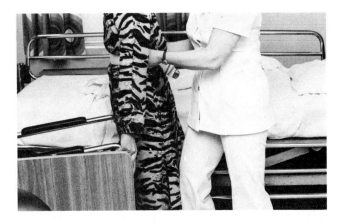

hands and arms under the patient's axillae, under the axillae and up on the upper back, or around the patient's waist. She may lock her knees against the patient's knees as she is

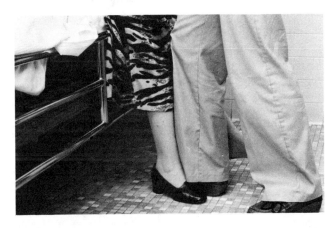

lifting or may place her foot in front of the patient's feet to prevent her from slipping as she rises and pivots.

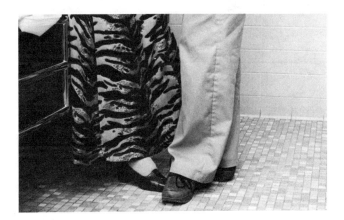

The important points to remember are that the nurse, as well as the patient, must feel secure in the method of lifting that is chosen and that the patient should never be allowed to grab the nurse around the neck. The patient should wear slippers or shoes with nonskid bottoms as a safety measure whenever she gets out of bed.

When helping the patient to stand, instruct her to bear no weight on the affected limb and to pivot or turn on the other leg until her back is toward the chair seat. She should be guided into the chair, which is parallel to the bed and locked into position.

Once the patient is seated comfortably it might be a good opportunity to get her out of her room and in contact with the world around her by wheeling her into the day room or hall. Frequently, older people remain more oriented when they are no longer confined to one room. However, once in awhile, a mentally alert patient objects to leaving her room, preferring the company of a roommate or the opportunity just to look out the window. Therefore, whenever possible, the patient should be consulted about what she would like to do.

Although the plan of care may be to have the patient remain up in a chair for several hours, she may be unable to tolerate this immobile position for longer than 1 or 2 hours and should not be expected to do so.

To encourage self-reliance, the patient can be assisted in doing things for herself, such as combing her hair or brushing her teeth. Putting on her glasses or hearing aid, if she has one, will help her develop interest in what is going on around her. The nurse who takes the time to involve the patient in this way shows that she cares and helps the elderly patient to increase her feelings of self-worth.

When the time comes to put the patient back to bed, the chair should be steadied and locked in place and the patient

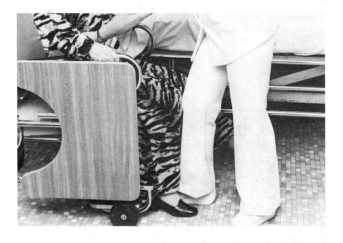

instructed to bend forward from the hips. Next she should be told to place her unaffected leg far backward into an acute angle. If she can flex the knee on her affected side and

place her foot flat on the floor, she can be helped to a standing position, with weightbearing on the uninvolved side. She can then be swung around with her back to the bed. Once again, if the patient shows signs of apprehension or unwillingness to cooperate, the nurse should ask another person to assist.

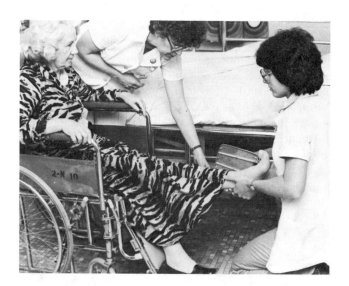

Remember, all of these procedures are made awkward by the patient's discomfort, stiffness, and apprehension. Using proper body mechanics lessens the strain of transferring a resisting patient.

Physical Therapy

Ambulating without weightbearing is ordered according to patient readiness and the surgeon's preference, but ambulation is generally begun about 3 days after surgery. As with all new endeavors, the patient needs a great deal of support. However, so does the therapist! This important fact is easily overlooked by a busy nurse.

Conferring with the therapist about the patient's general condition and response to treatment will produce insights into management. When the patient first goes to the therapy department, the therapist should know if she has recently been given a pain medication, laxative, or anything else that might affect behavior and stability.

Visiting the physical therapy department occasionally when the patient is there enables the nurse to offer encouragement and evaluate later complaints about being "tired out" or "worked too hard." Also, the patient feels that the nurse who comes to physical therapy to see her really "cares."

Activities in physical therapy, besides the shoulder and arm exercises mentioned previously, include walking between parallel bars. The patient must be reminded con-

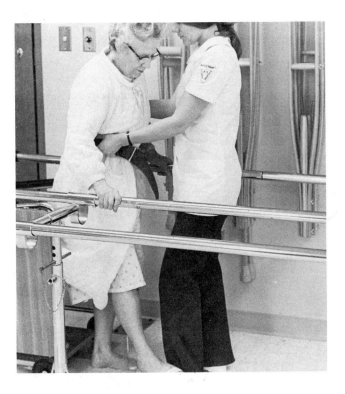

stantly not to bear weight on her affected leg. She is told to keep her foot on top of the therapist's. In this way the therapist "walks" the patient's involved leg.

Use of the walker is undertaken when the therapist judges that the patient has the stability and strength neces-

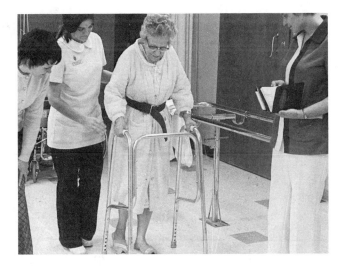

sary to handle it. Close communication between physical therapist and surgeon is essential at this stage of rehabilitation.

Moving a walker and bearing weight on only one leg often require much concentration, and the patient must be encouraged to stand up straight and look ahead.

Discharge Planning

Since the patient will not be allowed to bear full weight on the operated leg for 10 weeks to 3 months after she leaves the hospital, discharge planning with patient and family teaching should begin as soon as possible after admission. The nurse should work closely with the discharge planner or social worker in acquainting herself with family members and helping acquire and relay information. This often requires watching for visitors and making phone calls, because there may not be many relatives or people available with whom to discuss plans. After it is determined where the patient will go when she leaves the hospital, specific recommendations are possible.

If the patient is to return to her own home or that of a family member, there are many suggestions the nurse can offer to help eliminate frustration and avoid feelings of helplessness in those who are involved.

An informational booklet designed for the family is a useful tool and may be given to a family member long before the patient is ready for discharge. An example of such a booklet is "Going Home with the Patient Who Has Had a Hip Pinning" (p. 194–195). The discharge planner, staff nurse, and physical therapist should provide the input for such a booklet, and all three should assume responsibility for discussing the information with the patient's family.

Because insecurity and disability are related more to physiologic rather than chronologic age, the physical therapist and nurse must individualize instruction. There is no complete list of rules for everyone. A thin 80-year-old woman may be more agile with a walker at discharge than one who is 65 and obese. However, most older patients go home with a walker as an assistive device because they feel more secure.

Younger people who fracture their hips are frequently discharged from the hospital with crutches. The comprehensive approach to their care and discharge planning is, of course, modified accordingly.

Special Considerations For The Patient With a Femoral Prosthesis

Nursing Implications

Patients who have had a hip prosthesis inserted return from surgery with an abductor splint or pillow in place between their thighs. Although it is awkward to do nursing procedures around this supportive device, it does ensure proper position of the limb. But, if the patient becomes confused, she may attempt to remove it or twist her body in an effort to turn herself unassisted.

A word of caution about abductor pillows is advisable at this point. When at all possible, the straps should be fastened loosely. The proximal straps of the pillow may lie over

GOING HOME WITH THE PATIENT WHO HAS HAD A HIP PINNING*

Although it is necessary to make some changes in the home to accommodate the person who has had a hip pinning, it is not necessary — at least, not usually — to make an invalid out of someone who was previously active.

Therefore, while there is a lot of equipment (such as wheelchairs, and hospital beds) that could be purchased, do not turn the home into a hospital. Buy what you need to make life *safe* and *comfortable* for your relative, not what Uncle Harry bought or what the neighbors have.

The discharge planner and the physical therapist will help you decide what those needs are. Besides the fact that your relative has some limits on how much moving around he/she can do, things that affect what you need to change or buy are: height; the condition of other joints (is the patient stiff?), eyesight, and sleeping habits.

Arrangements in the Home . . .

It is most important to do the following:

1. Make wide, clear pathways.
2. Remove scatter rugs.
3. Do *not* wax floors.
4. Be sure there are no lamp cords where the bottom of a walker or crutch could catch on them.

Lighting . . .

The home should have plenty of lights in areas where your relative will do the most moving around. Also, leave a light on at night in the pathway that leads to the bathroom.

Chairs . . .

Keep chairs where they are easy to reach. It is good to place chairs near a favorite window, the bed, and the television set, and to leave them there. These chairs should have firm bottoms and good arm supports. Otherwise, your relative may need to use the walker as a support when getting out of the chair, and since a walker is not made for this purpose, it will tip over. A chair should not be so deep that the person has trouble getting out of it. If your relative has stiff elbows, you may want straight-backed chairs, so the seat can be used as a means to push up when rising.

The Bed . . .

Should be on the first floor. A special bed is usually not necessary.

Bathroom Facilities . . .

A raised toilet seat may or may not be necessary, depending on how tall the person is. A guard rail may be purchased that attaches to the toilet and is useful in getting up and down. The therapist, nurse, or discharge planner can show you pictures of these items if you would like to see the various types.

You may even want to keep a chair or stool in the tub on a bathmat for the patient to sit on while taking a shower. It is easier and safer to have an attachment for the bathtub faucet that allows your relative to shower, than it is for him/her to take a tub bath.

Activity . . .

Will be discussed in detail before you go home, and the physical therapist will give you all the instructions you need. Although it varies from person to person, full weight bearing on the operated side is usually not allowed for at least 8 to 10 weeks.

You can remember the following as general rules:

1. Encourage arm and shoulder exercises and deep breathing.
2. Remind your relative not to "shuffle" when walking. The physical therapist stresses this and will be grateful if you remember it also.

(continued)

GOING HOME WITH THE PATIENT WHO HAS HAD A HIP PINNING *(Continued)*

3. Bending way over should not be permitted, since it puts a strain on the hip joint.
QUESTIONS ABOUT AMBULATION or use of equipment used for walking can be answered by the physical-therapy department if you call the hospital. PAIN during weight bearing should be reported to the doctor.

Where to Buy Equipment . . .

The discharge planner will help you choose the things you need and advise you on the best ways to purchase them. For example, if it is something you do not need right away, you may prefer to order it out of a catalog. Sears has a catalog illustrating many types of equipment for home health care. Otherwise, many items may be purchased somewhere else in the city. Usually it is not necessary to purchase any items other than a walker or other assistive device and a raised toilet seat.

The discharge planner also has information on what Medicare covers.

Using Other People's Equipment . . .

Sometimes this is all right. But if you are going to borrow any assistive devices for walking, such as a walker, be sure you bring it in to the physical-therapy department for adjustment, *first.*

Tender Loving Care . . .

"TLC" is always important. It consists, first of all, in knowing that the elderly person who has broken a hip once may be fearful of doing so again. Even when the patient appears to be making great progress, he/she may feel helpless at times. Remember also that other limitations, such as poor eyesight, are harder to deal with when someone is trying to walk again. Have patience, and even though you, yourself, feel helpless at times, remember that giving moral support is one of the most important things you can do.

* Courtesy, Bellin Memorial Hospital, Green Bay, Wisconsin

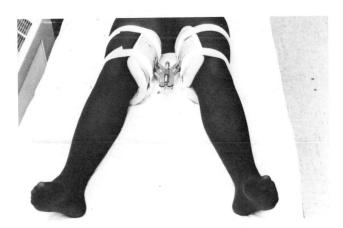

Abductor splint (Courtesy, Richards Manufacturing Co)

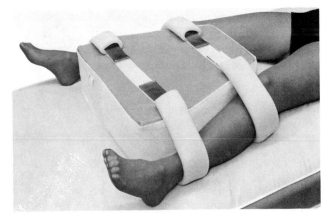

Abductor pillow (Courtesy, Zimmer Co, Warsaw, Ind)

the upper end of the fibula. This is especially true in the case of a patient with short, heavy legs. It is imperative that the nurse check every 3 hours to be certain that the patient's toes have sensation and motion and are not pointing toward the midline of the body, indicating pressure on the peroneal nerve.

One way to avoid pressure on the peroneal nerve is to position the abductor pillow further up between the patient's thighs. This creates problems too, since it makes using the bedpan awkward. However, on a patient with heavy legs for whom straps need to be tighter to make contact with the pillow, it may be desirable to have the pillow positioned where the straps are not directly over the superficial peroneal nerve.

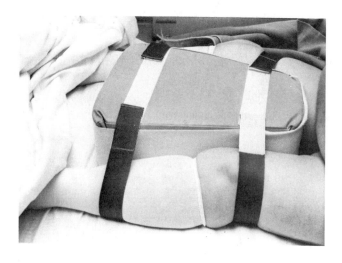

Implications for Ambulation

Since no healing of a fracture site is involved, weightbearing proceeds almost immediately after the patient has achieved balance when in a standing position between parallel bars. Whether the first visit to physical therapy occurs 2 or 5 days after surgery depends on the orders of the individual surgeon.

Surgeons permit the abductor splint or pillow to be removed *only* for daily skin care and physical therapy. The length of time it remains on the patient is a decision made by the physician on an individual patient basis.

General condition and the stability of the whole hip joint may dictate when these patients are allowed to get out of bed, but it is not unusual for the patient to be sitting in a chair 2 days postoperatively.

The abductor splint or pillow proves especially difficult at this time, because it is a cumbersome device in which to pivot. Thus, the patient needs *time,* and encouragement, and assistance to manage while the pillow is in place.

Discussion Questions

1. The following information is from a 7:00 A.M. shift report. What additional data is necessary in order for the nurse to make an assessment and plan care for the patient? Mrs. J. is an 80-year old patient who had a right hip pinning 8 days ago. She has been doing fine. But her temperature at midnight was 100.4°, and at 4:00 A.M. it was 99.6°. She was very restless part of the night but not really disoriented. Her oral intake was 150 ml, and her indwelling catheter output was 450 ml. On evening shift she kept complaining that her "legs hurt," but she seemed unable or unwilling to be more specific.

Consider. What are the possible causes of an elevated temperature at this point in time? Disorientation? What complications might be causing the patient's legs to hurt? Could some aspects of treatment and therapy be responsible for pain in the patient's legs?

2. Mrs. R. is an 84-year-old woman who enters the hospital with a diagnosis of "subcapital fracture of the right hip." Her daughter states that her mother "did not really fall" but slipped and "almost lost her balance" 2 days ago. Since then the patient was in and out of bed with discomfort in her hip. Today she saw her family physician, who took the x-ray films and admitted her to the hospital. What can the nurse tell the daughter about the following?

   a. The type of operative procedure likely to be done
   b. Routine postoperative regimen
   c. Progression of activities and ambulation

Consider. How do the following affect surgical treatment of hip fracture: Location of fracture? Time interval? What is the basic difference between planning care and rehabilitation for a hip pinning as opposed to insertion of a femoral prosthesis?

3 L. K. is a 53-year old school teacher who sustained an intertrochanteric fracture of his left hip in a fall while downhill skiing. He enters the hospital the same Sunday afternoon in severe pain and is emotionally distressed about his "clumsiness." The emergency-room physician has ordered that an orthopedic surgeon be asked to see the patient.

   a. What are the priorities in giving care for the remainder of the day?
   b. What factors must be taken into consideration in formulating both long-term and short-term goals?

Consider: What signs and symptoms need immediate attention? How might the patient's concerns change as the day progresses? How important is immediate contact with an orthopedic surgeon? From what standpoint? In what ways will the patient's lifestyle have implications for patient teaching and supportive care?

Bibliography

Allen S, Moschak V: Step by step . . . . Nursing '81 11:56–7, 1981

Arnold WD: The effect of early weight-bearing on the stability of femoral neck fractures treated with Knowles pins. J Bone Joint Surg (Am) 66(6):847, 1984

Barden RM: Osteonecrosis of the femoral head. Orthop Nurs 4(4):45, 1985

Bhuller GS: Use of the Giliberty bipolar endoprosthesis in femoral neck fractures. Clin Orthop 162:165, 1982

Brown R: Implants: Hip and knee arthroplasty. JORRI, 2:26, 1982

Brunner, N.A.: Orthopedic Nursing, 4th ed. St. Louis, CV Mosby, 1983

Burnett JW, et al: Prophylactic antibiotics in hip fractures. J Bone Joint Surg (Am) 62(3):457, 1980

Cameron HU: The results of early clinical trials with a microporus coated metal hip prosthesis. Clin Orthop, 165:188, 1982

Ceccio CM: Postoperative pain relief through relaxation in elderly patients with fractured hips. Orthop Nurs 3(3):11, 1984

Chaffee E. Lytle M: Basic Physiology and Anatomy, 4th ed. Philadelphia; JB Lippincott, 1980

Crenshaw AH (ed.): Campbell's Operative Orthopaedics, 6th ed. St. Louis, CV Mosby, 1980

Davis P: Nursing care study: A break from the bottle. Nurs Mirror 155(23):48, 1982

Derscheid G: Symposium on orthopedic nursing, rehabilitation of common orthopedic problems. Nurs Clin North Am 16:709, 1981

DeYoung M: Care of the acutely ill older adult: Planning for discharge. Geriatr Nurs 3(8):399, 1982

Duerksen J: Hip fractures: Special considerations for the elderly patient. Orthop Nurs 1:43, 1982

Durney E: Fractured hip: How to position and mobilize patients without undoing their surgery. RN 42:44, 1979

Evans E: Back on her feet again: how an elderly patient learned to be independent again after falling and fracturing her hip. Nurs Mirror, 155(23):48, 1982

Farrell J: Orthopedic pain: What does it mean? Am J Nurs 84(4):466, 1984

Garland DE, Miller G: Fractures and dislocations about the hip in head-injured adults. Clin Orthop 186:154, 1984

Godina E: Femur fracture in an elderly patient: Make or break. Nurs Mirror 153:32, 1981

Goss CM (ed.): Gray's Anatomy, 20th ed. Philadelphia, Lea & Febiger, 1973

Grant PM: Hospitalization and the elderly patient. Nurs Times 72:379, 1976

Hadden WA: Hip fractures of rheumatoid arthritis. Clin Orthop 170:252, 1982

Hanna A: Nursing care study: Make or break. Nurs Mirror. 155(15):59, 1982

Heppenstall R: Fracture Treatment and Healing. Philadelphia. WB Saunders, 1980

Heyse-Moore GH, et al: Treatment of intertrochanteric fractures of the femur: A comparison of the Richards screw plate with the Jewett nail plate. J Bone Joint Surg (Br) 65(3):262, 1983

Hilt N, Cogburn S: Manual of Orthopedics. St. Louis, CV Mosby, 1980

Hollinshead WH: Textbook of Anatomy, 3rd ed. Hagerstown, Md, Harper & Row, 1974

Jacobs B, Young M: Transferring patients. Nursing '81 11:64, 1981

Kenzora JE, et al: Hip fracture mortality: Relation to age, treatment, preoperative illness, time of surgery, and complications. Clin Orthop 186:45, 1984

Klasen HJ, Binnendijk B: Fracture of the neck of the femur associated with posterior dislocation of the hip. J Bone Joint Surg (Br) 66(1):45, 1984

Langley LL, et al: Dynamic Anatomy and Physiology, 5th ed. New York, McGraw-Hill, 1980

Larson C, Gould M: Orthopedic Nursing, 9th ed. St. Louis, CV Mosby, 1978

Lipson D: Hip fractures and the elderly—Can one predict the success of rehabilitation? Nursing Homes 30:18, 1981

Melton LJ, et al: Fifty-year trend in the hip fracture incidence. Clin Orthop 162:144, 1982

Mikhail SF, et al: Optimism in the management of hip fracture in elderly patients. J Am Geriatr Soc 26(1):39, 1978

Miller CW: Survival and ambulation following hip fracture. Bone and Joint Surg 60A(7):930, 1978

Mullendore JW: What goes on in physical therapy. RN 45(5):54, 1982

Oliver M: Have crutch, will travel . . . I fractured my hip. Am J Nurs 83(8):1228, 1983

Ort PJ, LaMondt J: Treatment of femoral neck fractures with a sliding compression screw and two Knowles pins. Clin Orthop 190:158, 1984

Owen RA: Colle's fracture and subsequent hip fracture risk. Clin Orthop 171:37, 1982

Portnoi VA, Koshes R: Institutionalization of patients with hip fractures. JAMA 249(10):29, 1983

Punton S: Activities of living: The struggle for independence. Burford: A model for nursing. Nurs Times 79(9):29, 1983

Raney RB, Brashear HR: Shand's Handbook of Orthopaedic Surgery, 9th ed. St. Louis, CV Mosby, 1978

Rao JP, et al: Treatment of unstable intertrochanteric fractures with anatomic reduction and compression hip screw fixation. Clin Orthop (175):65, May 1983

Rau FD, et al: Treatment of femoral neck fractures with the sliding compression screw. Clin Orthop 163:137, 1982

Regan WA: Decubitus ulcers in nursing home care. Regan Report on Nursing Law 22(9):4, 1982

Rockwood CA, Green DP: Fractures. Philadelphia, JB Lippincott, 1975

Spicer A: Nursing care study: Home from home. Nurs Mirror 157(14):44, 1983

Stephany, TM: That's our grandma. J Pract Nurs 32(4):34, 1982

Stephens SJ: Creative approaches to pressure sore problems. Orthop Nurs 4(4):40, 1985

Swiontkowski MF, et al: Fractures of the femoral neck in patients between the ages of twelve and forty-nine years. J Bone Joint Surg (Am) 66(6):837, 1984

White L, et al: Who is at risk? Hip fracture epidemiology report. J Gerontol Nurs 10(10):26, 1984

Wile PB, et al: Treatment of subtrochanteric fractures with a high-angle compression hip screw. Clin Orthop 175:72, 1983

Williams M, et al: Nursing activities and acute confusional states. Nurs Res 28(1):25, 1979

Wolfgang GL, et al: Treatment of intertrochanteric fracture of the femur using sliding screw plate fixation. Clin Orthop 165:188, 1982

6

Care of the Patient Who Has Undergone Hip Reconstruction

Whatever the future of joint replacement, there is no doubt that it has given many people with degenerative hip joint disease a new lease on life. A great number of people who have not ambulated without pain for years, or perhaps have not ambulated at all, are now able to do so. As a result of a joint replacement operation, many people walk with decreased joint discomfort, increased range of motion, and less dependence on assistive devices.

Joint re-replacement sometimes becomes necessary because cement failure or bone resorption can occur, causing loosening of the components, usually the femoral ones. Although this happens more frequently in active patients, the lifespan of an original procedure is variable.

Problems with the devices themselves have been identified, and the design of prostheses continues to evolve. Methods of fixation of the prosthesis into the skeleton are also the subject of ongoing research.

For the orthopedic nurse, the field of joint replacement continues to offer rewarding opportunities for patient care and education. Since hip joint replacement has become a common procedure, the average patient is somewhat familiar with the concept and probably knows at least one other person who has had total hip replacement. Nursing care plans and rehabilitation programs differ regionally and are based on the surgical approach and the surgeon's philosophy. The nurse often has to answer questions such as "Why did my friend in Washington have to stay in bed 4 days if I don't?" It is still true that joint replacement operations and the circumstances surrounding them are not all alike, and the nurse must constantly encourage the patient to rely on the physician or members of the nursing staff for answers to questions. Each individual may present a unique problem.

Assisting in the rehabilitation of a patient who has had hip joint replacement and hearing him marvel at his progress is stimulating and gratifying to the nurse. This has not changed; if anything, statistics on the success of the procedure have made it even more true.

Although the hip and the knee are the joints most commonly being replaced, it is not uncommon to replace shoulders, elbows, wrists, finger joints, and ankles. The principles of postoperative treatment are basically the same for all joint replacements and relate to restoring painfree motion and helping the patient regain strength in the operated extremity.

However, certain warnings are in order. These operations are no panacea for joint disease. Like all surgical procedures, they have contraindications, disadvantages, and complications. A realization of this should serve to prevent the development of a false sense of security in those who work in orthopedics. An added danger arises from the fact that when something is as successful as the total hip replacement, it is easy to lose sight of the patient as an individual.

Degenerative Disease of the Hip Joint

Mechanics of the Hip Joint

The hip is a weightbearing ball and socket joint. The forces

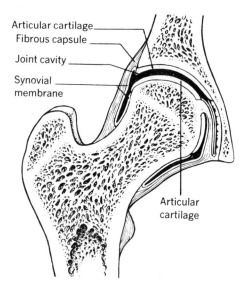

(Chaffee and Lytle: Basic Physiology and Anatomy, 4th ed. Lippincott, 1980)

across a normal hip, just in walking, consist of body weight plus the pull of abductor muscles. As the average person walks, he puts 2½ to 3 times his body weight on each hip.

In order for the hip to function properly under this stress, the head of the femur needs to be nearly spherical in shape, covered with smooth articular cartilage, and riding in an acetabulum that is a near-perfect match.

Factors Inducing Degenerative Disease

Anything that disturbs the normal relationship of the ball and socket may result in joint incongruity and friction, leading in turn to areas of wear, pain, and degeneration. Some factors involved in this process include the following:

1. Inflammation due to disease, such as rheumatoid arthritis or infection, or an injury, leading to the release of enzymes that cause degradation of the joint.
2. Irregularities that occur in the femoral head, following the healing of a fracture, Legg-Perthes disease, or slipped epiphysis.
3. Instability caused by dysplasia.
4. Irregularities of the acetabulum secondary to fractures of the pelvis.
5. Avascular necrosis of the femoral head secondary to alcoholism, Caisson's disease, and systemic diseases.
6. Miscellaneous factors, such as obesity, hormonal dysfunction, and menopause.
7. Physiologic changes in the articular cartilage due to aging, which hasten the degenerative process.

Clinical Picture

Pain that is increased by weight bearing is the major symptom of degenerative hip disease. It may be referred from the hip along the anterior and medial aspect of the thigh, as far down as the knee. This pain restricts motion. The patient also complains of stiffness after the hip has been at rest. When walking, he will shift his weight to protect the diseased hip, producing a protective limp.

As the disease progresses, motion becomes even more limited due to joint contracture. Pain is present at rest, as well as with function. Night pain becomes a common complaint. Severe joint changes eventually cause shortening of the extremity.

X-ray Findings

Major x-ray findings include narrowing or disappearance of the joint space, flattening of the femoral head, sclerotic changes, and osteophytes. In the x-ray film below, note the shortening of the neck of the femur and the sclerotic areas resulting from the bone's response to stress.

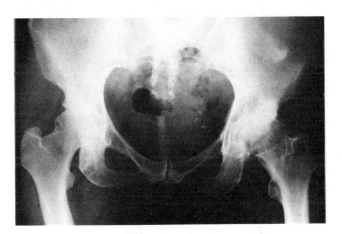

Total Hip Replacement

The complete replacement of a hip joint by acetabular and femoral components is the standard treatment for degenerative hip joint disease. The prosthesis most commonly used consists of a high-density polyethylene cup and a metal or metal-alloy femoral component, which produces a low-friction joint surface.

Each element is secured in place by a compound, methyl methacrylate, which has an elasticity comparable to that of bone. Variations in the basic design of plastic-cup and metal-femoral components are related to the size of the femoral head and the shape of the neck and stem and depend on the manufacturer.

Aluminum oxide ceramic has also been used in the construction of a prosthesis model. This prosthesis is generally used in cementless fixation techniques.

In the area of research and development, better methods of fixation are being pursued intensively in the hope of reducing the incidence of loosening and enabling surgeons to do hip joint replacement on younger patients. Prostheses that are porous-coated, fenestrated, or threaded, to provide places for bony ingrowth, are currently in use, and the

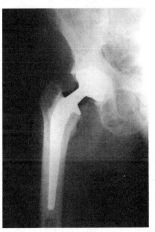 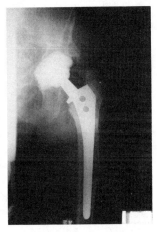

Common cemented total hip prosthesis.

Autophor ceramic-head cup. (Courtesy Osteo AG, Selzach, Switzerland)

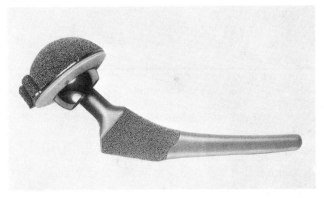

PCA porous-coated prosthesis. (Courtesy Howmedica, Inc, Rutherford, New Jersey)

search for a more physiological cement substance continues.

Engineers have also had to design femoral components for the patient who fractures a femur around and just below the femoral stem of a total hip replacement.

Perhaps the most obvious trend in hip joint replacement is that surgeons are placing more emphasis on alteration in life-style. Any hip replacement patient needs to keep his weight down and live with a measure of caution, keeping safety in his environment a priority so that the possibility of falling is kept to a minimum. Selection of the appropriate prosthetic system is the surgeon's responsibility, but care of the implanted unit is the lifelong responsibility of the patient.

Care of the Patient Undergoing a Total Hip Replacement

Rationale

The plan of care for total hip replacement as presented here is based on: (1) the fact that modern surgical techniques make it possible for the average patient to be out of bed and standing between parallel bars as early as the first postoperative day, and (2) the assumption that since immobility is undesirable, early ambulation is a common practice.

Candidates

The development of new designs and refinement of operative techniques have made total hip replacement the treatment of choice for patients of all ages and conditions for whom a painful hip has become intolerable. Ideal candidates are the elderly patient with osteoarthritis of one or both hips who is otherwise in good general health, and the younger patient with a degenerative hip condition due to trauma. Less favorable candidates include the patient with severe, crippling rheumatoid arthritis in many joints, some of which will eventually need reconstructive surgery, and the overweight patient with hypertension, diabetes, or Paget's disease. These patients may suffer setbacks not related to their hip replacement, or they may make slower progress in their physical-therapy program. Nevertheless, with time, care, and love, they will show marked improvement in their ambulation.

Regardless of the type of patient, the objectives remain the same for all patients—to eliminate pain and restore function.

Prognosis

In general, a patient having a total hip replacement is kept on bed rest a minimal amount of time, with the operated extremity in abduction by means of traction, an abductor splint, or an abductor pillow. Early ambulation is the key to reducing postoperative complications.

Once he is allowed out of bed, his progression in activities and ambulation is steady, so that discharge, perhaps with only one cane, is possible 9 or 10 days postoperatively. Weightbearing may be restricted with some cementless prostheses. Nevertheless, early discharge with walker or crutches is still the norm.

Overall, the prognosis for total hip replacement is excellent, and within 6 months, most patients have returned to a more active life than they had known before surgery. Their activities are not restricted, except for those postions that require extreme hip flexion, such as bending over to pick up an object from the floor. Reports of pain are rare.

PREOPERATIVE PREPARATION

Psychological Preparation

Fortunately, whatever the patient's condition and preoperative attitude and fears, success has made total hip replacement an "I told you so" operation, thereby facilitating the job of surgeon, nurse, and therapist.

Education for the operation begins in the physician's office. Patients should have a thorough explanation of what a "total hip" is and what the plan of treatment and care will be like following the operation.

In the hospital, an excellent teaching tool for both the patient and family is a photograph album containing snapshots of people, equipment, and procedures involved in the entire program, along with captions and paragraphs providing explanations. The inside of the recovery room, the application of Buck's traction, an abductor splint, an abductor pillow, exercise equipment, a picture of a prosthesis, the turning procedure, the hospital chaplain, and the discharge planner are examples of what should be included in the album.

In addition to the written explanations, the patient should meet the therapist and other personnel with whom he will have the most contact. The therapist visits the pa-

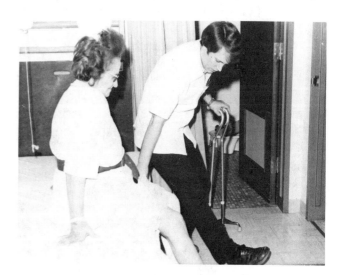

tient to establish rapport, obtain a history, evaluate the condition of the affected hip, determine the patient's ability to ambulate, and teach the basic elements of the rehabilitation program.

The therapist must also learn from the patient what effect pain and limitation of motion have had on activities of daily living, such as dressing, walking, and climbing stairs. He also questions the status of the patient's other joints to evaluate how they might affect the outcome of rehabilitation.

Evaluation of the patient's condition includes testing the strength of the hip by manual muscle test, determining endurance (how far the patient can walk with or without pain), and checking the range of motion of the hip. The knees are also checked for signs of contractures, and the patient's gait is evaluated, along with the ability to transfer from bed to chair. An example of a completed data base, such as might be used by a physical-therapy department, appears on page 202.

Once this evaluation is completed, the patient is "introduced" to the physical-therapy department to learn more about what will happen there. Three specific areas of the rehabilitation program are explained to the patient:

1. The *typical* postoperative course is described, along with those aspects of the program that will emphasize the patient's individual needs based on the therapist's evaluation. For instance, a patient with severe contractures may need more exercises to stretch flexors.
2. The various exercises are discussed, demonstrated when possible, and perhaps illustrated in drawings.
3. Finally, the patient is told about the precautions that will be taken when he is being moved and about those that he must take postoperatively, such as avoiding hip flexion and adduction.

Here, too, it is important to let the patient know that any modification of the general plan is only done by order of the surgeon.

In addition to meetings with the physical therapist, the patient most likely will receive a preoperative visit from the anesthesiologist for the purpose of explaining the type of anesthesia that will be used. Spinal anesthesia, in particular, can be frightening to a patient who has not been properly instructed. Surgeons who prefer spinal anesthesia do so because blood loss is less, cardiopulmonary problems are fewer, and the patient's immediate postoperative comfort is greater. Follow-up clarification and positive reinforcement by the nurse may be required if the patient still has anxiety and questions.

During all of this preparation, the nurse must consider the patient as an individual, recognizing when cooperation is due to understanding, and when the patient is agreeing automatically because of preoccupation with other concerns. Perhaps the most pressing problem on the mind of a 65-year-old woman is whether or not her 90-year-old mother will be properly cared for in her absence. In this instance, a perceptive nurse will realize the importance of regular communication between the patient and whoever is taking care of her mother.

Physical Preparation

A complete physical examination is necessary before surgery. For many surgeons it is routine to admit patients to the hospital a day early in order to have the physical examination done as close to the scheduled date of operation as possible. Owing to the average age of these patients, preoperative electrocardiograms are routine. Those patients with existing health problems may require evaluation of their status by an internist. Arthritics who have been taking aspirin need additional laboratory studies, such as prothrombin times, to determine whether or not bleeding might be a problem. In general, patients on anti-inflammatory drugs should have non-aspirin medications postoperatively. However, to shorten the period of hospitalization, patients frequently enter the hospital with most of their preoperative tests completed.

The goal of preoperative medical treatment is to have the patient in the best physiological condition possible prior to this major surgery.

Surgical preparation of the skin is done the day before the operation. The entire thigh and hip area is scrubbed at least twice with a germicidal solution. The skin is shaved with great care, so as not to inflict scratches or cuts and thus provide an entry site for bacteria. More and more surgeons are electing to have the shaving done on the day of surgery. Since postoperative infection in joint replacement is extremely serious, prophylactic antibiotics may be started orally the day before surgery.

Equipment and Room Preparation

It goes without saying that the bed should be equipped with a firm foundation under the mattress, a trapeze on the overhead frame, and an attachment to hold an intravenous solution.

After the patient goes to surgery, the bed is stripped and a complete change of linen is applied. Then, along with the bed, the equipment for providing abduction of the operated hip, traction, the abductor pillow or splint, and a pair of heel protectors can be sent to surgery.

POSTOPERATIVE CARE

Vital Signs

A patient who has had a total hip replacement frequently returns to the unit from the recovery room showing signs of pallor, chilliness, low blood pressure, and a rapid pulse. This is due to a combination of factors including the preoperative medication, spinal anesthesia, and blood loss during sur-

DATA BASE FOR PHYSICAL THERAPY*
TOTAL HIP PREOP EVALUATION (RIGHT/(LEFT))

Name _Jacobs, Henry_   Patient # _10865-3_   Date _4-10_

Physician _Dr. Smith_   Diagnosis _Left hip osteoarthritis, left THR 4-11_

Patient's understanding of why physical therapy was ordered, his/her receptivity to P.T., and response to preop instructions/precautions.

Pt. expressed concern over the precautions and needed reassuring. Somewhat apprehensive
regarding the exercise program he will need to do at home.

ROM:	INVOLVED	UNINVOLVED	Strength:	INVOLVED	UNINVOLVED
Flexion	$0°-90°$	$0°-106°$	Flexion	$Fair^+$	$Good^-$
Thomas position	$0°$	$0°-5°$	Extension	$Fair$	$Fair^+$
Abduction	$0°-10°$	$0°-25°$	Abduction	$Fair^-$	$Fair$
External rotation	$0°-8°$	$0°-30°$	External rotation	$Fair^-$	$Fair^+$
Knee ext./flex.	$0°/110°$	$0°/115°$	Knee ext./flex.	$Good^-/Good^-$	$Good^-/Good^-$

Anthropometric:	INVOLVED	UNINVOLVED	Leg Length:	
15 cm. above	48 cm	49 cm	Asis—lateral malleolus	_left 90 cm right 91 cm_
Knee joint line	41	42	Apparent (observed supine)	_left < right_

Independent/
Assistive devices/
Distance ambulating/
Note degree of
pain/Limp

GAIT

Pt. walks indep. short distances without assistive device. Obvious
limp; noted 2° pain left hip during stance phase.

Determine activities
for which the patient
is dependent upon
others; e.g., feeding,
dressing, bathing,
stairs, transportation

ACTIVITIES OF DAILY LIVING AND HOME STATUS

Pt. lives c̄ his wife in a ranch home c̄ only steps into the basement, which
has a rail. He depends on his wife to fix meals, laundry, housekeeping.
He dresses independently & is indep. in shower.

MEDICAL CONDITIONS — HEALTH STATUS

Good health status. Has history of SOB c̄ exertion.

Performance, length
of stay, back to
work, others

PATIENT'S EXPECTATIONS

Pt. expects a 10-12 day hospital stay. Plans on returning home to live
c̄ wife.

REMARKS

Medicare equipment form signed _✓_

M. Stuart _____, P.T.

* Courtesy Physical Therapy Department, Bellin Memorial Hospital, Green Bay, Wisconsin

gery. Until vital signs are stable, they must be monitored every 30 minutes to 1 hour, depending on their status. Once they have stabilized, they should be checked and recorded every 4 hours for 24 hours.

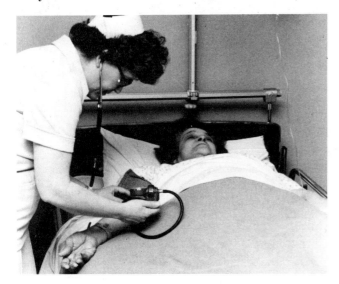

If ice bags are placed on the operative hip they make the patient feel cold; therefore, extra blankets should be added as covering.

Chest pain may be symptom of pulmonary embolism, as well as of atelectasis or a change in cardiac status. Daily auscultation of the lungs, recording of temperature, pulse, and respirations, every 4 hours for 48 hours will help detect developing complications. In conjunction with this, the nurse should know whether or not the patient has a history of cardiac problems and what the results are of any electro-cardiograms.

Every effort should be made to keep the total hip replacement patient on the orthopedic unit after surgery. This is important not only because of the specialized nursing care the orthopedic unit can provide but also because it reduces anxiety in both the patient and her family.

The modern orthopedic patient care unit should provide a method of monitoring the patient with cardiac problems. The orthopedic nursing staff must remain up to date in assessment skills.

Nausea and Vomiting

In the first 24 to 48 hours, some patients experience nausea and vomiting. Coffee-ground emeses are occassionally reported, but the cause is unknown. Some surgeons believe it is the combination of stress and the fact that many elderly patients have had gastric problems before surgery, some of which are due to taking large doses of aspirin for arthritis. Usually the condition is self-limiting and is no cause for alarm. If it persists, or if the patient becomes distended, a nasogastric tube must be inserted and gastric suction maintained as long as necessary.

Medication

Intravenous solutions of antibiotics may be administered continuously for 48 hours or for the period of time the patient remains on bed rest.

While the patient is receiving large doses of antibiotics parenterally or orally, observations must be made for allergic reactions, such as itching and rash.

Traction and Leg Support

Buck's traction may be applied to the operative leg for about 48 hours to reduce muscle spasm and keep the hip in abduction.

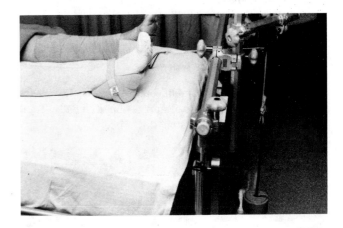

Abductor pillows or splints may be used in conjunction with or in place of Buck's traction. Russell's traction is preferred by some surgeons. A lot depends on the stability of the hip, the patient's orientation, and the surgeon's protocol. Whatever method is used, the principle is to keep the hip in abduction and out of internal rotation.

Elevation of the head of the bed is also a matter of the surgeon's preference. Patients in Buck's traction, who are only on bed rest for 48 hours, are normally allowed to have the head of their bed elevated 30 to 45 degrees for meals.

When traction is used, an elastic stocking is routinely placed on the opposite leg before or immediately following surgery. The patient with a pillow or splint should have a pair of elastic stockings on his legs. Elastic stockings remain on, except when the leg or legs are being cared for and inspected.

Routine Nursing Measures

While the patient is on bed rest, certain procedures and observations should be carried out every 3 hours. These nursing measures can be done at the same time and include the following:

1. The patient should be turned 45 degrees only to either side (unless otherwise ordered). A pillow should be placed between the legs when the patient is turned.
2. The back and buttocks are rubbed.

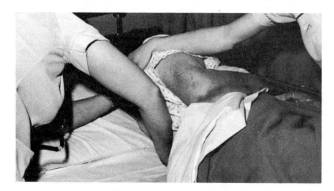

3. The dressing is checked for bleeding. A small amount of bloody drainage may be noted. Patients who have been on aspirin may bleed more than others. When it becomes necessary to reinforce a dressing, all but the last layer of dressing should be removed before new sterile dressings are applied. Otherwise, the dressing will become bulky and uncomfortable for the patient to lie on. Tape should be applied longitudinally. Total hip patients have postoperative edema in the thigh

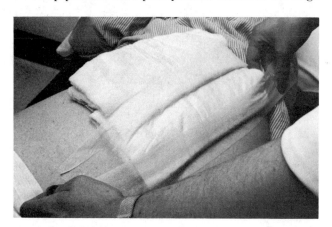

and a tendency to develop blisters from tape. Tape that is applied crosswise seems to "tighten up" and pull on the skin, thus increasing the chance of skin irritation and blisters. When the skin at the tape edges is reddened, the tape should be relocated and the skin irritation called to the surgeon's attention.

4. Wound drainage systems are sometimes used for a period of approximately 48 hours. They should be checked, along with the dressing, and emptied as necessary.

5. Icebags, if used, should be refilled and replaced.

6. The heel protectors must be removed and heels inspected and rubbed. Folded bath blankets under the calves of both legs keep the heels from digging into the mattress.

7. The traction should be checked to be certain it is in proper working order. If required, the elastic bandage is rewrapped. (Refer to Chap. 3 for care of the patient in traction.)

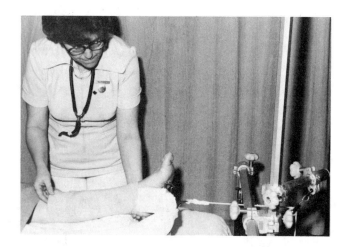

8. Nursing implications, when an abductor pillow or abductor splint is used, are discussed in Chapter 5.

9. Deep breathing, coughing, and movement of the uninvolved extremities are encouraged.

Since the trend in postoperative management of the patient with a total hip replacement is toward early ambulation, the measures just listed are adequate to promote circulation. However, active motion of the foot and ankle on the affected leg must be encouraged at more frequent intervals if the patient is to remain on bed rest longer than 48 hours.

Isometric exercises of the quadriceps and gluteal muscles will also be beneficial.

Intermittent positive pressure breathing treatments may be ordered four times a day until the patient is ambulatory. Or an incentive spirometer may be used, perhaps as long as the patient remains in the hospital. At any rate, it is important to promote lung expansion and avoid respiratory problems.

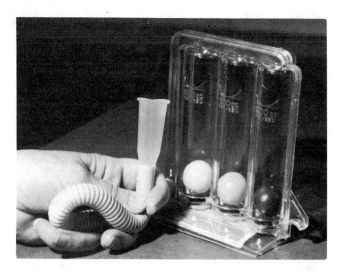

Nutrition

Normally the patient's diet is ordered as tolerated. Fluids should be encouraged orally as soon as possible.

Adequate nutrition in the postoperative period is extremely important. The patient should be offered extra nourishment during the day once the physical-therapy program has been initiated.

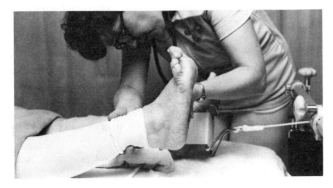

Special Skin Care

At least twice a day, the elastic stockings should be removed, the skin cared for, and the leg inspected for reddened areas that may indicate irritation or thrombophlebitis. The leg can be bathed daily. Lotions should be applied lightly, as needed and without massaging. Powder may be used intermittently because it helps in getting the stocking up on the leg.

Elastic stockings must not be allowed to roll down and act as "garters" on the patient's thighs. Therefore, when the nurse notes that a patient's stockings do tend to roll down easily, she should check the stockings every 3 to 4 hours to make certain they are in the proper place.

The elbows require inspection and rubbing on a routine basis if they become reddened or if the patient is inclined to lie quietly in bed most of the time. Undue and constant pressure on an elbow will cause paresthesias in the little and ring fingers that, if not relieved, will result in permanent damage to the ulnar nerve.

Voiding

Voiding may be difficult because of position, pain, and the spinal anesthesia. The fracture pan is easier to place than a regular bedpan. The patient can be turned 45 degrees to one side for this procedure with a pillow between the legs.

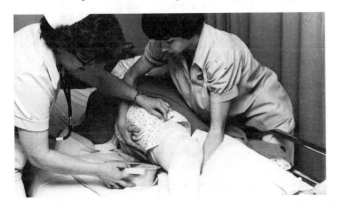

Since the patient is receiving intravenous fluids and usually taking oral fluids late on the operative day, voiding should occur within 8 to 10 hours. If the patient is unable to void after 10 to 12 hours, or if voiding is frequent and in small amounts, the surgeon may order an indwelling catheter to be left in place for several days.

Urinary infection may lead to deep wound infection; it may be preferable to try getting the patient out of bed and onto a bedside commode instead of resorting to catheterization. If nursing assessment indicates that the patient is alert enough and willing, the nurse should get an order from the surgeon. A word of caution: The nurse should have adequate assistance so that the patient can be transferred from bed to commode with a minimum of hip flexion. If the patient is in traction, the traction will have to be removed for this procedure and a pillow placed between the patient's knees.

Diuresis in the first 24 to 48 hours postoperatively is not uncommon. The major reason for this is probably the volume of intravenous fluids administered during surgery. Some surgeons order 2000 to 3000 ml of solution to increase the blood volume and help maintain blood pressure. Factors contributing to diuresis are: continuing intravenous solutions postoperatively, along with normal oral intake of fluids by the evening of the operative day. Since diuresis may result in sodium depletion, the nurse should consider disorientation in a normally lucid patient a warning sign, and report it to the surgeon.

Pain

Pain medication should be given as required. After the first 24 to 48 hours, injections may not be needed, and oral medication may be adequate. Muscle spasm is the source of much postoperative pain in total hip replacements for the first day or so, especially if the leg has been relatively lengthened. Muscle relaxants may be indicated.

Back pain, from having to remain relatively supine, is often a major source of discomfort to total hip patients while they are receivng intravenous fluids. Back rubs should be given at more frequent intervals when this is the case. Some guidelines for the assessment and management of pain are provided in the chart on page 206.

A typical nursing care plan for the patient with a total hip replacement is presented on pages 206–208.

NURSING CARE AFTER THE PATIENT IS OUT OF BED

When the surgeon orders physical therapy, the plan of care is somewhat altered. If traction was used, it is discontinued and an elastic stocking is applied to the operated leg. Patients may have splints or abductor pillows removed in physical therapy. The intravenous fluid may be discontinued at this time, although some surgeons continue intravenous antibiotic therapy for longer periods.

(text continues on page 208)

GUIDELINES FOR ASSESSING AND MANAGING PAIN IN THE PATIENT WITH A TOTAL HIP REPLACEMENT*

Expected Pain

1. Severe to moderately severe pain for about 24 hours.

Nursing Interventions

1. a. Offer IM analgesics on schedule.
   b. Ice to hip.
   c. NV checks toes q 4 hr to be certain pain is "normal" and not due to constriction of nerves and blood vessels.
   d. Keep extremity in neutral or slightly abducted position.
      Maintain traction, splint, or pillow as applied.
   e. Turn patient with pillow between legs for back care q 4 hr.

2. Amount of pain decreases steadily after first PO day.

2. Medicate p.r.n. and before PT.

Signs of Complications

1. Sudden severe pain in hip, any time postop, when attempting to move extremity. May not be able to move at all.

Nursing Interventions

1. a. Suspect dislocation of prosthesis.
   b. Compare hips as to appearance. Dislocated hip is in external or internal rotation. Hip also appears to be swollen.
   c. Notify surgeon immediately.

2. Usually after 2nd postoperative day. Increased pain on movement, may extend into thigh. Patient may complain "whole leg aches." Also may complain of tightness in hip.

2. a. Suspect hematoma.
   b. Inspect incisional area for swelling, discoloration, and drainage.
   c. Check elastic hose for fit.
   d. Call to physician's attention.

*These are very general guidelines and in all cases the total patient situation must be considered.

NURSING MANAGEMENT STANDARDS: TOTAL HIP REPLACEMENT

Potential Problems	Expected Outcomes	Deadlines	Preventive Nursing-Management
PRE-OP			
1. Standard*	1. Standard		1. a. Standard
			b. Provide with teaching book.
			c. Provide opportunity for patient to verbalize questions to assess level of understanding.
			d. Inform physical therapy department of patient's admission. Physical therapy will discuss exercise program.

NURSING MANAGEMENT STANDARDS: TOTAL HIP REPLACEMENT *(continued)*

Potential Problems	Expected Outcomes	Deadlines	Preventive Nursing-Management
POST-OP			
1. Standard†	1. Standard		1. Standard
2. Dislocation of prosthesis due to improper positioning.	2. Maintenance of proper alignment of extremity	Discharge	2. a. Check traction or abduction device for proper positioning q 6 hr (12−6−12−6) for first 2 days, or until traction discontinued. b. Place 1 pillow between legs while turning, if traction is used. c. Raise HOB no higher than 45° for 48 hr. Check q shift (6A−2P−10P). d. Transfer pt. from unaffected side.
3. Wound infection due to invasion by pathologic organisms.	3. Clean healing wound. Temp no higher than 99°*	Discharge	3. a. Inspect dressings or wound daily (10A). b. Check temperature q 4 hr for 48 hr (10−2−6− etc.) and bid (10−6) thereafter.
4. Shock due to excessive bleeding.	4. a. No bleeding b. Blood pressure stable for patient	24 hr	4. a. Apply ice to hip 48 hr continuously. b. Apply pressure to wound with sandbag if excessive bleeding (1 ABD saturated q 1 hr × 3). c. Check dressing q 4 hr for 24 hr (10−2−6−10−2−6). d. Check blood pressure q 4 hr for 48 hr. (10−2−6) then bid (10−6).
5. Impaired circulation or nerve damage due to surgical procedure, traction, or abduction device.	5. No circulatory deficit of operative leg compared to unoperative leg. No neurologic deficit.	48+ hr	5. a. Check color, motion, temperature, and sensation of operative leg q 1 hr × 6 then q 4 hr × 48 hr (10−2−6 etc.). b. Check pedal pulse q 1 hr × 6, then q 4 hr × 48 c. Check abduction device or traction for proper fit q 6 hr (12−6−12−6).
6. Thrombophlebitis or emboli due to venous stasis.	6. a. No calf pain (documented if it occurs). b. Negative Homans' sign if calf pain present c. Temperature ↓ 99°.	Discharge	6. a. Same as 5a. b. Apply antiembolism hose continuously if ordered. c. Report tenderness of calf or groin to M.D.; if tenderness present, check Homans' sign q shift. d. Cough and deep breathe q 4 hr for 48 hr (10−2−6 etc.). e. Check temperature bid* (10−6).

(continued)

NURSING MANAGEMENT STANDARDS: TOTAL HIP REPLACEMENT (continued)

Potential Problems	Expected Outcomes	Deadlines	Preventive Nursing-Management
PRE-OP			
7. Pulmonary emboli due to clot released in bloodstream.	7. a. No chest pain (documented if it occurs) b. Respiratory rate within +10 & -5 of pre-op rate c. Lungs clear on auscultation.	Discharge	7. a. Check BP, P, R, q 4 hr for 48 hr (10-2-6), then bid (10-6). b. Same as 6d. c. Patient up in chair 10-2-6 and assist with ambulation after physical therapy is ordered.
8. Abdominal distention due to slowed peristalsis.	8. Soft and nontympanic abdomen	48 hr post-op	8. a. Check for abdominal distention q 4 hr × 48 hr b. Increase diet from clear liquid to general as tolerated. c. Insert rectal tube or give suppository as needed.
9. Fat emboli due to fat globules released in the bloodstream.	9. a. No confusion that cannot be related to Rx or age b. Pulse between 60 and 100	3 days	9. a. Same as 7a. b. If patient becomes confused, evaluate cause; if thought to be due to fat emboli, notify M.D.
10. Difficulty with home management due to lack of understanding of home care.	10. Verbalization of understanding of home care‡	Discharge	10. a. Reinforce home programs of physical therapy and occupational therapy. b. Have patient verbalize understanding of home program.

* Hospital nursing management standard—all pre-ops

† Hospital nursing management standard—all post-ops.

‡ Part of Discharge Criteria

Initial Ambulation

A pain medication is given about 30 minutes before the patient is gotten out of bed. When the therapist gets the

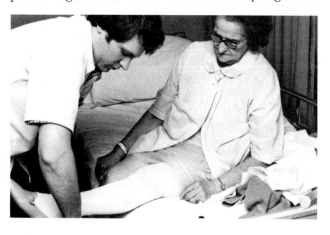

patient up for the first time, the nurse should be present to offer support, since the patient will feel weak, dizzy, apprehensive, and perhaps slightly nauseated. Flexion of the hip is kept to a minimum during this procedure. If the surgery was especially difficult, or if the patient was seriously incapacitated up to this time, the tilt table may be ordered for a day or two.

The nurse must assess the patient's physical and emotional state before the initial visit to physical therapy because the patient may find the activity exhausting. The patient, dressed in a robe and wearing slippers with nonskid soles, is allowed to sit in a wheelchair for a short time and then is helped to a standing position between parallel bars. This action is accompanied by incisional pain and may cause the patient some anxiety. When the patient is put back to bed, supportive care is necessary to offer assurance that the discomfort will pass as the operative area heals. A reminder

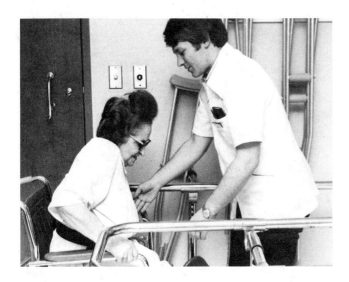

that the *joint itself* will not be very painful should be offered regularly during those first few days in physical therapy. This fact is the light at the end of the tunnel for total hip replacement patients.

Respiratory Status

Once the patient is out of bed, continued observation of respiratory status is not to be ignored, especially since pulmonary embolism can occur at any time. These patients may need to continue to use an incentive spirometer during their entire hospitalization.

Skin Care

The skin, especially over bony prominences, should be observed regularly, usually during bathing. Even though the patient is out of bed a few times a day, skin breakdown is still a possibility.

Pain and General Comfort

Patients with other arthritic joints have aches and pains that need to be considered. As a matter of fact, a patient will often complain *more* about pain in other joints than about pain in the operated hip. This is almost always the case with rheumatoid arthritics. The "installation" of a new hip joint sometimes means that the patient can assume a supine position with more ease and comfort. It may also mean added discomfort in other joints and muscles as progress is made in therapy.

Nurse and therapist alike need to remember that the total hip replacement patient is getting more exercise during the hospital rehabilitation program than has been possible for a long time preoperatively. It is essential that these patients get sufficient rest and sleep.

Positioning

Careful positioning when the patient is in bed is always a priority. The patient should be in good body alignment. Only minimal flexion of the knees and hips is allowed, and the patient should never be turned without a pillow between the legs. The bed should be flat when the patient is not engaged in activities that require a sitting position. This will help prevent pooling of blood in the pelvis and reduce the risk of clot formation and pulmonary embolism.

Elimination

Constipation may develop even though the patient takes fluids and food in sufficient quantities. Partial immobilization and pain medications are responsible, plus the fact that the older patient has some normal irregularity. Laxatives, suppositories, and enemas may be indicated. A stool softener daily or twice daily, depending on the patient's need, is an added aid to establishing regularity.

Complications

Infection. Skin irritation from the tape may prompt the surgeon to remove the dressing. Once the dressing is removed, the incision needs daily inspection. The breakdown of fatty tissue in patients with heavy thighs may result in a clear, yellow drainage. This must be distinguished from drainage due to infection.

Wound infection may spell disaster. Irrigation of an infected joint until cultures are negative is a long, unhappy process. Removing the components of a total hip replacement is a time-consuming and arduous task. Meticulous care must be taken to avoid irritation of the suture line, and the patient should be cautioned not to touch it.

Every effort should be made to prevent bladder infections in these patients. The septicemia that may occur can result in the development of an infection around the joint, which may not become symptomatic for months after surgery.

Dislocation of Prosthesis. Dislocation of the hip prosthesis, once healing of the tissues has taken place, is not likely and would only occur in the average patient as a result of

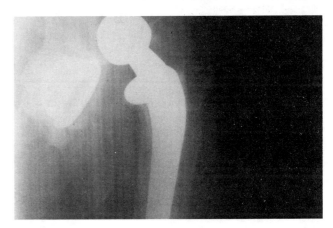

Dislocated prosthesis.

violent flexion on the hip joint. In the hospital, the patient should not be allowed to flex the hip past 90 degrees. The nurse must be especially vigilant of the patient who becomes confused at night. A pillow between the legs of a restless sleeper is an added precaution against adduction and subsequent dislocation.

Symptoms of a dislocated hip may appear when the patient attempts to turn or move about in bed. The affected extremity will be shortened. The patient may not be able to move it at all or to bear weight on it. The nurse should notify the surgeon immediately and not try to rotate the hip or have the patient do so in order to attempt further evaluation.

Physical Therapy

From the first time the total hip patient gets out of bed until the time of discharge, a program of planned exercise and ambulation is beneficial to progress. Such a schedule should be the result of coordinated efforts of the physical-therapy department and the nursing staff. There are individual differences in patients that must be considered, and surgeons vary in their approach to rehabilitation. However, a basic program should be written up and can be readjusted as necessary. The following program can serve as a model.

On the second postoperative day, the average patient is taken to physical therapy in a wheeelchair, by a therapist. There, the patient is assisted to a standing position between parallel bars. How soon and how far he walks between those bars depends entirely on his status.

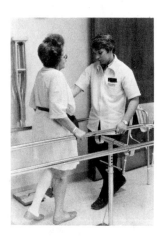 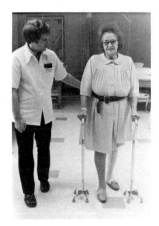

Generally, patient activity consists of transfer from wheelchair to bed and ambulation twice a day in the physical-therapy department. The goal is to be discharged ambulating with one cane. Patients progress from walker to quad canes, or two canes to one cane. The selection of an assistive device is a matter of the individual's ability to ambulate. Although canes provide the most natural gait pattern possible, some patients may need to be discharged with walkers.

Once the patient progresses from the parallel bars to either a walker or canes, he is allowed to be out of bed and to walk about the ward in the evening. However, he must have assistance, and he must wear a belt.

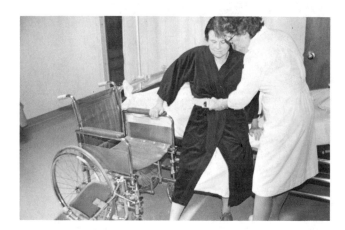

The patient begins using a bedside commode or a raised toilet seat when he is able to get out of bed with assistance from the nurse.

As early as the second postoperative day, depending on patient readiness, the therapist will begin teaching the patient exercises. These exercises will then be done each morning and afternoon in the therapy department. Many exercises are the same as those that are part of the home program, so it is logical that hospital physical therapy sessions may involve only those exercises in the discharge booklet (pp. 214–217).

Exercises and activities may include:

1. *Pendulum Flexion:* Tie a leather foot strap with rope to a pulley. Have the patient bend the knee, pulling the heel to the buttocks and then straightening the leg slowly and steadily.

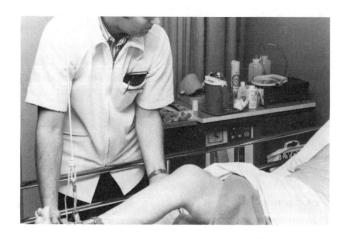

2. *Pendulum Abduction:* Tie a leather foot strap with rope to a pulley. Have the patient slowly push (with heel first) the leg outward, hold for a few seconds, and then pull back slowly and steadily.

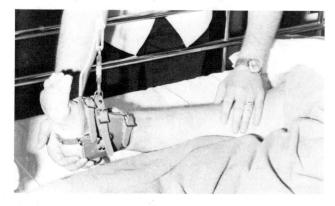

3. *Thomas Position or "Dangling".* Have the patient lie on his back (toward the operated side) near the edge of the table. Instruct the patient to flex the unoperated leg up as far as possible toward the chest and hold it in that position. Then flex the operated leg about two-thirds of the way up toward the chest. These two maneuvers flatten the back. Next, instruct the patient to keep the unoperated leg bent up as far as possible, foot flat on the table, and slowly lower the operated leg down and over the edge of the table. The patient should be forewarned that he will feel a "pull" in the front of his thigh, indicating the desired effect of stretching the hip flexors. Initially, the patient may require support, such as a pillow under the foot of the operated leg.

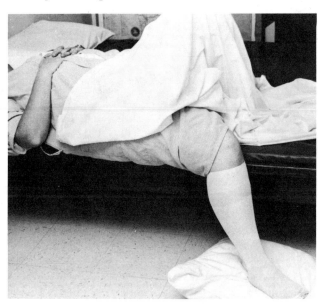

4. *Powderboard Flexion:* Have the patient lie with both legs resting on a powderboard. Instruct the patient to

flex the knee by sliding the heel towards the buttocks and then push the leg flat again, slowly and steadily. The unaffected leg may bend somewhat.

5. *Powderboard Abduction:* Have the patient rest both

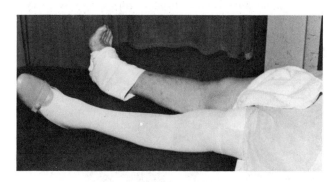

legs on a powderboard, Direct the patient to slide his heel outward and then pull back in slowly and steadily.

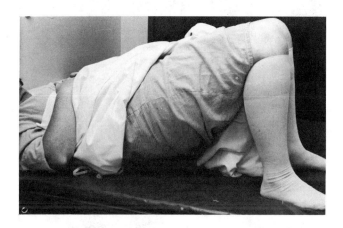

6. *Bridging or "Bedpan" Exercise:* The patient lies with knees flexed, feet and shoulders on the bed. Instruct the patient to raise his hips as if getting on a bedpan, and to hold for a few seconds and then lower back to bed.

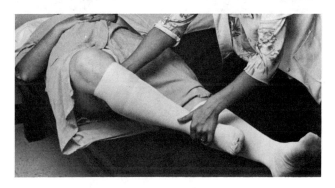

7. *Supine External Hip Rotation:* Instruct the patient to lie on his back on the table. Next, have him roll the

operated hip outward and draw the foot straight upward along the middle, or shin, of the unoperated leg as far as possible, allowing the knee to fall sideways. This is difficult for a patient with hip contractures, and he must be reminded not to draw the operated leg up toward the chest.

8. *Spring Extension:* Hook a foot strap to a spring and a pulley. Have the patient pull his foot to the powderboard (or powdered sheet) and lift his leg back up slowly and steadily. Do *not* let leg bounce up and down.

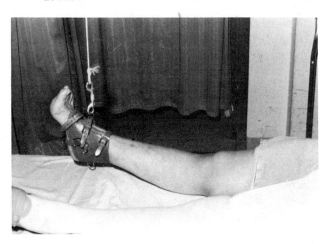

9. *Sitting External Hip Rotation:* Instruct the patient to sit with feet dangling over the edge of the table. Ask the patient to roll the operated hip outward, drawing the foot straight upward along the shin of

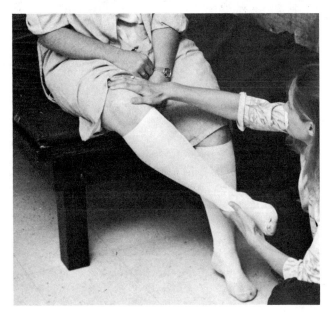

the unoperated leg as far as possible. The patient should be told *not* to bend the operated hip so that there is more than a 90-degree angle between the

hip and trunk. The simplest instruction is to tell him to keep the lateral aspect or "outside" of the affected thigh as close as he can to the tabletop.

10. *Straight Leg Raising:* The patient should lie on his back with the knee of the unoperated leg flexed and the bottom of the foot resting on the table. Next, instruct the patient to keep the knee of the operated leg straight and raise the leg up toward the ceiling.

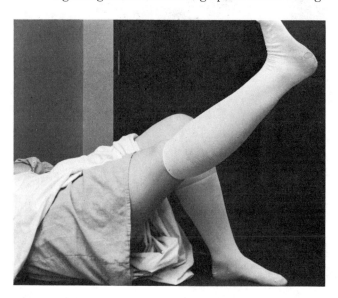

11. *Hip Abduction:* Instruct the patient to lie on the unoperated side with a pillow between the legs to keep the operated leg in a neutral position. The unoperated leg should be flexed slightly for balance. The patient is then instructed to raise the operated

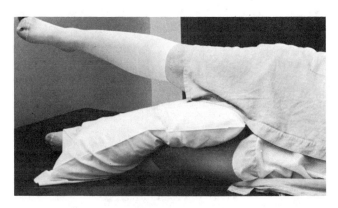

leg straight up toward the ceiling as far as he can, keeping the knee straight. Then the leg should be lowered slowly to the pillow, parallel with the table. The patient must be cautioned to stay on his side and not bring the leg horizontally toward the chest — in other words, forward — over the unoperated leg.

At this point, it should be emphasized once more that some patients have difficulty mastering certain exercises and should be given all the help and encouragement they need to remain cooperative and optimistic. The patient will also need assistance and practice in climbing stairs until both he and the therapist become confident in his ability to do so safely.

The physical therapist will determine the date on which the patient is to start the program and the rate at which he is to progress.

Obviously, the physical-therapy department and the nursing staff need to communicate regularly to maintain an effective rehabilitation program for each patient. A therapy department that is located on the same floor as the orthopedic ward is a tremendous advantage in terms of communication among therapists, staff, and orthopedic surgeons. It is also helpful in making observations of patient progress. Another advantage is that it is possible for patients to wheel themselves back and forth, holding quad canes in their laps, getting arm exercise, conversing with other patients and staff as they "travel," and prolonging the period of time when they are out of bed and part of the environment.

OCCUPATIONAL THERAPY

The goal of the occupational therapist is to ensure that the patient who has undergone total hip replacement remains independent in activites of daily living while adhering to the restrictions in movement taught by the physical-therapy department. In other words, the occupational therapist will teach the patient how to put on and remove shoes, stockings, and pants without flexing the hip more than 90 degrees.

When the activity and sitting tolerance of the patient have reached the level at which lower extremity dressing training is possible, the occupational therapist enters the rehabilitation picture. This usually occurs 7 to 10 days after the operation and is determined by the physical therapist. The occupational therapist explains the program and

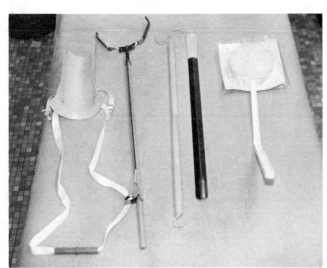

presents the adaptive equipment that will be used while reviewing the basic safety precautions in regard to posture and movement.

Simple instruction on postions for sexual relations should be included because patients are frequently reluctant to ask for this type of information. This might be written: "During sexual relations, it is best that you use positions that avoid raising your knees higher than your hips or bending at the hips more than 90 degrees. You should also try to avoid side-lying. Be sure that you are not tired before the activity. It is also recommended not to have sexual relations after eating or other activities." (Courtesy "Hip Info" Bellin Memorial Hospital Occupational Therapy Department, Green Bay, Wisconsin)

A teaching booklet is valuable from two aspects; (1) as an overview of the program, and (2) as a set of instructions and information for use after discharge. The therapist should explain the purpose of the booklet and ask the patient to read it prior to their next encounter.

In subsequent sessions with the occupational therapist, the total hip patient learns how to use the adaptive equip-

---

ONE LAST WORD FOR THE PATIENT WHO HAS HAD TOTAL JOINT REPLACEMENT*

PLEASE remember to:

1. make your appointments with the doctor and with the physical therapy department. Your nurse will help you if necessary.
2. take your prescriptions with you.
3. take home your Home Exercise Program booklet from physical therapy. If you have had a total hip replacement, you also have a booklet of instructions and some self-help equipment from the occupational therapy department.

IT IS IMPORTANT for you to know that bacteria in your bloodstream can get into your new joint and cause infection. Therefore:

1. any infection you get, in your teeth, throat, bladder, or wherever, *must* be treated.
2. YOU WILL ALWAYS NEED ANTIBIOTICS when you have dental work done.
3. you should tell your family doctor, or any other doctor who takes care of you in the future, that you have a total joint replacement. Then when you have problems or treatments, you will be given antibiotics as necessary.

The doctor who put your new joint in place will answer any questions you have about these instructions.

* Courtesy Bellin Memorial Hospital, Green Bay, Wisconsin

ment safely and with as much efficiency as possible. Patients with rheumatoid arthritis may requre equipment with built-up handles. Other adaptations are made as necessary, based on individual needs. The patient will need to use adaptive equipment for lower-extremity dressing and bending activities until the surgeon allows him to assume positions with more than 90 degrees of hip flexion.

Because the prevention of infection is imperative in any patient who has had a joint replacement, the total hip patient is given specific discharge instructions by the surgeon as to what information he must present to anyone giving him medical treatment in the future. The instructions may be part of a "last word" general instruction card as shown on p. 213.

The major share of discharge planning for the total hip replacement patient is the responsibility of the physical therapy department. The home exercise program is demonstrated and begun well in advance of discharge. A booklet, with photos as pictured on pages 214–217, illustrates and describes exercises that should be done. While the booklet is basically the same for each patient, exercises are crossed out if not appropriate for the individual patient. A schedule of hours and times is also decided upon by therapist and patient and noted in the booklet. A list may also be included, along with a set of photos illustrating the "Do's and Don'ts." A discharge evaluation is done, using the admission data base for a comparative study. (See data base chart on page 202.)

The therapy department should have a scheduled "hip clinic" for these patients to visit at regular intervals for a specific period of time. The purposes of such a clinic are to assess and evaluate the patient's progress and to see

(text continues page 217)

HOME EXERCISE PROGRAM FOR THE TOTAL HIP PATIENT*

1. *Hip tightening.* Tighten your "seat": Tighten the muscles in your buttocks, then relax. You may do this exercise lying on your back, on your stomach, or in a sitting position.

2. *Leg out to side.* Lie on your back with a pillow between your legs. Slide your operated leg out to the side as far as you can. Return to a neutral, midline position. Do not cross toward your unoperated leg.

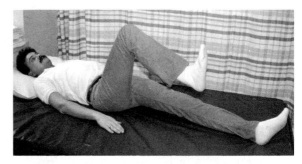

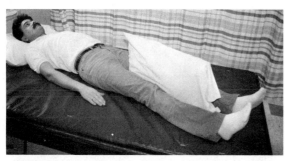

4. *Beginning hip rotation.* Lie on your back. Allow your operated hip to roll outward and slide your _____ foot up the inside of your unoperated leg. Lower your operated leg. (Be sure not to cross your operated leg over the midline of your body.)

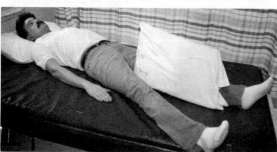

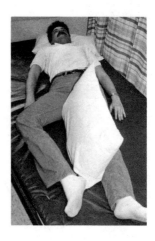

3. *Hip bending.* Lie on your back. Bend your hip and knee slowly up toward your chest. Return to starting position. Do not try to exceed the amount of bend pictured below.

* Courtesy of Physical Therapy Department, Bellin Memorial Hospital, Green Bay, Wisconsin

(continued)

HOME EXERCISE PROGRAM FOR THE TOTAL HIP PATIENT *(continued)*

5. *Bridging exercise.* Lie on your back with your hips and knees bent and the bottom of your feet resting on the bed. Straighten your hips and lift up your buttocks as though you are going to sit on a bed pan. Hold this position for 5 counts and then relax.

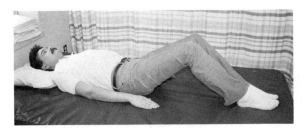

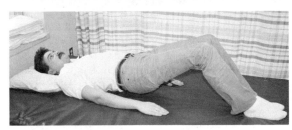

6. *Straight leg raise.* Lie on your back with the knee of your unoperated leg bent and the bottom of that foot resting on the bed. Keeping the knee of your operated leg straight, raise your leg up toward the ceiling. Return to starting position. Repeat ____ times.

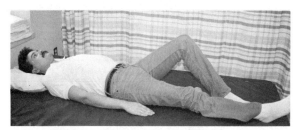

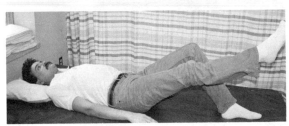

7. *Side-lying leg raise.* Lie on your unoperated side with a pillow between your legs to keep your operated leg in a neutral position. Your unoperated leg should be slightly bent for balance. Raise your operated leg *straight* up toward the ceiling as far as you can, keeping the knee straight. Slowly lower to the pillow, par-

allel with the table. Make sure you stay on your side and do not bring the leg forward toward your chest. Repeat _____ times.

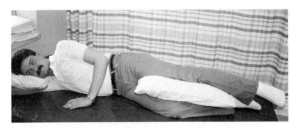

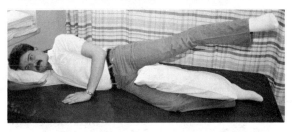

8. *Dangling.* Lie on your back near the edge of the bed (toward your operated side). Now bend your unoperated leg up and rest that foot flat on the bed. Keeping your unoperated leg in that position slowly lower your operated leg down over the edge of the bed. You will feel a pull in front of your operated thigh. Stay in this position for _____ minutes or as comfortably tolerated.

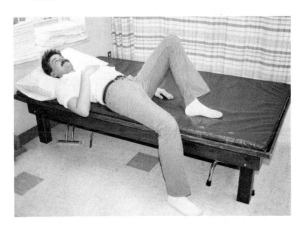

9. *Stomach-lying.* Lie on your stomach with your feet over the edge of a table. When assuming this position, be careful not to cross your operated leg toward your unoperated leg. You will need to use a pillow to keep legs separated. Initially, you will be most comfortable rolling onto your unoperated leg. Stay in this position for _____ minutes or as comfortably tolerated.

(continued)

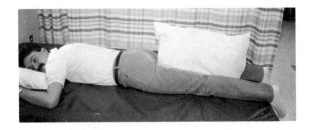

10. *Hip extension.* Lie on your stomach and bring your operated leg *straight* up toward the ceiling. Lower your operated leg back to starting position. Repeat _____ times.

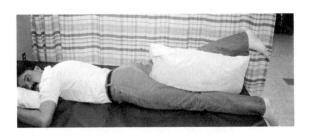

11. *Knee straightener.* Sitting in a straight-backed chair, slowly straighten your operated leg's knee as far as you can. Slowly lower.

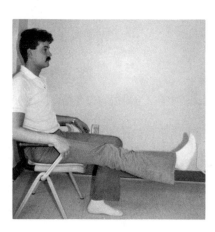

12. *Hip rotation.* Sitting in a straight-backed chair with feet on floor, roll your operated thigh outward and bring your foot straight up along the inside of your unoperated leg. This exercise is to achieve more outward rotation to allow donning of shoes and socks.

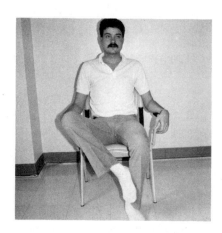

13. *Bicycle peddling.* Adjust seat height so that you can peddle without causing more than a 90° angle between hip and trunk. To get on the bike, approach from the unoperated side and place the unoperated leg over the bar onto the opposite pedal. Step up. To get down place the operated leg on the floor and dismount to that side.

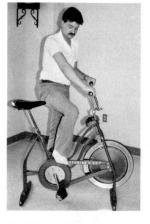
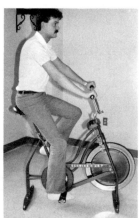
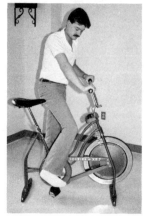

14. *Stairs*

A. To climb up stairs, bring your unoperated leg up first, then the cane and your operated leg.

B. To descend, put the cane down first, then the operated leg and then the unoperated leg.

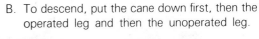

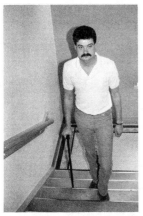 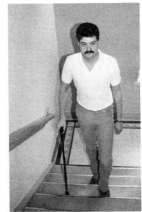 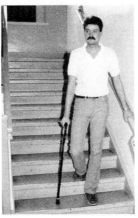 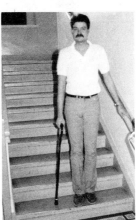

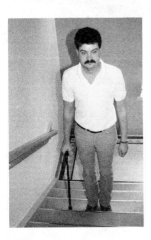

whether or not the exercises are being done correctly. Questions are answered and the opportunity is there for patients to offer each other encouragement and insights. An alternative to a regular "hip clinic" is the practice of scheduling the total hip replacement patient for a visit to the hospital physical-therapy department in the hour prior to his first postoperative visit to the surgeon. This allows the therapist to evaluate the patient's progress and provide reinstruction and clarification, and it gives the patient an updated report to bring to the surgeon's office.

Throughout the hospitalization, the patient and nurse must be sensitive to total patients needs. For instance, if the patient is a diabetic, then at some point during his hospital stay, the nurse should have evaluated his knowledge of his disease and determined whether or not any teaching or review of previous teaching was needed. An example of this type of individualized nursing care is provided in the chart on page 222.

Even if a patient has had an "uneventful" recovery and appears ready and willing to go home, he may still have questions about his rehabilitation program. The nurse should be present when the surgeon gives the final instructions and prescriptions. If the patient has been encouraged to write down any questions he has beforehand, he will not forget to ask them, and the nurse will not have to find answers or call the physician at the last minute.

(text continues page 223)

TOTAL HIP REPLACEMENT INSTRUCTIONS/PRECAUTIONS

Your new hip is designed to eliminate pain and increase function. However, there are certain movements that place too much stress on your new hip; for your safety these should be avoided for as long as your doctor recommends.

Do's and Don'ts

CAUTION #1

Don't move your operated hip toward your chest (flexion) any more than 90 degress or a right angle.

Do keep your hip at a 90-degree angle.

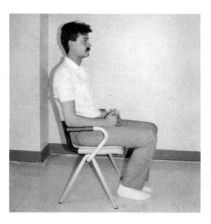

Don't lean forward when getting up from a chair or toilet seat.

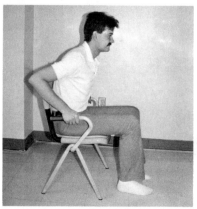

Do use a raised toilet seat.

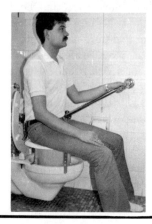

TOTAL HIP REPLACEMENT INSTRUCTIONS/PRECAUTIONS *(continued)*

Do use a chair with arms. Place your operated leg in front and your unoperated leg well under you when getting up. *Do* grasp chair arms to help you rise safely to standing position. Place extra pillow(s) or cushion(s) in your chair so that you do not bend your hip more than 90 degrees.

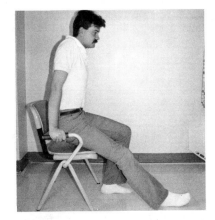

Don't bend way over to pick up objects or put on shoes and stockings.

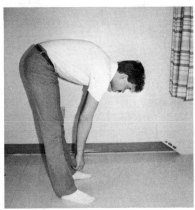

Do pick up objects from the floor like this. Place your operated leg well behind you. Your therapist may show you another way.

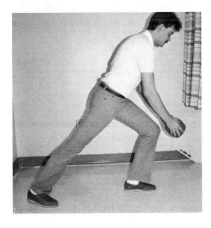

(continued)

TOTAL HIP REPLACEMENT INSTRUCTIONS/PRECAUTIONS *(continued)*

Do use equipment from your occupational therapist to put on your shoes and stockings.

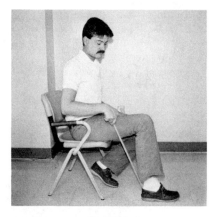

Don't pull up blankets like this.

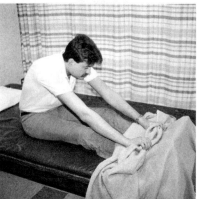

Do use a long-handled reacher to pull up sheets or blankets or do so as directed by your therapist.

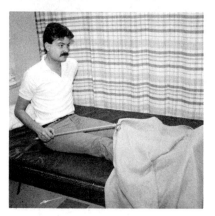

HOME EXERCISE PROGRAM FOR THE TOTAL HIP PATIENT *(continued)*

CAUTION #2

Don't cross your operated leg across the midline of your body.

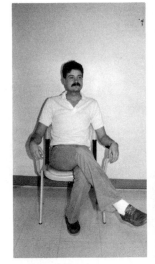 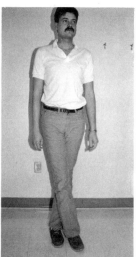

Do keep operated leg away from midline of your body.

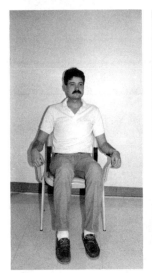 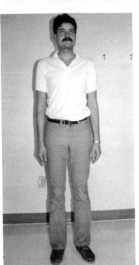

Don't lie without a pillow between your legs.

Do keep a pillow between your legs when lying or rolling onto your side.

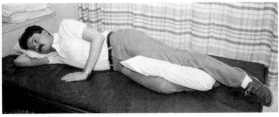

(continued)

TOTAL HIP REPLACEMENT INSTRUCTIONS/PRECAUTIONS *(continued)*

CAUTION #3

Don't turn the knee of your operated leg inward.

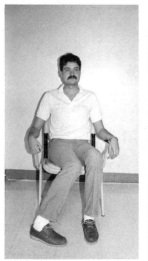 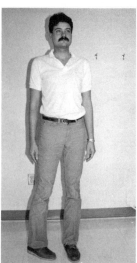

THE TOTAL HIP REPLACEMENT PATIENT: INDIVIDUALIZING NURSING CARE

Significant Data: E.K. is a 71-year-old female patient who had a left total hip replacement. Six months ago she had a cholecystectomy. She is 5'3" tall and weighs 176 lb. She had a B.P. of 154/100 on admission. She is on medication for her hypertension. She also has varicose veins. She states that when she had her cholecystectomy, she was told that she was a "borderline diabetic." On this admission her preoperative fasting blood sugar was 124 and her urine showed a trace of sugar.

Standard Postoperative Nursing Orders*

1. Check dressings
2. Take vital signs
3. Apply ice to incision
4. CMTS, pedal pulses both feet, compare
5. Stir-up
6. Check for abdominal distention
7. Provide back and heel care
8. Turn with pillow between legs.
9. Elevate head of bed 45 degrees only
10. Check traction and re-wrap elastic bandage q 6 hr
11. Remove stocking for skin care q shift

Additional Nursing Implications†

1. Provide convoluted bedpad to prevent skin breakdown.
2. Check elastic hose q 3 hr to be certain it is not rolling down or wrinkling.
3. Check calves for tenderness q 3 hr shift.
4. Check Homans' sign q shift.
5. Check urine for sugar and acetone tid a.c.
6. Have dietician see patient about diabetic diet, no salt added.
7. Evaluate patient's knowledge of diabetes and self-care required to prevent associated problems and instruct as needed.
8. Continue to take B.P. b.i.d.
9. Evaluate patient's knowledge

about her antihypertensive medicine.
10. Consult with physical therapist and make aware of observations relative to thrombophlebitis if symptoms occur.

Rationale

1. Due to her weight, patient will move about in bed more slowly. Diabetes necessitates care to maintain integrity of skin.
2,3. Past history makes her an
4,10. excellent candidate for thrombophlebitis.
5,6,7. Borderline diabetic. Has hypertension.
8,9. On B.P. medication.

* 1 through 7 will be done on a 3-hr schedule due to patient's weight, general condition, and past history. The normal would be to order these routines q 4 hr. These orders will be reviewed in 48 hr.

† Evaluations and teaching will be done later in postoperative period, depending on condition and readiness.

Discussion Questions

1. For postoperative care of the total hip replacement patient, identify the nursing actions that should be taken in each of the following situations.

    a. 4 hours postoperatively, the patient complains of chest pain.

    b. 8 days postoperatively, the patient states he must be getting a cold because he has a cough.

    c. 12 hours postoperatively, the patient has lost sensation in the toes on the operated leg.

Consider: (a) How much time has elapsed since surgery? What happens in O.R.? Patient history? (b) Causes of cough? Importance of time it occurs? (c) All the causes of loss of sensation in the toes? Is the time important? What is his position status at this time.

2. The following information is given at the 7:00 A.M. shift report. What are the priorities in nursing assessment?

D.C. is a 63-year-old patient who had a left total hip replacement 3 days ago. He was up yesterday in PT and did fine. He slept well during the night, but at 6:00 A.M. this morning he complained of much pain in his incisional area. Up until now he has been moving very well and turns almost without help. The dressing is off, the area is slightly swollen but not inflamed. His temperature is 100.2°.

Consider: Is there necessarily a relationship between the temperature and the pain? How significant, by itself, is the fact that the hip is swollen? What does the patient's level of activity tell you?

Bibliography

Adair F: Nursing care study: Hip replacement. Nurs Mirror, 158(5):39, 1984

Blake S: Noncemented femoral prosthesis: Intraoperative focus. Orthop Nurs 4(1):40, 1985

Brantley P: Orthopedic innovations: Porous coated hip implant. Today's OR Nurs 6(10):8, 1984

Brown R: Implants: Hip and knee arthroplasty. JORRI 2:26, 1982

Brunner NA: Orthopedic Nursing, 4th ed. St. Louis, CV Mosby, 1983

Buchholz HW, et al: Antibiotic-loaded acrylic cement: Current concepts. Clin Orthop 190:96, 1984

Chaffee E, Lytle I: Basic Physiology and Anatomy, 4th ed. Philadelphia, JB Lippincott, 1980

Clayton ML, Stringer TL: Total hip arthroplasty with a new long-stem prosthesis: Two-to five-year follow-up evaluation. Clin Orthop 173:140, 1983

Crenshaw AH (ed): Campbell's Operative Orthopaedics, 6th ed. St. Louis, CV Mosby, 1980

Crutchley C: Trends in orthopedic surgery. Today's OR Nurs 6(12):22, 1984

Derscheid G: Symposium on orthopaedic nursing. Rehabilitation of common orthopedic problems. Nurs Clin North Am 16:709, 1981

Doheny M: Porous coated femoral prosthesis: Concepts and care considerations. Orthop Nurs 44(1):43, 1985

Dohr LD, et al: Total hip arthroplasties in patients less than forty-five years old. J Bone Joint Surg 65(4):474, 1983

Dohr LD, et al: Classification and treatment of dislocations of total hip arthroplasty. Clin Orthop 173:151, 1983

Engh CA: Hip arthroplasty with a Moore prosthesis with porous coating. A five-year study. Clin Orthop 176:52 1983

Engineering a new hip. Newsweek, 12(99):78, Apr 1982

Fox JA: Revision arthroplasty of the hip: Some current methods for reducing failure in this branch of surgery. Nurs Times, 76(44):1930, 1980

Freeman MA, et al: Cementless fixation of prosthetic components in total arthroplasty of the knee and hip. Clin Orthop 176:88 1983

Glynn MK, Sheehan JM: An analysis of the causes of deep infection after hip and knee arthroplasties. Clin Orthop 178:202 1983

Harris WH, et al: Detection of pulmonary emboli after total hip replacement using serial C1502 pulmonary scans. J. Bone Joint Surg 66(9):1388 1984

Hilt N, Cogburn S: Manual of Orthopedics. St. Louis, CV Mosby, 1980

Hollinshead WH: Textbook of Anatomy, 3rd ed. Hagerstown, Harper & Row, 1974

Hoogland T, et al: Revision of Mueller total hip arthroplasties. Clin Orthop Rel Res 161:180 1981

Kaye G: The cementless total hip arthroplasty. Physiotherapy 68(12):394 1982

Klenerman L: The management of the infected endoprosthesis. J Bone Joint Surg (Br) 66(5):645 1984

Langley LL, et al: Dynamic Anatomy and Physiology, 5th ed. New York, McGraw-Hill, 1980

Larson C, Gould M: Orthopedic Nursing, 9th ed. St. Louis CV Mosby, 1978

Leeman EK: Deep venous thrombosis in total hip replacement. JAMA, 251(23):3081 1984

Macek C: Bony ingrowth holds new joints in place. JAMA 247(12):1680, 1982

Mendes DG, et al: Reconstruction of the acetabular wall with bone graft in arthroplasty of the hip. Clin Orthop 186:29, 1984

Menzies J: The whole team won . . . a successful outcome was achieved for an elderly patient undergoing a total hip replacement. Nurs Mirror 154:47, 1982

Merkow RL, et al: Total hip replacement for Paget's disease of the hip. J Bone Joint Sur 66(5):752, 1984

Morscher EW: Cementless total hip arthroplasty. Clin Orthop 181:76 1983

Mourad L: Nursing Care of Adults with Orthopedic Conditions. New York, John Wiley & Sons, 1980

Murray WR: Use of antibiotic-containing bone cement. Clin Orthop 190:89 1984

Nelson CL, et al: One day versus seven days of preventive antibiotic therapy in orthopedic surgery. Clin Orthop 176:258, 1983

Olerud S, Karlstrom G: Hip arthroplasty with an extended femoral stem for salvage procedures. Clin Orthop 191:64, 1984

Orpwood J: Bilateral hip arthroplasty: Two hips for old. Nurs Mirror 153:8, 1981

Parks S: Total joint revision surgery. Today's OR Nurs 4(11):16, 1983

Pavlik MD: An efficient patient teaching tool. Orthop Nurs 2(1):23, 1983

Pierron RL: Pulmonary embolism in total-hip patients. Clin Orthop 188:310, 1984

Seeger MS: Adaptive equipment used in the rehabilitation of hip arthroplasty patients. AJOT, 36:503, 1982

Spindler CE: Audiovisual preoperative teaching for the total hip patient. Orthop Nurs 3(1):30, 1984

Stinchfield FE: The evolution of total hip replacement. Surg Technol 15(3):16, 1983

Surin VV, Sundholm K: Survival of patients and prostheses after total hip arthroplasty. Clin Orthop 177:48, 1983

Swanson RL, Evarts CM: Dual-lock total hip arthroplasty: A preliminary experience. Clin Orthop 191:224, 1984

Tullos HS, et al: Total hip arthroplasty with a low-sodium porous-coated femoral component. J Bone Joint Surg 66(6):888, 1984

Wolfgang GL: Total hip arthroplasty: Picking the right candidate helps determine success. Consultant 24(3):209, 1984

Wong S, et al: Total hip replacements: Improving post-hospital adjustment. Nurs Manag 15(7):34C, 1984

7

Care of the Patient Undergoing Knee Repair or Reconstruction

Sports sections of newspapers devote considerable coverage to knee injuries sustained by professional athletes. Yet the world is *full* of people who, at one time or another, have been hospitalized for treatment of a "bad knee." Just as all fractures and casts are not alike, all knee injuries and operations are not alike. These patients require special, individualized care.

Knee surgery, if it is not a joint replacement, is frequently dismissed as "minor" by hospital personnel. This is so for at least two reasons. First, people are able to undergo arthroscopic surgery either as outpatients or one-day care patients. Second, patients who have open knee repairs are often young athletes and are hospitalized for only a few days.

Knee surgery is never minor to the owner of the knee, in question. The nurse has an important role in providing psychological care, supporting the patient during rehabilitation, and preventing complications. Any knee surgery traumatizes tissue and immobilizes the extremity to some extent. A nurse has only to see one knee-repair patient develop a pulmonary embolism while waiting to be discharged to become a believer in comprehensive care for all knee patients.

Knee injuries do not all require surgical treatment or even hospitalization. The duration of a rehabilitation period largely depends on the type and extent of the injury. Furthermore, physicians do not all have the same approach to treatment or postoperative regimens.

An understanding of the types and treatments of knee injuries, and of the consequences of neglect (such as erosion of the articular cartilage due to the torn edge of a meniscus), will enable the nurse to give more intelligent care to the hospitalized patient. Of course, such knowledge also carries the fringe benefit of preparing the nurse to be a more effective teacher of health in the community, because the advice of the neighborhood nurse is better tolerated, and sometimes even followed, if it appears to be based on facts.

Anatomy of the Knee

The Knee Joints

The knee is the largest joint in the body. It is formed by the distal end of the femur, the proximal ends of the tibia and fibula, and the patella or kneecap. Within the knee joint there are practically no isolated structures. They all work together to stabilize the knee in all positions. The knee is also the most complex joint in the body, being actually three articulations in one.

Two condyloid joints, one on the lateral side of the knee and one on the medial side, are formed by the condyles of the femur, the menisci, and the condyles of the tibia. The femoral condyles are not the same shape. The lateral femoral condyle is more ball-like in shape, while the medial femoral

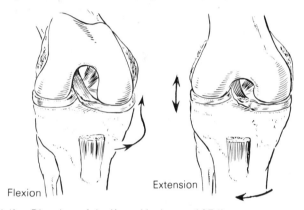

Flexion   Extension

(Helfet: Disorders of the Knee. Lippincott, 1974)

condyle is elongated. This means that the articulations of which they are a part are likewise asymmetrical and yet must work in unison. The articulating surfaces of the femur and tibia are covered by cartilage.

The patella lies in the intercondylar notch and is part of a sliding joint. The undersurface of this bone has condyles that articulate with the femur in various positions of flexion and extension. The patella also serves as protection for the front of the knee joint and as a fulcrum for the quadriceps muscle in providing it with leverage in extending the leg. In flexion, the knee is like a hinge. However, as it is extended, the lateral part of the joint packs and checks, and the femur slides back medially on the tibia with a corkscrew motion. This action locks the knee in position.

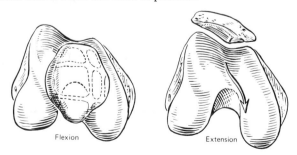

Flexion   Extension

(Helfet: Disorders of the Knee. Lippincott, 1974)

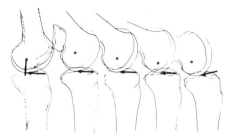

(Helfet: Disorders of the Knee. Lippincott, 1974)

The Menisci (Semilunar Cartilage)

Two cartilage pads attached on top of the tibia act as shock absorbers and deepen the sockets for the femoral condyles. They are the menisci or semilunar cartilages. The menisci have smooth surfaces and migrate to some extent during the gliding movements of the femoral condyles.

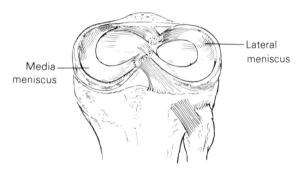

(Helfet: Disorders of the Knee. Lippincott, 1974)

Ligamentous Structures of the Knee

Although a number of ligaments and tendons support the knee, all of which are important, some are more commonly associated with knee problems and repair than others. These are the following.

The *cruciate ligaments*, two in number, are so named because they cross (X) between the femur and the tibia. They are thick, strong ligaments, called anterior and poste-

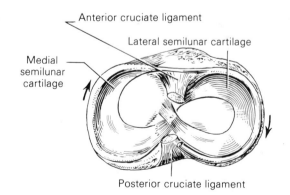

(Helfet: Disorders of the Knee. Lippincott, 1974)

rior according to their attachment on the tibia. The anterior cruciate limits extension of the knee and rotation of the tibia on the femur. The posterior cruciate prevents backward displacement of the tibia on the femur. They are the main stabilizing ligaments of the knee.

The two *collateral ligaments* are located one on either side of the knee. They are the fibular collateral and the tibial collateral ligaments, and their function is to prevent lateral dislocation of the knee.

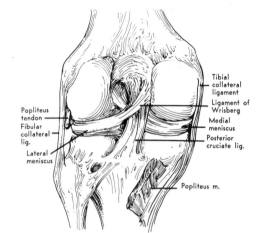

(Turek: Orthopaedics, 3rd ed. Lippincott, 1977)

The *patellar ligament* attaches the patella to the tibia. It extends from the central part of the quadriceps tendon, and is referred to in many orthopedic textbooks as the patellar tendon, rather than ligament.

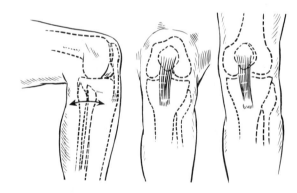

(Helfet: Disorders of the Knee. Lippincott, 1974)

The Capsule

The articular capsule, enclosing the joint space, is composed of thin, strong, fibrous membrane. Reinforcing bands from the fascia lata, along with tendons around the joint, are an inseparable part of the fibrous capsule.

The *synovial membrane*, or inner lining of the fibrous capsule, is the most extensive synovial membrane in the body. In lining the capsule, it also excludes the cruciate ligaments from the interior part of the joint.

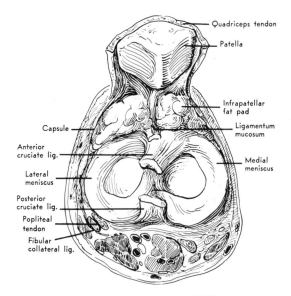

(Turek: Orthopaedics, 3rd ed. Lippincott, 1977)

An infrapatellar fat pad separates the synovium from the patellar ligament or tendon.

Bursae

Numerous bursae around the knee joint provide protection between skin and bone and permit muscles and tendons to glide smoothly over the bony surfaces. The prepatellar bursa, located between the patella and the skin, is prone to an inflammatory condition known as "housemaid's knee."

Major Nerves and Blood Vessels

The posterior structure of the knee joint is a complex of nerves and blood vessels and is generally considered a surgeon's nightmare.

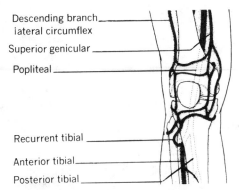

Arteries in area of the knee. (Chaffee and Lytle: Basic Physiology and Anatomy, 4th ed. Lippincott, 1980)

The main blood vessels in this area are the popliteal artery and vein. Running down the middle of the posterior compartment of the knee is the large tibial nerve. The peroneal nerve runs posterior and lateral.

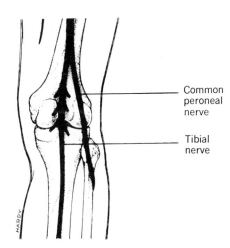

(Chaffee and Lytle: Basic Physiology and Anatomy, 4th ed. Lippincott, 1980)

Predisposing Factors in Knee Problems

Are some people more prone to knee injuries and problems than others? From a structural standpoint, there are several factors that should be mentioned. Because the female has a wide pelvis and parallel tibias, her knees are in a slightly valgus (knock-knee) position. This fact, along with the ligamentous laxity normal in a female, predisposes her to patellar instability.

The child with the combination of knock-knees (genu valgum) and back-knees (genu recurvatum) is a candidate for ligament problems if this condition persists into adolescence.

The prevalence of genu varum or bowlegs in males may be one reason they are subject to medial meniscus injury more frequently than females.

A "which-came-first" discussion may follow these questions. Is overweight a factor? Are obese people prone to knee instability, or do young people become obese because unstable knees curtail their activities?

A very tall, thin boy will most probably injure his knee if he plays football. A lack of coordination associated with this type of body build is partly responsible.

Does the reverence accorded professional athletes put pressure on them, as well as the youth of the nation, to compete and excel even with injured knees? It often appears that way.

Whatever theories on cause of knee disorders one subscribes to, one fact seems clear. The knee sends more people to surgery than any joint in the body.

Diagnostic Examinations

Patients who are hospitalized with knee injuries or pain in the knee joint may eventually undergo additional diagnostic examinations. Therefore, the nurse should have some basic knowledge of what kinds of procedures can be done.

Occasionally patients doubt the necessity for undergoing examinations, especially if their problem is one that comes and goes, or if they seem to be "getting better." Nearly any patient can be convinced of the worth of a thorough knee examination once he has been told that a knee does not *simply* wear out with age. It is destroyed by mechanical factors or disease over a period of time. Early diagnosis and treatment of disorders may keep the knee joint in working condition for many years.

Symptoms

Pain, swelling, mechanical dysfunctions (buckling, clicking, locking) stiffness, and limping are symptoms of a knee problem. However, sometimes pain in the knee is referred from the hip and is related to problems of the hip joint rather than the knee.

Clinical Examination

When the knee is examined it is evaluated as to appearance, the way it feels, and the way it moves. This is done with the patient lying first on his back and then on his abdomen. The knees are constantly compared during an examination. On visual inspection, color, scars, wasting, swelling, lumps, and position of the knee are observed.

Feeling the knee may help determine the presence of lumps and also localizes tenderness. Ligamentous structures and bony prominences are identified and the condition and size of the quadriceps noted.

The knee is tested for normal and abnormal movements and for those movements that produce pain or grating.

Instability of the cruciate ligaments may be evidenced by having the patient lie down and flex his knee at a 90-degree angle. The examiner stabilizes the patient's foot and then grasps the leg below the knee, pushing forward and backward. Movement within the knee indicates instability of the cruciate ligaments.

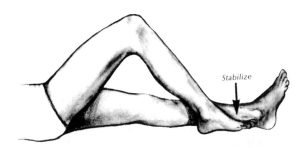

Method of testing for instability of the cruciate ligaments. (Bates: A Guide to Physical Examination, 2nd ed, Lippincott, 1979)

A test of collateral ligament tears includes having the patient extend his knee, at which point the examiner stabi-

lizes the femur with one hand and grasps the ankle with the other while attempting to adduct and abduct the leg at the knee.

The major test for localizing a meniscus injury is McMurray's test. The knee is externally and internally rotated in various degrees of flexion. At a certain point, a click may be felt or heard, the patient may experience pain, and the cartilage may protrude.

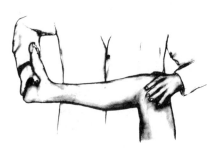

McMurray's test for localizing a meniscus injury. (Bates: A Guide to Physical Examination, 2nd ed. Lippincott, 1979)

X-Rays

The bones and their density, along with the position of the joint, can be seen on x-ray film. Ligaments and tendons, however, are not visible. Typical x-ray findings include fractures, a displaced patella (see below, left), loose bodies (see below, right) exostoses, and arthritic changes. *Loose bodies* in a joint are small pieces of bone, usually attached to cartilage, that are generally the result of disease or trauma. *Exostoses* are benign protrusions of bone, characteristically covered by growing cartilage.

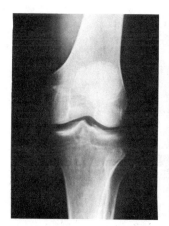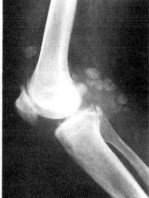

(*Left*) Displaced patella. (*Right*) Loose bodies.

Arthroscopy

By definition, *arthroscopy* is a visual examination of the interior surface of a joint, primarily the knee. The instrument used is an arthroscope, sometimes referred to as a needlescope.

The size of the needle varies up to 6 to 7 mm, but with an instrument that is 1.7 mm in diameter, it is possible to inspect about 95% of the knee joint with one puncture. This is true because at 45 degrees of flexion, the knee is at its most unstable point. It can be opened by exerting varus and valgus strain so that there is about ⅛ inch between the tibial and femoral condyles. The size of the instrument permits the surgeon to view the patellar surfaces and the entire back of the knee joint.

The normal field of the scope is revealed below on the left. The field of the scope on the right shows a tear in the meniscus.

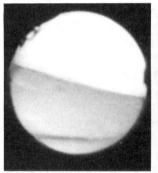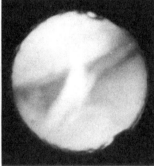

(*Left*) Normal field of arthroscope. (*Right*) Torn meniscus.

The examination is performed as a sterile surgical procedure in the operating room, and under local anesthesia. The patient receives a barbiturate before the examination. A tourniquet is used to reduce blood flow to the extremity, and the arthroscope is inserted into the joint medial to the patellar tendon, just lateral to the anterior cruciate and immediately above the meniscus. A surgeon may elect to use epinephrine in the saline solution rather than a tourniquet on the thigh.

Arthroscopy has greatly reduced diagnostic error and allows the surgeon about 30% more visibility in the knee joint than an arthrotomy. Also, it can be done on an outpatient basis. The use of general anesthesia, like larger needles and tourniquets, is a matter of surgeon's preference.

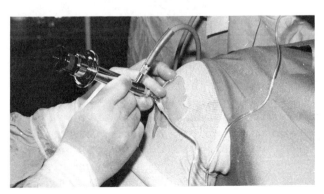

Arthrotomy

An arthrotomy, or opening of the joint, is technically an exploratory procedure. When it appears on a surgical schedule, it does not tell the nurse what additional procedure will be carried out on the patient's knee. Sophisticated use of an arthroscope has eliminated the necessity for the use of this procedure as a diagnostic aid.

Arthrography

An arthrogram is a roentgenological examination of a joint following the injection of radiopaque dye. When the knee is examined by this method, the menisci are outlined and tears may become visible. This examination is most valuable in visualizing the junction of the posterior and middle third of the medial meniscus. In the lateral-view arthrogram shown below, the white areas are caused by the opaque dye.

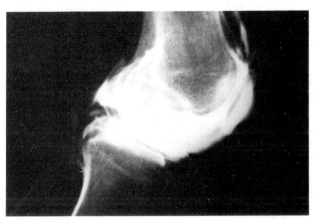

Arthrogram of knee.

Mechanisms and Treatment of Knee Injuries

The following discussion of the various types of knee injuries and treatment provides background information that helps to clarify the principles of nursing care. Rehabilitation of the patient with a knee injury or operation is discussed in more detail in a separate section on pages 240–242.

Menisci Injuries

A twisting movement when the knee is flexed and the foot is firmly planted on the ground may result in a torn meniscus. This is a frequent injury in football, skiing, and other activities in which a twisting motion occurs, such as may happen when a duck hunter, with his boots "stuck" in marshy ground, suddenly rises from a crouched position, twisting his body in the process.

A medial meniscus can tear when the femur is internally rotated on the fixed tibia while the knee is in flexion and abduction. In the reverse situation, the lateral meniscus is torn. Tears may occur in either the anterior or posterior horn of a meniscus. The medial meniscus is more likely to tear than the lateral, because it is less mobile. For the same reason, a "bowstring" or "bucket-handle" tear, or longitudinal splitting, is usually confined to the medial meniscus.

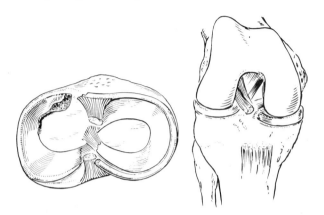

Torn medial meniscus showing retracted medial horn. (Helfet: Disorders of the Knee. Lippincott, 1974)

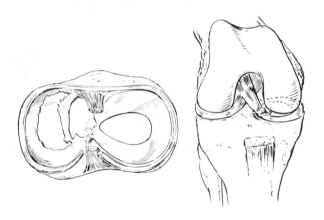

"Bowstring" or "bucket-handle" tear of the medial meniscus. (Helfet: Disorders of the Knee. Lippincott, 1974)

Symptoms. Pain, mild effusion, and tenderness in the anterior joint after prolonged activity may be the most prominent symptoms. The patient may complain of sensations of snapping, clicking, or jerking. If the torn cartilage becomes displaced, it may get jammed between femur and tibia, thus preventing extension. This is called a "locked" knee.

Treatment and Rehabilitation. When a torn meniscus is suspected or definitely diagnosed, one should obviously avoid any activity that causes symptoms. A "locked" knee is treated by manipulation. One method is to have the patient lie on the table while the knee is hyperflexed with valgus strain until the cartilage slips back into place. The knee is then extended. The patient may be instructed to limit his activity by staying off the leg for several weeks, after which the meniscus is surgically removed before it has an opportunity to lock once more. Alternatively, the patient's leg may

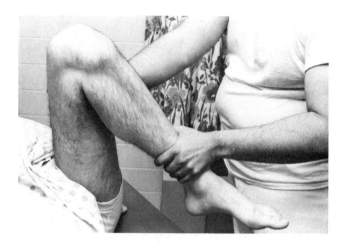

be immobilized in a splint or compression bandage to help avoid further injury until the operation. Quadriceps setting exercises may be done in the preoperative period to maintain muscle strength.

A *meniscectomy*, or removal of a meniscus, is indicated for a knee that locks, or for a torn cartilage that causes recurrent pain and limitation of motion.

Many surgeons are becoming reluctant to remove the whole meniscus, preferring to excise only the portion that is torn loose. Subsequent arthroscopy examinations on these knees have shown that a pseudomeniscus may grow to replace the cartilage that has been removed, although the blood supply to the meniscus is in the outer rim or part that is attached to the tibia. Leaving the undamaged part of the meniscus intact in the knee joint also salvages some of the shock-absorbing effect that a normal meniscus has. A closed meniscectomy is the procedure of choice.

Closed Meniscectomy. The closed meniscectomy utilizes the arthroscope for visualization of the torn meniscus. The arthroscope is inserted into the joint through a puncture wound. A saline solution enters the joint through tubing in a second puncture wound. A cannula is inserted into the joint through still another puncture site and is used as a portal of entry for cutting instruments and as a means of exit for the saline solution, which carries tiny particles of cartilage as they are more or less "chewed away" by the surgeon's knife.

The patient who has had a closed meniscectomy is usually ambulatory on crutches by the evening of the operative day. Weight bearing is only restricted if the knee becomes swollen. The initial dressing is removed and adhesive strips are applied to the puncture sites on the day after surgery, and the patient is discharged. Postoperative discomfort is minimal. After a follow-up visit to the surgeon 7 to 10 days postoperatively, the patient will usually be allowed to return to normal activities and exercise as tolerated. The closed meniscectomy, like all arthroscopic surgery, is becoming an outpatient or "short stay" procedure.

Collateral Ligament Injury

The tibial or medial collateral ligament may easily rupture when force is applied to the lateral side of the knee while the foot is anchored on the ground. The best known example of this type of injury comes from "clipping" in football. Extreme adduction of the leg is usually necessary to injure the fibular or lateral collateral ligament.

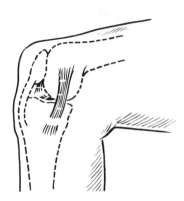

Ruptured collateral ligament. (Helfet: Disorders of the Knee. Lippincott, 1974)

Symptoms. Violent rupture of the ligament results in swelling and a hematoma. Frequently, the only symptom is pain over the ligament that is aggravated by weight bearing.

Treatment and Rehabilitation. The extent of the injury determines the method of immobilization and the length of time that the patient will be on crutches. An elastic bandage, immobilizer, or a long leg cast will be applied. If the leg is casted, it is first placed in a slightly flexed position.

Gross instability of the knee requires that the ligament be sutured. After surgery, a long leg cast may be applied for 5 to 6 weeks.

Rotatory instability of the knee may be improved by a pes anserinus transfer, or Slocum procedure. In this operation the lower two-thirds of the pes anserinus, or conjoined ten-

don of the sartorius, gracilus, and semitendinosus muscles, is reflected proximally and secured to the tibia. The anticipated result is medial support for the joint. Following surgery on a knee ligament, the length of hospitalization averages 5 days, but much depends on the patient's general comfort and how soon he becomes independent on crutches.

Quadriceps-setting exercises, followed by weight-resistive exercises after the pain subsides, are generally prescribed for all patients who have had collateral ligament injuries. Those who have had surgical repair of a ligament(s) require a gradual and intensive program of exercises to restore adequate functioning of the quadriceps and the knee joint once the tissues have healed.

Cruciate Ligament Injury

Violent trauma is normally required to rupture the cruciate ligaments. Such trauma includes a force that drives the femur backward while the knee is flexed and the tibia fixed, dislocation of the knee, hyperextension, and exteme rotation. The common areas of cruciate ligament tears as indicated in the following figure are: (*A*) anterior cruciate from the femoral attachment (posterior view); (*B*) subsynovial tears of anterior cruciate (anterior view); (*C*) midportion tear of anterior cruciate (posterior view); (*D*) tear of tibial attachment of anterior cruciate (anterior view); and (*E*) detachment of the bony insertion of the posterior cruciate to the tibia (posterior view).

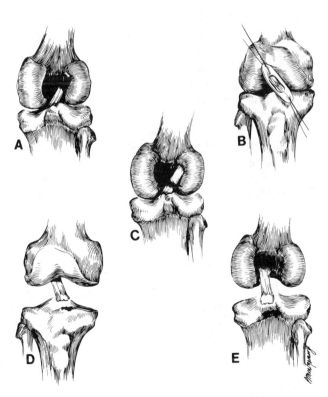

Common areas of cruciate ligament tears. (Rockwood and Green: Fractures. Lippincott, 1975)

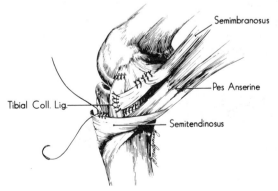

Slocum procedure. (Rockwood and Green: Fractures. Lippincott, 1975)

Symptoms. Severe swelling and instability of the knee joint follow rupture of a cruciate ligament. The tibia will be displaced forward if the anterior cruciate is involved, and backward when the knee is flexed if the posterior cruciate is involved. Gross instability is present when both ligaments are injured.

Treatment. For an older, less active person, immobilization of the slightly flexed knee in a cast for a few months, followed by a knee brace, may be the treatment of choice. However, in an active young adult, surgical repair is perhaps the best treatment, followed by application of a long leg cast in about 30 degrees of flexion. Methods of repairing or replacing the anterior cruciate ligament are the subject of considerable research and debate. An acute rupture of the posterior cruciate is normally treated by surgical repair.

The length of hospitalization may be 5 to 7 days. The patient will be non-weightbearing on crutches for 6 weeks or longer, depending on the extent of the injury.

Multiple Injuries

Violent rupture of one ligament is often accompanied by damage to other ligaments. Repeated trauma, such as might occur in football, is one cause of multiple injuries. The "unhappy triad," as it is sometimes called, consists of a tear in the medial meniscus and rupture of the tibial collateral and anterior cruciate ligaments.

Symptoms and Treatment. Pain, swelling, and instability are the clinical features of this injury. A meniscectomy and surgical restoration of the other two ligaments has been successful in treatment of this condition. The patient may be in the hospital 5 to 7 days with the leg casted in about 30 degrees of flexion. Crutches may be necessary for 6 to 8 weeks.

Rehabilitation. Patients with cruciate ligament injuries and repairs need a vigorous program of resistive exercises during the rehabilitation period to build up the quadriceps muscle. When this starts and how it progresses is decided by the surgeon and is suited to the individual patient.

Tendon Rupture

Avulsion of the *patellar tendon* is an injury common in young people engaged in strenuous athletic activity. As indicated in the following figure, a ruptured patella tendon is reflected by (*1*) upward displacement of the patella and (*2*) a palpable depression below the patella.

The *quadriceps tendon* may be ruptured in older people as a result of a forcible flexion of the knee when the quadriceps is contracted, as may occur when a person falls down the stairs. Rupture of the quadriceps tendon may be accompanied by swelling of the knee joint due to bloody effusion. There is also a tender depression above the superior margin of the patella.

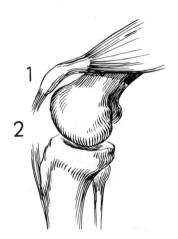

Disruption of patellar tendon indicating (*1*) high patella and (*2*) patella tendon defect. (Rockwood and Green: Fractures. Lippincott, 1975)

Treatment and Rehabilitation. In both cases of tendon rupture, surgical repair of the affected tendon is indicated. The leg is immobilized in extension for 6 to 8 weeks. Following this a program of physical therapy that includes a progression of flexion exercises is beneficial.

Recurrent Dislocation of the Patella

As mentioned earlier, instability of the patella is more common in females because of genu valgum (knock-knee). In this situation, the line of pull exerted by the quadriceps tends to displace the patella laterally. Traumatic dislocation is due to outward torsion of the leg while the knee is in full extension.

Recurrent dislocation may be due to the following factors:

1. Abnormal development of the patella. For example, one that is too small.
2. A shallow femoral groove.
3. Ligaments allowing hyperextension of the knee.
4. Weakness of the vastus medialis.

Repeated displacement of the patella eventually damages its articulating surfaces and those of the femoral condyle. Slipping or subluxation of the patella is not as obvious as complete dislocation but perhaps does even more harm to the undersurface of the patella.

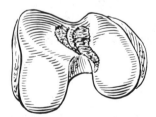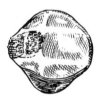

Erosion of the patella. (Helfet: Disorders of the Knee. Lippincott, 1974)

Symptoms. Sharp pain follows dislocation, and the patient may fall. Some swelling due to effusion may be present. Once the patella has dislocated, the patient may complain of feeling insecure about exercising.

Treatment. Extension of the knee and flexion of the hip will cause the patella to slip back into place. Since the condition is recurrent, surgery is recommended.

Many cases of chronic dislocation of the patella may be corrected by a closed operation under arthroscopy. In this procedure, the retinaculum of the lateral quadriceps is released from the patella. The patient will return from surgery with the leg wrapped in an elastic bandage and a small foam rubber pressure pad over the lateral incision. Crutchwalk-

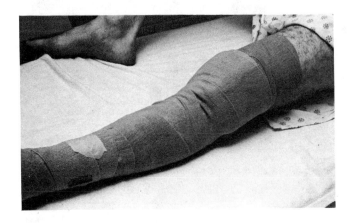

ing, quadriceps setting, *gentle* flexion, and straight leg raising may be initiated on the first postoperative day, and the patient is discharged on the first or second day. The purpose of gentleness in flexion is to avoid the possibility of bleeding into the joint. The "lateral release" may be done in conjunction with a chondrectomy. A patellar tendon transplant, which consists of removing the distal end of the tendon along with its bony attachment and transplanting it in a medial location, is rarely indicated.

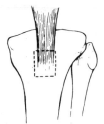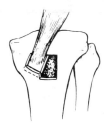

Tendon transplant. (Helfet: Disorders of the Knee. Lippincott, 1974)

After a patellar tendon transplant, the patient's leg is immobilized in extension in a knee immobilizer or a cylinder cast. The patient is in the hospital for about 5 days, with crutchwalking beginning as soon as tolerated. Exercises to strengthen the quadriceps are begun about 4 weeks after

surgery, and the patient spends about 6 weeks altogether on crutches. The recommendations in the section on general nursing care of the patient with a knee repair also apply to the care of the patient with a patellar tendon transplant (pp. 234–239).

Chondromalacia Patellae

Hypertrophic degenerative changes of the articulating cartilage of the patella may follow recurrent dislocation or subluxation, repeated minor injuries, major trauma, or friction in the femoral groove. When symptoms are severe enough to cause serious pain and disability, a chondrectomy is the procedure of choice.

A chondrectomy (patellar shaving), or removal of degenerative cartilage, is an arthroscopic procedure in which the underside of the patella is shaved. The end of the femoral condyle may also be shaved. A small television camera is placed over the eyepiece of the arthroscope after it has been introduced into the joint. A second puncture wound is made

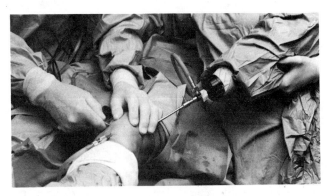

for the tubing, through which normal saline enters and expands the joint capsule. An instrument that contains a shaving device and allows the return flow of saline solution along with the pieces of cartilage into a large container is introduced through a third puncture wound. The surgeon performs the operation by observing his actions on a television screen.

The chondrectomy patient returns from surgery with a small elastoplast dressing or elastic bandage and dressing on the knee. This dressing is removed and replaced by adhesive strips on the evening of the operative or first postoperative day, and the patient is discharged. Full range of motion and ambulation begin on the operative day as tolerated. The use of crutches is optional. The nursing management standards for arthroscopic surgery given on page 235 may be used as the basis of care planning for these patients.

Loose Bodies

In the knee joint, loose bodies of cartilage and bone may be present due to injury, inflammation, degeneration, or unknown causes. They are removed only when they cause symptoms. Whenever possible, loose bodies are removed under arthroscopy.

Care of the Patient Undergoing Knee Repair

Preoperative Preparation

Data Collection

Before any planning or instruction can begin, the nurse should inspect the patient's knee and get an accurate description of the amount of pain and disability present. The problem knee should be compared to the normal knee and the comparison described on the data base. Comparison parameters include appearance (swelling), range of motion in the knee, pedal pulses, and neurovascular status of the foot.

Many patients enter the hospital for knee repair immediately after an injury occurs or a problem develops. Others have long histories of recurrent pain or injuries. Patients who have lived with a knee disorder for any length of time may have second thoughts about the advisability of surgery. Therefore, it is necessary to learn how the patient feels about impending surgery and how much information the physician has provided. Then the patient's immediate physical and psychological needs can be identified and a plan of care established that will help meet these needs. During the preoperative period, the nurse should identify potential postoperative problems and take measures to prevent them (see chart, p. 236).

Patient Teaching

An orthopedic nurse must have basic knowledge about the operative procedure and expected outcomes. Without this background it is difficult to reinforce and clarify what the surgeon has told the patient about the procedure, length of hospitalization, and progression of activities. For example, as was previously discussed, the amount of flexion and weight bearing allowed following a meniscectomy differs from that following a ligament repair. Furthermore, stability on crutches is somewhat determined by the method of immobilizing the knee. A cast will be less awkward if the leg is in a flexed position. A knee immobilizer is more cumbersome than a dressing.

Finally, the nurse should be familiar with the particular surgeon's approach to patients. Some physicians have a "wait and see" attitude, and prescribe and explain physical therapy and ambulation on a day-to-day basis. Others discuss treatment thoroughly and set goals while the patient is in the office. It is confusing to a patient if the surgeon has told him that he could be up with crutches the day after surgery "if he feels like it," only to have the first nurse he talks to after admission say quite positively that no one ever gets up before the second postoperative day.

Use of Trapeze

Although a patient having a knee repair is only partially immobilized, and sometimes only for a matter of hours, it helps if he knows how to use a trapeze. Because the patient is not helpless, it is easy to forget to put a trapeze on the overhead frame postoperatively and to teach the patient how to use it. To eliminate this oversight the trapeze should be in place preoperatively as a matter of routine. In this way it will be there the first time the patient needs it for independent movement.

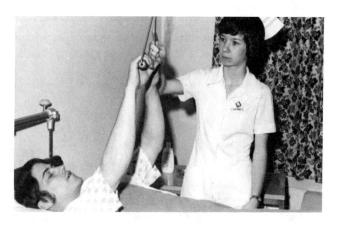

Exercises and Crutchwalking

Quadriceps-setting exercises should be taught if the patient has not been doing them as part of a conservative treatment program. This exercise may be demonstrated on the unaffected leg if the affected knee is painful. The patient is asked

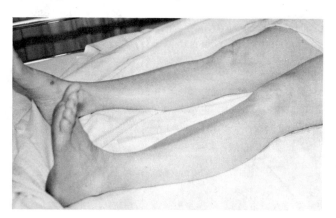

to straighten his leg on the bed, pull his toes forward, and then either "pull his kneecap up into his thigh" or press the back of his knee into the mattress, whichever direction seems easiest for him to follow. He should be instructed to observe his quadriceps tighten as he does this, and then to place his hand on the muscle to feel the contraction. The nurse also places her hand just above the patient's knee during the exercise to evaluate strength of muscle response.

NURSING MANAGEMENT STANDARDS: ARTHROSCOPY/ARTHROSCOPIC SURGERY*

Potential Problems	Expected Outcomes	Deadlines	Preventive Nursing Management
PRE-OP			
1. Standard.*	1. Standard.		1. a. Standard. b. Provide opportunity for patient to verbalize questions to assess level of understanding. (Normally not documented.)
POST-OP			
1. Standard.†	1. Standard.		1. Standard.
2. Wound infection due to invasion by pathologic organisms.	2. Clean wound. Temperature no higher than 100°F.	Discharge	2. a. Inspect dressing or wound daily (10 A.M.). b. Check temperature q 4 hr until HS day of surgery (10−2−6−*etc.*) and bid (6−6) thereafter.
3. Severe swelling due to trauma of procedure.	3. Swelling of operative knee less than 1½ times other knee (would be documented as minimal).	Discharge	3. a. Apply ice to knee q 4 hr (10−2−6−10−2−6) for 24 hr. b. Check knee q shift for 24 hr. c. Elevate leg continuously for 24 hr.
4. Thrombophlebitis due to venous stasis.	4. No calf pain (documented if pain occurs). Negative Homans' sign if calf pain present. Temperature below 100°F.	Discharge	4. a. Check CMTS of operated leg q 4 hr until HS day of surgery (10−2−6−*etc.*). b. Report tenderness of calf or groin to M.D. If tenderness present, check Homans' sign q day. c. Cough, turn, and deep breathe q 4 hr until HS day of surgery (10−2−6−*etc.*). d. Check temperature bid (6−6).
5. Difficulty with home management due to lack of understanding of exercises and how to prevent swelling.	5. Demonstration of ability to do exercises and verbalization of knowledge of how to prevent swelling.	Discharge	5. a. Instruct in straight leg raises, quadriceps setting. b. Instruct to elevate leg when lying or sitting, or for 1 hr if swelling occurs.

* Hospital nursing management standards—all pre-ops.
† Hospital nursing management standards—all post-ops.

The patient should understand that straight leg raising will follow "quad setting" after surgery (p. 239) and that both may be painful. He must have reassurance that he will be provided with physical and moral support when he begins moving his leg postoperatively, and that analgesics will be given as ordered.

If weight lifting will be part of his program while he is in the hospital, it will be done in the physical-therapy department and should be explained by the therapist.

One idea that has merit is admitting the patient to the hospital early enough the day before or of surgery to permit the physical therapist to instruct him in the use of crutches.

THE PATIENT UNDERGOING KNEE REPAIR:
IDENTIFYING AND PREVENTING POTENTIAL POSTOPERATIVE PROBLEMS

Significant Patient Data: J. F. is a 26-year-old male who injured his knee skiing 2 days ago. He enters the hospital to have surgery for the ''unhappy triad'' (a tear in the medial meniscus and rupture of the tibial collateral and anterior cruciate ligaments). He is 6'2" tall and weighs 160 lb. He has no other health problems and denies any allergies. This is his first hospitalization. His orthopedic assessment is negative except for slight swelling and bruising of the left knee. He has a severe amount of pain on movement. His biggest concern seems to be the fact that he will be in a cast that will not have a walker on it. He knows he must be in the hospital 5 to 7 days but hopes he can go home sooner. He is pleasant, cooperative, but ''jumpy.''

Data Concerning the Procedure: J. F. will return from surgery with his leg casted in 30 degrees of flexion with ankle slightly inverted. The surgery will be extensive. Postoperative pain may be severe for at least 48 hr.

Potential Problems

I. General discomfort due to improper body alignment
II. Anxiety may
    a. Increase his pain
    b. Prevent him from resting
    c. Cause problems voiding
    d. Inhibit communication

Nursing Implications

I. Find him a longer bed.
II. Identify and take measures to prevent possible sources of anxiety.
    a. Evaluate knowledge of what is happening to him. How much does he remember of what surgeon has told him? Provide instruction and clarification.
    b. Tell him that discharge will depend on how soon he is independent on crutches. Appropriate steps to achieve this follow:
        1. Keep leg properly elevated postoperatively to decrease swelling, which dictates when he can be out of bed.
        2. Instruct him in quadriceps setting and straight leg raising for unaffected leg to maintain strength to do work for both legs.
    c. Discuss management of postoperative pain.
        1. Determine if he has any ''fear'' of needles.
        2. Stress importance of having pain medications prn.
    d. Review hospital routines as they will affect him.
        1. How does he make special requests for food, drink?
        2. Does he sleep late? Watch TV?
        3. Explain that he will need to use a urinal for a day or two.
    e. Provide him with hospital ''shorts'' and tell him he can wear them postoperatively in bed. (Hospital gowns will not be adequate clothing because of his height, and this may cause him embarrassment and reluctance to move about in bed.)
    f. Make Kardex note to discuss the importance of postoperative fluids with him, perhaps on the first postoperative day, in order to prevent voiding problems and constipation. To do so at the present time could create more anxiety.

It makes sense to learn the mechanics of crutchwalking before the advent of postsurgical pain or the application of an immobilizer or cast. This practice will also facilitate early discharge.

Postoperative Care

Dressings, Immobilizers, Casts

The type of knee surgery will dictate whether the patient is to return from surgery with a dressing, a knee immobilizer, or a cast (straight-legged, flexed, or cylinder).

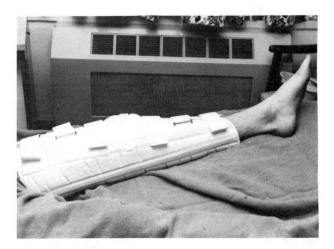

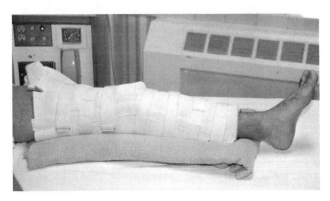

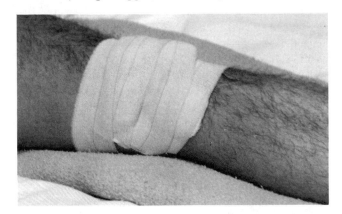

Dressings and Drainage. The type of dressing that is applied to the knee will depend on the procedure and the surgeon's preference. Dressings for patients having arthroscopic surgery may be Elastoplast or elastic wrap over gauze pads. Observable drainage is rare, except in the occasional patient who has a residual drainage of saline from the continuous irrigation (p. 233) of his knee joint. The dressing may have a small to large amount of dark pink drainage, which could alarm the patient unless he is told that a drop of blood goes a long way in a few ounces of saline. Dark red drainage should be carefully evaluated to determine if it is "old" or "new," and if there is more than a minimal amount, it should be reported to the physician. Complaints of pressure in the knee, or increased pain, may indicate that some bleeding is occurring. These same complaints may mean that the dressing is simply too tight. An elastic bandage should be loosened and rewrapped when it constricts to the point of causing pain, or swelling of the foot. Bulky dressings with or without posterior plaster splints may be used on the knee to provide compression or temporary immobilization. These require the same observations as smaller dressings.

Knee Immobilizers. Knee immobilizers may be used following surgical procedures in which immobilization is crucial to healing, such as a patellar tendon transplant. They are also frequently used to immobilize a knee with a damaged ligament diagnosed by arthroscopy. Various styles are manufactured by orthopedic supply companies. They hold

the leg in extension or flexion and are normally more comfortable than a cast. Still, they tend to be a bit awkward. Patients who must wear immobilizers frequently make the following complaints: (1) They are warm. (2) The strap over the knee can cause pressure if there is any amount of swelling. (3) They may slip down or feel as if they are slipping down once the patient is up on crutches. To overcome some of these problems, sheet wadding can be placed under the immobilizer and the straps readjusted. Cornstarch applied lightly to the skin under a knee immobilizer helps keep the skin dry and decrease irritation. The nurse must also remember that the purpose of an immobilizer is to immobilize, not apply pressure; therefore, it can be fastened loosely while the patient is in bed. When the patient complains of burning, the immobilizer should be opened, and the skin checked for irritation and skin breakdown due to the combination of perspiration and padding. Depending on the protocol of the surgeon, this may or may not require a written order, and the nurse should be clear on this point.

Casts. Casts are generally required following *cruciate ligament repair or multiple ligament repair.* A cylinder cast that does not extend over the ankle and foot and is straight-legged or flexed may be used when a long period of strict immobilization of the knee in extension or slight flexion is essential to the healing of its structures.

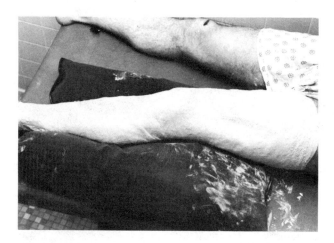

When the cast is applied some provision must be made for it to stay in place. To keep the cast from slipping, tincture of benzoin may be applied to the skin before the stockinette is put on. Or two dents can be made over the anterior thigh portion of the cast. A nurse who is not aware that these dents are deliberate may become anxious over the appearance of the cast and the condition of the extremity. These dents more or less follow the contour of the muscle and do not lie over bony prominences. Some ligament repairs or reconstructions require immobilization of the leg in flexion with the foot casted and inverted.

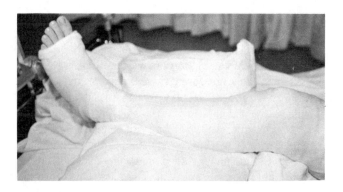

Patients wearing casts following knee surgery are subject to all the cautions and considerations of cast care, as discussed in Chapter 2.

Leg Position and Comfort

As a general rule, following knee surgery the foot of the bed should be elevated so that the patient's feet are as high as the heart. This will reduce swelling. If the patient returns from surgery without a cast or knee immobilizer, his leg must be kept in full extension. For this reason, placing pillows under the leg is undesirable, since the combination of a pillow and soft dressing causes flexion of the knee and compression of nerves and blood vessels.

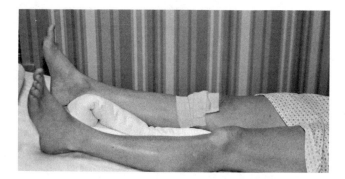

Unfortunately, even with the foot of the bed elevated, the patient can still seek the more comfortable position of flexion and external rotation — a "frog leg." Therefore, his leg position should be checked every 3 hours.

If a knee immobilizer has been applied, the leg will be automatically extended, but the foot of the bed still needs to be elevated for 24 hours. If a cast has been applied, the casted leg is elevated on pillows until the plaster is dry and should be left open to the air. The foot of the bed may be elevated slightly if pillow elevation is not sufficient to reduce symptoms of swelling in the operative knee. However, the foot of the bed must be lowered if the patient complains of discomfort in the lower back. When the knee is casted in slight flexion, place pillows under the flexed area to provide adequate support.

Ice bags are used for 24 to 48 hours to reduce swelling. How they are placed over a dressing or immobilizer depends on the patient's tolerance. Remember, an ice bag will dent a damp cast if it is placed directly on top of it.

Neurovascular Checks

Following knee surgery, the condition of the patient's extremity is of immediate concern to all of those involved in his care. The toes should be reasonably warm and pink, and the patient should be able to move each one in response to a stimulus. The pedal pulse should be present and checked periodically.

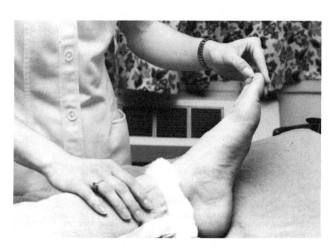

A decrease in sensation over the dorsum of the foot or the inability to dorsiflex the toes or evert the foot may indicate compression of the peroneal nerve in the area of the knee where the bandage or cast is. Numbness and pain may also mean impaired circulation. A patient who has complaints of this nature may obtain relief if his dressing is loosened slightly. Any of these symptoms that persist should be called to the surgeon's attention as soon as possible.

Checking neurovascular status should continue to be a regular postoperative routine while any wrapping remains on the knee.

Pain and Analgesics

An accurate evaluation of the type and location of pain that is present must be emphasized. The extent of surgery is one clue to the amount of pain the patient may have, but care must be taken to see that the dressing is not too tight or that the cast does not cause compression or circulatory problems. The nurse must make certain not to overlook a complaint of *calf pain* by assuming that all pain is in the surgical area. Pain in the calf may be an indication of thrombophlebitis. The patient with a leg casted, knee flexed, and foot inverted often complains of severe muscle spasms for 24 to 48 hours. The nurse must distinguish spasms from early postoperative pain, and if necessary, obtain a physician's order for a muscle relaxant.

Athletes and some large men are sometimes reluctant to ask for pain medication. The nurse must stress the importance of being comfortable in order to tolerate exercise and ambulation. Oral pain medication, as soon as the patient can take food and fluids, is often more acceptable than injections and sometimes seems to have a more lasting effect.

Voiding Problems

Although surgical patients are generally expected to void within 8 to 12 hours following surgery, the patient undergoing knee surgery may be allowed more time if no abdominal distention or distress is present. Voiding into a bedpan or urinal with an elevated leg is difficult. Yet good nursing judgment often aids in avoiding catheterization. Giving the patient an analgesic, if possible, when he first feels the urge to void and cannot, may enable him to relax. The orthopedic nurse with foresight will get a postoperative order (before the problem arises) to stand a male patient at the bedside to void, if necessary. For a female patient who cannot use the bedpan with any success, it is wise to obtain an order that will allow her to be assisted to a bedside commode or taken to the bathroom in a wheelchair with the operated leg elevated. Some of these actions require more time and patience than doing a catheterization but are better for the patient. Granted, some patients do have distended bladders before they are able to stand at a bedside or sit on a commode. But no patient in good general health who has undergone a knee repair should have to be catheterized more than once.

Arthroscopic Surgery: Nursing Implications

For the most part, the patient who has had knee surgery under arthroscopy requires the same nursing care routines as other knee patients. However, this type of patient frequently "feels so good" that he may try to get out of bed by himself when he needs to void or wants something he cannot reach. For this reason, the nurse should make it clear in the immediate postoperative period that for his own safety, he needs standby assistance, at least the first time he gets up.

Exercise and Ambulation

Specific exercises and plans for rehabilitation are discussed briefly in the section describing treatment of various disorders of the knee. *Most* patients who have undergone surgical repair of the knee begin quadriceps-setting exercises as soon as they are fully awake. Straight leg raising is also initiated as soon as the patient can tolerate it.

This exercise is most effectively accomplished the first time if the nurse assists the patient. The unaffected leg should be flexed with the foot flat on the bed to ease strain on the lower back. The nurse places her hand under the heel of the operated leg and instructs the patient to relax while she lifts the leg up to 60 to 90 degrees of hip flexion. Then the nurse asks the patient to lower the leg slowly, by himself, while she holds her hand just below the heel. After a short rest period the same procedure is repeated, and this time the patient might be requested to "hold" the leg up for a few seconds before attempting to lower it back down to

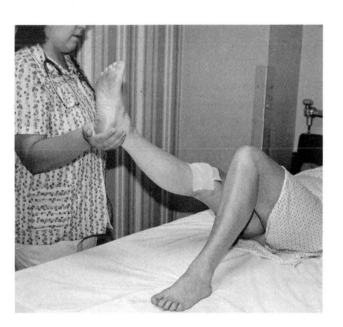

the bed. The patient is given the amount of support he requires, and it may take several sessions before he progresses to independent straight leg raising.

An alert nurse will note that the first few times the patient raises his leg independently, he may rotate it slightly internally or externally. This is a protective maneuver and decreases the pain of movement. Although this is *not* what he should be doing, it is not harmful. The nurse should allow him to rest a few seconds, explain to him what is happening, and encourage him to "try again." Gentleness, as well as persistence, praise, and reassurance, helps motivate the patient and lessens his apprehension. At this point the patient must be instructed to do a "quad set" prior to doing each straight leg raise. Supervision of this exercise is necessary until the patient does it correctly.

Since straight leg raising is very important in the development of quadriceps power, it is ideal if the patient can gradually work up to doing it at least five times every hour.

Ways the nurse can help a patient ease into the routines of straight leg raising are to tell him to do the exercise every time the television program changes or someone comes into the room. Some physicians will not permit the patient to begin crutchwalking until straight leg raising can be done well.

Knee immobilizers and long leg casts are obstacles in performing this exercise. Flexing the unaffected knee with the foot on the bed and using the trapeze will help prevent strain on the lower back.

A reminder at this point: Before starting any exercises, the orthopedic nurse should know the limits of exercise allowed following the various surgical procedures on the knee.

A progressive physical-therapy department will have discussed rehabilitation with the patient before surgery. Ambulation on crutches varies according to the procedure and may begin as soon as the patient has recovered from anesthesia.

Psychological Considerations

Although it is the responsibility of the surgeon to explain his surgical approach to a knee disorder to the patient, it is the responsibility of the nurse to support this instruction. However, the nurse must also deal with concerns the patient may develop during hospitalization. The sheer number of people who have knee surgery means that there are usually several patients in the physical therapy department or walking in the hallway at the same time, as well as sharing the same room. They compare casts, dressings, and postoperative complaints. When a patient does have a question about a knee operation, the nurse should encourage him to communicate with his surgeon for clarification.

It may come as a surprise to the nurse to learn that males are as concerned as females about scars on their knees. There is nothing a nurse can do about a scar, but knowing that it may be a source of concern to the patient keeps a nurse sensitive to individual needs.

A young, athletic person may not be thoroughly convinced he or she will regain complete use of a knee. In addition, the prospect of spending a few months on crutches, even when total rehabilitation is expected, is not pleasant. When encountering an anxious patient the nurse would do well to stop and consider what adjustments a knee disorder would necessitate in her own life.

Complications

Remember, knee surgery is not necessarily minor. Damage to blood vessels or nerves is not impossible. Pulmonary embolism has been known to occur after a meniscectomy, just as it may after any other operation on the lower extremity. Thrombophlebitis, wound infection, and hematomas are other possible, if infrequent, complications. The source of patient complaints, especially of pain, must always be identified.

Rehabilitation

The physical therapist and the surgeon will discuss goals with the patient and plans for attaining them. Length of rehabilitation, including progression of activities while in the hospital, depends on patient readiness and the type of surgery that was done. At least 6 to 8 weeks, including hospitalization may be required to regain normal function after the simplest surgical procedure.

The patient who has had a knee repair may do all of his exercises independently at home, or he may require treatment in physical therapy as an outpatient. Patients who have had arthroscopic surgery generally require basic instruction in exercises that will strengthen the quadriceps muscle and aid in terminal extension or straightening the leg completely. Since hospitalization time is minimal, preprinted exercise instructions are recommended for discharge. A sample of such instructions is on page 241.

Sometimes the chondrectomy patient will need assistance in regaining freedom of motion and strength, especially if he was relatively inactive preoperatively due to discomfort caused by certain activities, such as climbing stairs. The exercise bicycle is a valuable aid in this endeavor.

In all rehabilitation programs for knee repair patients, it is important to check and maintain strength in other muscle groups. For instance, if the ankle has been casted along with the knee following a ligament repair, planned exercise of this joint may be necessary once the cast is removed.

Physical therapy departments frequently use an isokinetic machine for knee rehabilitation programs. These machines assist the patient in gaining strength, endurance,

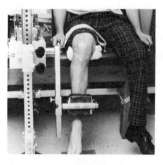 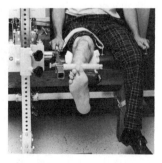

KNEE EXERCISES: ARTHROSCOPIC SURGERY*

1. *Quad Set*
   Frequency:
   In hospital _____
   At home _____

   - Lie on your back with knee straight.
   - Pull your toes and forefoot toward you.
   - Tighten the muscles on the top of your thigh—
     Your knee should straighten.
   - Hold 5 seconds, then relax. Repeat _____ times.

   Quad set

   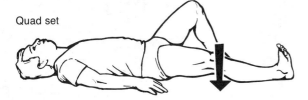

3. *Knee Bending*

   - Do in bed or sitting in chair.
   - Gently bend back as far as possible.
   - Stop when you experience minimal discomfort.
     Repeat _____ times.

   Knee bending

   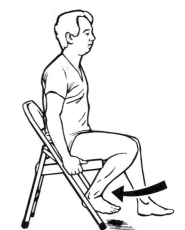

2. *Straight Leg Raise*

   - Lie on your back with good leg bent.
   - Do a quad set as above.
   - Lift leg slowly, keeping knee straight.
   - Hold 2 seconds.
   - Slowly lower and relax. Repeat _____ times.

   Straight leg raise

   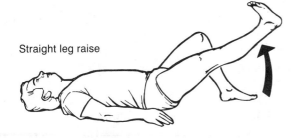

* Courtesy of Physical Therapy Department, Bellin Memorial Hospital, Green Bay, Wisconsin.

and power by offering resistance the entire time he is going through a motion.

Ligament Repair. To avoid straining a repaired ligament exercises are planned so that the patient can progress at his own tolerance. The patient is encouraged to get what motion he can without forcing himself, and in general all of his exercises will be active.

Weightbearing may be limited during rehabilitation for the patient who has had an anterior cruciate ligament repaired. He will not be allowed to do exercises that involve going from knee flexion to extension. Quadriceps setting, straight leg raising, isometrics, and working on an exercise bicycle may constitute his entire program. Some surgeons use continuous passive motion following some procedures; this is discussed on p. 251.

Nursing Responsibilities in Rehabilitation

The nurse gives reinforcing instructions about crutchwalking once the patient leaves the hospital, emphasizing safety factors and stressing the importance of following the orders of both physician and therapist. Athletes, in particular, are anxious to return to the sport that injured them in the first place. Remind the eager patient that a knee may feel good to its owner before the quadriceps is ready for strenuous activity. Finally, to help prevent anxiety after discharge, patients should be told that some numbness may persist around the operative area for a time after surgery.

Knee Reconstruction

It is appropriate to mention again that the knee is no simple hinge joint. Any reconstruction procedure must take into consideration the traveling axis of motion in each position of flexion, and the four distinct articular surfaces.

Factors in Degenerative Knee Joint Disease

Degenerative joint disease most commonly affects the knee. The following disorders may be precursors to this disease.

1. Injury to the articular surfaces. This is due to fractures, the abrasive effects of torn menisci, recurrent dislocation or subluxation of the patella, and the presence of loose bodies.
2. Malalignment, such as genu varum (bow-legs) or genu valgum (knock-knees), in which body weight is not transferred normally through the joint. As a result, increased stress is placed on the weightbearing surfaces of one compartment. Consequently, that part of the joint becomes worn down.
3. Chronic inflammation due to disease, such as rheumatoid arthritis or tuberculosis. Joint incongruity results from the destruction of surfaces.
4. Other disorders include vascular faults in the bone, which may cause the overlying cartilage to deteriorate, and chondromalacia, which results in erosion of the femoral condyles and eventually those of the tibia.

Clinical Picture

The chief symptoms of degenerative disease of the knee joint are pain that is aggravated by use of the joint, and stiffness that is present after the knee has been at rest. There may also be swelling of the joint. Varus deformity is more common than valgus. The articular margins may be tender when they are examined by the physician, and movement may be limited and painful, if forced. Grating on motion may be another symptom, and occasionally the patient will complain of the knee giving away or locking. When the disease is in a fairly advanced stage, there may be wasting of the quadriceps muscle.

X-Ray Findings

A decrease in all or part of the joint space may be evident on x-ray film. The tibiofemoral joint space is diminished with one side (medial or lateral) more affected than the other. In the x-ray film shown below, the left knee reveals degenerative changes in the medial compartment and absence of joint space.

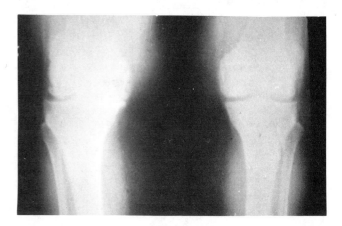

The patellofemoral joint space may also be involved. Other findings may be present, such as loose bodies or osteophyte formation. Osteophytes are bony outgrowths caused by stress.

Surgical Procedures for Degenerative Knee Disease

Debridement and Synovectomy

These procedures are done together and consist of removing as much diseased cartilage, soft tissue, synovium, and osteophyte buildup as possible. Most surgeons consider this temporary treatment, and consequently, it is not very common.

Postoperative Regimen. Following surgery, a compression bandage or immobilizer may be applied. Full extension and lateral rotation of the leg are the objectives of postoperative care. Quadriceps-setting exercises are started on the first or second postoperative day, with flexion exercises beginning about one week after surgery. However, the knee should be in extension when it is not being exercised. The patient's progress to crutchwalking and weight bearing as ordered by the surgeon and may depend on the extent of surgery and the general physical condition of the patient.

Decortication (Abrasion Arthroplasty)

Decortication may be indicated in the surgical treatment of the arthritic knee. Patients undergoing decortication are usually younger than the average candidate for a total knee replacement. Because they must use crutches and remain nonweightbearing for 8 weeks postoperatively, the surgeon must be very selective in his choice of patients in terms of mental acuity and physical ability.

Procedure. Decortication is a shaving of the denuded areas, those *completely devoid* of articular cartilage, until multiple bleeding points are demonstrated. This procedure is done as arthroscopic surgery using a motor-driven, encased, high-speed burr. After approximately 8 weeks of nonweightbearing, maturation of fibrous tissue occurs, and the patient has a fibrocartilage joint surface.

Nursing Considerations. The patient who has undergone decortication in the knee joint is rarely in the hospital longer than 48 hours. The postoperative dressing is similar to that for other arthroscopic surgery procedures and the nursing care is the same. The most important aspect of nursing care is reinforcement of the surgeon's instructions to remain on crutches and nonweightbearing for the prescribed 8-week period.

Exercises. Exercises for these patients are taught in the physical therapy department and are described on p. 241.

Osteotomy

A tibial osteotomy may be the procedure of choice when the patient is young and appears to have one healthy articular surface as indicated by x-ray examination. The technique involves removing a wedge of bone from the tibia and shifting the weight bearing to the opposite side.

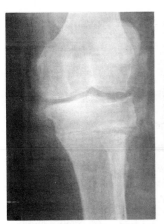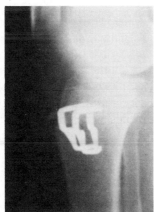

Tibial osteotomy. *(Left)* without staples. *(Right)* with staples.

Postoperative Regimen. As a general rule a patient who undergoes an osteotomy returns from surgery in a long leg cast or plaster splint with a bulky dressing. The nurse should realize that there may be a large amount of bloody drainage through the cast for about 48 hours unless a wound drainage system has been used. These are generally removed by the second postoperative day. Routine nursing care for knee repair as described on pages 234 to 239 is

indicated. The hospitalization period is about 5 days, with crutchwalking beginning as early as the second postoperative day.

If the osteotomy patient's foot has been casted, he usually needs a lift on the shoe for the unoperated leg. The nurse may instruct the family to have this done as soon as possible. Then when the physical therapist teaches the patient crutchwalking, he will be learning with the shoe on that he will be wearing when he returns home.

Patients discard their crutches as they become able to do without them. The cast is generally removed approximately 8 weeks after surgery and may be changed during this period. Patients who have soft dressings and splints require casting before discharge from the hospital. Some surgeons prefer continuous passive motion as an alternative to immobilization (pp. 251). The surgical procedure in these cases requires an appropriate means of internal fixation.

The patient will need to do exercises that will help him to regain strength in his quadriceps and range of motion of the knee joint. He may need to be on an outpatient program in the physical therapy department.

Arthrodesis

Surgical fusion of the knee joint completely and permanently eliminates pain, but the creation of a stiff knee is an inconvenience to the individual who must use it. An arthrodesis might be done if there has been complete failure of a knee prosthesis.

Following arthrodesis of the knee, a long leg cast is applied. The patient proceeds with nonweightbearing on crutches, as condition permits. Four weeks postoperatively the patient may begin bearing weight on a walking cast. Much of the treatment following this procedure depends on the circumstances that preceded it, and how active the patient was prior to surgery.

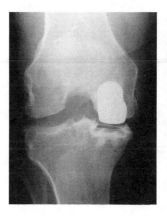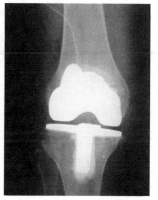

Total Knee Replacement

The most common surgical treatment of advanced degenerative joint disease in the knee is hemi- or total knee replacement. Bone and articulating surfaces are replaced by artificial components that are inserted to realign the joint and correct the existing deformity. Two basic types of prosthesis are commonly used.

1. The condylar prosthesis basically consists of metal femoral implants and high-density polyethylene tibial implants with or without metal backing. It is designed to replace the degenerated surfaces of the condyles and is available in unicondylar or duocondylar models. The creation of smooth joint surfaces permits pain-free motion and weight bearing. The bone cement methyl methacrylate is used for fixation. There are many models of knee prostheses. Some of the features that may be incorporated into the basic designs include the patellar component, the various types of tibial projections (stems and pegs), and porous coating. As in the total hip replacement, porous coating is utilized in the hope that it will improve fixation.

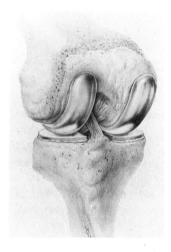

(Top) Marmor modular knee system. (Courtesy Richards Manufacturing Co., Memphis, Tenn.). *(Bottom)* PCA porous-coated prosthesis. (Courtesy Howmedica, Inc., Rutherford, NJ.).

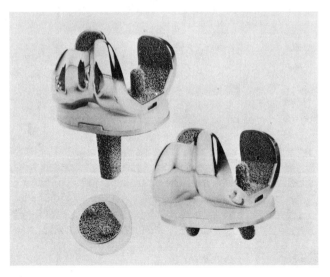

2. The hinged-knee prosthesis is used when joint destruction is extensive enough to include the collateral ligaments, thereby eliminating stability altogether.

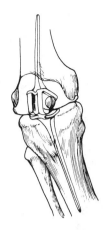

Hinged-knee prosthesis. (Drawing from Patient Care, Mar 15, 1972. Miller and Fink Corp., Darien, Conn.).

There are various types of prostheses that provide a hinge-type action. Most of them require methyl methacrylate for fixation.

Although the results of total knee replacement have been remarkable, research to design a more anatomically correct prosthesis continues because, while total knee prostheses come in standard sizes and shapes, the human knee does not. Each knee is to some degree unique, not only in construction, but also in motion. Knee re-replacements necessitated by wear and loosening are a fact of life.

Care of the Patient Undergoing Total Knee Replacement

Indications

Surgical intervention is indicated in a knee that does not respond to ordinary medical management, rest, immobilization, heat, and quadriceps exercises.

Sometimes a tibial osteotomy will be the procedure of choice. However, the patient who has severe pain, joint contractures, and swelling that does not permit extension and flexion will need total knee replacement.

Preoperative Preparation

Patient Teaching

Admission to the hospital is preceded by a thorough discussion of the operative procedure with the orthopedic surgeon. Nevertheless, the patient who is about to undergo a total knee replacement has mixed feelings of anxiety and relief. A photograph album, similar to the one described for the total hip replacement, will be a valuable aid in preoperative instruction. An understanding of the postoperative routines will help ensure patient cooperation following surgery. Unless every surgeon who does total knee replacements in a particular hospital uses continuous passive motion postoperatively, preoperative teaching of the protocol should be provided under separate cover.

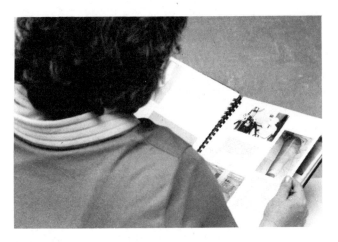

A visit from the physical therapist provides an opportunity to teach the patient postoperative exercises and identify other problems the patient may have in reaching rehabilitation goals. The patient is able to express fears about exercising and to receive reassurance. Thus the program itself can begin on a positive note, when that point in time is reached.

During the preoperative visit, the physical therapist can measure the amount of flexion and extension in the knee and compare it with that of the other knee. The patient can

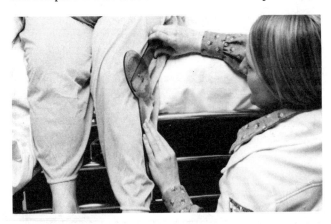

also be questioned about the amount of pain present in the knee and how much ambulation increases that pain. How well the patient walks is also evaluated. The condition of other joints in the body is discussed in order for the therapist to evaluate what effect their functioning may have on the total rehabilitation of the patient. The exercise program is described in detail, and the patient is shown how to use equipment to perform some of these exercises.

The physical therapy department may have its own data base for use with total knee replacement patients. An example of such a data base is on p. 248.

The anesthesiologist should also make a preoperative visit to explain the type of anesthesia that will be administered.

As a general rule, and in contrast to total hip patients, total knee replacement patients are not easily compared to one other. If the patient comments on the "luck," good or bad, that friends may have had with total knees, he is probably seeking reassurance that he is doing the right thing and that his "luck" will be good. The nurse should take the time to explain that there are many kinds of prostheses and some require more extensive surgery than others. A patient should also know that individuals who come to the hospital for this operation are in different stages of mobility. Thus, the amount of pain and progress in total knee replacement patients varies a great deal.

Physical Preparation

Preparation of the patient involves a complete physical examination, bloodtyping, and crossmatching. Some surgeons require their patients to have preoperative tests done on an outpatient basis to shorten the hospitalization. A great number of these patients take large amounts of aspirin. Appropriate laboratory studies should be done to determine bleeding tendencies. The extent of blood loss during surgery may mean the patient will need replacement.

The "family doctor" or an internist may need to be consulted if the patient is on antihypertensives or corticosteroids, because adjustments in the administration of these medications will have to be made, at least temporarily.

Oral antibiotics may be started. These will be discontinued from midnight on the day of surgery until the patient is able to tolerate them after surgery.

Preparation of the knee should include three 10-minute germicidal scrubs. Two scrubs are done at established intervals depending on the time of admission. After the leg is shaved and the patient has showered, the third scrub is done.

Postoperative Care

The nursing management standards appearing on pages 246–247 may serve as guidelines for formulating postoperative nursing-care plans for total knee replacement patients. Priorities in postoperative assessment are presented in the chart on pages 250–251.

Since the total knee replacement patient often is elderly and has other medical problems, the orthopedic nurse must maintain up-to-date assessment skills in order to identify developing complications. When an orthopedic patient care unit has a system for monitoring caridac status, patients who would otherwise need to recover in an intensive care setting are able to remain on the orthopedic ward. There is a definite psychological advantage in this.

Immobilization of the Knee

Patients who have total knee replacements may return from surgery with the knee immobilized in a position of exten-

NURSING MANAGEMENT STANDARDS: TOTAL KNEE REPLACEMENT

Potential Problems	Expected Outcomes	Deadlines	Preventive Nursing Management
PRE-OP			
1. Standard.*	1. Standard.		1. a. Standard. b. Provide with Total Knee Replacement teaching book. c. Provide opportunity for patient to verbalize questions to assess levels of understanding. d. Inform physical therapy of patient's admission. Physical therapy will discuss exercise program.
POST-OP			
1. Standard.†	1. Standard.	Discharge	1. Standard.
2. Wound infection due to invasion by pathologic organisms.	2. Clean healing wound. Temp. no higher than 99°F.	Discharge	2. a. Inspect dressing or wound daily (10 A.M.). b. Check temperature q 4 hr for 48 hr (10−2−6−*etc.*) and bid (10−6) thereafter.
3. Shock due to excessive bleeding.	3. No bleeding. Blood pressure stable for patient within 10 mm of admission BP.	24 hr	3. a. Apply ice to knee 48 hr continuously. b. Check wound drainage system q 4 hr (10−2−6−10−2−6). Empty p.r.n. If 400 ml or more in 4 hr, notify physician. c. Check blood pressure q 4 hr for 48 hr (10−2−6−10−2−6), then bid (10−6).
4. Impaired circulation or nerve damage due to surgery or casting.	4. Color, motion, temperature, sensation (CMTS) normal.	48 hr	4. a. Check CMTS of operative leg q 1 hr for 6 hr, then q 4 hr for 48 hr (10−2−6−*etc.*), then daily. b. Check pedal pulse q 4 hr for 48 hr (10−2−6−*etc.*).
5. Thrombophlebitis or emboli due to venous stasis.	5. No calf pain (document if pain occurs). Negative Homans' sign if calf pain present. Temp. below 99°F.	Discharge	5. a. Check CMTS of operative leg q 1 hr for 6 hr, then q 4 hr for 48 hr (10−2−6−*etc.*), then daily. b. Apply anti-embolism hose continuously. c. Report tenderness of calf or groin to M.D. If tenderness present, check Homans' sign q shift. d. Stir up q 4 hr for 48 hr (10−2−6−*etc.*). e. Check temperature bid (10−6).
6. Pulmonary emboli due to clot release in bloodstream.	6. No chest pain (document if pain occurs). Respiratory rate within +10 and −5 of pre-op rate.	Discharge	6. a. Check BP−P−R q 4 hr for 48 hr (10−2−6−*etc.*), then bid (10−6). b. Stir-up q 4 hr for 48 hr (10−2−6−*etc.*). c. Up in chair 10−2−6 and assist with ambulation after physical therapy is ordered.

NURSING MANAGEMENT STANDARDS: TOTAL KNEE REPLACEMENT *(continued)*

Potential Problems	Expected Outcomes	Deadlines	Preventive Nursing Management
7. Abdominal distention due to slowed peristalsis.	7. Soft and nontympanic abdomen.	48 hr	7. a. Check for abdominal distension q 4 hr (10–2–6–*etc.*). b. Increase diet from clear liquid to general as tolerated. c. Insert rectal tube or give suppository as needed.
8. Fat emboli due to fat globules released in the bloodstream.	8. No confusion that cannot be related to medication or age (assumed absent unless documented).	3 days	8. a. If patient becomes confused, evaluate cause, and if thought to be due to fat emboli, notify M.D.
9. Difficulty with home management due to lack of understanding of home care.	9. Verbalization of understanding of home care.	Discharge	9. a. Reinforce home exercise program of physical-therapy department. b. Have patient verbalize understanding of home program.

* Hospital nursing management standard—all pre-ops.
† Hospital nursing management standard—all post-ops.

sion. Two of the most common methods of immobilization are the commercial knee immobilizer, of which there are as many different styles as there are orthopedic supply companies who manufacture them, and the cylinder cast.

The problems that patients encounter with knee immobilizers are identified on page 237.

If a cast has been applied, general cast care and observations are carried out as discussed in Chapter 2. However, some specific problems do arise for patients wearing a cast following a total knee replacement. As might be expected, pain and pressure occur in the operative area. To offset this discomfort, the cast is usually split in the recovery room.

Thereafter it may be spread as necessary. Added discomfort may be caused by the ends of the cast. The Achilles tendon rests against the cast edge resulting in frequent complaints about a "sore heel." The top of the posterior side of the cast may also be somewhat irritating. One method of relieving pressure on the Achilles tendon is to make several longitudinal cuts with a cast saw and then bend the strips out in a "fishtail" effect.

Vital Signs

Very frequently, the patient returns from the recovery room chilly and pale, with a low blood pressure and rapid pulse. As

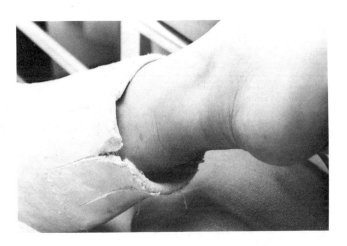

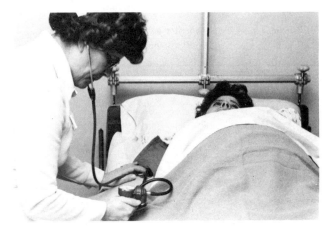

DATA BASE FOR PHYSICAL THERAPY*
TOTAL KNEE PREOP EVALUATION ((RIGHT) /LEFT)

Name_ *Smith, Jane* _____ Patient # _*42506-9*_____ Date_*6-15-86*_____
Physician__*Dr. Jones*_____ Diagnosis__*Right knee osteoarthritis, right TKR 6-16-86*

Patient's understanding of why physical therapy was ordered, his/her receptivity to P.T., and response to preop instruction.
   Pt. responded favorably to preop P.T. instructions. Receptive to the exercise & gait training which will take place BID post-op
   in P.T. Dept.

Rom	*Involved*	*Uninvolved*	**Anthropometric**	*Involved*	*Uninvolved*
JOINT					
Knee-sitting	*20°–90°*	*0°–115°*	15 cm. above	*48½ cm.*	*49 cm.*
Knee-supine	*5°–85°*	*0°–110°*	5 cm. above	*43*	*44*
Quad lag	*15°*	*0°*	Joint line	*41½*	*43½*
Thomas Position	*0°*	*0°–10°*	5 cm. below	*37*	*39*

Strength	*Involved*	*Uninvolved*
Quadriceps	*Fair⁺* → $Fair^+$	*Good*
Hamstrings	*Good⁻* → $Good^-$	*Good⁺* → $Good^+$

Independent/Note degree of pain/Assistive devices/Distance ambulating/Limp

GAIT
   Pt. uses a single point cane for indep. gait. Moderate c/o pain p̄ ambulating distances of 1 block or
   more. Antalgic limp c̄ poor knee extension during stance, poor flexion in swing phase.

Determine activities for which the patient is dependent upon others; e.g., feeding, dressing, bathing, stairs, transportation

ACTIVITIES OF DAILY LIVING AND HOME STATUS
   Pt. is widowed & lives with her son in a 1 story home which has 2 outside steps without a rail.
   Presently is independent in all ADL's. Depends on son for transportation.

MEDICAL CONDITIONS—HEALTH STATUS
   Good health status, no past surgeries.
   Obese

Performance, length of stay, back to work, others

PATIENT'S EXPECTATIONS
   Pt. expects a 10-day hospital stay. She is retired but wishes to return to light housekeeping
   tasks and independent living.

Remarks

   Pt. is pleasant and cooperative.
   Resistive right knee movements elicited pain.

Medicare equipment form signed_✔_____

                                    W. Erickson _____P.T.

* Courtesy Physical Therapy Department, Bellin Memorial Hospital, Green Bay, Wisconsin.

is true with total hip replacement, this is due to preoperative medication, spinal anesthesia and blood loss.

Vital signs must be checked and recorded every 30 minutes until they are stable. Then they need only be monitored every 4 hours for 24 hours.

For about 3 days after surgery, a moderate elevation in body temperature is not too unusual. If such an elevation persists, it should be called to the attention of the surgeon.

Positioning

The operated leg should always be elevated high on pillows for about 48 hours to reduce swelling. The foot of the bed may be elevated but should be lowered if the patient complains of discomfort in the lower back. A folded bath blanket

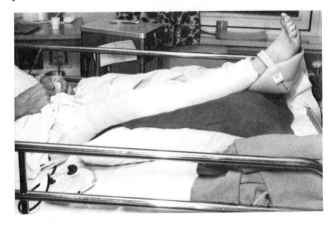

under the calf portion of the cast or immobilizer should keep the heel off the bed, but heel protectors are an added precaution against circulatory impairment and skin breakdown. A "dark" heel develops rapidly from prolonged pressure. An elastic stocking on the uninvolved leg is routine.

Special Skin Care

Because the total knee patient spends so much time in the supine position, back care should be given every 3 to 4 hours while he is awake. For the same reason, the elbows need close inspection at least every shift. Whenever possible, the patient should be encouraged to rub his elbows with lotion when they feel irritated. This routine may need to be written as a nursing order if redness and irritation are a persistent problem. When the patient is resting on his elbows more than is good for his skin, the ulnar nerve is in danger of compression. The nurse needs to question this type of patient for complaints of numbness, tingling, or pain in the ring and little fingers.

Once the patient is out of his cast or immobilizer, elastic hose may be ordered for the operated leg. These stockings need to be removed every shift and the leg(s) inspected, cleansed as necessary, and lotion or a powder applied gently. The tops of elastic hose must not be allowed to roll down and create a constricting effect. This will impair circulation and predispose the patient to thrombophlebitis.

Neurovascular Status

Every 3 or 4 hours for the entire time the leg is in a cast or immobilizer, the toes should be checked for color, motion,

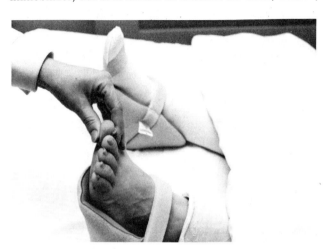

temperature, and sensation, and a pedal pulse should be taken.

Bleeding

Closed wound suction is routine for about 48 hours. Bloody drainage from the knee may total up to 500 ml for the first 24 hours. Ice bags, propped against the sides of the knee, are refilled as needed for 48 hours.

Fluid Therapy and Medication

Parenteral fluids are ordered for 2 or 3 days, chiefly as a route for antibiotics. These, along with the oral antibiotic, constitute a heavy dosage, and the patient must be observed for allergic response.

Voiding

In the first 24 to 48 hours, total knee patients may have diuresis as a result of intravenous fluids administered during surgery to maintain blood volume. Outputs up to 2000 ml in 8 hours are not unusual. Sodium depletion may occur, resulting in mental confusion. Such signs should be reported to the surgeon.

If the patient has difficulty in voiding because of the anesthetic or position, urine output should be checked and measured for as long as the difficulty lasts.

Nausea and Vomiting

Nausea and vomiting may occur and are usually self-limiting.

Respiratory Status

"Stirring up" the patient, by encouraging coughing, deep breathing, and moving the unaffected extremities, is a priority while the patient is flat in bed with intravenous fluid running into one arm. An incentive spirometer is effective in

TOTAL KNEE REPLACEMENT PATIENT: PRIORITIES IN POSTOPERATIVE ASSESSMENT

Significant Admission Data: B. R. is 69 years old, 5'9" tall, and weighs 193 lb. He enters the hospital to have a left total knee replacement for osteoarthritis. He has an "old" back injury and occasionally sees a chiropractor for treatment. Complains of some shortness of breath on exertion but denies any history of heart problems. (His admission ECG will show no significant findings.) He has an admission blood pressure of 154/88. He is pleasant and cooperative.

Operative Day: 10:00 P.M. Assessment Data

1. Vital signs: B.P. 118/76, T. 98, P. 74, R. 20

2. Total closed wound suction drainage since noon 510 ml.

3. Neurovascular status of toes satisfactory. Toes slightly cool.

4. Taking water and clear liquids only. 420 ml since surgery. Has had several episodes of nausea.

5. Receiving IV fluids with antibiotics. Total for shift: 950 ml.

Re-Assessment and Intervention

1. Check at 2:00 A.M. as scheduled. Flow sheet indicates range of BP to be 118/76–130/84. Lowest readings follow IM analgesics.

2. Notify surgeon. This is probably no cause for alarm, considering vital signs and patient size. Also operative report indicates procedure took almost 3 hours, but surgeon may want Hgb and Hct sooner than previously ordered, so notify now.

3. Check if needs more toe "cover." Encourage foot movement.

4. Check events preceding nausea. Does it follow pain medication? Taking fluids?

5. IV infusing at proper rate. About 1000 ml q 8 hr as ordered.

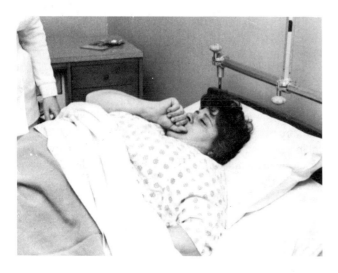

promoting lung expansion and can be used during the entire hospital stay.

Pain

The patient who has undergone a total knee replacement seems to have more pain, for a longer period, than does the patient with a total hip replacement. Once the exercise pro-

gram is started, a pain medication should be given for as many days as is necessary before activity in physical therapy is begun. Added pain may be experienced in the other knee if it is arthritic. In fact, it may be more painful than the tissue around the operated joint. Guidelines for assessing and managing pain in the patient with a total knee replacement are provided on page 256.

Nutrition

The patient with a total knee replacement is usually able to have a normal diet as tolerated, with fluids given frequently. Adequate nutrition is essential not only in maintaining physical health but also in maintaining mental acuity. The dietitian should visit the patient periodically.

Sometimes a patient will suffer from digestive upsets as a result of the large doses of oral antibiotics. This must be called to the attention of the surgeon.

Elimination

Maintaining adequate fluid intake and good nutrition reduces the problems of constipation. But many elderly patients will suffer from this condition to some degree. A stool softener given once or twice daily will be helpful in establishing a fairly normal elimination pattern.

TOTAL KNEE REPLACEMENT PATIENT *(continued)*

6. Has voided twice. 120 and 160 ml. Not concentrated. Does not appear distended and does not complain of distress.

6. Abdomen must be checked again and more often during night. Patient is a heavy man, and distention may be difficult to diagnose. Has had 1370 ml total intake. Does he have retention with overflow? Report indicates urine not concentrated.

7. Skin dry and color good, "cheeks pink."

8. Came back from OR with oxygen at 6 1/m because he had been slightly cyanotic. Has refused to use it since 4:00 P.M.

9. Denies chest pain or shortness of breath at present. Is somewhat restless but alert and oriented. Lungs clear on auscultation.

7,8,9. Appearance of patient at present indicates no need for oxygen, except that patient is slightly restless. Instruct him to report respiratory distress or chest pain. Admission note mentions back problem. Is this making him restless?

10. Last IM analgesic given at 9:00 P.M.

10. Evaluate effectiveness of analgesic at this point. Patient is a big man and has had medication q 3 hr since surgery. Important to be specific about location of pain, again because of back problem. Total knee patients commonly have positional back pain; and when asked if they have pain, their response may be affected by how the back is feeling. Give back care q 2 hr during night if necessary.

11. Cylinder cast. Foot of bed is elevated. Leg is elevated on two pillows. Cast was split in surgery. Is complaining of some tightness in knee.

11. Check leg elevation to be certain pillows are not "sinking" into each other. May need to elevate foot of bed higher and reposition pillows. Pinpoint tightness. Is it normal postoperative edema or a pressure point? May need to spread cast if tightness persists or neurovascular status of toes changes significantly.

Continuous Passive Motion

Description. Continuous passive motion is supplied by an electrically controlled unit that is placed on the patient's

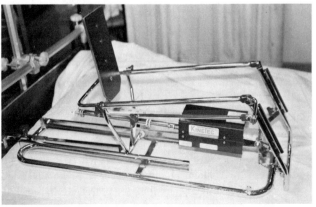

KineTec continuous passive motion unit. (Courtesy Richards Manufacturing Co., Memphis, Tenn.)

bed. The unit consists of an adjustable frame, supportive padding, and the power supply. The frame is constructed to fit the lower extremity and move it from 110 degrees of flexion to 0 degrees of extension, or any combination in between, at a rate that can also be regulated.

The usual procedure is to begin continuous passive motion (CPM) with flexion set at 40 to 50 degrees and extension at 0 to 5 degrees. The flexion is increased 10 degrees daily, according to patient tolerance, and usually does not exceed 90 degrees. However, the extent of flexion depends on the surgeon's preference and the patient's progress. The rate of motion is generally very slow—ten to fifteen minutes per flexion-extension maneuver.

Purpose. Although the continuous passive motion device was originally developed to aid in healing joint cartilage, it is currently being used in the postoperative treatment of total knee replacement patients to:

1. Prevent adhesions
2. Restore range of motion
3. Prevent phlebitis
4. Reduce pain, swelling, and inflammation

Many surgeons place the operated leg in the device immediately after surgery, whereas others begin the use of continuous passive motion 2 or 3 days postoperatively or when the wound drainage system has been removed. The machine is used continuously or intermittently for hours at a time, for a period of days that depends on patient progress and tolerance.

General Nursing Implications of Use. The orthopedic nurse must know:

1. The protocols of the surgeons who use the device
2. How to activate and adjust the controls on the unit
3. How to adjust the frame and fit the patient's extremity
4. How to recognize and deal with problems

Because continuous passive motion is not used by all surgeons, the nurse is well advised not to place two total knee replacement patients in the same room unless their postoperative regimes are similar.

Nursing Care of the Total Knee Replacement Patient in a Continuous Passive Motion Device

Preoperative Psychological Preparation. The patient must be psychologically prepared for the use of the continuous passive motion unit. The nurse should explain what the machine is supposed to accomplish, how it should fit, and how it will work.

An immediate concern of many patients is the inability to comfortably maintain a supine position. The question often asked is: How am I going to sleep on my back? The nurse should routinely reassure every patient who is to be placed in a continuous passive motion device that he will be turned and given back care as often as required, and that after a couple of days he will be out of bed often enough to alleviate the discomfort caused by lying in one position.

Preoperative Physical Preparation. Preoperatively the device must be adjusted to fit the patient's extremity. Since several such machines are available, only general directions can be given here.

The pads should be positioned and applied to support the leg during measurement. They can be adjusted once the leg is situated. The thigh length should be measured first and is best measured if the frame is at 90 degrees of knee flexion, with the thigh part perpendicular to the bed. The tibial length is adjusted by moving the footpiece. The pads are

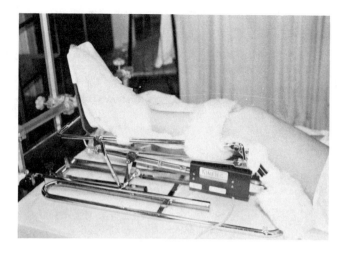

then adjusted so that the leg is comfortable and well supported.

The patient's foot is generally most comfortable if the footpiece is positioned in slight plantar flexion. The continuous passive motion device should be placed on the bed so that the extremity will be in slight abduction. This is a more natural and comfortable position.

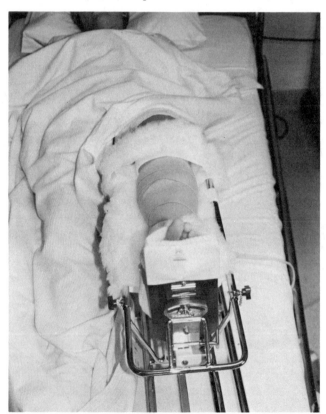

The nurse may want to try placing a fracture pan at this point, so that the patient has an idea of where it should be and knows how it should feel when it is properly placed.

Several points must be emphasized to the patient once he and the machine have been "tried" together. These are:

1. The knee must remain at the angle of the machine. The patient needs to know that he can move up or down and that the nursing staff can move the machine to maintain this position.
2. The leg should not turn sideways (frogleg) in the device, since this may cause pressure on the peroneal nerve. Sometimes patients get themselves in this position from shifting the buttocks in search of comfort.
3. Continuous passive motion should not restrict the mobility of the rest of the body.

Immediate Postoperative Observations. If the continuous passive motion device is applied in surgery, the nurse should make an initial assessment of the situation immediately after the patient returns to the room. The rate and amount of flexion and extension should be documented. The position of the leg in the machine and the position of the machine and of the patient in the bed should be checked and, if necessary, changed according to the previous instructions. The tubes from the wound drainage system must be checked to be certain they are not kinked or caught in any part of the device.

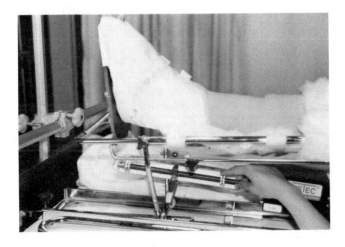

Routine Assessment. At regular intervals (every 4 hours is a proper initial order) and when the patient offers a complaint of discomfort, the nurse should assess the relationship of the machine to the leg and the relationship of the patient to both.

Because improper alignment of the patient can cause problems between the leg and the passive motion device, assessment begins with observation of the patient as a whole. Is he lying perpendicular to the ends of the bed with the involved leg slightly abducted? Is he resting with his weight equally distributed on both buttocks?

Once the patient's overall alignment has been checked and corrected, the position of the leg can be evaluated. Begin with a hip to knee-joint inspection. Is the proximal thigh sufficiently padded if it rests on the end of the frame?

Is the thigh pad taut enough to provide support? The knee joint should be well padded without undue pressure on the popliteal space and positioned at the angle of the frame. The lower leg must also be properly padded and supported. Continuous passive motion devices may be equipped with padded straps to secure the lower leg in position, and these should always be checked to be certain they are not too tight. The foot must be comfortable and resting against the footpiece. Sheet wadding is effective for securing a foot that wants to slide sideways or as a buffer when the patient complains that the pad is too warm. The purpose of a foot pad is to secure the foot in position and provide comfort. Therefore it should be adjusted accordingly. All disposable pads with continuous passive motion machines can be cut and used where they are needed.

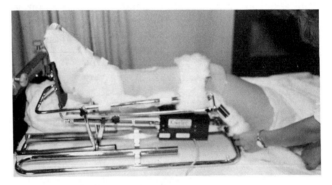

Once every 8 hours the nurse should observe the leg as it moves through a flexion-extension-flexion cycle.

Other Potential Problems. The nurse must be aware of the surgeon's expectations about the management of the continuous passive motion device. May the patient have the machine turned off for short intervals if it "bothers" him? Who will increase the flexion, and when?

Each time the head of the bed is elevated, the patient will slide into or against the machine. Therefore, when the head of the bed is being lowered, the patient should be instructed to grasp the trapeze, flex the uninvolved leg and plant the foot flat on the bed, and move toward the head end until the knee is at the correct position in the device.

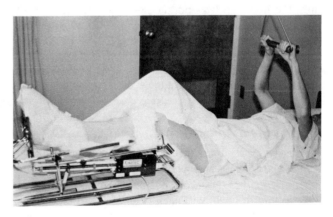

Since the action of the machine may make placement of a tray table difficult, the machine should be turned off at mealtimes.

Most nursing routines, such as giving skin care and encouraging deep breathing and coughing, are no more difficult for this type of patient than for the total knee replacement patient in a long leg cast or immobilizer.

Changing Linen. The bottom bed linen is changed in the following manner. Raise the siderail on the involved side and with the help of another nurse on *that* side, assist the patient in turning toward the machine. The linen can be rolled almost completely under the patient except for the operated leg. The patient is turned back onto his back. Then assist him in turning the top half of his body so that the linen can be pulled through. The continuous passive motion device only has to be slightly lifted or tipped from side to side and the remainder of the linen can be worked underneath.

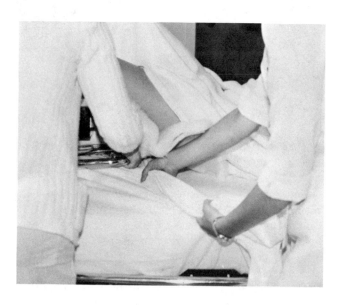

When the Patient Gets Out of Bed. Most total knee replacement patients are out of bed in 48 hours. The machine should be turned off when the leg is in extension. One nurse lifts the operated leg and another nurse can remove the machine from the bed. Depending on the size of the patient, it may be just as easy to move the leg off the machine and the whole patient over to one side of the bed. The nurse must remember that continuous passive motion does not replace foot exercise, moving extremities with deep breathing and coughing, or physical therapy.

Exercise and Ambulation

Exercises for the total knee replacement patient can begin as early as the first postoperative day. However, many surgeons agree that the second postoperative day is an appropriate time to begin with quadriceps setting, straight leg raising, and flexion-extension exercises. By this time,

bleeding as reported in the drainage device has usually ceased and the suction tubes have been removed. The patient is able to move about in bed with the aid of the trapeze. Initial dressings, casts, or immobilizers may be removed for wound inspection. A light dressing may be applied and secured with tape or an elastic bandage. A fishnet type of tubular gauze is useful for the patient who has sensitive skin, or who may require dressing changes.

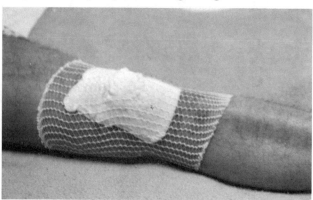

The physical therapy program for the total knee patient is very individual in terms of tolerance and progression. Therefore, while all of the exercises are encouraged and their importance is stressed, patients progress through their rehabilitation programs at different rates.

On the first visit to the physical therapy department the patient will learn how to transfer into a chair. The operated leg will require support during any transfer until the patient has sufficient quadriceps power to stand on the leg and lift it in and out of bed. Twisting of the knee should be avoided. The patient will be assisted to a standing position between parallel bars and will begin to ambulate as tolerated. A knee immobilizer is recommended for walking until the patient can do a straight leg raise. (The patient who has difficulty keeping his leg straight may also require an immobilizer during the night to prevent him from sleeping with the knee in flexion.)

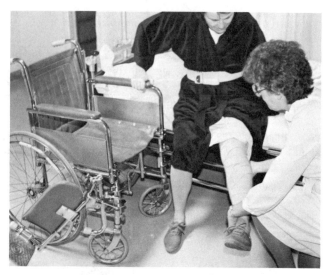

Total knee replacement patients go to the physical therapy department twice a day. Hospital exercise programs for these patients are largely based on the same exercise programs they will be expected to follow at home. By simplifying instructions, the therapist saves time and helps reduce the length of hospitalization. A logical progression of exercises follows.

1. *Quadriceps Setting (Backlying)* This exercise is extremely difficult for the average total knee patient because of contractures and the trauma of the surgical procedure. Therefore, it is usually not possible for the patient to push his knee down into the bed to obtain the desired contraction in the quadriceps muscle. An alternative to this method is to place a rolled towel under the knee or heel before encouraging the patient to push his knee down. This measure not only modifies the exercise but provides a feeling of "pushing" that may be encouraging to the patient. Many total knee patients work hard and long to get a "good" quadriceps contraction and need constant moral support.

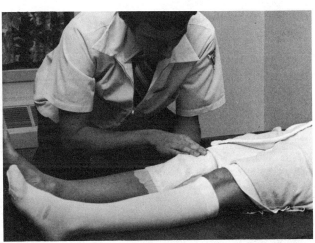

2. *Sling-Assisted Straight Leg Raise* A sling is placed under the mid- to distal calf area of the leg. The spring is pulled down and a clip is attached to it. The patient then lifts his leg up holding the knee straight

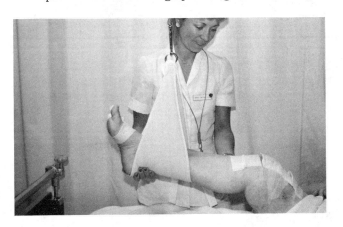

and tightening the quadriceps as much as possible. Toes should be pointed straight up (not rolled out to side).

3. *Sling-Assisted Knee Flexion* A sling is placed under the mid- to distal calf of the leg and a clip and spring are attached. The patient then pulls the heel toward the buttocks, bending the knee to tolerance. The patient then straightens his leg slowly and steadily to touch the entire posterior portion of the leg to the bed. Repeat.

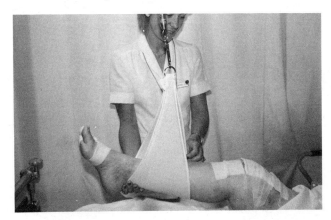

"Slings and springs" exercises can be done in the patient's room once the physical therapist informs the nurse that the patient has learned them. These exercises may be discontinued in the department in favor of more active range of motion and strengthening exercises.

4. *Independent Straight Leg Raise* Without using a sling and spring, the patient bends the noninvolved leg with his foot resting flat on bed. He then lifts the involved leg, keeping the knee straight, and lowers it slowly and steadily. Most patients require assistance in doing this exercise for several days.

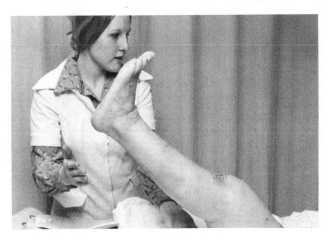

5. *Supine Knee Flexion* The patient lies on his back and flexes the operated knee as far as he can by sliding the heel up a powderboard toward his buttock.

GUIDELINES FOR ASSESSING AND MANAGING PAIN IN THE PATIENT WITH A TOTAL KNEE REPLACEMENT*

A. Expected Pain

1. Severe to moderate 24–48 hr post-op. May be associated with pressure.

2. Moderate pain after each PT exercise session.

3. Amount and type of pain post-op after 48 hr varies depending on extent of surgery, condition of extremity, and patient in general.

Nursing Interventions

1. a. Offer IM analgesics on schedule.
   b. Neurovascular checks toes q 4 hr.†
   c. Ice to knee.
   d. Elevate leg "toes higher than nose."

2. a. Offer pain medication *before* PT (30 min).
   b. Encourage elevation of leg.
   c. Encourage to continue active exercise as this will eventually help decrease pain.

3. a. Check any dressings or elastic hose at regular intervals. Must not be too tight. Stockings must not be allowed to roll like garters.
   b. Analgesics p.r.n.
   c. Keep knee in extension when not exercising. In immobilizer at night.

B. Signs of Complications

1. In early post-op period (24–48 hr) pain unrelieved after medication. May be associated with pressure.

2. Anytime in post-op period: pressure pain, "tightness" in knee joint. Patient may have more difficulty in flexing knee (if the knee is no longer in rigid dressing).

3. Pain extending below posterior knee joint into calf.

Nursing Interventions

1. a. Increase NV checks.
   b. Increase elevation.
   c. Check if wound suction device is functioning.
   d. Notify M.D. if *a* and *b* offer no relief.
   e. Split and spread cast about 1 inch if NV status of toes becomes unsatisfactory, or loosen immobilizer.

2. a. Suspect hematoma.
   b. Check knee for swelling, ecchymosis, incisional drainage.
   c. Call to M.D.'s attention.

3. a. Suspect thrombophlebitis.
   b. Check Homans' sign.
   c. Inspect calf for redness, tenderness.
   d. If *b* and *c* are positive (or just *b*), notify M.D. immediately; otherwise, report on rounds.

* These are very general guidelines, and in all cases the total patient situation must be considered.

† If unsatisfactory, elevate leg higher—may decrease feeling of pressure.

6. *Sitting Active Knee Extension/Flexion* The therapist helps the patient to a sitting position on the table and places a towel roll under the involved knee. The patient is encouraged to lift his lower leg until it is straight and then lower it again.

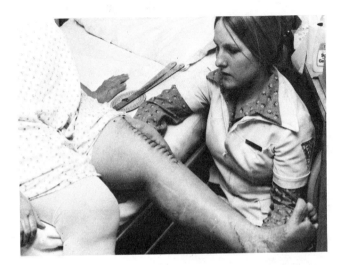

7. *Terminal Extension* With the patient supine on the table, one or two rolled towels or a small pillow is placed under the knee to support it in 30 to 40 degrees of flexion. The patient is directed to lift his foot off the table and straighten the lower leg. The total knee patient often finds it difficult to regain terminal extension because of contractures or weakness of the medialis muscle.

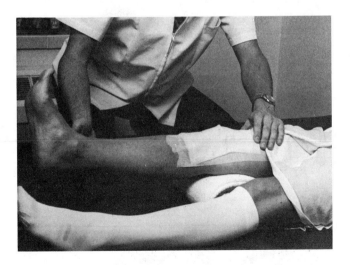

8. *Anti-Gravity Abduction (Leg Raise-Sidelying)* The patient is instructed to lie on his unaffected side and flex hip and knee slightly for balance. Next, he is asked to raise the affected leg straight up toward the ceiling, keeping the knee straight. He should try to hold this position for a count of five and lower his leg slowly.

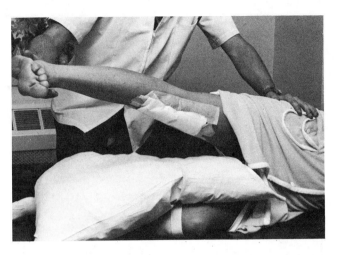

9. *Prone Flexion* On his abdomen, the patient is asked to flex his operated knee as far as possible. When incisional pain makes this position uncomfortable, a rolled towel may be placed under the thigh to keep pressure off the incision.

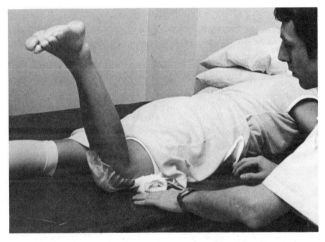

In ambulating, the patient progresses from parallel bars to a walker to two canes, to one cane or quad canes, according to his individual readiness. Patients are also taught how to go up and down stairs.

The key to progression of activity is obtaining 90 degrees of flexion.

A preprinted home exercise plan is desirable. An example of appropriate information, with photographs and written instructions appears on pages 258–261.

The physical therapist may do a discharge evaluation of the patient's status, using the admission data base as a comparative study.

Psychological Considerations

Many patients who have had total knee replacements become discouraged because they have a tendency to compare their progress with that of others. This occurs daily when

(text continues on p. 261)

HOME EXERCISE PROGRAM FOR TOTAL KNEE REPLACEMENT PATIENT*

1. *Quad Sets*
   - Lie on your back with your legs out straight.
   - Pull your toes toward your knee.
   - Tighten your thigh muscles by straigtening out your operated knee very hard.
   - If you do this right, the back of your knee should go down towards the table, and your heel should rise.
   - Hold 5 seconds. Relax. Repeat.
   - This exercise can also be done when standing or when sitting with the leg straight.

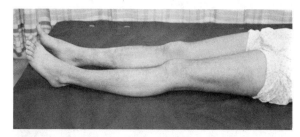

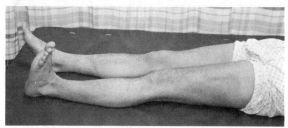

2. *Straight Leg Raise*
   - Lie on your back with your unoperated knee bent and your operated knee straight.
   - Do a quad set, and keep your operated knee straight.

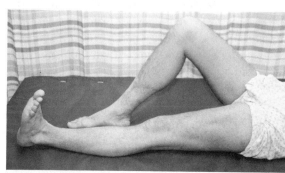

   - Raise your leg, but only as high as your opposite knee.
   - Slowly lower to starting position, keeping knee as straight as possible.
   - Relax. Repeat.

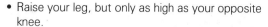

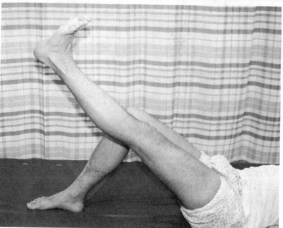

HOME EXERCISE PROGRAM FOR TOTAL KNEE REPLACEMENT PATIENT* *(continued)*

3. *Knee Straightening With Roll*
   - Lie on your back with operated knee bent over pillow or rolled towel.
   - Slowly straighten your knee, keeping your thigh down on the pillow.
   - Hold 5 seconds, then slowly bend knee back to starting position.
   - Relax. Repeat.

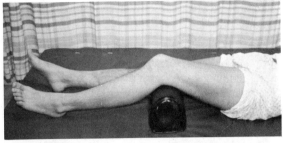

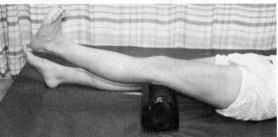

4. *Back-Lying Knee Bending and Straightening*
   - Lie on your back.
   - Bend your operated knee up as far as you can, sliding your heel along the bed.
   - Hold, then slowly straighten operated knee out.
   - Relax. Repeat.

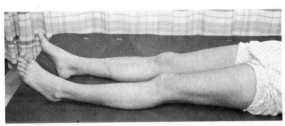

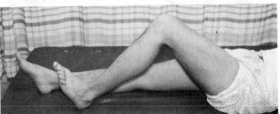

(continues)

HOME EXERCISE PROGRAM FOR TOTAL KNEE REPLACEMENT PATIENT* *(continued)*

5. *Stomach-Lying Knee Bend*
   - Lie on your stomach with your feet over the bottom edge of the bed.
   - Bend your operated knee as far as you can, keeping your hips down on the bed.
   - Hold, then slowly straighten your knee out.
   - Relax. Repeat.

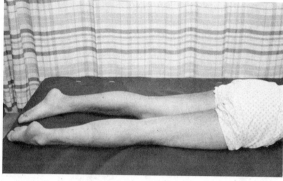

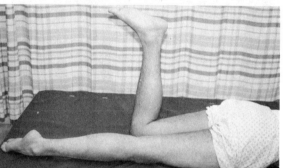

6. *Sitting Knee Bending and Straightening*
   - Sit with your thigh supported on the bed or chair.
   - Put a folded towel under your thigh.
   - Straighten out your operated knee as far as possible.
   - Hold.
   - Then lower your foot, bending your knee as far as you can.
   - Repeat.

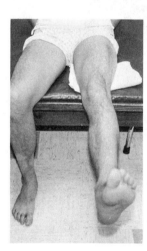

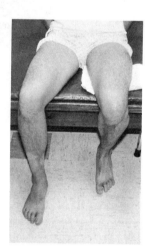

HOME EXERCISE PROGRAM FOR TOTAL KNEE REPLACEMENT PATIENT* *(continued)*

7. *Stairs*
   - To climb up stairs, bring your unoperated leg up first, then the cane and then operated leg.
   - To descend, put the cane down first, then the operated leg, and then the unoperated leg.

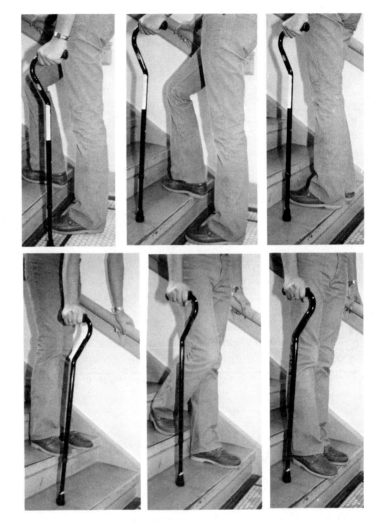

* Courtesy of Physical Therapy Department, Bellin Memorial Hospital, Green Bay, Wisconsin

---

several patients are exercising in the physical therapy department at the same time. Very often, patients start out with comparatively good knee flexion during exercise, and then as the area around the incision becomes tender and painful, they either advance more slowly or reach a plateau for a couple days. When they reach this point, they become disheartened. They may need a great deal of encouragement and support to continue exercise and ambulation.

Swelling and discoloration of the knee with serosanguinous drainage from the incision is quite common because of the early postoperative exercise. Sometimes this is alarming to the patient, and the nurse must make an effort to convince him that it is normal. Apprehension, depression, and anxiety are manifested in many ways. Anorexia is one. Unfortunately, anorexia is also a symptom of good old-fash-ioned homesickness! Elderly ladies often miss their own cooking when they are in the hospital. When the patient apparently understands what is happening, in terms of recovery and rehabilitation, and still does not respond positively to reassurance, try a little extra kindness.

Preventing Complications

Pulmonary embolism, which may be due to impaired circulation caused by the tourniquet during surgery, by immobility, or by both, is a real danger.

Elastic stockings are believed to aid in preventing thrombophlebitis and perhaps lessening the threat of embolism.

The patient should be encouraged to exercise his feet as soon as he can in the postoperative period. He should be instructed to move his feet "back and forth and around" because this will increase his circulation and decrease his discomfort. If an alert patient is made aware that clotting results from inactivity, he will require little supervision in doing foot exercises.

Keeping the patient reasonably active and establishing the cause of complaints of "leg pain" are part of the nursing-care plan as long as the patient is hospitalized. Remember, it is easy to overlook calf pain, swelling, and tenderness in the presence of the same symptoms in the area of the knee joint.

Another possible complication to prevent is infection. Any appreciable elevation in the patient's temperature after the first 72 hours should be reported to the surgeon. Drainage from the wound should be inspected carefully to be certain it is not purulent.

Discharge Planning

The physical therapist will make many suggestions as to how the patient can best carry out a schedule of exercises. For example, plastic bleach bottles with handles make good weights when partially filled with water and tied around the foot. Or, a hot water bottle filled and weighed can be laid across the foot to act as a weight. Clear directions as to what activities the patient can resume or attempt ("Can I scrub the floor?") must be given before discharge.

The same general instructions given total hip replacement patients can also be given to total knee patients (p. 213).

Discussion Questions

1 What nursing assessment is necessary in each of the following?
 a. First postoperative day, a meniscectomy patient states that he cannot "feel" all of his toes.
 b. Three days postoperatively, a patient who has had a ligament repair complains of a "burning" pain.
 c. Seven days postoperatively, a total knee replacement patient does not want to exercise her feet because this makes her leg "ache."

Consider: In all three examples the patient's description of feeling, the time element, the location of symptoms.

2 T. J. is a 75-year-old female, 5'4" tall, who weighs 140 lb. She has severe "arthritis" in her left knee. She enters the hospital to have a left total knee replacement. She states she has "a little rheumatism in all my joints," for which she takes alfalfa tablets. She is slightly hard of hearing and wears glasses and dentures. Her closest relative is a daughter who has brought her to the hospital. Mrs. J. also takes a "water pill," which she has brought to the hospital with her. She is cheerful and softspoken.

 a. What additional assessment is necessary?
 b. Identify potential problems.
 c. Write initial nursing orders.

Consider: What information must be obtained from the daughter? How important is physical assessment of her extremities? What other health problems may be present? What will be the relationship between her orthopedic problem, present health status, and potential problems of immobility? What kind of health teaching and discharge planning can be considered this early?

Bibliography

Andrews JR, Axe MJ: The classification of knee ligament instability. Orthop Clin North Am, p. 69, Jan 1985.

Andrews JR, et al: The anterior cruciate ligament, part II. Orthop Clin North Am, April 1985

Andrish J, Komisarz J: Chrondromalacia of the patella. Orthop Nurs 3(3):26, 1984

Arnoczky SP: Blood supply to the anterior cruciate ligament and supporting structures. Orthop Clin North Am, p. 15, Jan 1985

Bae KK, et al: Unicompartmental knee arthroplasty for single compartment disease: Clinical experience with an average four-year follow-up study. Clin Orthop 176:233, 1983

Bates B: A Guide to Physical Examination 2nd ed. Philadelphia, JB Lippincott, 1979

Bayne O, Cameron HU: Total knee arthroplasty following patellectomy. Clin Orthop 186:112, 1984

Bejui H: Concerning acquired valgus instability after knee replacement. Clin Orthop 162:311, 1982

Bergstrom R, et al: Comparison of open and endoscopic meniscectomy. Clin Orthop 184:133, 1984

Bianchi M: Acute tears of the posterior cruciate ligament: Clinical study and results of operative treatment in 27 cases. Am J Sports Med 11(5):308, 1983

Brewster CE: Rehabilitation for anterior cruciate reconstruction. J Orthop Sports Phys Ther 5(3):121, 1983

Brown R: Implants: Hip and knee arthroplasty. JORRI 2:26, 1982

Brunner NA: Orthopedic Nursing, 4th ed. St. Louis, CV Mosby, 1983

Burnett QM, Fowler PJ: Reconstruction of the anterior cruciate ligament: Historical overview. Orthop Clin North Am, p. 143, 1985

Cameron HU, Hunter GA: Failure in total knee arthroplasty: Mechanisms, revisions, and results. Clin Orthop 170:141, 1982

Chaffee EE, Lytle IM: Basic Physiology and Anatomy, 4th ed. Philadelphia, JB Lippincott, 1980

Chen SC, Ramanathan EB: The treatment of patellar instability by lateral release. J Bone Joint Surg (Br) 66(3):344, 1984

Cloutier JM: Results of total knee arthroplasty with a nonconstrained prosthesis. J Bone Joint Surg (Am) 65(7):906, 1983

Coventry MB: Upper tibial osteotomy. Clin Orthop 182:46, 1984

Crenshaw AH (ed): Campbell's Operative Orthopaedics, 6th ed. St. Louis, CV Mosby, 1980

Crutchley C: Trends in orthopedic surgery. Today's OR Nurs 6(12):22, 1984

Dandy DJ: Arthroscopic surgery. J Bone Joint Surg (BR) 66(5):627, 1984

Dandy DJ: Arthroscopy of the Knee. Philadelphia, Lea & Febiger, 1984

Dandy DJ, O'Carroll PF: The removal of loose bodies from the knee under arthroscopic control. J Bone Joint Surg (Br) 64(4):473, 1982

Dandy DJ, et al: Arthroscopy and the management of the ruptured anterior cruciate ligament. Clin Orthop 167:43, 1982

Daniel D, et al: The diagnosis of meniscus pathology. Clin Orthop 163:218, 1982

DeHaven KE: Arthroscopy in the diagnosis and management of the anterior cruciate ligament deficient knee. Clin Orthop 172:52, 1983

DeLee JC: Acute posterolateral rotatory instability of the knee. Am J Sports Med 11(4):199, 1983

Dorr LD, et al: Factors influencing the intrusion of methyl methacrylate into human tibiae. Clin Orthop 183:147, 1984

Ellison AE, Berg EE: Embryology, anatomy, and function of the anterior cruciate ligament. Orthop Clin North Am p. 3, Jan 1985

Farrell J: Deciphering diagnostic studies: Arthroscopy. Nursing (Horsham) 12(5):73, 1982

Feagin JA, Jr, Lambert KL: Mechanism of injury and pathology of anterior cruciate ligament injuries. Orthop Clin North Am, p.41, Jan 1985

Freeman MA, et al: Cementless fixation of prosthetic components in total arthroplasty of the knee and hip. Clin Orthop 176:88, 1983

Friedman MJ, et al: Preliminary results with abrasive arthroplasty in the osteoarthritic knee. Clin Orthop 182:200, 1984

Funk FJ, Jr: Osteoarthritis of the knee following ligamentous injury. Clin Orthop 172:154, 1983

Gillquist J, Oretorp N: Arthroscopic partial meniscectomy: Technique and long-term results. Clin Orthop 167:29, 1982

Gleason TF, et al: Can carbon fiber implants substitute for collateral ligament? Clin Orthop 191:274, 1984

Glynn MK, Sheehan JM: An analysis of the causes of deep infection after hip and knee arthroplasties. Clin Orthop 178:202, 1983

Gollehon DL, et al: Acute repairs of the anterior cruciate ligament — past and present. Orthop Clin North Am, p. 111, Jan 1985.

Gomes E, Marczyk LR: Anterior cruciate ligament reconstruction with a loop or double thickness of semitendinosus tendon. Am J Sports Med 12(3):199, 1984

Goodfellow JW: Closed meniscectomy. J Bone Joint Surg (Br) 65(4):373, 1983

Grana WA: Arthroscopy to diagnose knee disorders. AORN J 27:823, 1978

Grana WA, et al: Arthroscopic evaluation and treatment of patellar malalignment. Clin Orthop 186:122, 1984

Grana WA, et al: Partial arthroscopic meniscectomy: A preliminary report. Clin Orthop 164:78, 1982

Guhl JF: Arthroscopic treatment of osteochondritis dissecans. Clin Orthop 167:65, 1982

Halperin N, et al: Anterior cruciate ligament insufficiency syndrome. Clin Orthop 179:179, 1983

Hamberg, P, et al: Suture of new and old peripheral meniscus tears. J Bone Joint Surg (Am) 65(2):193, 1983

Helfet A: Disorders of the knee. Philadelphia, JB Lippincott, 1974

Hendler, RC: Arthroscopic meniscal repair: Surgical technique. Clin Orthop 190:163, 1984

Hershman EB, et al: Intrameniscal approach for arthroscopic resection of tears of the posterior one-third of the medial meniscus. Clin Orthop 190:245, 1984

Hilt N, Cogburn S: Manual of Orthopedics. St. Louis, CV Mosby, 1980

Holden DL, Jackson DW: Treatment selection in acute anterior cruciate ligament tears. Orthop Clin North Am, 99, Jan 1985

Hollinshead WH: Textbook of Anatomy, 3rd Ed. Hagerstown, MD. Harper & Row, 1974

Hungerford DS, Kenna RV: Preliminary experience with a total knee prosthesis with porous coating used without cement. Clin Orthop 176:95, 1983

Hunter SC, et al: Disruption of the vastus medialis obliquus with medial knee ligament injuries. Am J Sports Med 11(6):427, 1983

Ikeuchi H: Arthroscopic treatment of the discoid lateral meniscus: Technique and long-term results. Clin Orthop 167:19, 1982

Indelicato PA: Non-operative treatment of complete tears of the medial collateral ligament of the knee. J Bone Joint Surg (Am) 65(3):323, 1983

Insall JN, Dethmers DA: Revision of total knee arthroplasty. Clin Orthop 170:123, 1982

Jackson RW: Arthroscopic surgery. J Bone Joint Surg (Am) 65(3):416, 1983

Jackson RW, Burdick W: Unicompartmental knee arthroplasty. Clin Orthop 190:182, 1984

Jackson RW, Rouse DW: The results of partial arthroscopic meniscectomy in patients over 40 years of age. J Bone Joint Surg (Br) 64(4):481, 1982

Johnson LL: Impact of diagnostic arthroscopy on the clinical judgment of an experienced arthroscopist. Clin Orthop 167:75, 1982

Jokl P, et al: Non-operative treatment of severe injuries to the medial and anterior cruciate ligaments of the knee. J Bone Joint Surg (Am) 66(5):741, 1984

Keene JS, Dyreby RR, Jr: High tibial osteotomy in the treatment of osteoarthritis of the knee: The role of preoperative arthroscopy. J Bone Joint Surg (Am) 65(1):36, 1983

Knee injuries: Multiple ligament tear. Hosp Med 19(10):109, 1983

Komisarz JM: Chondromalacia patella. Orthop Nurs 3(3):24, 1984

Langley LL, et al: Dynamic Anatomy and Physiology, 5th ed. New York, McGraw-Hill, 1980

Larson C, Gould M: Orthopedic Nursing, 9th ed. St. Louis, CV Mosby, 1978

Larson RL: Augmentation of acute rupture of the anterior cruciate ligament. Ortho Clin North Am p. 135, Jan 1985

Laskin RS: Total knee replacement. AORN J 36:577, 1982

Lombardo JA: The athlete's knee: An orderly exam, part 1. Emerg Med 16(14):34, 1984

Losee RE: Diagnosis of chronic injury to the anterior cruciate ligament. Orthop Clin North Am, p. 83, 1985

Lotke PA, et al: Indications for the treatment of deep venous thrombosis following total knee replacement. J Bone Joint Surg (Am) 66(2):202, 1984

Macek C: Bony ingrowth holds new joints in place. JAMA 247(12):1680, 1982

Mallory T: A plastic intermedullary plug for total hip arthroplasty. Clin Orthop Rel Res 155:37, 1981

Mallory TH, et al: Total articular replacement arthroplasty: A clinical review. Clin Orthop, 185:131, 1984

Maquet P: Valgus osteotomy for osteoarthritis of the knee. Clin Orthop 120:143, 1976

Marmor L: Lateral compartment arthroplasty of the knee. Clin Orthop 186:115, 1984

McBride GG et al: Arthroscopic partial medial meniscectomy in the older patient. J Bone Joint Surg (Am) 66(4):547, 1984

Mercier LR: Practical Orthopedics. Chicago, Year Book Medical Publishers, 1980

Metcalf RW: An arthroscopic method for lateral release of subluxating or dislocating patella. Clin Orthop 167:9, 1982

Mooney V: A few lessons in orthopedics. JAMA 247(11):1606, 1982

Morrissy RT, et al: Arthroscopy of the knee in children. Clin Orthop 162:103, 1982

Mott HW: Semitendinosus anatomic reconstruction for cruciate ligament insufficiency. Clin Orthop 172:90, 1983

Mourad L: Nursing Care of Adults with Orthopedic Conditions. New York, John Wiley & Sons, 1980

Nelson CL, et al: One day versus seven days of preventive antibiotic therapy in orthopedic surgery. Clin Orthop 176:258, 1983

Northmore-Ball MD, Dandy DJ: Long-term results of arthroscopic partial meniscectomy. Clin Orthop 167:34, 1982

Northmore-Ball MD, et al: Arthroscopic, open partial, and total meniscectomy: A comparative study. J Bone Joint Surg (Br) 65(4):400, 1983

Norwood LA: Treatment of acute anterolateral rotatory instability. Orthop Clin North Am, p. 127, Jan 1985

Noyes FR, et al: The variable functional disability of the anterior cruciate ligament-deficient knee. Orthop Clin North Am, p. 47, Jan 1985

O'Donaghue DH: Treatment of Injuries to Athletes, 3rd ed. Philadelphia, WB Saunders, 1976

Ogilvie-Harris DJ, Jackson RW: The arthroscopic treatment of chondromalacia patellae. J Bone Joint Surg (Br) 66(5):660, 1984

Oglesby JW, Wilson FC: The evolution of knee arthroplasty. Results with three generations of prostheses. Clin Orthop 188:96, 1984

Parks S: Total joint revision surgery. Today's OR Nurs 4(11):16, 1983

Paterson FW, Trickey EL: Meniscectomy for tears of the meniscus combined with rupture of the anterior cruciate ligament. J Bone Joint Surg (Br), 65(4):388, 1983

Pritsch M, et al: Ankle arthroscopy. Clin Orthop 184:137, 1984

Raney RB, Brashear HR: Shand's Handbook of Orthopaedic Surgery, 9th ed. St. Louis, CV Mosby, 1978

Rockwood CA, Green DP: Fractures. Philadelphia, JB Lippincott, 1975

Rovere, GD, Adair, DM: Anterior cruciate-deficient knees: A review of the literature. Am J Sports Med 11(6):412, 1983

Rushton N, et al: The clinical, arthroscopic and histological findings after replacement of the anterior cruciate ligament with carbon-fibre. J Bone Joint Surg (Br) 65(3):309, 1983

Schank MJ: Evolution of a patient teaching project: Total knee replacement. J Rehab 48:59, 1982

Simpson LA, Barrett JP, Jr: Factors associated with poor results following arthroscopic subcutaneous lateral retinacular release. Clin Orthop 186:165, 1984

Sledge CB, Walker PS: Total knee arthroplasty in rheumatoid arthritis. Clin Orthop 182:127, 1984

Sprague NF III: Arthroscopic debridement for degenerative knee joint disease. Clin Orthop 160:118, 1981

Strans EL, Johns JL: Nursing care of the patient treated with continuous passive motion following total knee arthroplasty. Orthop Nurs, 3(6):27, 1984

Suman RK, et al: Diagnostic arthroscopy of the knee in children. J Bone Joint Surg (Br) 66(4):535, 1984

Terry GC, Hughston JC: Associated joint pathology in the anterior cruciate ligament. Orthop Clin North Am, p. 29, 1985

Thompson MB: An overview of arthroscopy. Today's OR Nurse 4(11):9, 1983

Turek SL: Orthopaedics, 3rd ed. Philadelphia, JB Lippincott, 1977

Vaughan-Lane T, Dandy DJ: The synovial shelf syndrome. J Bone Joint Surg (Br) 64(4):475, 1982

Walker RH, Schurman DJ: Management of infected total knee arthroplasties. Clin Orthop 186:81, 1984

Walsh C: Total knee arthroplasty: Biomechanical and nursing considerations. Orthop Nurs 4(1):29, 1985

Warren RF: Primary repair of the anterior cruciate ligament. Clin Orthop 172:65, 1983

Warren RF, Levy IM: Meniscal lesions associated with anterior cruciate ligament injury. Clin Orthop 172:32, 1983

Whipple TL, et al: Arthroscopic meniscectomy: An interim report at three to four years after operation. Clin Orthop 183:105, 1984

Wredmark T, Lundh R: Arthroscopy under local anaesthesia using controlled pressure-irrigation with prilocaine. J Bone Joint Surg (Br) 64(5):583, 1982

8

Care of the Amputee

The refinement of surgical techniques and the development of sophisticated prostheses have contributed to the efficient nursing care of an amputation stump and rehabilitation of an extremity. But what about the amputee? What contributes to his or her *total* rehabilitation?

Patient education and supportive care are paramount, but cannot even begin until the nurse understands what effect amputation has had upon the *individual* patient's feelings of competency and self-esteem. The value of such insight may be explained by the following example.

A middle-aged woman lost a finger as result of a crushing hand injury and was hospitalized for a week. On an orthopedic ward where bigger and better business was caring for people with joint replacements and multiple fractures, her habit of constantly removing the dressing on her hand to "look at it" was irritating to the staff, besides being contrary to physician's orders. One day, while her dressing was being replaced for the third time, she began to cry over the loss of her finger. Her exasperated nurse, in an attempt to be supportive, reminded her that the injury *was* healing and that she could have lost her entire hand. To this the patient replied, "But it was part of my body!"

This reaction, whether typical or not, emphasizes the point that each person responds differently to the loss of any part, or all, of a limb. Awareness of this fact should be a baseline for planning and delivering comprehensive nursing care for the amputee. Otherwise, such nursing amounts to meeting the needs of a stump instead of an individual.

Psychological Considerations

Response to the psychological trauma of suddenly being "handicapped" depends on the individual patient — his age, his emotional stability, the prognosis concerning any related disease, and the circumstances surrounding the amputation. In the most ideal situation, in which the patient has been thoroughly prepared for the amputation and given extensive psychological support, adjustment will be difficult. In instances in which accident precipitates the amputation, the sudden emotional shock may be overwhelming.

Whatever the circumstances, the patient is faced with an irreplaceable loss, and as in any instance of loss, he can be expected to grieve for that which is gone forever. No matter how useless a diseased extremity may be, it still gives the impression of "wholeness." When the limb is gone, the amputee must live out the remainder of his life with the aid of crutches, a walker, a prosthesis, or perhaps a wheelchair. Compensating for a lost limb is a tremendous adjustment for any individual; for an older person in poor health, it may easily increase feelings of inadequacy or uselessness.

Initially, it may be difficult for an amputee to even look at his stump. He needs time to accept it himself before he can participate in his rehabilitation.

The use of the word "stump" in reference to the residual limb is controversial. As one amputee put it, hearing people talk about his stump made him feel "like part of a tree." On the other hand, many health care personnel who are extensively involved in the rehabilitation of amputees believe that "stump" is a realistic term and avoiding the use of it serves no therapeutic purpose.

At any rate, adjusting to the change in body image and the limitations on mobility and dexterity, with all the social, economic, and psychological ramifications implied, is a monumental task for any person and requires the support of all those involved in the patient's rehabilitation.

For the nurse, having as much knowledge as possible about the anxieties and adjustments confronting the amputee is the best preparation for being equal to the task. One thing is clear: sympathy with the amputee is not therapeutic or realistic. The condition is irrevocable. Nothing can replace the missing limb. The best medicine for the patient is candid discussion of his potential problems and the fears he might have, along with thorough education as to the functional use of a prosthesis.

Psychological comfort is derived from different sources for different people. For the patient plagued by feelings of "Why me?" spiritual assistance may be helpful. For a patient who is apparently close to members of his family, emotional support can be provided by the family, especially if they are kept informed of his reactions and progress. For a

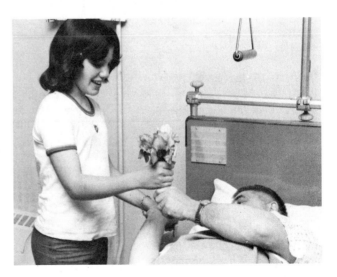

patient who is extremely independent at the outset and wants to get back to normal as soon as possible, it is important that a relationship with the physical therapist and prosthetist be established at an early date. He needs to know that healing of the stump and preparing and making a prosthesis take time. For the patient overwhelmed by feelings of inadequacy and depression, psychotherapy may be required.

In many of these instances the nurse may help by doing what nursing instructors term "the little extras." Taking the patient out of doors in a wheelchair is one such "extra" that may prove satisfying to both nurse and patient.

Whatever the patient's psychological state, most can benefit from contact with a rehabilitated amputee. An orthopedic nurse should have the names of amputees who showed high motivation during their rehabilitation and therefore might be interested in helping others build independence. The result of this sort of effort can be very gratifying, especially if the nurse maintains contact with the patient throughout the period of rehabilitation. For example, it is rewarding to find out that an amputee has accepted the loss of an arm to such a degree that he will ask to meet another amputee with whom he can share a pair of gloves. Recounting such an experience to a new amputee helps him to be more receptive to a nurse's suggestions, because it indicates that the nurse has a genuine interest in the individual.

Actually, once an amputee has become accustomed to the loss of a limb, he may regard the use of a prosthesis as incidental. The problem then becomes how to deal with those who think he is incapacitated. There will always be those people who stare sympathetically at an arm or leg prosthesis, as well as those who avoid looking at it altogether. Furthermore, an amputee may encounter difficulty with activities that were previously routine, such as having a driving license renewed. A well-informed nurse or a rehabilitated amputee can help prepare the patient for many of these situations before they arise. Such measures may help make the adjustment smoother.

Indications for Amputation

Most civilian amputations are the result of peripheral vascular disease. However, circulatory inadequacy is just one of many causes for amputation, as indicated by the following list.

1. *Trauma.* An extremity that has been severely damaged as a result of a crushing injury, explosion, or armed conflict is likely to require amputation.
2. *Thermal Injuries.* Injuries from frostbite or burns may necessitate amputation.
3. *Infection.* An uncontrolled infection, such as gas gangrene or osteomyelitis (bone infection), may ne-

cessitate amputation of a limb.
4. *Gangrene.* Vascular disease due to diabetes or arteriosclerosis may result in an inadequate blood supply to the tissues, causing a gangrenous limb.
5. *Congenital Deformity.* Persons who have congenital deformities of limbs that do not respond to other corrective surgical procedures frequently require amputations.
6. *Tumors.* The possibility of metastases in the case of a malignancy makes amputation of the affected limb desirable.
7. *Pain.* An extremity may be painful because of a circulatory problem. If relief is not obtainable any other way, amputation may be indicated.

Types of Amputation

Generally speaking, there are two types of amputation procedures: the open or "guillotine" method and the closed or "flap" method.

Open Amputations

An open amputation is generally performed in the presence of infection or when infection is probably inevitable due to the circumstances surrounding the amputation. In this procedure the tissues are divided and allowed to retract. The bone is then divided at this point so that all of the open edges are at the same level. The skin flaps are not sutured to enclose the stump end, thereby allowing for open drainage of any purulent exudate. The stump end is then covered with a bulky soft compression dressing.

Since infection is the determining factor in this type of amputation, antibiotic therapy is an integral part of treatment. In addition, it is imperative that aseptic technique be used when dressings are changed or stump care is administered.

Healing is prolonged in a guillotine amputation and occurs as granulation covers the bone end and scar contractures cover the edges of the skin. The resulting stump is conical in shape and satisfactory for prosthetic fitting.

In many instances of open amputation, skin flaps may be prepared and inverted for future closing of the amputation stump, or the stump may be revised to create skin flaps for closure.

Skin Traction. To prevent retraction of the skin and muscles following open amputation, skin traction can be applied. Several methods may be employed. One common type involves the use of three or four strips of adhesive tape which are applied longitudinally above the dressing on the lateral, anterior, and posterior sides of the thigh. They are attached to a spreader made of either wood or wire. A rope runs from the spreader through a pulley over the end of the bed. Five pounds of weight is generally applied to stump traction.

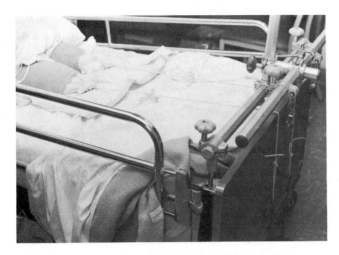

In the second method, strips of vented foam rubber, instead of adhesive, may be secured to the lateral aspects of the thigh by an elastic bandage. Suction provides the means of adherence to the skin.

A third method employs the use of stockinette. The skin above the dressing is coated with an adherent substance. A piece of stockinette, long enough to extend well past the end of the stump, is applied over the adherent. Depending on the condition of the patient's skin, it may be preferable to secure the stockinette with elastic bandages.

Closed Amputation

In a closed or myoplastic amputation, the muscles are divided at least 2 inches distal to the level of intended bone

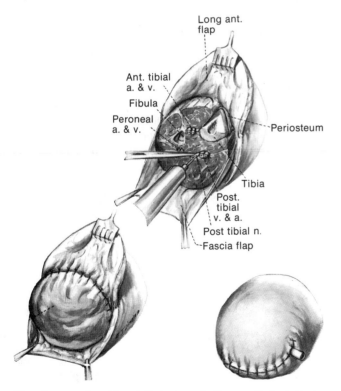

Closed amputation. (Thorek P. Anatomy in Surgery, 2nd ed. Lippincott)

section. They are then sutured under tension to the bone or opposing muscle groups. Drains are placed in the wound, to remain for 48 to 72 hours, and brought out through the suture line. The skin is sutured with just enough stress to cause the ends to meet. Suturing is done so that the incision line is not directly in the area that will bear weight.

In some instances, the stump is covered with a plaster cast so that a temporary prosthesis can be applied immediately in the operating room. In other instances, a compression dressing, consisting of large soft gauze dressings secured in place by an elastic bandage, is used to reduce edema and begin the process of molding the stump for application of a prosthesis at a later date.

Proponents of the myoplastic method believe that muscle function in the stump is improved, because the muscles will contract isometrically as they would normally do during the act of walking. The amputee is thereby provided with sensory feedback that enables him to have better control of his prosthesis, regain a sense of balance, and establish a more acceptable gait.

Sites of Amputation

The function of the part as well as muscle balance must be considered when selecting an amputation site. An adequate blood supply for the stump is also imperative. If a prosthesis is to be worn, the stump must be of optimal length for proper fit and control. Naturally, the surgeon wishes to preserve as much of the limb as he can.

Foot. Loss of balance and possible deformity must be considered when part of a foot or toes are removed. Therefore, as much muscle as is feasible should be left, along with a heavy skin flap to serve as protective covering.

Ankle (Syme). This amputation removes the foot at the ankle, and can be a very satisfactory operation, since it produces a stump that is ideal for weight bearing.

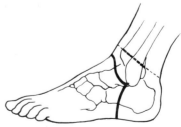

Syme amputation (Turek: Orthopaedics, 3rd ed. Lippincott, 1977)

Below the Knee (BK). An ideal stump for prosthetic fitting should include 5 to 7 inches of the tibia. Inadequate circulation may cause problems in a stump that is much longer and stump fitting can be a problem.

Knee Disarticulation. The patella is either removed, with the quadriceps tendon brought over the end of the femur, or else the patella is fixed to a cut surface between the condyles. the latter procedure is called the Gritti-Stokes amputation.

Above the Knee (AK). Three inches above the knee joint usually provides a good length for control of a prosthesis, although in lower extremity amputation all efforts are made to amputate below the knee to avoid the disabling effects frequently resulting from an above the knee amputation.

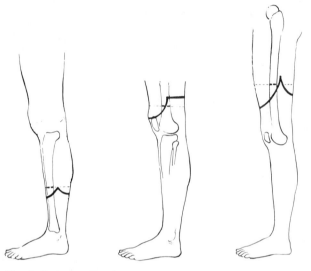

(Turek: Orthopaedics, 3rd ed. Lippincott, 1977)

Hip Disarticulation. Amputation through the hip or pelvis is a rare operation and is used in instances of malignant tumors and extensive injuries or gangrene.

Hemipelvectomy. Removal of the entire extremity and half of the pelvis is a shocking procedure and is done rarely even in the case of a malignancy.

Fingers. When any part or all of a finger is removed, the stump must be designed so it will not interfere with the function of other fingers. Also, a thick flap must cover the end of the stump to protect it from pain due to constant contact with objects and surfaces.

Wrist Disarticulation. This amputation results in a stump that is easily fitted with a prosthesis.

Below the Elbow (BE). About 7 inches from the elbow, or the junction between the middle and lower thirds of the forearm, is the ideal site for this amputation.

Above the Elbow (AE). In this type of amputation, as much length as possible is saved, in order to preserve arm strength.

Elbow Disarticulation. These amputations are infrequently done because the shape of the end of the humerus does not lend itself to good prosthetic fitting.

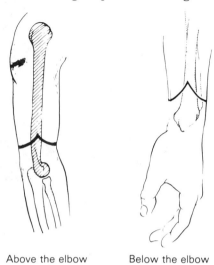

Above the elbow   Below the elbow

(Turek: Orthopaedics, 3rd ed. Lippincott, 1977)

Shoulder Disarticulation. This operation, like hip disarticulation and hemipelvectomy, is rarely done because it is so disabling and traumatic.

Care of the Patient With Amputation of the Lower Extremity

TRAUMATIC AMPUTATION

Since most lower extremity amputations are the result of vascular disorders, there generally is time to prepare the patient psychologically and physically for the impending operation. However, in the instance of traumatic amputation, there is no such opportunity so that the approach to patient care takes a different course.

A motorcycle, snowmobile, or "souped up" automobile is very often part of the scene when traumatic amputation of the lower extremity occurs. As long as high-speed vehicles are part of the American way of life, traumatic amputations, especially among young people, will be part of it also.

The majority of these patients are young males who begin their period of hospitalization bitter, hostile, and often uncooperative. Occasionally, the nurse will encounter a young amputee whose first reaction is almost one of euphoria. This must not be confused with acceptance. Perhaps he has suddenly become the center of attention, with a multitude of visitors and a hovering, sympathetic girl friend. Who knows? This may be an unfamiliar role for him, and he cannot help but enjoy it, at least temporarily. In this environment, he may even convince himself, again temporarily, that he may "never have to work again."

The point is that the behavior of a new amputee is not predictable. Until it is understood, however, the nurse cannot help him to help himself. The young amputee who regains consciousness after an accident and finds he has a limb missing requires time and tolerance to work through his feelings and to make adjustments.

A realistic approach by the nurse is best. How can we help you? Where do we start? These are the concerns that should manifest themselves in all aspects of nursing care. Sympathy serves no useful purpose.

In the hospital, the nurse and therapist can help the patient regain independence by encouraging him to set and attain his own goals in self-care, exercises, and ambulation. In this way he will be able to convince others that his is not totally incapacitated or disabled.

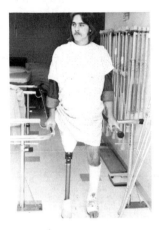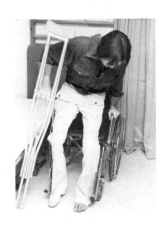

ELECTIVE SURGERY: PSYCHOLOGICAL PREPARATION

Notwithstanding the improvements in techniques in vascular surgery and in early diagnosis and control of diabetes, these diseases still claim the lower extremities of many elderly people. In such instances, amputation becomes the alternative to a painful, useless limb or perhaps death. However, since amputation bears the connotation of being destructive, most people find it extremely difficult to accept the idea of losing a limb, even when, as in the case of elective amputations, the operation may be a life-saving measure or the first step toward regaining some degree of function. If the nurse can help the patient to understand that the operation is a beginning rather than an end, it will be easier for both to work toward positive rehabilitation goals.

Many times the patient has already undergone amputation at a lower level on the affected limb, amputation of the *other* limb, or various procedures and treatments related to his disease. Such a patient may become extremely depressed. He may feel as though he is "doomed." A "one day at a time" attitude coupled with a giant dose of patience may be the nurse's best approach.

It is extremely important that the patient have an opportunity to express his fears and anxieties about the impending amputation. If he is not encouraged to ventilate his feelings preoperatively, his postoperative progress may be severely hampered. While a positive outlook is one of the goals of psychological adjustment, the nurse should be careful not to allow her own enthusiastic expectations to overshadow the patient's feelings. He must feel free to express his own negative emotions no matter how depressing and hopeless they may be. It is futile if he is forced to assume a false smiling facade as a means of fulfilling the nurse's expectations.

The nurse should observe interactions between the patient and other family members to evaluate family reactions to the impending amputation. A wife may exhibit feelings of anger and subsequent guilt because she "put off going places" with her husband until the children were grown, and now she feels that traveling will be impossible. Families often hover over the patient as if to be present to fulfill every need. The atmosphere in the patient's room is frequently similar to that surrounding a dying patient. On the other hand, some relatives will discuss everything but the impending amputation, leaving it "all in the doctor's hands."

Whatever the reaction of family members, loss of a limb may elicit feelings of inadequacy in those who will live with the amputee as well as in the amputee himself. It is not an exaggeration to say that the family's emotional adjustment will greatly influence the adjustment of the patient.

It is during this preoperative period that a visit from a rehabilitated amputee can be most helpful. The sight of a capable functioning amputee can serve as an encouraging

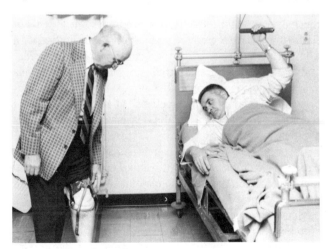

example and provide living proof of the positive points the nurse has been stressing. Moreover, since most elective amputations are performed on the elderly, optimism about "the future" is a difficult frame of mind to acquire. It could very well be that contact with a rehabilitated elderly amputee may be the only sign of hope that the patient is able to see.

Patient Teaching

As a further step toward reducing the patient's anxiety postoperatively, the nurse should prepare the patient for what to expect once the operation is over. Undoubtedly, the surgeon has already outlined some aspects of the operation and the postoperative regimen to the patient. In this regard, it is important that the nurse know what the surgeon has told the patient in order to avoid the possibility of providing conflicting information.

A patient who is about to undergo an amputation should know the level at which the limb will be amputated as well as the postoperative routines of the hospital. Whether or not a patient should be forewarned of the possibility of "phantom limb" sensations is questionable. Some surgeons, on the basis of their observations and experience, believe that the patient will have less phantom pain if he is not forewarned about it.

There are numerous theories about what causes so many patients to experience the feeling that the amputated limb is still there. These include interruption of sensory pathways, "memory" of the limb, or suppressed feelings of denial, anger, grief, and depression. Phantom limb pain is usually more severe in the immediate postoperative period. Patients may describe such pain as burning, cramping, or throbbing. In general, phantom pain subsides with time. When it persists, it causes mental and physical discomfort. Phantom limb sensations of itching and tingling, however, may come and go for years.

EXERCISE PREPARATION

Since exercise and rehabilitation are important aspects of the postoperative regimen, a preoperative consultation with a physical therapist will initiate rapport between patient and therapist. During this introductory meeting the various aspects of postoperative positioning, exercise, and ambulation can be discussed and practiced. At the same time, the therapist can make an initial assessment of the patient's abilities and motivation.

A series of preoperative exercises may be started if the patient's condition warrants it. However, it is important to remember that a painful limb may make it difficult for the patient to carry out some of these activities.

Since the patient's arms must be strengthened for crutchwalking or another means of ambulation, a trapeze should be placed on the overhead frame and the patient instructed as to its use in helping him to move about in bed. The patient should be taught that lifting his body off the bed holding on to the trapeze and then easing himself down again is a relatively easy exercise for strengthening the arms in preparation for using assistive ambulation devices. To further increase wrist strength, he should also be encouraged to tighten and then relax his grip on the trapeze.

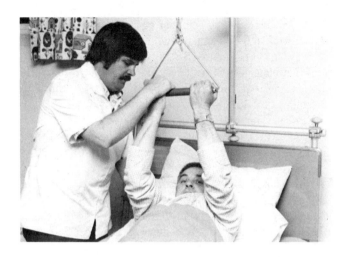

If the patient's condition permits he may be encouraged to do arm pushups while lying prone. However, older patients suffering with painful limbs will be very reluctant to comply and should not be forced beyond their limits. They may even find it difficult to perform an easier pushup exercise — sitting in bed and pushing down on the mattress with their hands to strengthen their arms. For such patients another alternative for triceps strengthening is use of the "weighted wand." Weights are secured in the middle of a

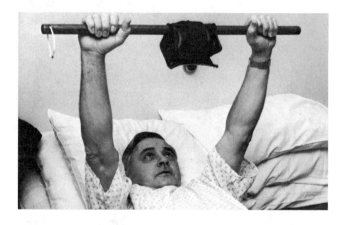

sturdy stick, and the patient is taught to raise and lower the wand with both arms in a pushup maneuver.

Arm exercises may also be carried out while the patient is in a wheelchair. Such exercise includes lifting the body by pushing down on the arms or seat of the chair or just maneuvering the chair routinely by means of its wheels.

The technique of walking with crutches or a walker may also be demonstrated and practiced preoperatively along with various muscle and stretching exercises necessary for the prevention of contractures. Gluteal muscle and quadriceps settings, along with straight leg raising, should be encouraged.

If a patient is a candidate for a prosthesis, the prosthetist should be brought in to answer questions. Although not all elderly amputees are candidates for prostheses, many of

---

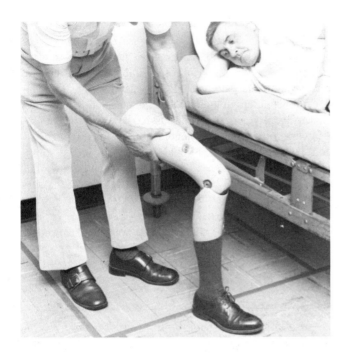

them will be able to ambulate postoperatively to some extent and therefore should be given some form of preoperative preparation. The importance of ambulation should be stressed on the basis that inactivity in the geriatric patient leads to grave problems of immobility.

Since loss of self-esteem is common in the geriatric amputee, the nurse and therapist must reassure him that every effort will be made to help him do the best he can with the limbs he has left.

Physical Preparation

During the preoperative period emphasis is placed on physical preparation of the total patient. Chronic diseases such as diabetes must be under control, and adjustments must be made in diet and dosage of insulin in anticipation of postoperative intravenous fluids. The debilitated or dehydrated patient may be treated preoperatively with intravenous fluids and fortified with vitamin preparations. Diets high in minerals, vitamins, and protein are indicated if the patient has a fairly good appetite. Blood transfusions may be ordered preoperatively for the anemic patient and will most likely be needed following surgery, for all patients.

Evaluation of the patient's vascular status is only indicated when it is thought that the limb might be saved by vessel surgery. Therefore, this procedure would have been done before any routine preoperative preparation is begun.

POSTOPERATIVE CARE

Much of patient care following an amputation depends on whether a temporary prosthesis is to be applied immediately in the operating room or on a delayed basis several weeks or months after surgery. Although the immediate fitting procedure is considered by some surgeons to be more promising, many patients with severe vascular or systemic disease must be treated by the delayed fitting method. Immediate postoperative fitting of a lower extremity is discussed on pages 286–287. The discussion that follows here deals with delayed fitting.

Vital Signs and Bleeding

In the immediate postoperative period, following lower extremity amputation, vital signs should be taken and recorded every 30 minutes until the condition of the patient is stable. Dressings, which are usually soft and bulky, should be checked for drainage every time the vital signs are taken

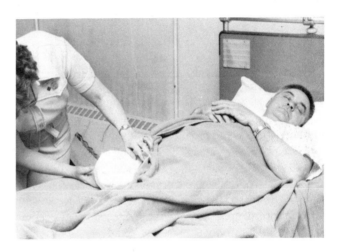

until the patient's condition is stable, and then every 3 hours thereafter. Drains in the incision are routinely left in place for approximately 48 hours, so bloody drainage may seep through the dressing. The dressing should be checked more frequently when the drainage appears to be increasing.

Bright red bleeding is not normal and may indicate that a ligature has become loose. When bright red bleeding is noted, a pressure dressing should be applied immediately and the stump should be elevated by raising the foot of the bed. The surgeon should also be notified immediately. Vigilant observation of vital signs and the dressing allows the nurse to take preventive measures before serious bleeding occurs.

When a pressure dressing is not sufficient to stop oozing, the wound is reopened by the surgeon, the bleeding controlled, and the incision re-sutured.

Since a hematoma resulting from accumulation of fluid postoperatively provides a culture medium for bacteria, aspiration may be indicated.

Swelling

Since the dressings are applied for compression, the proximal end of the extremity should be observed for swelling. A dressing that is too tight may produce ischemia in the end of the stump. The value of icebags on a stump to reduce swelling is a matter of debate among surgeons. Vascular surgeons may consider them undesirable since they may only decrease already inadequate circulation. In the case of the traumatic amputation, an orthopedic surgeon may want to use ice for 24 hours as a preventative measure to reduce swelling. The nursing implication is clearly that icebags should not be applied to an amputation stump without an order.

The foot of the bed may be elevated for 24 to 48 hours to lessen edema in the stump. Pillows should not be used because they contribute to the development of contractures.

If an open amputation has been done because of preoperative infection, and skin traction has been applied, it is important to see that the traction is continuous.

Infection

Infection may be present because of the injury or may develop postoperatively as a result of bleeding in the stump or a stitch abscess. The nurse should be alert for any odor indicating infection and should inform the surgeon when such odor is present.

Antibiotics, elevation of the stump by elevating the foot of the bed, and hot packs may be sufficient when the infection is not deep. Incision and drainage may be necessary in the case of a stitch abscess. Since the danger of a developing osteomyelitis is present, wounds are opened for inspection and appropriate treatment when infection persists. Reamputation at a higher level may be necessary.

Pain

Since the incision is not subject to the stress of an incision over a movable joint, such as the knee or hip, postoperative pain is not a major problem. The patient can be positioned and nursing care given without the nurse exerting any pressure against the incisional area.

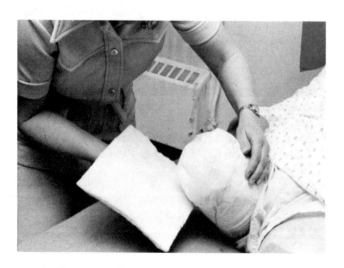

Phantom pain may be of more concern than pain in the operative area. Attempts to deal with this condition are often not very successful. Pain medications may be required for a few days, along with intensive supportive nursing care. Encouraging the patient to describe, in detail, the sensations in his phantom limb may be beneficial in finally "laying the limb to rest." When discussing this with the patient, it is wise to refer to the phenomenon as "phantom sensation" rather than pain. Should severe pain in the stump continue for more than a day or two, it may be a sign of infection and should be called to the attention of the surgeon.

A neuroma that forms at the end of a severed nerve can also be responsible for pain. If the nerves are allowed to retract during the amputation procedure, a neuroma need not be a source of pain due to pressure at the operative site. Treatment of a painful neuroma is by excision.

Respiratory Measures

Because of the age and health of the average patient with an elective amputation, postoperative measures to promote circulation are doubly important. Deep breathing and coughing should be encouraged at frequent intervals. An incentive spirometer may also be helpful. The patient must be assisted in moving the extremities. If general health permits, the patient is allowed out of bed a day or two after surgery, to reduce the risk of pulmonary embolism.

Skin Care and Elimination

Skin breakdown is a potential problem in patients with circulatory conditions. Inspecting and rubbing the back, buttocks, elbows, and heel, at 3- to 4-hour intervals from 6 A.M. to midnight is wise.

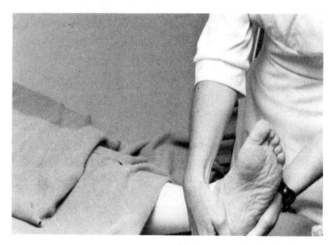

In caring for the elderly or debilitated amputee, the nurse must make frequent observations to determine if the patient has been incontinent of urine or feces. Immediate and thorough cleansing and drying of the perineal area, thighs, and buttocks should be done in order to avoid skin breakdown. When a bandage or dressing becomes soiled, it should be changed promptly to prevent contamination of the wound. The bedpan or urinal should be offered every 3 hours if the patient is the least bit disoriented.

Ulcerations about the incision may develop due to infection, hemorrhage, the drain, poor circulation, or improper compression by the bandage.

Nutrition

Fluids and diet are generally ordered as tolerated, with special attention given to individual needs when the patient has diabetes or another ailment requiring diet considerations.

Nursing responsibilities relative to the medical condition responsible for the diseased limb should be understood and incorporated into the nursing care plan. For example, if the patient is diabetic, the nurse must instruct the team members to be alert for symptoms of problems arising from temporary adjustment in diet and insulin dosage or other medication.

Position and Exercise

The position of the patient following surgery is extremely important at all times to prevent contractures. Pillows are never used under an above-knee stump, under the knee in a below-knee stump, or between the thighs. Unfortunately, hip flexion, hip abduction, external rotation, and knee flexion are positions assumed by the patient for comfort and protection of the wound; all of these positions contribute to contracture formation. Contractures make proper fitting and use of a prosthesis very difficult.

Prolonged periods of sitting, either in or out of bed, will flex the stump and therefore should be avoided. To avoid these potentially damaging positions the following "do's" should be instituted.

1. First of all, a firm bed is essential. A sagging mattress is a factor in contracture formation.
2. When the patient is in a supine position, he should be completely flat except for the pillow under his head. Observe the stump to make certain it is flat on the bed.
3. As soon as possible postoperatively the patient should be encouraged to lie on his stomach for 30-minute periods at 3- to 4-hour intervals. Achieving this position is difficult and somewhat painful at first. The patient requires assistance in turning and, for the first day, may experience severe discomfort maintaining his pelvis flat on the bed. He needs much encouragement to "do the best he can." When he is lying on his stomach, his head should be turned away from his affected side. At the same time, and as tolerated, the patient can be instructed to pull the stump close to the

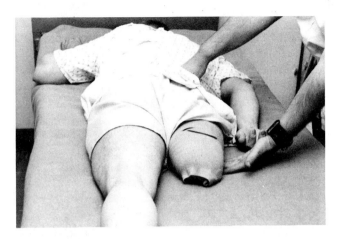

other leg and to lift the stump and contract the gluteal muscles. During this exercise, the foot of the normal leg should be over the edge of the bed. The patient who cannot tolerate stomach-lying can remain on his back and be instructed to push the posterior surface of his residual limb down against the mattress, contracting the gluteal muscles.

4. For below-knee amputations, another effective resistive exercise can be performed while the amputee is on his abdomen. A pillow or large towel is made into a tight roll and placed under the distal end of the residual limb. The patient pushes down against the pillow to strengthen the muscles of the thigh. this exercise is begun when the patient starts lying on his stomach, preferably the day after surgery.
5. Additional exercises can be initiated on the second day after surgery. The above-knee amputee can be taught to squeeze his thighs together, rolling them

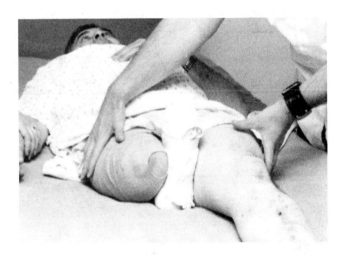

inward. This exercise in internal rotation aids in preventing a position of external rotation.
6. Isometric exercises of the gluteal and quadriceps muscles and assistive range of motion of the stump

are standard, as are range of motion exercises for the other limbs. At least five times a day, at 3-hour intervals, the nurse or therapist should assist the amputee in doing these exercises. As his condition improves and his apprehension about moving his stump lessens,

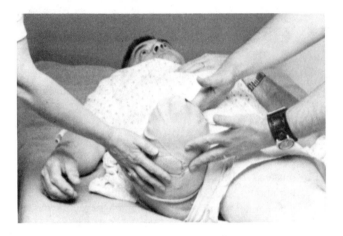

he may be motivated to do more exercise independently. Conscientious nursing care in regard to exercise routines, whether assistive or supportive, eliminates the need for a footboard.

7. The patient may also begin ambulating with an assistive device 4 days postoperatively, testing his balance first at the parallel bars. When the patient begins crutchwalking he should be instructed to avoid holding the stump in a flexed position to prevent a permanent flexion deformity. Instead he should move the stump back and forth while he is walking.

8. Resistive exercises are initiated when the sutures are removed. A "sling and spring" apparatus for resistive exercise can be provided for the patient to use in the hospital and at home after discharge. The stump is placed in the sling, which is suspended from the overhead frame by a spring. The amputee exercises by pushing the stump down against the sling.

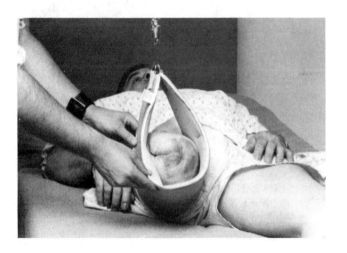

Throughout the period of hospitalization, the nursing staff will need to coordinate efforts with the physical therapists, and both should continue to assess patient ability and evaluate progress.

Stump Conditioning

Stump Wrapping. Stump wrapping for proper shaping begins at the surgeon's discretion. This could be as early as the first postoperative day. It is important that the stump be shaped to ensure proper fitting of the prosthesis. Correct bandaging limits edema while the stump is in a dependent position and maintains the muscle in as firm a state as possible. Improper bandaging or failure to bandage will result in a bulky, flabby stump.

Elastic bandages of 4- and 6-inch widths are used, depending on the size of the residual limb. For above-knee amputees, the bandage is started on the front of the thigh and brought down to secure the distal end first.

Pressure is used during wrapping in order to compress the stump at the bottom and work the edema to the proximal end of the limb. Compression should be decreased gradually during the wrapping procedure.

When the stump is healing, this compression force must be light enough so that it will not cause any discomfort. All of the skin is covered, special attention begin given to the ends of the distal stump to avoid formation of "dog ears."

Above-Knee Wrapping. Although there are many effective methods of bandaging a stump, the following procedure for wrapping an above-knee stump is less awkward than others.

The patient is lying either supine, with stump fully extended, or on the unaffected side with knee and hip flexed for stability and the stump kept in hyperextension through-

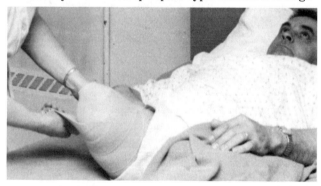

out the procedure. (As the patient learns to do his own bandaging he will have to assume a semi-sitting position.) The following directions on limb wrapping, with appropriate photographs, can be made into instruction booklets for amputees and their families.

1. The bandage is started on the diagonal on the anterior surface of the stump just inferior to the level of the inguinal ligament.

2. The bandage is passed over the distal end of the stump on the medial side.

3. The diagonal turn is anchored by crossing over the end of the bandage. As the stump is wrapped, the figure-eight turns are begun on the medial side and run posteriorly to the lateral side. This is important for the later steps of the procedure, because when the hip spica phase of the wrapping begins (steps 6–8) the bandage must run from lateral to medial on the anterior surface.

4. The bandage is brought down around the end of the stump and up again by means of an oblique or a modified figure-eight turn. Never use circular turns that are not oblique because they tend to constrict circulation.

5. The bandage is brought well up into the groin area to eliminate all possibility of the adductor muscle forming a roll over the bandage. To facilitate conical shaping, compression of the stump should be greatest at the distal end and should decrease gradually as wrapping proceeds in a proximal direction.

6. The hip spica portion of the wrapping serves the dual purpose of anchoring the bandage and covering the tissue high in the groin and the lateral surface of the hip. This eliminates any possibility of bulges forming in this area, a problem that frequently occurs when the hip spica is not used. The spica is started from the anterior lateral aspect of the stump and runs medially across the anterior surface of the stump in the inguinal region.

7. The bandage is carried around the body at the level of the iliac crest and returned to the stump.

8. The wrapping is completed by means of oblique turns on the stump.

9. The bandage is then anchored with safety pins over the lateral and anterior surfaces of the stump, and high in the anterior groin area.

For photographs illustrating this procedure, see pages 276–277.

Below-Knee Wrapping. In below-knee wrapping, the mass of the gastrocnemius and soleus muscles must not be pulled toward the medial aspect of the tibia. Care must also be taken not to compress the popliteal area. The knee should be in extension and the bandage should extend onto the thigh. The below-knee prosthesis will extend over the femoral condyles, and it is essential that this part of the limb be shaped.

A simple procedure for wrapping a below-knee stump is as follows:

1. With the patient in a sitting position, the end of the bandage can be secured under the thigh. When the patient does his own bandaging, this will free both hands to do the work.

2. The bandage is brought posterior to anterior and pulled firmly over the distal end of the residual limb and above the knee.

3. Next, the bandage is drawn medially and posteriorly to begin a diagonal wrap.

4. Wrapping can be done from the proximal end of the residual limb to the distal end. However, extreme care must be taken to *begin* with light pressure and increase the amount of compression as bandaging continues in a distal direction. The patient must understand the importance of this procedure.

5. Two or three figure-eights are made over the distal end of the stump for medial and lateral compression.

6. The remainder of the bandage is wrapped in diagonal turns, again with less and less compression in the proximal direction.

7. Safety pins should be used to secure the anterior and lateral aspects of the bandage.

An illustrated guide for this procedure is shown on page 278.

Routine Stump Care. The stump should be bandaged four to six times a day with clean bandages. Two sets of bandages are needed to alternate so that after each day they can be washed in warm soapy water, thoroughly rinsed, and allowed to dry on a flat surface. Hanging an elastic bandage may result in stretching. Bandages should also be rolled snugly, but not stretched. As soon as possible the therapist or nurse should teach the patient to wrap his own stump. If the patient is unable to do so, the person responsible for his care at home should learn the wrapping procedure.

A stump shrinker, similar to a heavy stockinette sock, is sometimes prescribed for the amputee who has difficulty keeping a bandage in place.

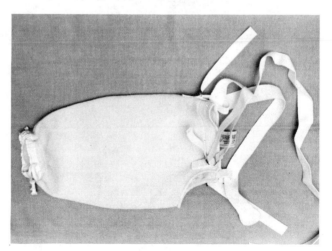

WRAPPING AN ABOVE-KNEE RESIDUAL LIMB

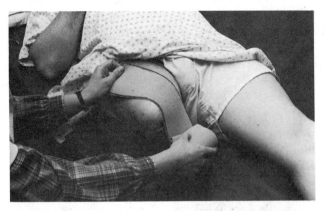

The bandage is started on the diagonal on the anterior surface of the residual limb just below the level of the inguinal ligament and is passed over the distal end of the residual limb on the medial side.

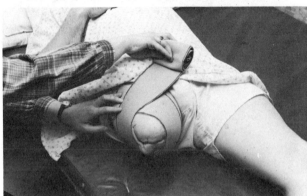

The diagonal turn is anchored by crossing over the end of the bandage.

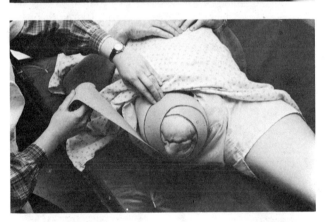

As the residual limb is wrapped, the figure-eight turns are begun on the medial side and run posteriorly to the lateral side. This is important for the later steps of the procedure because when the hip spica phase of the wrapping begins, the bandage must run from lateral to medial on the anterior surface.

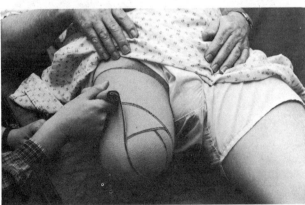

The bandage is brought down around the end of the residual limb and up again by means of an oblique or a modified figure-eight turn. Never use circular turns that are not oblique because they tend to constrict circulation.

WRAPPING AN ABOVE-KNEE RESIDUAL LIMB *(continued)*

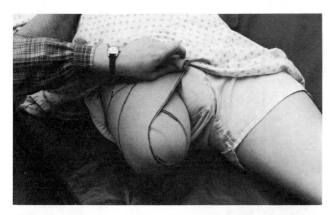

The bandage is brought well up into the groin area to eliminate all possibility of the adductor muscle's forming a roll over the bandage. To facilitate conical shaping, compression of the residual limb should be greatest at the distal end and should decrease gradually as wrapping proceeds in a proximal direction.

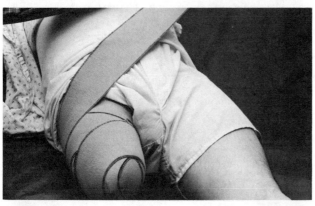

The hip spica portion of the wrapping serves to anchor the bandage and to cover the tissue high in the groin and the lateral surface of the hip. This prevents bulges from forming in this area, a problem that frequently occurs when the hip spica is not used. The spica is started from the anterior lateral aspect of the residual limb and runs medially across the anterior surface of the residual limb in the inguinal region. The bandage is carried around the body at the level of the iliac crest and returned to the residual limb.

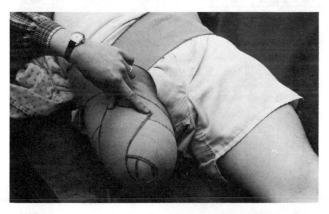

The wrapping is completed by means of oblique turns on the end of the residual limb.

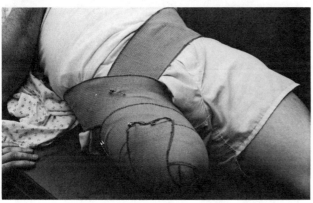

The bandage is then anchored with safety pins over the lateral and anterior surfaces of the residual limb.

WRAPPING A BELOW-KNEE RESIDUAL LIMB

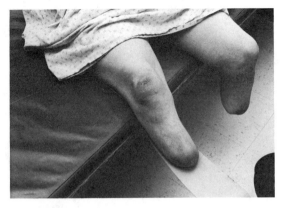

1. With the patient in a sitting position, the end of the bandage is secured under the thigh. When the patient does his own bandaging, this will free both hands to do the work.

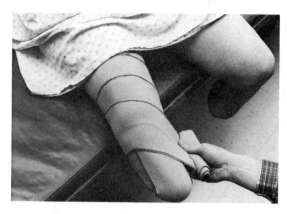

4. Wrapping can be done from the proximal end of the residual limb to the distal end. However, extreme care must be taken to *begin* with light pressure and increase the amount of compression as bandaging continues in a distal direction. The patient must understand the importance of this procedure.

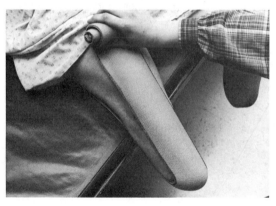

2. The bandage is brought posterior to anterior and pulled firmly over the distal end of the residual limb and above the knee.

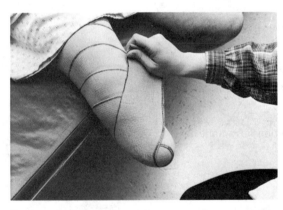

5. Two or three figure-eights are made over the distal end of the residual limb for medial and lateral compression. The remainder of the bandage is wrapped in diagonal turns, again with less and less compression in the proximal direction.

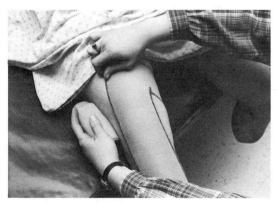

3. Next, the bandage is drawn medially and posteriorly to begin a diagonal wrap.

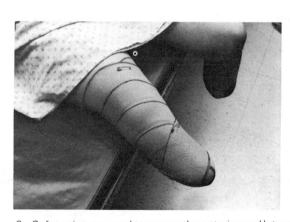

6. Safety pins are used to secure the anterior and lateral aspects of the bandage.

Elastic wrapping bandages are warm and may cause perspiration. Therefore each time the bandage is removed, the skin should be inspected, cleansed, and dried thoroughly. Powder that contains a drying agent, or cornstarch, may be applied lightly. Dry skin should be rubbed with a petrolatum-base lotion.

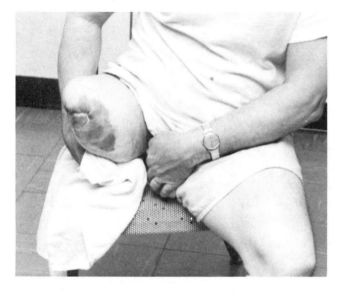

Heat in the form of light cradles or ultraviolet or infrared lamps is not usually ordered. However, when it is, it must be used very carefully to avoid burning the stump. An incisional line that appears reddened may benefit from the application of radiant heat.

Massage in stump conditioning has a psychological as well as physiological effect. Handling the stump helps the amputee recognize the reality of the amputation and may reduce phantom sensations. In addition, physical massage stimulates circulation, relieves muscle spasm, and can be done after the stump has been cleansed and before the bandage is reapplied.

Another measure that is often successful in reducing phantom sensation is to place a large bath towel over the end of the stump, medial to lateral, lengthwise, and have the patient hold the ends so that he can "feel" the end of his

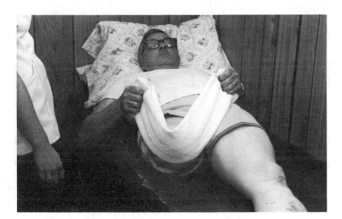

residual limb in the towel. As postoperative discomfort lessens, he can increase the pressure of the towel on the stump and repeat the procedure of pushing into the towel and then relaxing as often as desired.

Circumferential measurements of the stump should be taken regularly to note the amount of shrinkage that has occurred.

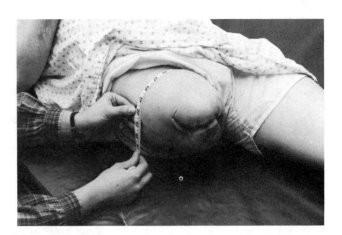

The "Difficult" Amputee: Nursing Implications

The patient who faces particularly complex and difficult problems as a result of an amputation requires special support. An example of a realistic nursing approach to problem solving is presented on pages 280–281.

Psychological Considerations

In the elderly amputee, all the problems of aging become more intense: poor eyesight, lack of coordination, and diminished mental acuity. The patient may also be afraid that he will lose his other limb to the same disease. Younger amputees have such questions as: How do I look to others? How do I look to myself? Will I get a job because someone feels sorry for me? Will I lose a job because I can't handle it? Self-image and sexuality, a very real concern to many amputees, is discussed in Chapter 11.

Discharge Teaching

Anything an elderly amputee is taught about how to care for his stump at home should be presented simply and repeated several times. Following the procedure, his comprehension of what has been taught should be evaluated. Confusion can easily occur, as indicated by the following example. A 70-year-old man with an above-knee amputation was readmitted to the hospital for an unrelated condition 3 months after his surgery. The nurse who admitted him discovered that he had not taken a complete bath since leaving the hospital because "someone" had told him not to touch the scabs on the incision.

THE "DIFFICULT" AMPUTEE: REALISTIC APPROACH TO PROBLEM SOLVING

Significant Data: E. D. is an obese 57-year-old female with severe, uncontrollable diabetes. She had a right below-knee amputation 3 years ago. At that time her physician told her that if she did not keep her diabetes under control she would lose her left leg. She ignored his warning and as a result had to undergo an above-knee amputation of her left leg. She lives with her husband and her three sons, and they run a farm as well as a country tavern. E. D. did most of the bartending because she could "get around" on a barstool that had small wheels. She has a prosthesis for her right leg but does not wear it. Her husband and sons are all tall and very thin.

Nursing Diagnoses

1. Knowledge deficit: Related to lack of motivation to participate in own care or take responsibility for own care, and to ineffective coping patterns (depression)
2. Self-concept, potential disturbance in: Related to loss of body parts
3. Coping, ineffective individual: Related to depression in response to identifiable stressors
4. Self-care deficit: Related to inability or unwillingness to bathe, dress, and groom self
5. Mobility, impaired physical: Related to alterations in lower limbs (loss of both lower limbs)
6. Alteration in comfort—Pain: Related to surgical incision, pressure of bandages, handling during treatment
7. Skin integrity, impairment of, potential: Related to immobility and obesity
8. Family processes, potential alterations in: Related to illness of a family member
9. Diversional activity deficit: Related to monotony of confinement, immobility, lack of interest in usual activities

Problems: 2nd Week of Hospitalization	Factors to Consider in Nursing Assessment and Care	Possible Nursing Actions
1. Can give her own insulin and do urine testing but does not like to.	1.&2. Has she had a problem with giving own insulin and testing urine in the past? Does she "fear" needles? Is this part of denial of her disease? Does she really understand her diabetes?	1.&2. Evaluate patient and family knowledge of disease and treatment and provide needed instruction. Observe interactions between patient and family. Talk to them as a family unit to try to assess their feelings and fears as well as capabilities. Also note if E. seems willing to let them help her. Investigate possibility of a family member learning how to give insulin. Discuss likes and dislikes in food with whole family to evaluate feelings about food and weight in general. Bring dietician into frequent conferences, if necessary, with family unit.
2. 1200 calorie diabetic diet. But her family brings her food, even though the staff explains why they should not. "They seem apathetic" (staff comment).	Do her husband and sons fully understand her disease and its treatment? Does the fact that they are thin make it difficult for them to understand or *believe* in the need for diet restrictions? Are they denying the existence of her disease? Are they apathetic or do they believe that there is nothing they can do? In fact, does E. allow them to be any other way?	
3. Does not like to do any self-care.	3. What would the patient like to do for herself? Would E. be more receptive to doing self-care at some other time of day?	3. Adjust nursing care schedule if at all possible to patient preference. Continue to encourage her to do own bath. Suggest possibility of having something done to her hair.
4. Elastic wrapping will not stay on residual limb for more than 30–60 minutes.	4. Size of patient and "fat" stump prevent satisfactory regular wrapping for any sizable period of time.	4. Call on prosthetist for ideas on creating a special stump wrap or sock. Check with hospital linen room on what a seamstress can put together in way of stump sock. Perhaps a partial body sock, which will incorporate both stumps?

Problems: 2nd Week of Hospitalization	Factors to Consider in Nursing Assessment and Care	Possible Nursing Actions
5. Complains that her stump "hurts all the time."	5. Is on oral pain medication. Healing stitch abscess. Incisional area being treated with hot packs. Complaints of pain seem out of proportion and continuous. Did she have a problem with previous amputation? What was her experience with phantom pain? What does she say about her limbs? Observe if she looks at them.	5. Evaluate effect of pain medication. Continue present regimen. Ask her for precise description of pain, touching stump when possible. Increase frequency of skin care routines and change in position.
6. Does not like to move or be moved.	6. Because she is obese, moving may be difficult. Skin breakdown is a potential problem. She is on convoluted bedpan.	6. Evaluate ways patient is being moved. She is gotten out of bed by Hoyer lift.
7. Difficult to evaluate her complaints because she "whines a lot," according to staff. Not interested in the crocheting she brought with her and has little interest in television. Depressed?	7. Who comes to see her? What are her relationships with family? Was she accustomed to a lot of conversation as a bartender? Does she need different diversion? She may be deeply concerned over how she will get around when she goes home. Has talked about getting a wheelchair since she has four men to "lift me around."	7. Again, observe interactions between patient, family, and visitors. Ask family and visitors for suggestions for diversion. Check if there are other ambulatory patients who might like to play cards or other games with her. Rotate staff often when assigning her care in order to evaluate her. However, if she becomes attached to anyone, this must be taken into consideration.
		Begin discharge planning from the perspective that E. D. will probably spend the remainder of her life in a wheelchair.
		It is very likely that even the most comprehensive nursing care will not modify this patient's behavior or improve her emotional status. However, daily conferences with staff to document and share actions and approaches that are proving effective may be beneficial.
		Maintaining a positive attitude in the nursing staff even when results are not evident will be very important. Acceptance of "what will be" may make E. D. feel cared about . . . and less "difficult."

To prevent such misunderstanding an amputee should be taught that once the sutures have been removed, the stump should be cleansed like any other body part. The proper time to start this instruction is when stump conditioning begins. Whenever possible, a responsible person who will be closely associated with the amputee should be given clear directions on stump care, bandaging, and exercises.

How much the stump shrinks depends on the original size of the thigh. But it must be shrunk before the prosthesis is fitted, to ensure a proper fit. Usually it is 2 to 3 months before the stump is well-healed and molded so that the fitting can take place.

In the interim between discharge from the hospital and prosthetic fitting, there should be physical therapy follow-up either on an outpatient basis or in the home. The therapist thereby follows the amputee's progress in terms of exercises, gait training, posture, and stump wrapping. Visiting nurse services may be part of the preprosthetic program to supervise care of the stump. All of the instructions given by the therapist before discharge should be reinforced by the nurse.

For the amputee who will not be able to wear a prosthesis, or for the double amputee, there are wheelchairs designed to compensate for the loss of body weight in such a way that the amputee will not tip over backwards.

The patient who is going to an extended care facility must take with him a comprehensive account of his responses to specific nursing intervention and rehabilitative efforts. The nurse who plans his discharge is responsible for setting the guidelines for continuity of care.

Ideally, nursing care should not terminate just because the amputee has been dismissed into the care of a family member. Providing the name of a specific nurse, along with the hospital telephone number, will reassure the family and the amputee that the orthopedic nurse has an ongoing commitment and is available to offer suggestions and provide emotional support.

LOWER EXTREMITY PROSTHESES

Selecting a Prosthesis

When shrinkage of the stump is controlled, the physician prescribes a prosthesis. Shrinker bandages are still applied to the stump to help maintain the desirable shape while the prosthesis is being constructed. Many factors must be considered before an amputee is matched with a prosthesis. These include:

1. *Age.* A young person needs a prosthesis that is durable, whereas an elderly person might need a prosthesis that will provide stability.
2. *Intelligence.* Some prostheses are more complex than others. However, average intelligence is required to handle any prosthesis.
3. *Occupation.* A farmer or any other type of laborer will need a heavy-duty prosthesis.
4. *Weight and Agility.* A prosthesis must be constructed to withstand the stress placed on it by an obese person or one who lacks agility.
5. *Economic Factors.* Prostheses are very expensive.
6. *Health Status.* Poor vision, poor balance, and cardiac problems are examples of conditions that might influence how much an amputee would use a prosthesis.
7. *Motivation.* This is the magic word. Rehabilitative efforts on the part of the orthopedic personnel and prosthetist are pointless if the amputee lacks the will or determination to use his prosthesis once he has it.

The level of amputation and the age of the patient determine the complexity of the prosthesis and the units that will be used. There are a variety of prostheses in use; those described in the following sections are probably the most common ones. Being familiar with the various types of prostheses helps the nurse become aware of the prosthesis as a device that is as individual as the amputee to whom it is attached.

Above-Knee Prostheses

The nurse will encounter some patients using above-knee prostheses with wooden sockets. However, most prostheses are now constructed with plastic laminate sockets. These sockets are made from plaster molds of the residual limb. A critical factor in the construction of any prosthesis is the proper fit of the residual limb to the socket. The best-fitting mold for an above-knee limb is made by using a metal casting brim for the proximal end. The size of the brim used is determined by the circumferential measurement of the residual limb at the ischial tuberosity. The remainder of the limb is casted in a conventional manner.

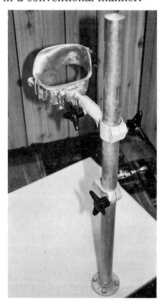

Two examples of above-knee prostheses are:

1. For the conventional above-knee amputee, or the one whose residual limb will probably undergo changes due to weight or activity, a prosthesis with a hip joint and pelvic belt is usually the choice (shown below at left). This prosthesis has a Bock safety knee that locks by friction when weight is applied, preventing the knee from buckling. Most knee units are also designed so that friction created within them during the swing phase of walking limits the distance the heel rises from the floor and provides smooth extension before the heel touches the floor. This prosthesis has a SACH (Solid Ankle Cushion Heel) foot.

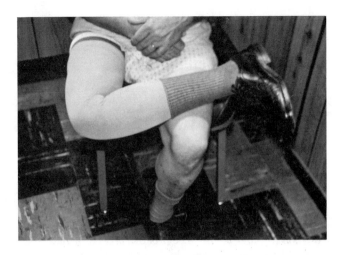

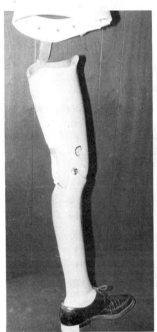 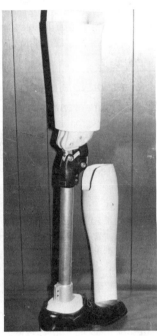

2. The suction socket prosthesis, pictured below, has total contact, meaning that it touches all aspects of the stump. It has a modular polycentric knee joint. The four-bar linkage design can be adjusted to the

individual patient's requirements for greater knee stability at heel strike. The adjustable design enables more physiological function of the prosthetic leg. Polyurethane foam material, which is used to form the shape of the leg, is soft and fleshlike in appearance. For an active above-knee amputee, the suction socket prothesis has an advantage, since the wearer feels "closer" to and in better control of the artificial limb. The suction effect is created by pulling the stump into the socket by means of a long piece of stockinette. This stockinette is pulled on, well up to the top of the thigh. The prosthesis is put in place with the remainder of the stockinette extending out an

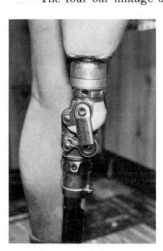 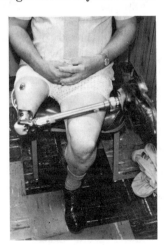

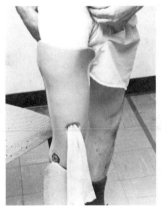 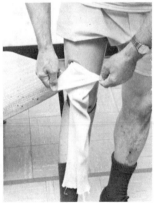

opening near the knee joint, which serves as a valve. The amputee grasps the distal end of the stockinette and pulls it through the opening with a twisting motion so that the stockinette, which tends to stretch, pulls down evenly on all sides of the stump. This procedure works the stump into close contact with the socket. When the stockinette is pulled through the opening, the vacuum created is maintained by installing the valve.

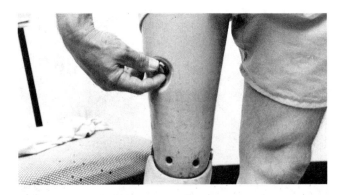

The Below-Knee Prosthesis

The most popular below-knee prosthesis is constructed for patellar tendon weight bearing. Construction of the prosthesis begins with the application of a plaster cast over the stump. The cast is removed and a modified cast (pictured with attached pole) is made by pouring plaster into the original cast. The soft insert is also pictured. The next illustration shows the soft insert, the "set up," and the finished

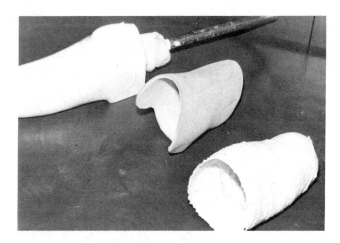

prosthesis, with a condylar cuff, SACH foot, and attachment for waist belt. In the "set up" the pylon tube can be

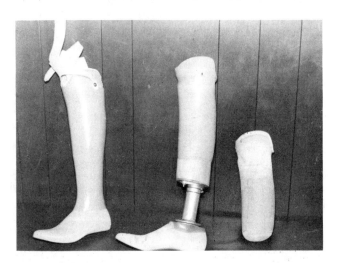

adjusted for trial walking. The prosthesis for the Syme amputation allows weight bearing on the end of the tibia. The stump is placed in the prosthesis by way of an opening

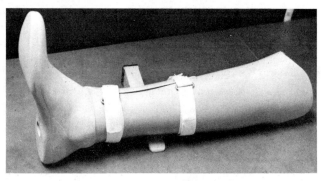

in the shank. The prosthesis incorporates a SACH foot with sponge rubber in the heel to absorb the impact caused by stepping.

Orientation to a Prosthesis

How fast a new amputee adjusts to his prosthesis and how well he learns to use it depends partly on his age and general condition, as well as the condition of the stump. As noted earlier, motivation is the most important factor and should be reinforced by physical and mental preparation for the experience.

The various types of prostheses should be described to an amputee as well as the reasons why a particular type will best suit his needs. Such explanation helps develop confidence in the prosthesis and in those involved in the prosthetic training. The procedure for making the prosthesis should be discussed, along with the potential problems and their effects on the period of adjustment.

Hopefully, by the time the prosthesis is ready for the amputee, the stump is ready for the prosthesis. If the patient has been conscientious about stump conditioning, then prosthesis training can start immediately. The amputee should have been instructed to inform the prosthetist and therapist of any problems such as edema or contractures of the stump. This eliminates the need for "last minute" treatment before prosthetic training begins.

The prosthetist will fit and instruct the amputee on how to put it on and how to remove it. For an above-knee pros-

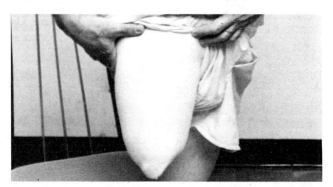

thesis, the first step is to apply a stump sock. The stump is then settled into place in the prosthesis and the belt or harness fastened. After learning to balance himself on the prosthesis, the amputee takes a few steps so that the prosthetist can determine whether or not adjustments are necessary. Usually, the amputee is asked to visit the prosthetist 1 month after receiving the artificial limb, or sooner if problems arise. From that time on, inspection of the prosthesis as to fit and wear is scheduled every 6 months.

Once the prosthetist and the amputee have agreed that the prostesis is the proper fit, gait training will begin under the supervision of the physical therapist who has been conducting post-amputation exercises.

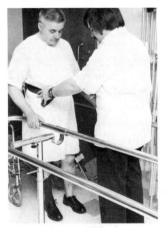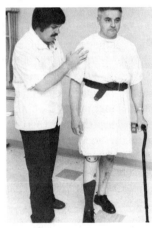

At times, female amputees face certain problems in dealing with male prosthetists. Although women generally accept, as routine, examinations by male physicians, the prospect of having a male prosthetist measure for and fit a leg prosthesis may be embarrassing. It was a revelation to this author to discover that an elderly female amputee would not return to the prosthetist for a much needed adjustment of her prosthesis because there was "no one but men in the place," and it seemed like a "machine shop." She may have been unusually modest, but the experience prompted a visit to the orthopedic appliance center and research into how and where prostheses are made. Knowledge of the procedure provided insights into the apprehensions a female amputee might have and was the basis for making suggestions and offering support to other amputees, both male and female.

Care of the Prosthesis

A prosthesis should receive the attention given any other mechanical device. Periodic checks are in order to determine whether or not parts need repair or replacement. Signs of malfunction in a prosthesis include joint clicks, foot creaking, a "heavy feeling" and changes in the way the stump looks or feels.

For general care, the amputee can be taught how to take

the bolts out of squeaky knee or hip joints and how to grease them. Repairs beyond this procedure should not be attempted without specific instructions from the prosthetist.

A wooden socket requires refinishing about every 6 months. However, the amputee is instructed not to "finish" the prosthesis with stain or varnish and to refrain from getting it water-soaked. The socket of the prosthesis may need frequent cleansing and should be washed carefully with mild soap and water and then dried completely. How often this is necessary should be discussed with the prosthe-

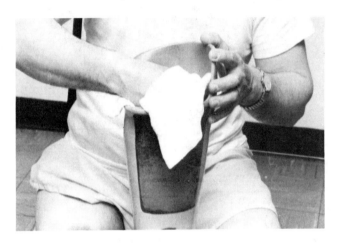

tist. Socket liners and inserts can be replaced when they become excessively soiled or worn. Regular sponging of these components with soap and water is advised.

To keep stockings in place, garters are preferable to adhesive tape. Some prosthetists recommend taking small

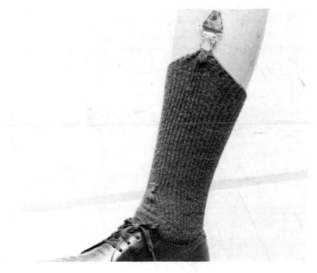

garter snaps, such as those on a woman's garter belt, and attaching them to the prosthesis with screws.

Finally, attention must be paid to the condition of the shoe. Any change in shoe height needs to be approved by the prosthetist, and shoes should be replaced before they become completely worn out.

Stump Care and the Prosthesis

An amputee should understand that his stump needs to be washed daily with mild soap and water, dried, and inspected for skin irritation. No extra cleaning agents, lotions, or

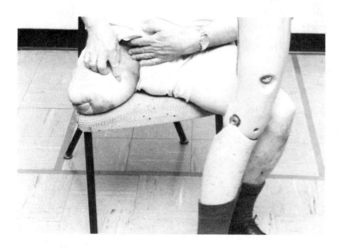

creams are necessary. However, cornstarch may be used in very warm weather.

After removing the prosthesis and stump sock, the amputee should check the general appearance of the stump. The imprint of the sock pattern may help identify any pressure areas caused by the prosthesis. Eczema, blisters, and calluses are associated with a poorly fitted prosthesis or improper care of a stump. It is especially important to identify stump problems and report them to the prosthetist as they develop. Neglect will lead to difficulty in securing the proper fit of a prosthesis.

When stump socks are worn, the amputee should have an ample supply to allow for a daily change. In the past, stump socks were usually made of pure virgin wool, because this material was considered most durable. However, stump

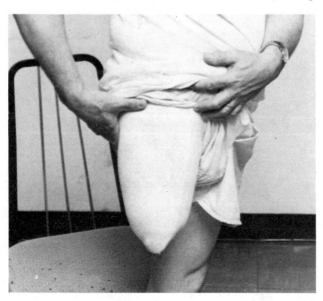

socks made of more washable materials are becoming increasingly popular. Any stump sock should be discarded when it develops rough spots or holes.

The correct size of the sock is determined by measuring the circumference of both the upper rim of the socket and the distal end of the stump, plus the length of the stump from the distal end of the stump to the place where the upper rim of the prosthesis rests against the leg. Several inches are added to allow for a "cuff" over the end of the socket. Socks that are not the correct size may wrinkle or sag causing poor contact, or no contact at all, between the end of the stump and the prosthesis. This could result in edema.

Frequently, amputees make the mistake of applying more than one stump sock when the stump continues to shrink over several years. They would rather not "bother" the prosthetist with the problem of a loose prosthesis. The amputee may also try to fill in the space produced by stump shrinkage with other material like wads of cotton or washcloths. This emphasizes once again the importance of thoroughly instructing the amputee at the time the prosthesis is fit to visit the prosthetist periodically for any necessary adjustments. In the case of an elderly amputee who may not be able to care for himself, it is wise to provide the person responsible for his care with detailed information on the care of the stump and prosthesis.

EARLY POSTOPERATIVE FITTING OF A LOWER EXTREMITY PROSTHESIS

The Procedure

For some patients with below-knee amputations, early functional use of the limb is considered to be preferable to delayed prosthesis fitting. These patients are fitted with a prosthetic unit in the operating room through the cooperative efforts of surgeon and prosthetist. This procedure is called an immediate postoperative fitting. An intermediate postoperative fitting is one that is done about 2 weeks after surgery, to allow the surgeon the opportunity to observe healing of the incision. The following technique is used for both.

The fluffy dressing on the stump is protected by a sterile stump stocking, and felt pads are placed over bony prominences. A plaster-of-Paris dressing, incorporating the support strap for later use with a waist belt, is then applied over the stump. An adjustable prosthetic unit, consisting of a pylon tube and a foot, is attached to the cast by means of additional plaster when the cast is dry.

An infection, or potential infection, is probably the main contraindication for this type of prosthesis. However, patients who are senile or afflicted with disabling diseases do not make good candidates for the immediate postsurgical prosthetic fitting.

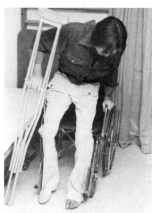
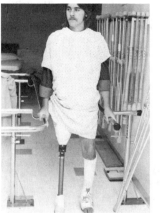

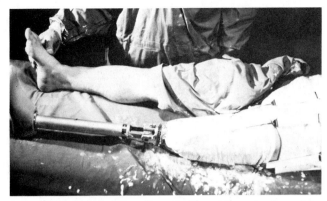

Immediate prosthetic fitting. (From Smith and Germain: Care of the Adult Patient)

Advantages and Disadvantages

The advantages of immediate prosthetic fitting are perhaps a matter of opinion, but they include:

1. Prevention of edema in the stump, thus accelerating healing and molding of the stump
2. Decreased phantom pain
3. Earlier ambulation
4. Shorter hospitalization
5. Improved psychological adjustment
6. Decreased financial burden due to shortened hospital stay
7. Earlier rehabilitation with definitive prosthesis

The main disadvantages of the procedure may be sloughing of the skin due to early weight bearing and problems associated with a cast.

Nursing Implications and Rehabilitation

The nurse should be alert to odors about the cast that signal infection and should report any persistent pain within the cast. If the cast becomes loose, the surgeon must be notified so that irritation of the skin or edema can be avoided by proper removal of the cast and application of a new cast. If the cast falls off, the nurse should immediately rewrap the stump with an elastic bandage until the surgeon can reapply a new cast. After 48 hours, the drain from the incision is removed through a window in the cast.

The first postoperative day, the patient will stand and bear weight under supervision, and as tolerated. Usually this first effort lasts only a few minutes. The patient progresses according to his own tolerance and under surgeon's orders, from parallel bars to crutches or a walker, then to a cane, and finally to no assistive device at all. The length of time required to accomplish this goal depends on the individual, but it may take several months. Active assistive exercises of the hip joint also begin the day after surgery.

Early rehabilitative goals for the patient consist of regaining strength and gaining control of the prosthesis. Weight bearing is limited for the first 2 or 3 weeks while

healing takes place. Although the patient may become confident as he progresses to crutches, he should never be allowed to walk without supervision. He may need to be reminded frequently of this limitation if he becomes enthusiastic over the prospect of early ambulation. The nurse and therapist must provide encouragement with the right amount of restraint.

The cast is changed approximately 10 days after surgery. The stitches are usually removed at this time, and another cast, extending to midthigh, is applied. About 10 days later, or sooner if shrinkage of the stump causes loosening, this cast is removed. Then a very short cast, which will allow for knee flexion, is applied and remains on the stump until the prosthesis is ready. The mold for a permanent prosthesis may be made 3 to 4 weeks postoperatively.

Since the amputee's progress in the rehabilitation program depends to a certain degree on a good working relationship with the therapist and prosthetist, the nurse should remind the amputee, before discharge, of the importance of maintaining this relationship.

Use of a Postoperative Air Boot

Another alternative in preparing the below-knee amputee for early ambulation with a prosthesis is the Jobst Post-Op Air Boot. This plastic air boot is applied in the operating room or the recovery room in the following manner. A piece of stockinette is slipped over the surgical dressing and the residual limb to prevent contact between plastic and skin.

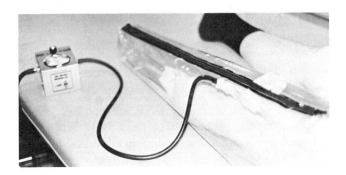

The boot is applied and an air pressure control unit with a foot pump is attached for the purpose of inflating the boot up to 25 to 30 mm Hg pressure. The air boot provides compressive pressure that will control and decrease edema in the stump while allowing visualization of the dressing. The plastic garment is worn continuously and opened for dressing changes. Ambulation with the boot and a metal cylinder is usually started 7 to 8 days postoperatively. The metal cylinder is positioned over the deflated boot, at a level

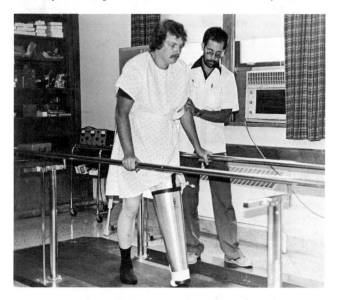

that will equalize leg lengths. Following that, the boot is inflated once more, to 45 to 50 mm Hg pressure.

Because the plastic material is subject to puncture, the air boot is designed for use in the hospital or the home. This means that the amputee will still require gait training without a prosthetic leg before discharge from the hospital.

Contraindications to the use of the Jobst boot include senility, confusion, cardiac or neurologic disability, communication problems, and known inadequate life expectancy.

Care of the Patient With Amputation of the Upper Extremity

In a highly mechanized society, traumatic amputation of the upper extremity is a fact of life. The cornpicker and power table saw are two of the culprits often responsible for the loss of hands or arms. Vascular disease rarely requires amputation of the arm.

Postoperative Care

Usually, then, the orthopedic nurse is confronted with a patient who has had some emergency surgery following a traumatic amputation. For this reason it is rare for an immediate prosthetic fitting to be used, because any complica-

tions following trauma could go unnoticed if a rigid dressing were applied. Furthermore, equipping the patient with an immediate prosthetic hook may not be as psychologically helpful as some contend. In fact, it might intensify the emotional trauma, especially since in many instances the state of shock noted in these patients is more psychological than physiological. At any rate, vital signs must be closely monitored until they are stable.

Intravenous Therapy

Parenteral fluids containing antibiotics may be administered as prophylactic treatment against infection. How long this therapy continues will depend on the cause and extent of the initial injury. The nurse must realize that giving intravenous fluids limits the use of the unaffected arm and serves to create even greater feelings of helplessness in the patient. The nurse must anticipate his needs when planning patient care during this period.

Dressings

The dressing on the residual limb should be checked regularly to make certain it is not too tight. A drain may be left in the operative area for 2 to 3 days. Considering the trauma to the arm, this area must not be too tightly compressed, which would result in discomfort and swelling in the upper arm. Dressings are intended to provide support, not to shrink the arm. They are usually soft and bulky and are secured in place by an elastic bandage. The dressing should also be dry.

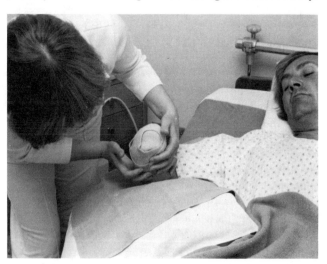

Pain

Pain is present and persists in varying degrees while the patient is hospitalized. Arm amputees often report rather severe intermittent pain for 2 or 3 months after an amputation. Part of this pain may be due to phantom sensations, simulating the pain of a cramped hand or a thumb pressing into the palm.

The possibility of pain should be discussed with the patient before discharge from the hospital. However, there is no need to cause unnecessary alarm. On the other hand, if pain occurs without some forewarning, the patient may become discouraged and stop exercising.

Positioning and Exercise

Anticipation of pain may lead to "muscle splinting" or contraction of the muscles as a protective mechanism. In turn, muscle rigidity makes movement difficult. To avoid this complication, the residual limb should be positioned and supported so as to promote muscle relaxation. In addition, the patient should be encouraged to relax his arm to avoid muscle fatigue and subsequent discomfort. For a below-the-elbow amputee, a sling may be helpful. The end of the stump must extend out of the sling to avoid pressure on the operative area.

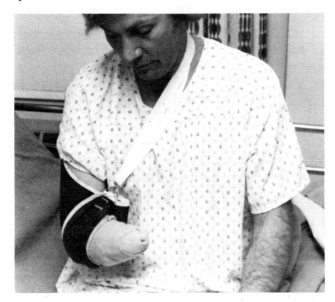

Exercises begin on the first postoperative day and are mostly assistive at first. If the patient has suffered a shoulder injury along with amputation of the upper extremity, he may be reluctant to exercise independently and

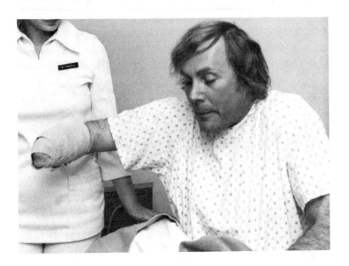

therefore must be encouraged and assisted in doing his exercises. For an above-the-elbow amputation, range of motion of the shoulder is carried out. In the instance of a below-the-elbow amputation, both range of motion of the shoulder and extension of the elbow become important aspects of exercising. Shrugging the shoulders and breathing deeply are important for all upper extremity amputees. Exercises should be done with help or supervision several times a day.

Arm amputees are up and around early in the recovery period, at which time posture should be noted. How does the patient hold the residual limb when he walks? Is it rigid, flexed? Is his shoulder hunched? It must be remembered that some deviation in posture will occur due to loss of the weight of the arm and is manifested by a tendency to tilt the trunk away from the amputated side while tilting the head toward the amputated side (see photo below, on left). The result could be foreshortening of the shoulder girdle. If this consequence is explained to the patient, he may make a more conscious effort to walk and stand straight, as shown in the photo on the right. The end result of such effort, of course, is ease in the fitting and wearing of a functional prosthesis.

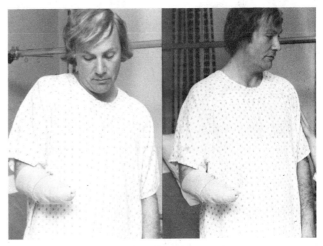

Psychological Considerations

What are some fairly typical worries and adjustments that the arm amputee faces? One of the biggest concerns may be how to relearn the activities that were done with the lost hand or hands. Writing, eating, carrying bundles, selecting coins, taking care of personal hygiene, using a can opener, tying a tie, driving a car are only a few of the activities that the amputee may have to relearn. If he has lost his dominant hand, such retraining may require a tremendous amount of time. The awkwardness of doing everything with one hand can prove very frustrating. In some instances, a temporary or even permanent change in occupation may be necessary and can be truly disastrous in terms of income and supporting a family. Supportive nursing care includes allowing the patient to ventilate his feelings and express his worries.

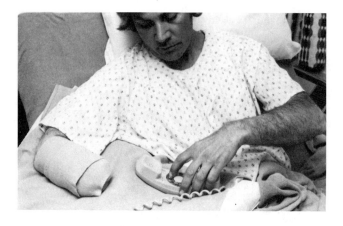

Molding the Stump

Bandaging to mold the upper extremity stump begins when the stitches are removed. The elastic bandage is secured at the proximal end of the limb with wrapping beginning at the

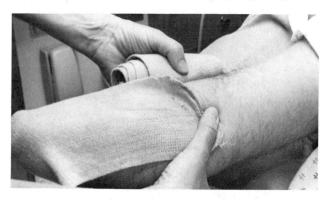

distal end. The wrap must be smooth and applied in such a way as to prevent circular constriction while providing compression without discomfort. Methods of wrapping the stump of a lower extremity can be adapted for use on the arm.

When the residual arm is being wrapped, compression is greatest at the distal end, being gradually decreased as the bandage is applied in a proximal direction. Keeping the bandage in place becomes a problem if the stump is short.

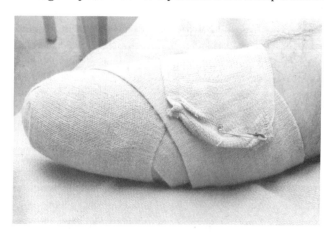

Since wrapping the stump can be awkward or nearly impossible for the amputee, a family member or some available person should be taught the bandaging procedure.

The time required to mold a residual arm is about 3 months. An arm stump will usually shrink less than a leg stump, unless the arm is very fat.

UPPER EXTREMITY PROSTHESIS

Preparation for a Prosthesis

In addition to having the stump molded, the patient requires physical preparation before a prosthesis is fitted. Regular visits to a physical therapy department are necessary to be certain that the exercises are keeping the arm in the best condition possible. Both shoulders should be exercised to maintain a mobile shoulder girdle, because the amputee uses both in operating the prosthesis. Emphasis on posture remains important, since "round" shoulders make prosthetic fitting difficult. The patient with an above-the-elbow amputation should be instructed to practice contracting the biceps during the exercise periods. Doing this exercise strengthens the biceps muscle and decreases the amount of excess tissue in the stump.

The amputee must be psychologically prepared for the fact that the prosthesis cannot totally replace the hand. Although some of the functions of the hand can be reproduced, the amputee should be aware that it takes time to become accustomed to the lack of sensation.

All physical and psychological preparation for an upper extremity prosthesis should begin in the hospital, since planning is the major part of the work that goes into a prosthesis. Remember, planning includes promoting and maintaining a positive attitude in the amputee, and is the responsibility of the entire orthopedic team.

The Body-Powered Arm Prosthesis: Components and Control

In general, prostheses for the upper extremity function by means of a terminal device that is powered by a control cable. The terminal device commonly used is the split hook. It is simple, sturdy, and easy to maintain. The most popular hook is designed to open voluntarily by a control cable, and then close by heavy rubber bands. Essentially, the function

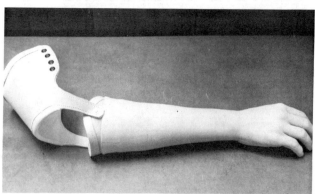

of the hook is to grasp and carry objects. A cosmetic hand offers less manual dexterity than the hook and may be used as a "dress" hand only.

The principal components of upper extremity prostheses depend on the level of amputation. Besides the terminal device, they include a socket and various arm sections made of plastic laminates, plus the wrist unit and the elbow unit, which are both made of metal.

A harness suspends the prosthesis from the shoulders and transmits power by means of control cables, to provide substitute functions for those that are missing.

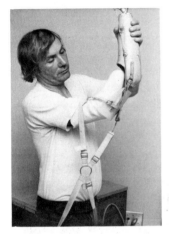
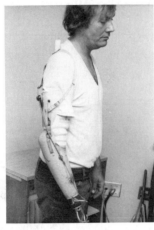

Since the level of amputation also determines the number of functions that are lost, it is logical that the control system of a prosthesis becomes more complex at each succeeding level. For instance, an above-elbow amputee must master elbow joint function so that he can place his hand at a desired position in space. This involves both flexing and locking the elbow.

The main source of power in upper extremity amputees is the shoulder girdle and the residual limb. This power is transmitted through the control cable to a terminal device in the below-elbow amputee. In the above-elbow amputee, this power serves a dual purpose. It will flex the elbow and open the terminal device. Two control cables may be used.

The shoulder prosthesis depends on scapular abduction, adduction, and shoulder elevation to provide power for terminal device operation, forearm flexion, and locking and unlocking of the elbow joint. There is no satisfactory mechanical substitute for shoulder joint motion. A friction joint in the shoulder region allows the amputee to position the shoulder joint as required for specific uses.

The Externally Powered Arm Prosthesis

The most common externally powered arm prostheses in use today are electrical. These electrically powered limbs operate by switch or myoelectric control. A myoelectric system uses the electrical signal generated by muscle contractions to control the functioning components of a prosthesis such as the terminal device. The advantages of a myoelectric prosthesis are the following:

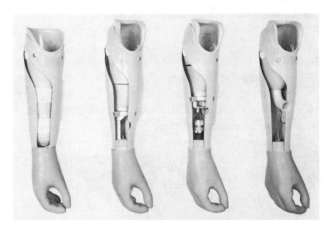

1. Control of the terminal device is more physiologically natural because the muscles that are used to control the prosthetic hand are the same muscles that are used to open and close the natural hand.
2. Less energy is required to activate the terminal device as compared to the conventional type of prosthesis.
3. The myoelectric prosthesis is more desirable from a cosmetic standpoint because there is no visible harnessing — gross body movements are not required and the prosthetic hand appears natural.
4. The muscles in the stump are used for control, and this improves circulation, which results in a "healthier" residual limb.
5. There is a greater range of operation than is possible with the body-powered prosthesis.

The myoelectric arm as developed by Otto Bock (Myobock System) is a prosthesis that may be used in cases of trauma, disease, or congenital anomaly. At present, it is primarily used for the below-elbow amputee.

The electric or motorized elbow prosthesis is a newer development for the above-elbow amputee.

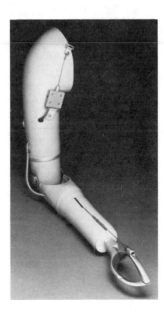

NYU-Hosmer electric elbow. (Courtesy Hosmer Dorrance Corp.)

Training the Amputee

The amputee must begin his training program by establishing a man-machine relationship. He must learn about his prosthesis: how to put it on, how to take it off, and how it functions. Following this, the first lesson in operation concerns use of the terminal device. More muscle strengthening exercises may be necessary. The above-elbow amputee must also learn how to operate the elbow lock and forearm lift. The emphasis in training is on skills that require two hands, such as tying shoelaces.

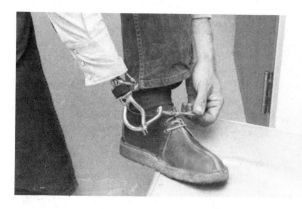

Motivation is the major determining factor in whether or not an amputee succeeds in reaching his maximum level of self-sufficiency in activities of daily living. Goals should be set according to individual needs, and may be partially based on the amputee's capabilities in relation to his former occupation.

Care of the Arm Prosthesis and Stump

The stump must be bathed daily with mild soap and water and inspected for skin problems. For amputees who take daily baths or showers the stump is simply bathed like the rest of the body.

The plastic socket should be cleansed with soap and water both inside and outside at least once a day. However, water must not be allowed to get into the mechanical components. The harness should be washed when soiled.

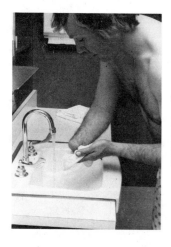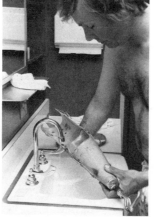

Any problems with stump or prosthesis require immediate attention of the prosthetist.

Trends in Prosthesis Design

Designers and manufacturers are constantly striving to create prostheses that are more serviceable, versatile, and cosmetic. Flexible suction sockets and vacuum-forming casts for the below-knee amputee are two examples of innovations gaining the attention of prosthetists.

Discussion Questions

1. Suggest possible approaches in planning supportive care for the following patients.

   a. B. A. is a very attractive, single, 22-year-old female who lost her right leg in a motorcycle accident. She had an AK amputation. She is a passive patient with few requests. On her sixth postoperative day she says that she no longer wants any nursing student to take care of her.

   b. L. M. is an 82-year-old widowed woman of Norwegian descent. She lives with her only daughter and her husband in an apparently harmonious arrangement. She has had an AK amputation of her right leg due to vascular disease. Her left leg is "good." She is alert and cheerful. The nursing staff calls her a "doll." PT has arranged an arm exercise program for her because she is determined to be independent, use crutches, and eventually get a prosthesis. Upon learning about the exercise program and the patient's intentions, the physician states that it is all a "waste of time because of her age." He does not believe a prosthesis is advisable. The daughter does "not know what to think."

Consider: a. What must you know about this patient's relationships with others? What clues might you look for to help determine how her amputation has affected her self-image? Of what significance is her age, marital status? Will it be of any value to know about her occupation and interests? Why? What feelings might she have about students? Why? What information must be obtained from students who have been assigned to her care? b. Who has the problem in this situation?

2. Write a plan of assessment and care for the following patients.

   a. M. D. is a 30-year-old milk truck driver whose left lower leg was crushed when his truck skidded on the ice and struck a telephone pole. He had a BK amputation of the leg. He also suffered a fractured right tibia and right radius. Both right extremities are in short plaster casts. This is his sixth postoperative day and the day the nursing staff is beginning to note that "he sleeps too much." He has a wife and two children, ages 5 and 6.

b. D. K. is a 16-year-old boy who lives on a farm. He is the oldest of four children. He lost his right arm, below the elbow, and the tips of his left middle, ring, and little fingers in a cornpicking accident. His residual limb has been surgically treated, and he has returned to the orthopedic unit. There is a bulky compression dressing on the residual limb and his three injured fingers. An intravenous solution with antibiotics is infusing in his left arm. His parents plan to stay with him "all night."

Consider: For both patients: What are their physical limitations in regard to self-care? How can the environment be adapted to their needs? What interaction with family members will be most helpful? What might the psychological needs of the family members be? In (a), of what significance is the fact that the patient is sleeping so much? For (b), what immediate postoperative assessment is important?

Bibliography

Bennett D: Activities of living: A problem of mobility, part 5. Nurs Times 80(24):46, 1984

Bourne BA, Kutcher JL: Amputation: Helping a patient face loss of a limb. RN, p. 38–45, Feb 1985

Brunner NA: Orthopedic Nursing, 4th ed. St. Louis, CV Mosby, 1983

Buckwalter KC, et al: Musculo-skeletal conditions and sexuality, part 2. Sex Disabil 5(4):195, 1982

Clark GS, et al: Rehabilitation of the elderly amputee. J Am Geriatr Soc 31(7):439, 1983

Clarke-Williams MJ: Problems of lower limb amputee. NJ Pract 220(1319):703, 1978

Conine TA, Evans JH: Sexual reactivation of chronically ill and disabled adults. J Allied Health 11(4):261, 1982

Connolly J: Phantom and stump pain following operation. Psychotherapy, 65(1):13, 1979

Crenshaw AH (ed): Campbell's Operative Orthopaedics, 6th ed. St. Louis, CV Mosby, 1980

Datta PK: Lower limb amputations: The last report. Nurs Mirror 54:41, 1982

Dealing with emergency amputations. Nurs '80 10(4):82, 1980

Dixon D: An erotic attraction to amputees. Sex Disabil 6(1):3, 1983

Ebbage SL: Lower limb amputation following peripheral vascular disease. Nursing (Oxford) 2(26):773, 1984

Farrell J: Helping the new amputee. Orthop Nurs 1(3):18, 1982

Frank RG, et al: Psychological response to amputation as a function of age and time since amputation. Br J Psychiatry 144:493, 1984

Furst L, Humphrey M: Coping with the loss of a leg. Prosthet Orthot Int 7(3):152, 1983

Gandy ED, Veigh G: Help the amputee stand on his own again. Nursing (Horsham) 14(7):46, 1984

Hankes DD: Self-care: Assessing the aged client's need for independence. J Gerontol Nurs 10(5):26, 1984

Hilt N, Cogburn S: Manual of Orthopedics. St. Louis, CV Mosby, 1980

Howard DL: Group therapy for amputees in a ward setting. Milit Med 148(8):678, 1983

Jackson RW, Davis GM: The value of sports and recreation for the physically disabled. Orthop Clin North Am 14(2):301, 1983

Karcher WC: Anxiety reduction in lower limb amputees. Rehabil Nurs 8(4):15, 1983

Kashani JH, et al: Depression amoung amputees. J Clin Psychiatry, 44(7):256, 1983

Larson C, Gould M: Orthopedic Nursing, 9th ed. St. Louis, CV Mosby, 1978

Lockstone G: A lower limb amputee. Nurs Times 79(33):23, 1983

McNaughton D: The physical and social adjustment problems of amputees. Cona J 5(2):20, 1983

Meador R: Learning to live with a new leg. Am J Nurs 79:1393, 1979

Meinhart NT, McCaffery M: Pain: A Nursing Approach to Assessment and Analysis. Norwalk, CT, Appleton-Century-Crofts, 1983

Merkley R: Nineteen, and facing a right below-elbow amputation. Cona J 5(2):14, 1983

Moyer K: Nursing management of a patient undergoing medical amputation . . . involves freezing of the affected extremity. Crit Care Update 19(7):7, 1983

Pasnau RO: Psychologic aspects of postamputation pain. Nurs Clin North Am 11:679, 1976

Patricelli J, et al: Adapted knife for partial hand-amputation patients. Am J Occup Ther 36:193, 1982

Pfefferbaum B: Postamputation grief. Nurs Clin North Am 11:687, 1976

Plombon M: Teaching plan for amputation. Diabetes Educ 8(4):34, 1983

Postop needs of the amputee: RN Master Care Plan. RN, p. 46, Feb 1985

Quinn L: It's worth the effort–I know! RN p. 57, Oct 1976

Raney RB, Brashear HR: Shand's Handbook of Orthopaedic Surgery, 9th ed. St. Louis, CV Mosby, 1978

Reinstein L, et al: Sexual adjustment after lower extremity amputation. Arch Phys Med Rehabil 59(11):501, 1978

Roon AJ, et al: Below-knee amputation: A modern approach. Am J Surg 134(1):153, 1977

Rubin G, Fleiss D: Devices to enable persons with amputation to participate in sports. Arch Phys Med Rehabil 64(1):37, 1983

Ruby LK: Acute traumatic amputation of an extremity. Orthop Clin North Am 9(3):679, 1978

Rutan FM: Preprosthetic program for the amputee. Orthop Nurs 1(3):14, 1982

Scott J: Peter's challenge . . . osteosarcoma. Nurs Mirror 155(18):56, 1982

Shine MS: Discharge planning for the elderly patient in the acute care setting. Nurs Clin North Am 18(2):403, 1983

Solomon GF, et al: A burning issue. Phantom limb pain and psychological preparation of the patient for amputation. Arch surg 113(2):185, 1978

Southcombe A: Hindquarter amputation . . . Nurs Times 78(45):1889, 1982

Stoudemire A: The onset and adaptation to cancer: Psychodynamics of an ill physician. Psychiatry 46(4):377, 1983

Stratmann DT, et al: Determination of ideal body weight and nutritional requirements post amputation. Orthop Nurs 3(3):37, 1984

Thompson DM, Haran D: Living with an amputation: The patient. Int Rehabil Med 5(4):165, 1983

Thorek P: Anatomy in Surgery, 2nd ed. Philadelphia, JB Lippincott, 1962

Turek SL: Orthopaedics: Principles and Their Application, 3rd ed. Philadelphia, JB Lippincott, 1977

Tursay A, Sonuvar B: Emotional aspects of arm or leg amputation in children. Can J Psychiatry 28(4):294, 1983

Walters J: Coping with a leg amputation. Am J Nurs 81:1349, 1981

Wedman B: Nutrition for the amputee. Diabetic Educ, 8(4):29–31, Winter 1983

Wiley L (ed): Battered body: A teenage amputee taught us four tips for better long-term care. Nursing '78 78(8):36, 1978

Wiley SD: Structural treatment approach for families in crisis. A challenge to rehabilitation. Am J Phys Med 62(6):271, 1983

9

Special Orthopedic Surgery: Nursing Implications

There are many surgical procedures in orthopedics in which postoperative care is based primarily on general principles of orthopedic nursing involving the neurovascular status of an extremity and methods of immobilization. However, the particulars of nursing care are determined by the specific situation and the individual patient. For example, though many patients undergoing these procedures have similar dressings or casts, their pains and problems are not necessarily the same. Therefore, the nursing observations and care are not entirely the same. The discomfort experienced by the patient who has had a carpal tunnel release is different from that of one who has undergone release of a Dupuytren's contracture. Yet both patients may have bandages on the wrist and hand. Similarly, nursing the patient with a triple arthrodesis is basically the care of a patient with a casted extremity, but unless the nurse knows what the procedure entails, it is difficult to determine whether or not drainage on the cast is "normal."

Other orthopedic surgical procedures that might be considered "special" are those joint replacements that are not as common as total hips and knees and digital replantation techniques.

One goal of this chapter is to define various common orthopedic conditions, identify corrective surgical procedures, provide insights into specific nursing problems that may arise, and establish some guidelines for patient teaching. The second is to discuss selected procedures that reflect trends in orthopedics and to present general principles of nursing care.

Foot Surgery

Common Problems and Corrective Procedures

Regardless of its size or shape, the foot bears the weight of the human body on its bony structure during such activities as walking, running, skipping, jumping, dancing, and so on. Like other complicated bony structures, the foot with its multiplicity of muscles and tendons is prone to numerous disorders and malfunctions, whether from disease, trauma, congenital conditions, or structural breakdown. Many conditions within each of these categories are subject to surgical correction. However, since our purpose here is to deal with the more common types of problems encountered in a hospital's orthopedic department, the discussion will briefly cover such conditions as hallux valgus, hammertoes, Morton's neuroma, and foot instability requiring triple arthrodesis.

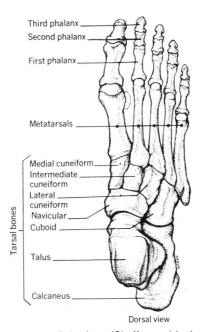

Bony structure of the foot. (Chaffee and Lytle. Basic Physiology and Anatomy, 4th ed. Lippincott, 1980)

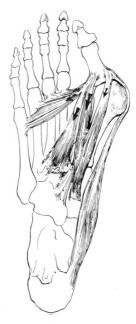

Bunion formation. (Turek: Orthopaedics, 3rd ed. Lippincott, 1977)

Hallux Valgus

This deformity is characterized by lateral deviation of the large toe at the metatarsophalangeal joint. The medial side of the first metatarsal head is usually enlarged. A bony prominence covered by a bursa may develop over this area and is known as a *bunion*.

Hallux valgus deformity is primarily congenital in nature, although arthritis of the first metatarsophalangeal joint may be a predisposing factor. Whether or not shoes that are too narrow or short are factors in the development of bunions is debatable, although bunions do seem to be more common in women. Pain is the reason for surgical removal.

Operative Procedures. The operative treatment of disabling and painful bunions can be simple or complex, depending on the extent of deformity. A simple *bunionectomy* involves removing the bony growth and bursa.

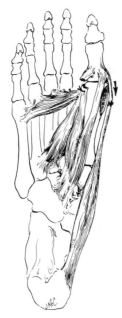

Bunionectomy. (Turek: Orthopaedics, 3rd ed. Lippincott, 1977)

A more complex procedure is *metatarsal osteotomy*, which involves removing a wedge at the proximal end of the first metatarsal bone. Other osteotomies may be done also. For example, in the Keller operation, the proximal one-half of the first phalanx is also resected and a Kirschner wire is sometimes inserted longitudinally through the great toe and into the first metatarsal. If a wire is inserted, it will protrude through the end of the toe. In other surgical procedures, such as McBride's, tendons are transplanted.

Various procedures may be combined or modified to suit the individual case, since some foot deformities are associated with other abnormalities.

Postoperative Regimen. Depending on the type of procedures used to correct the hallux valgus, a compression dressing or a short cast may be applied. The period of hospitalization ranges from several days to a week.

The amount of weight bearing allowed, and therefore the period of crutchwalking, also varies according to the surgical procedure. When osteotomies are done, the patient may not be permitted to bear weight for 4 to 6 weeks. In the McBride operation, in which the soft tissues are primarily involved, the patient may be allowed to walk on his heels several days after surgery, with gradual resumption of normal activities after the sutures have healed.

Nursing assessment and interventions applicable to the bunionectomy patient are summarized on pages 298–300.

Hammertoes

A hammertoe is a dorsiflexion of the metatarsophalangeal joint with plantar flexion of the proximal interphalangeal joint of the second toe. This condition is often associated with a bunion. As a result of a hammertoe, corns may develop on the dorsum of the flexed proximal interphalangeal joint and on the end of the toe due to irritation from the shoe. A callus may develop on the plantar surface of the foot over the prominent metatarsal head. Patients may complain of burning on the bottom of the foot and pain and difficulty in walking when wearing shoes.

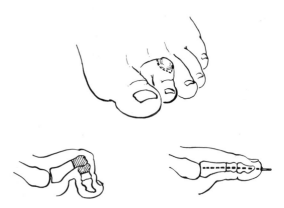

Surgical correction of hammertoe. (Turek: Orthopaedics, 3rd ed. Lippincott, 1977)

Surgical Treatment. Some surgeons begin by removing the corn, although others consider this step unnecessary since the corns disappear after the deformity has been corrected and pressure from the shoe has been relieved. The main steps in correcting a hammertoe involve resecting the base of the middle phalanx and the head of the proximal phalanx and bringing the raw ends of these bones together. The corrected position is maintained by fixation of a Kirschner wire.

Postoperative Regimen. Following surgery to correct a hammertoe, a compression dressing is usually applied. The patient will be crutchwalking as soon after surgery as he is able, and weight bearing is permitted in 2 weeks. The wire is removed in 3 to 4 weeks.

Morton's Neuroma

Morton's toe, also known as perineural fibrosis, is a neuroma, usually in the web space, subjecting the third or fourth toe to sudden sharp attacks of pain, as well as burning sensations. Hyperesthesia may be present on the opposing surfaces of the two affected toes. The treatment is surgical removal.

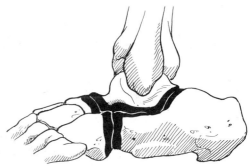

Triple arthrodesis (Turek: Orthopaedics, 3rd ed. Lippincott, 1977)

The procedure involves removing the articular cartilage along with wedges of bone and fitting the bone ends together. Dead space is packed with bone chips taken from the

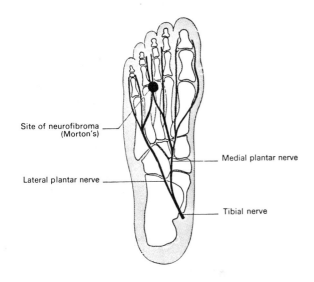

Site of neurofibroma (Morton's)

Lateral plantar nerve

Medial plantar nerve

Tibial nerve

Morton's neuroma. (Brunner and Suddarth: Textbook of Medical-Surgical Nursing, 4th ed. Lippincott, 1980)

Postoperative Regimen. A compression dressing is usually applied to the foot following surgery. Ambulation is permitted in the immediate postoperative period with full weight bearing allowed as soon as the wound is healed.

Foot Instability: Triple Arthrodesis

Instability of the foot requiring surgical correction may be due to fractures of the calcaneus or other joint bones in the foot; muscle imbalance, irritative changes in the joint (resulting from rheumatoid arthritis, osteoarthritis, tuberculosis of the bone, or trauma); rigid spastic flat foot; or congenital defects in the union of the bones.

Surgical Correction. The operative procedure that is most often recommended in these instances is a triple arthrodesis, which creates a fusion of the talocalcaneal, talonavicular, and calcaneocuboid joints and eliminates inversion and eversion at the subtalar joint.

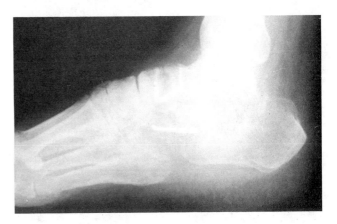

joint itself. Staples are often used to hold the bones together more securely.

Some forms of foot instability may be corrected without disrupting the joint space by inserting dowel grafts from the iliac crest between the joint bones to create fusion and stabilize the foot. However, this procedure does add the risk of another potential infection site since it necessitates a separate incision to obtain bone grafts.

Postoperative Regimen. Following a triple arthrodesis, a plaster cast is applied to immobilize the foot while fusion takes place. The period of hospitalization is about 4–5 days but depends on the amount of discomfort the patient is having and his adjustment to crutchwalking. Sutures are removed in about 2 weeks. The patient may be on crutches for 1 month to 6 weeks without weight bearing, depending on the procedure that was done. A walking cast may be applied 6 weeks after surgery and worn for 3 months. Many times corrective surgery on a foot is based on a very individual problem. Surgery of this kind may involve transferring tendons. The nurse should be aware of how much motion the surgeon expects in the toes and whether or not it should be checked at all.

THE PATIENT WHO HAS HAD A BUNIONECTOMY: PROBLEM SOLVING

Significant Data: S. F. is a 27-year-old Physical Education teacher who is single and lives alone. She is 5′7″ tall and weighs 125 lb. This is her first hospitalization, and she has had a bunionectomy with a metatarsal osteotomy. She has no other medical problems or allergies. It is the first week in June, and she has no definite summer plans for when she is released from the hospital. She will not be allowed to bear full weight on her foot for 4 weeks after discharge from the hospital. She is in a ''slipper'' cast that does not cover her malleoli. She has a Kirschner wire through her great toe, and the end of the toe and the wire are protected by a metal splint in the cast.

7 A.M. Third Post-operative Day	Ongoing Assessment	Data Collected	Nursing Interventions
1. S. F. states she was awake for long periods during the night, although this was not evident on nursing rounds.	1. Has she any concerns that might be keeping her awake? Remember, this is her first hospitalization. Is she constipated? How did she respond to using the bedpan? Is immobility making her restless? What is her normal sleep pattern and evening routine? What might the evening shift do to make her routines more normal? She is ''lean''—does she need more backrubs over bony prominences?	1. Is slightly constipated and ''hates'' bedpan. Runs every evening. Retires at 11 P.M. on school nights. Evening hospital routines are ''fine.'' ''Loves'' backrubs. Being immobile is not difficult except for ''now when I ache all over.''	1. Encourage the patient to ask for assistance when getting up to go to the bathroom on crutches. Reinforce necessity for fluids and proper diet. Stool softener or laxative. Walk in hall with crutches and assistance, late in evening as tolerated. ''Extra'' backrub at bedtime.

NURSING CARE AFTER FOOT SURGERY

Dressing and Casts

After a simple surgical procedure on the foot, such as a simple bunionectomy or removal of a Morton's neuroma, the foot will be wrapped in a bulky dressing and the toes will be partially hidden. Bloody drainage is not normally present on the external wrapping.

For more complex or multiple procedures a short leg cast or foot cast will be applied. The amount of drainage on the cast will depend on the extent of the surgical procedure. A

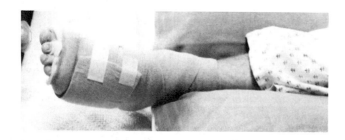

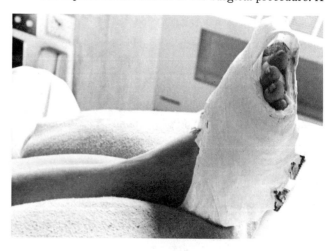

7 A.M. Third Post-operative Day	Ongoing Assessment	Data Collected	Nursing Interventions
2. She was medicated for pain at 3 and 6 A.M. Still complains of much pain in foot and muscle cramps in both legs. Calves were not tender or reddened. Homans' sign is negative. Can move her four toes. Toes are warm to the touch. Temperature is normal.	2. She was up on crutches yesterday. Is this contributing to her discomfort? Anxiety? Reassess neurovascular status of foot and check calf again. Identify exact locations of pains and discomforts.	2. Feels crutchwalking may be cause of discomfort. "Never thought it would be so tedious!" Neurovascular status of foot still satisfactory. Calves ache slightly now but no more than rest of her legs. Homans' sign still negative. No redness or tenderness.	2. Visit her before and after physical therapy to provide moral support regarding crutchwalking. Give assurance that she is making progress.
3. She also seems withdrawn or depressed this morning.	3. Does she have enough diversional activities? Is being on crutches affecting her self-image? Does she anticipate problems getting around? Are her expectations concerning her recovery and rehabilitation realistic? What are her attitudes about pain?	3. Has enough to do, is catching up on her reading. "Hates" being slow. Wonders about carrying a purse. Has had little experience with pain and did not believe it would be as great as it is. Did not "know" such a small cast could be so "clumsy." Has a small car. Worries about getting self and crutches into car.	3. Confer with therapist about patient's concerns. Check on possibility of having patient assigned to a physical therapist who is close to her life situation, single, female, athletic. Should have instructions and simulated practice getting in and out of car. Give pain medications p.r.n. Reassure her that pain is normal.

moderate to large amount of bloody drainage is to be expected on the cast of a patient with a triple arthrodesis. Cast care as discussed in Chapter 2 is part of the nursing care of these patients.

Checking Neurovascular Status

Normally, for most patients in a leg or foot cast, the neurovascular status of the toes is checked by (1) noting skin color as evidenced by the blanching test (the nail of the big toe is gently compressed between the fingers; upon release of the toe, the color should quickly change from white to pink); (2) evaluating the patient's ability to wiggle or exercise his toes; (3) feeling the toes to ascertain temperature; and (4) determining the amount of sensation present, as indicated by any patient complaints of numbness, paresthesias, or lack of feeling as each toe is slightly pinched.

However, in patients who have undergone foot surgery,

assessment of the neurovascular status of the foot may be incomplete for various reasons, including the type of procedure performed. For example, a patient who has undergone a Keller bunionectomy or correction of a hammertoe, may have pins extending through the ends of one or more toes, or a protective splint extending over the end of the foot. In such instances, moving the toes as a test of neurovascular status may be almost impossible. In addition, in most foot patients, toe discoloration from the solution used in routine preoperative preparation in the operating room makes it difficult to check circulation by means of skin color. As a result, testing the temperature of the skin by feeling the toes becomes the major means of assessing circulation in the foot and toes of these patients. As for sensation in the toes, postoperative pain in the foot may make it difficult for the patient to distinguish between pain from the operation and pain due to nerve pressure or circulatory impairment.

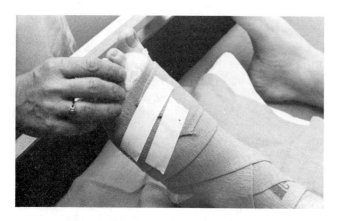

Promoting Comfort

The foot should be elevated with the heel off the bed. To prevent discomfort from swelling, icebags may be applied. For a patient in a cast following triple arthrodesis, icebags are used saddle style over the operative area for 24 to 48 hours. Keeping ice on the toes becomes a challenge. One solution is to use rubber gloves filled with crushed ice. They are fairly light and flexible and may be secured to the foot by

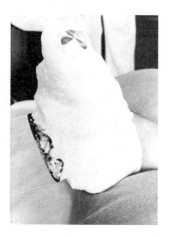 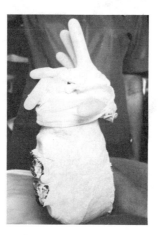

a roll of gauze, adhesive, or paper tape. The nurse must remember that the ice-filled rubber glove may "sweat" and add more moisture to the damp cast. A washcloth under the

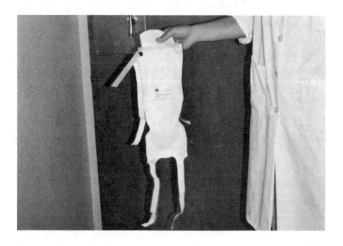

glove will absorb such moisture. Disposable icebags that are long, narrow, and have ties may work in some situations. The patient may require pain medications every 3 hours for the first 24 to 48 hours.

Problems in Ambulation

Depending on the type of surgery that was performed, pain or throbbing in the foot may be experienced when the patient begins ambulating with or without crutches. The patient with a bunionectomy is very apprehensive about bumping the toes and will tend to walk on the heels. As a result, pain in the ankles and calves becomes an added complaint. Hard-soled postoperative shoes, which are available in many sizes, provide good toe protection and a stable base for ambulation for the patient in a soft foot dressing. The shoe should fit so that the patient's toes do not come all the way to the front end.

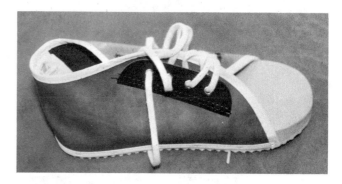

After a walking heel or irons are applied to a foot or short leg cast, the source of pain, when the patient is standing, must be identified to evaluate whether it is from the operation or due to pressure from the cast.

Patient Teaching

The nurse should reinforce instructions given by the therapist if the patient is to use crutches. To do this, the nurse must know whether or not the patient had any special problems when learning to crutchwalk. Once patients are able to ambulate without crutches, they are often reluctant to stand straight or walk with proper weight distribution. They need to be reminded that correct posture will help prevent muscle fatigue.

Patients who are discharged with a cast should be instructed in the particulars of cast care. For the patient who has undergone a triple arthrodesis, a large area of the cast may be brown in color due to old bloody drainage. If the sight of this is distressing to the patient, the nurse should wrap that part of the cast with a roll of wet plaster before discharge. The patient should be advised that there is some odor associated with this type of drainage on a cast.

The patient should also be instructed about the importance of frequent rest periods with the foot elevated during the convalescent period.

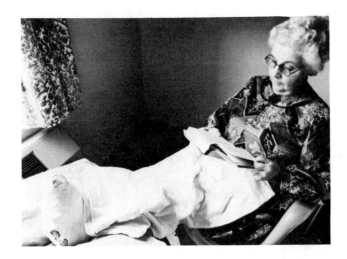

Hand and Wrist Surgery

Basic Principle

Hand repair and reconstruction procedures are not uncommon. Surgical procedures to correct problems due to injury, disease, or congenital deformities, may involve one or several digits. Many patients having surgery of this kind are in the hospital less than 24 hours. The nurse should have specific orders about elevation, application of ice, and assessment of neurovascular status for each patient who is scheduled for hand surgery other than carpal tunnel, Dupuytren's contracture release, or removal of a ganglion.

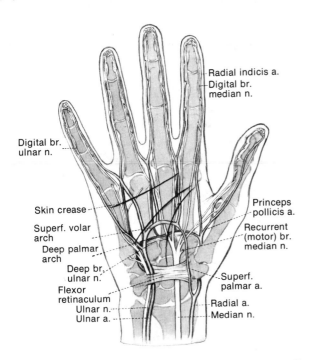

Nerve distribution in the hand. Compression of median nerve in area of the carpal tunnel (flexor retinaculum) produces carpal tunnel syndrome. (Thorek: Anatomy in Surgery. 2nd ed. Lippincott.)

Carpal Tunnel Syndrome

The carpal canal in the wrist is formed by the carpal bones and the transverse carpal ligament contained within the flexor retinaculum. The median nerve and the long flexor tendons pass through this narrow and inelastic space.

Any injury or disease that produces edema, bony deformity, or thickening of the tendon sheaths or ligament may cause compression of the median nerve or its blood supply. The resulting symptoms are called the carpal tunnel syndrome. They include tingling pain and numbness in the area of median nerve distribution. Symptoms are frequently worse at night and the patient will complain of being awakened by burning or aching pain and a "pins and needles" feeling. The pain may radiate up the forearm. If the condition is allowed to go untreated, a serious disability will result from median-nerve paralysis. The syndrome is more common in women and may be bilateral.

Treatment. Cortisone injections and splinting may provide temporary relief, but the treatment is usually a complete section of the transverse carpal ligament.

Postoperative Treatment. A splint is usually applied and covered with a pressure dressing. The patient is only in the

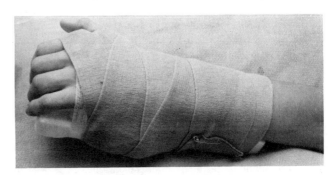

hospital for 24 – 48 hours. After 1 week a smaller dressing is applied, and normal use of the hand is encouraged. Sutures are removed 10 to 14 days after surgery.

Nursing Care. *Each* finger must be assessed separately for color, motion, temperature, and sensation (CMTS). The dressing, along with discoloration due to the solutions used in surgical preparation, may be obstacles to this routine. However, it should be carried out regularly to the extent that it is possible.

Generally, a patient who undergoes a carpal tunnel release has less pain postoperatively than preoperatively. Only occasional pain medication is required. The dressing covering hand and wrist is bulky, and swelling is not usually a problem. Therefore, icebags are not indicated.

Instruction and Exercise. The patient who has had a carpal tunnel release should be informed that numbness and tingling may persist for a short period. Once the skin is healed, hand and wrist movement should present no problems.

Dupuytren's Contracture

This common condition is characterized by a slowly progressive fibrosis contracture of the palmar fascia that usually begins in line with the ring finger at the distal palmar increase.

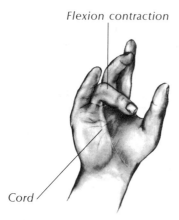

Flexion contraction

Cord

Dupuytren's contracture. (Bates: A Guide to Physical Examination, 2nd ed. Lippincott, 1979)

The contracture results in a flexion deformity, most frequently of the ring or little finger. The etiology is unknown. The main complaint of the patient is that the deformity interferes with function of the hand. It often occurs in families, usually in the older males, and can be bilateral.

Treatment. The treatment for Dupuytren's contracture is surgical release. The extent of the surgery depends on a number of variables: the degree of contracture; the age, occupation, and general health of the patient; the condition of the palmar skin; and whether or not the patient has arthritis. The operation most frequently used is a partial or selective fasciectomy. A drain is inserted following the procedure.

Postoperative Treatment. A splint and pressure dressing are applied. Gentle movement of the fingers is encouraged

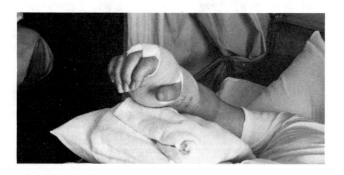

as soon as possible after surgery. Hospitalization time depends on the extent of surgery and may be only 24–48 hours. The splint and drain may be removed in 3 to 7 days and a dressing reapplied. Sutures are removed in 10 to 14 days.

Nursing Care. To prevent edema following release of Dupuytren's contractures, elevation of the hand is necessary. When elevation on pillows is not adequate, stockinette may be applied over hand and wrist, secured by tape and tied by the distal end to an attachment on the overhead frame. Icebags may be attached in a similar fashion. The arm must

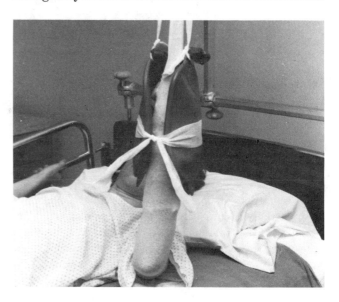

be observed for constriction due to bandaging. If the patient's arm is resting on the bed, the elbow needs to be rubbed frequently and the patient encouraged to shift position often to avoid pressure on the elbow. Ideally, the elbow should be off the mattress.

As well as possibly causing skin breakdown, pressure on the elbow may result in ulnar nerve compression. Therefore, careful evaluation of the sensation in each finger is important. Numbness or coldness in the fingers or a poor blanching sign in the fingernails indicates compression of blood vessels and requires that the bandage be loosened.

The patient may ambulate with hand and wrist resting on top of his head to decrease edema and discomfort.

Following release of a Dupuytren's contracture, active and passive exercises of the hand should be begun as soon as the skin has healed. Exercising the hand in warm water may be easier.

Ganglion

A *ganglion* is a cystic structure overlying a joint or tendon sheath, most often on the back of the wrist. The etiology is thought to be colloid degeneration of the synovial tissue during the development of the capsule or the tendon sheath.

The swelling may appear, disappear, and recur. Pain or discomfort is often present in the joint or tendon after prolonged use of the wrist. Ganglia occur most frequently in the 15-to-50 age group.

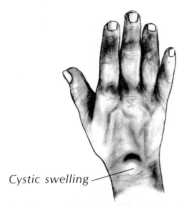

Cystic swelling

Ganglion formation. (Bates: A Guide to Physical Examination 2nd ed. Lippincott, 1979)

Treatment. The current treatment is surgical excision, with the patient being discharged from the hospital on the same day. The wrist may be immobilized in a relaxed posi-

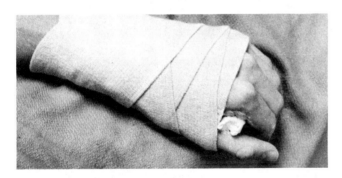

tion in a plaster splint, where it will remain for several weeks. The slight limitation of motion in the wrist is temporary. Recurrences are common.

Shoulder Surgery

Recurrent Dislocation of the Shoulder

Although the shoulder is traditionally viewed as a ball-and-socket joint with articulation primarily at the scapulohumeral (glenohumeral) joint, in actuality it is composed of four joints—the sternoclavicular, the acromioclavicular, the scapulohumeral (glenohumeral), and the thoracoscapular (scapulothoracic).

Although the sternoclavicular, acromioclavicular, and glenohumeral joints are subject to sprains, subluxations, and dislocations, one of the most common conditions encountered by the orthopedic nurse working in a hospital setting is dislocation of the glenohumeral (head of the humerus) joint.

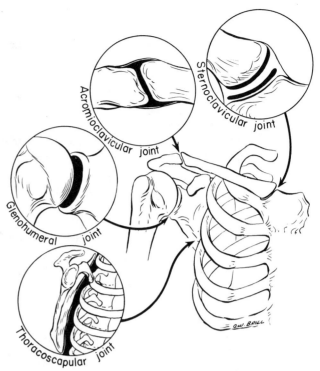

Joints of the shoulder. (DePalma: Surgery of the Shoulder, 2nd ed. Lippincott, 1973)

Since this joint is a round ball articulating with an almost flat plate (glenoid cavity of scapula), dislocation is fairly common and usually occurs in an anterior direction. Traumatic anterior dislocation is usually caused by severe forces applied to the hand, forearm, and elbow, resulting in hyperabduction.

Many patients afflicted with this condition are young adults. The symptoms of dislocation include excruciating pain and a rigidly immobile arm held in a position of abduction. The shoulder does not have its normal rounded appearance, and the upper arm appears longer than the one on the uninvolved side.

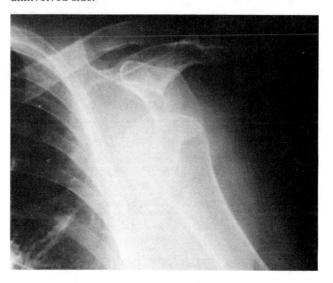

Once the shoulder joint is damaged, weakness of the musculature and relaxation of the capsular ligaments contribute to repeated dislocations. These can occur following minor movements involving abduction of the shoulder. Even sneezing has been reported as a cause of dislocation in people with severely compromised shoulders.

Treatment. The treatment for recurrent dislocation is surgical. One of the commonly used procedures is the Bristow shoulder repair. In this operation the origin of the short ends of the biceps and coracobrachialis muscles are transferred from the coracoid process to the scapular neck, medial to the anteroinferior rim of the glenoid cavity. These muscles serve as a band across the head of the humerus when the arm is in an abducted position, thus preventing dislocation.

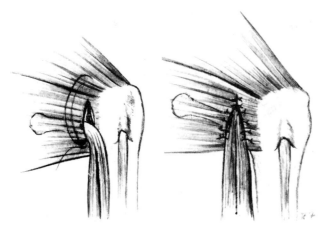

Bristow shoulder repair. (DePalma: Surgery of the shoulder, 2nd ed. Lippincott, 1973)

Postoperative Regimen. A dressing is applied and a thick cotton pad is placed in the axilla. A shoulder immobilizer is applied with an arm cuff attached at the side and a wrist cuff attached in front. The cuffs maintain the arm and shoulder in a set position. After 7 to 10 days the dressing and sutures are removed.

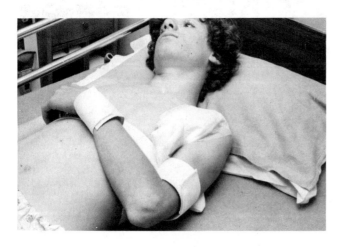

Rupture of Tendons

The shoulder is a very mobile joint and depends to a large extent on many tendons and muscles for its stability. Frequently one or more of these tendons are ruptured as a result of trauma. Degenerative changes in the musculotendinous cuff of the shoulder, which is partially formed by the infraspinatus, supraspinatus, and teres minor and is located beneath the subacromial bursa, also predispose it to ruptures in older people. Pain and limitation of motion accompany this injury.

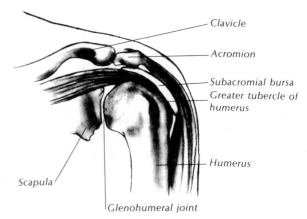

Anterior view of the shoulder. (Bates: A Guide to Physical Examination, 2nd ed. Lippincott, 1979)

Symptoms. The patient experiences pain and tenderness just below the acromion and along the greater tubercle of the humerus. Because of the tear the patient is unable to abduct his arm. Attempts to do so result in a shoulder shrugging that is characteristic of the rupture.

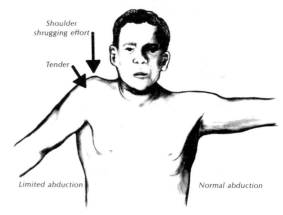

Shoulder shrugging seen in rupture of shoulder tendon. (Bates: A Guide to Physical Examination, 2nd ed. Lippincott, 1979)

Treatment. If the rupture is complete or extensive, surgical repair is indicated. For most repairs of the rotator cuff, external immobilization by means of a sling is adequate postoperatively. Pendulum exercises are started as soon as tolerated, and more active exercises are begun in 3 to 4 weeks.

NURSING CARE AFTER SHOULDER SURGERY

Vital signs should be checked every hour until stable, and the dressing should be inspected every 3 hours. Drainage is not normally visible on the dressing. If edema occurs ice-bags can be used.

As soon as the patient responds well to verbal stimuli and can evaluate the "fit" of the shoulder immobilizer, some adjustment may be necessary. For instance, if the hand is not positioned properly, the edge of the strap may cut into the wrist. If the strap over the upper arm is slipping down, circulation may be impaired at the elbow. The chest strap of the shoulder immobilizer can be another source of discomfort to the patient if it is fastened too tight.

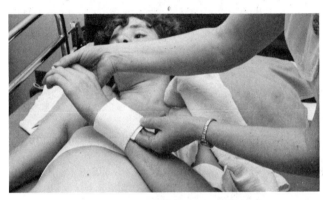

The neurovascular status of the hand should be checked every 3 hours for as long as designated by the patient care standards.

Pain

The amount of pain these patients experience is related to the extent of the procedure and the structure of the arm. A heavy arm means more tissue to incise and operate around

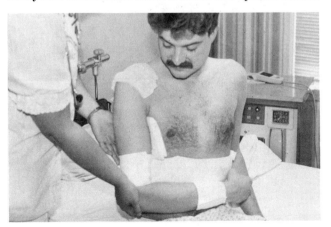

and, consequently, more postoperative pain. An arm in a shoulder immobilizer tends to fall back when the patient is lying in bed. Therefore, when assessing a complaint of pain, the nurse should check the position of the arm. Frequently, moving the arm slightly forward will relieve stress on the shoulder joint and decrease discomfort.

Psychological Considerations

The patient is often surprised at how much he depended on the affected arm to aid him in activities of daily living, even if it is not the arm he uses most. Because of awkwardness caused by the injury, he may "jar" his shoulder, causing pain, by trying to get out of bed alone too soon after the operation. The nurse should advise him, prior to any ambulation order, that he must ask for assistance the first few times he gets out of bed. To avoid undue strain, the bedside unit should be placed where it can be easily reached.

Postoperative Exercises

The immobilizer is on for 1 month and then gentle pendulum exercises may be done by the patient for several months.

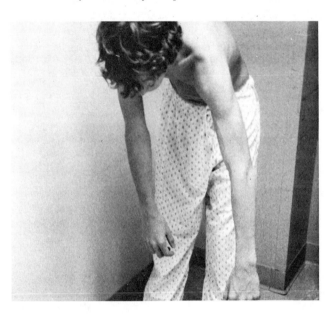

Pendulum exercises are carried out by leaning forward, allowing the arm to hang down, and then slowly swinging the arm back and forward and from side to side. The exercise program varies from surgeon to surgeon. Some advocate nothing more than gradual resumption of normal activities 3 to 4 months after surgery.

Instructions for Discharge

There are many ways in which the nurse can offer helpful suggestions when the patient is ready to be released from the hospital. In the area of skin care, she can forewarn the patient that skin irritation under the immobilizer is probably inevitable, especially in hot weather. The surgeon will usually tell the patient he may open the wrist strap, exercise his wrist, move his lower arm, and wash his hand, but that he should not move the shoulder. The nurse must reinforce this instruction and demonstrate as necessary. Perspiration

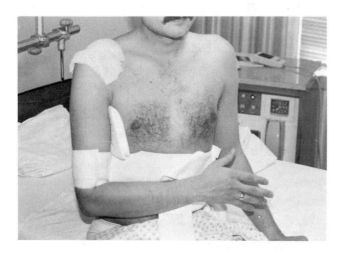

may create an odor, but the immobilizer should not be completely removed without explicit directions from the surgeon. Since spray or stick deodorant may be impossible to use under the affected arm, alcohol may be applied with a cotton ball, or a cream deodorant or commercially prepared deodorant pad can be used. Upon discharge the patient should be reminded to keep the axilla padded. Skin immobilized against skin is subject to irritation and breakdown.

To help the patient avoid undue discomfort, the nurse can point out that riding a long distance in an automobile may be uncomfortable because of the motion. Therefore, frequent stops are advisable.

Finally, the nurse should discuss with the patient the importance of adhering to the physician's orders about follow-up visits for the purpose of beginning an exercise program.

Joint Replacement

Goals

The goals of any joint replacement procedure are to decrease pain and increase function. The surgeon selects an implant that will allow him to do a reconstructive operation without resecting more than a minimal amount of bone.

Selection Criteria

The general criteria for the selection of patients who receive joint implants include the following:

1. Good general health
2. A positive outlook and willingness to cooperate
3. Satisfactory neurovascular status in the affected extremity

4. Sufficient bone stock in the joint to receive and support the implant
5. Supporting structures that have the possibility of function

Complications

Certain complications may develop that directly involve the prosthesis or implant. These include loosening, bending, fracture of the device, and dislocation. Fractures may occur in the bone around the prosthesis. The patient may have adverse reactions to the implant itself or to the bone cement. Other risks are similar to those that exist in any surgical procedure; namely, infection, bleeding, thromboembolic disease, and reactions to anesthesia, blood transfusions, or medications.

Postoperative Treatment

Joints that have been replaced are immobilized for varying periods, depending on the structures that were involved in the surgical procedure. Exercise programs are begun when the joint has "settled down" or adequate healing has taken place to allow motion.

Nursing Care of the Joint Replacement Patient

The nursing care plan for the joint replacement patient is based on maintaining the proper position of the extremity in order to promote healing and prevent complications. Close observation of the neurovascular status of the extremity is critical in the first 24 to 48 hours. Icebags are applied and the extremity is elevated. Proper position of the part must be maintained as comfortably as possible, and the nurse must remember that immobilization means restriction, not constriction. Dressings should be checked routinely for signs of drainage and should be reinforced as required. Complaints of pain and pressure must be evaluated in detail.

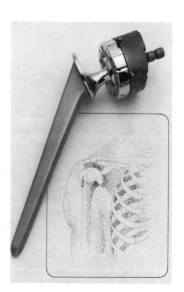

Once an exercise program is begun, the role of the nurse includes encouraging the patient and reinforcing the instructions of the physical therapist. The patient must be made aware that the responsibility for the "care" of the new joint is his and that he must make the recommended adjustment in his life-style.

Types of Joint Replacement

Shoulder Joint Replacement. Indications for this procedure include the following:

1. Rheumatoid arthritis
2. Osteoarthritis
3. Chronic and uncorrected dislocations
4. Bone necrosis
5. Joint destruction due to chronic gout
6. Loss of muscles that stabilize the humeral head in the glenoid cavity
7. A resectable tumor of the proximal humerus

Elbow Joint Replacement. The indications for this procedure are a painful, arthritic, or unstable joint. Some prostheses are designed for use when the bone of the distal humerus is gone or involved in a pathological fracture.

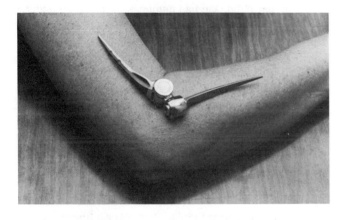

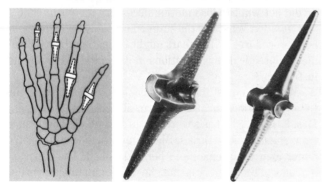

Swanson design. Dow Corning Wright Co.

Finger Joint Replacement. Implants for finger joint replacements are available in various designs. Two examples of such implants are (1) those designed for total joint replacement and (2) condylar replacements. Indications for finger joint implants include unstable or painfully stiff joints, usually due to rheumatoid arthritis. Post-traumatic disability is also an indication for this type of reconstuctive surgery.

Total Ankle Replacement. Fusion of the ankle is regarded as a desirable procedure, especially in the young and active patient, because it has a high success rate. However, total ankle replacement is an alternative to fusion or may be done when a fusion has failed. Replacement is generally indicated in cases of severe rheumatoid arthritis, osteoarthritis, or traumatic arthritis.

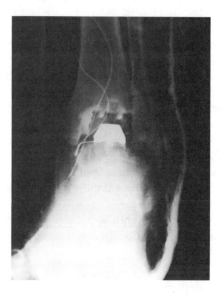

Digital Replantation

Indications

Digital replantation is done in a specially equipped center. This type of procedure is most often indicated when any of the following occurs:

1. The thumb is the amputated digit.
2. Amputation is incomplete.
3. There are multiple-digit injuries.
4. There is a solitary amputation, and the hand has been previously compromised.

Influencing Factors

The decision to attempt replantation is also influenced by many factors. They are as follows:

1. Age
2. Occupation
3. General health
4. Hand dominance
5. The presence of associated injuries
6. Time and cooling factors

7. Type and level of injury
8. Psychological factors
9. Financial status
10. Availability of microsurgery facilities
11. Microscopic assessment of the injured tissue in the operating room

Preoperative Care

The initial care of an amputated digit is critical. After 6 hours it will have irreversible muscle damage. Cooling the digit to 4°C (15.6°F) increases its tolerance to anoxia. The digit should be placed in a sterile towel moistened with Ringer's lactate or a saline solution. It should then be sealed in a plastic bag and placed on ice or in ice water. Freezing must not be allowed to occur. To avoid further tissue injury, debridement should not be attempted in spite of the fact that success of replantation also depends on the amount of contamination. When the amputation is incomplete, the injured digit should be placed in proper alignment and immobilized to prevent further damage to vessels. The extremity should be elevated.

Documentation of the exact time and mechanism of the accident is essential along with the time of the onset of cooling. All documentation, as well as the amputated part, should be kept with the patient during transport to surgical facilities.

Emergency nursing care also includes administering tetanus prophylaxis or antibiotics and initiating intravenous therapy as ordered.

Psychological Aspects

To prevent added emotional trauma, the patient and the family should not be told anything about the possibility of replantation other than the fact that such a decision will be made in the operating room.

Procedure

Microsurgical procedures are long and meticulous. Basically, the bone is shortened and the ends are joined by internal fixation. Microvascular repair involves at least one artery and two veins. A primary repair of nerves and tendons is then attempted.

Nursing Responsibilities

Precise positioning and monitoring of circulation in the hand is the primary nursing responsibility. The arm is elevated only slightly on pillows to reduce the chance of compromising arterial inflow while preventing edema. Elbow flexion is minimal to decrease the risk of compromising venous return. Color, temperature, and capillary filling should be checked every 15 minutes to 1 hour for the first 24 hours. Pallor and coolness are signs of arterial insufficiency; increased edema alerts the nurse to venous insufficiency.

All changes in the status of the hand must be recorded accurately and reported as necessary. Dressings on the hand are big and bulky and should only be changed by the surgeon. Since every effort must be made to keep pressure off the hand, the nurse must be alert to complaints of constriction caused by the dressing.

Rehabilitation

Rehabilitation of the hand may be started 3 to 4 weeks postoperatively; a highly individualized program is followed. Exposure to cold should be avoided along with stimuli that act as vasoconstrictors.

Discussion Questions

1. What nursing assessment is necessary in each of the following situations?
   a. First postoperative day — 7:00 A.M. — a 25-year-old patient with a carpal tunnel release is having "problems with pain." She has had intramuscular pain medication every 3 hours during the night, and the last one has not seemed to be effective. Besides pain in her hand, she has numbness in her little finger.
   b. Second postoperative day — 7:00 A.M. — a 42-year-old male with a Bristow shoulder repair had a 4 A.M. temperature that was 100.2°. Has moderate discomfort in shoulder. Fingers slightly cool.

Consider: (a) What is the real problem — pain or the medication? How significant is the size of the patient? What exactly is her pain like? What are the possible causes of the pain? Is it related to the numbness in her little finger? (b) Is an elevated temperature significant at this point? What other systems require assessment?

2. Discuss supportive care and discharge planning for a 47-year-old farmer and former professional baseball player who chose a total ankle replacement over a fusion because he did not want to lose motion necessary for farm work.

Consider: What has the surgeon probably told him about both procedures? What fears might the patient have? What are the practical considerations in discharge planning and instruction?

3. What data must the nurse have before she can help the following patient make long-term plans for rehabilitation? Mrs. E. is 53. She has severe loss of function in both hands from rheumatoid arthritis. She enters the hospital to have finger joint replacements in her right hand. The expected outcome of the surgery is that she will regain function in her hand.

Consider: The status of her other joints. How important is her motivation? In what ways has she altered her life-style to adapt to her disability? With whom will the nurse need to communicate besides the patient?

Bibliography

Antrobus JN: The primary deformity in hallux valgus and metatarsus primus varus. Clin Orthop 184:251, 1984

Bartell L: Bunionectomies. Orthopaed Nurs 4(1):21, 1985

Bassett RW, Cofield RH: Acute tears of the rotator cuff: The timing of surgical repair. Clin Orthop 175:18, 1983

Bateman JE: Surgery of the Shoulder. St. Louis, CV Mosby, 1984

Bates B: A Guide to Physical Examination, 2nd ed. Philadelphia, JB Lippincott, 1979

Bauman TD, et al: The acute carpal tunnel syndrome. Clin Orthop 156:151, 1981

Berger MR: Bunions: An overview. Orthop Nurs 3(5):17, 1984

Berger MR: Morton's neuroma. Orthop Nurs 1:31, 1982

Blair WF, et al: Metacarpophalangeal joint arthroplasty with a metallic hinged prosthesis. Clin Orthop 184:156, 1984

Blair WF, et al: Metacarpophalangeal joint implant arthroplasty with a Silastic spacer. J Bone Joint Surg (Am) 66(3):365, 1984

Borovov M, et al: Laser surgery in podiatric medicine—present and future. J Foot Surg 22(4):353, 1983

Bowens BA: Carpal tunnel syndrome. J Neurosurg Nurs 13(3):129, 1981

Boyes JH: Bunnell's Surgery of the Hand, 4th ed. Philadelphia, JB Lippincott, 1964

Brunner NA: Orthopedic Nursing, 4th ed. St. Louis, CV Mosby, 1983

Carlisle PS: Those miraculous digital replantations. RN 45:36, 1982

Cass JR, Morrey BF: Ankle instability: current concepts, diagnosis, and treatment. Mayo Clin Proc 59(3):165, 1984

Chaffee EE, Lytle IM: Basic Physiology and Anatomy, 3rd ed. Philadelphia, JB Lippincott, 1974

Chana GS, et al: A simple method of arthrodesis of the first metatarsophalangeal joint. J Bone Joint Surg (Br) 66(5):703, 1984

Cofield RH: Total joint arthroplasty: The shoulder. Mayo Clin Proc 54(8):500, 1979

Cohen BE, Aaronson S: Microvascular reconstructive surgery: Free tissue transfer. AORN J 38(4):602, 1983

Connolly JF: Shoulder subluxations and dislocations. Emerg Med 15(7):69, 1983

Coughlin MJ, et al: The semiconstrained total shoulder arthroplasty. J Bone Joint Surg (Am) 61(4):574, 1979

Crenshaw AH (ed): Campbell's Operative Orthopaedics, 6th ed. St. Louis, CV Mosby, 1980

Cushin B: The role of the nurse in microsurgical procedures. J Plast Reconstr Surg Nurs 1:93, 1981

DePalma A: Surgery of the Shoulder, 2nd ed. Philadelphia, JB Lippincott, 1973

Dryer RF, et al: Proximal interphalangeal joint arthroplasty. Clin Orthop 185:187, 1984

Evans GA, et al: Acute rupture of the lateral ligament of the ankle. To suture or not to suture? J Bone Joint Surg (Br) 66(2):209, 1984

Ewald FC, Jacobs MA: Total elbow arthroplasty. Clin Orthop 182:137, 1984

Freeing a frozen shoulder. Emerg Med 16(9):98, 1984

Gamble PC: The OR nurse and microsurgery. Today's OR Nurse 5(9):33, 1983

Gelberman RH, et al: The carpal tunnel syndrome: A study of carpal canal pressures. J Bone Joint Surg (Am) 63(3):380, 1981

Goss CM (ed): Gray's Anatomy, 20th ed. Philadelphia, Lea & Febiger, 1973

Graham CE, Graham DM: Morton's neuroma: A microscopic evaluation. Foot Ankle 5(3):150, 1984

Greenfield J, et al: Morton's interdigital neuroma: Indications for treatment by local injections versus surgery. Clin Orthop 185:142, 1984

Guiloff JR, et al: Morton's metatarsalgia: Clinical, electrophysiological and histological observations. J Bone Joint Surg (Br), 66(4):586, 1984

Hilt N, Cogburn S: Manual of Orthopedics. St. Louis, CV Mosby, 1980

Hollinshead WH: Textbook of Anatomy, 3rd ed. Hagerstown, Harper & Row, 1974

Horne G, et al: Chevron osteotomy for the treatment of hallux valgus. Clin Orthop 183:32, 1984

Inglis AE: Revision surgery following a failed total elbow arthroplasty. Clin Orthop 170:213, 1982

Kaplan EG, et al: Triple arthrodesis. J Foot Surg 15(3):93, 1976

Kilfoyle RM, et al: Nonexcision triple arthrodesis of the foot. Orthop Clin North Am 7(4):841, 1976

Lachiewicz PF, et al: Total ankle replacement in rheumatoid arthritis. J Bone Joint Surg (Am) 66(3):340, 1984

Langley LL, et al: Dynamic Anatomy and Physiology, 5th ed. New York, McGraw-Hill, 1980

Larson C, Gould M: Orthopedic Nursing, 9th ed. St. Louis, CV Mosby, 1978

Lindgren U, Turan I: A new operation for hallux valgus. Clin Orthop 175:179, 1983

Mercier LR: Practical Orthopedics. Chicago, Year Book Medical Publishers, 1980

Meuli H: Arthroplasty of the wrist. Clin Orthop 149:118, 1980

Miller BK: How to spot—and treat—carpal tunnel syndrome early. Nursing (Horsham) 10(3):50, 1980

Miller BK, Gregory M: Carpal tunnel syndrome. AORN J 38(3):525, 1983

Morrey BF, Bryan RS: Infection after total elbow arthroplasty. J Bone Joint Surg (Am) 65(3):330, 1983

Nalebuff EA: The rheumatoid hand: Reflections on metacarpophangeal arthroplasty. Clin Orthop 182:150, 1984

Nelson-Harvey C, Guyon B: Microvascular surgical repair of severed limbs. Crit Care Nurse, 3(5):113, 1983

Newton SE III: Total ankle arthroplasty, clinical study of fifty cases. J Bone Joint Surg (Am) 64A(1):104, 1982

Nissen KI: An explanation of Morton's metatarsalgia. Practitioner 227(1381):1179, 1983

Norwood LA: Treatment of acute shoulder dislocations. Ala Med 54(6):30, 1984

Nugent GR: Carpal tunnel syndrome. Hosp Med 19(3):31, 1983

O'Donaghue DH: Treatment of Injuries to Athletes, 3rd ed. Philadelphia, WB Saunders, 1976

O'Neill T: Microsurgery. Nursing (Oxford), 1:1449, 1982

Orgel MG: Experimental studies with clinical application to peripheral nerve injury: A review of the past decade. Clin Orthop 163:98, 1982

Patterson DC: Musculoskeletal examination. Occup Health Nurs 32(7):356, 1984

Pearson A: Replantation of a hand: The use of microsurgery today. J Plast Reconst Surg Nurs 2:71, 1982

Post M, et al: Rotator cuff tear: Diagnosis and treatment. Clin Orthop 173:78, 1983

Prilook ME: Coping with carpal tunnel syndrome. Patient Care 15(8):135, 1981

Pyle KL, et al: Carpal tunnel syndrome: Case data and nursing implications. J Neurosurg Nurs 16(6):292, 1984

Raney RB, Brashear HR: Shands' Handbook of Orthopaedic Surgery, 9th ed. St. Louis, CV Mosby, 1978

Rosenberg GM, Turner RH: Nonconstrained total elbow arthroplasty. Clin Orthop 187:154, 1984

Ross DG: Frozen shoulder. Orthop Nurs 2(2):45, 1983

Rowe CR, et al: Recurrent anterior dislocation of the shoulder after surgical repair: Apparent causes of failure and treatment. J Bone Joint Surg (Am) 66(2):159, 1984

Sadler C: New techniques in orthopaedic surgery. Nurs Mirror 153:ii, 1981

Scranton PE, Jr: Principles in bunion surgery. J Bone Joint Surg 65(7):1026, 1983

Sermeus SM: Digital replantation — the nurse's touch. Crit Care Nurse 4(33):956, 1984

Sermeus SM: Reconstructive microsurgery — high tech, high touch nursing. Orthop Nurs 3(2):10, 1984

Simonet WT, Cofield RH: Prognosis in anterior shoulder dislocation. Am J Sports Med 12(1):19, 1984

Stauffer RN: Salvage of painful total ankle arthroplasty. Clin Orthop 170:184, 1982

Stauffer RN: Total joint arthroplasty: The ankle. Mayo Clin Proc 54(9):570, 1979

Strauch B, Terzis JK: Replantation of digits: Microvascular surgery and limb replantation. Clin Orthop, 133:35, June, 1978

Szabo RM, et al: Sensibility testing in patients with carpal tunnel syndrome. J Bone Joint Surg (Am) 66(1):60, 1984

Thro E: Instrumentation for microsurgery. JORRI 2:7, 1982

Tubiana R, et al: Location of Dupuytren's disease on the radial aspect of the hand. Clin Orthop 168:222, 1982

Turek S: Orthopaedics: Principles and Their Application, 3rd ed. Philadelphia, JB Lippincott, 1977

Weiker GG: At the shoulder: This sporting arm. Emerg Med 15(14):152, 1983

Weiland AJ, et al: Vascularized bone autografts: Experience with 41 cases. Clin Orthop 174:87, 1983

When to look into a shoulder. Emerg Med 16(5):71, 1984

Zechman JS: Stress fracture of the second metatarsal after Keller bunionectomy. J Foot Surg 23:63, 1984

10

Care of the Patient With Chronic Bone or Joint Disease

Perhaps the most frustrating aspect of orthopedic nursing is caring for the patients with chronic bone or joint disease. This is easily understood when one considers that orthopedic nursing most often involves working with patients who have had constructive, even creative, procedures done for the purpose of repair or reconstruction. The nursing management of these patients promises immediate satisfaction and reward. The patient recovers "before your very eyes." Patient education is exciting for a nurse who can base instruction on the knowledge that the patient will have improved function and relief of pain in a predictable length of time. But what can a nurse promise a patient with multiple myeloma or rheumatoid arthritis?

Many chronic medical problems do not necessarily "show" on patients or affect their mobility and independence to a significant degree. However, most of the time victims of bone or joint disease lose function and mobility and also undergo obvious changes in appearance.

Learning to live with pain, disfigurement, and restricted activity requires that an individual and those who care about him develop and maintain a tremendous supply of inner resources such as hope, courage, and determination. One way of approaching the nursing care of the patient with a chronic bone or joint disease is to consider it a commitment to helping strengthen and increase those inner resources. From that viewpoint, this kind of nursing becomes very constructive, more challenging, and deeply rewarding.

Review: The Structure and Function of Bone

Definition of Bone

Bone is a dynamic tissue in that it is constantly remodeling in response to the demands of the body for support and locomotion. Older bone is replaced by new bone that is laid down in organized patterns to withstand stress and strain. Bone is classified as a form of connective tissue because (1) its chief constituents are intercellular material, and (2) it provides support of epithelium and other tissues. The inter-

cellular substance of bone is composed of collagenous, or protein, fibers embedded in a solid matrix. These fibers reinforce bone in much the same way as steel rods reinforce concrete.

Although bone seems to be a rigid tissue, it is slightly elastic. This property enables it to tolerate a substantial degree of stress.

Gross Anatomy

Bone is called *osseous tissue*. It is either cancellous (trabecular) or compact. *Cancellous bone* is a spongy structure that is located in the interior portion of a bone. It is composed of slender bony processes called *trabeculae* and concentric rings of bony tissue known as *lamellae*. Most of the cancellous tissue in long bones is located at the proximal ends. Flat bones and short bones, like the sternum, ribs, cranial bones, and vertebral bodies, are primarily made up of cancellous, or spongy, bone tissue. The exterior portion of a bone is composed of compact tissue that is dense and feels hard, like ivory; it is called the *cortex*, or cortical bone.

Bone cavities and canals are lined with a loosely woven vascular membrane known as *endosteum*. Periosteum is the tough, fibrous membrane that covers all bone surfaces except those that go into the construction of joints. Periosteum is incorporated into the tendons and ligaments that are attached to bone by perforating fibers.

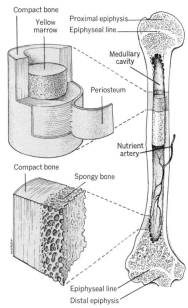

(Chaffee EE, Lytle IM: Basic Physiology and Anatomy, 4th ed. JB Lippincott, 1980)

The cavities in bone contain connective tissue called *marrow*. The medullary cavities in long bones are filled with yellow marrow that is mainly composed of fat cells and a few myelocytes. Red marrow, which is myeloid tissue, is found in cancellous bone and contains mostly immature red blood cells.

Neurovascular Supply

Bone has an extensive vascular network. Blood vessels in the periosteum enter and leave the compact bone through many minute canals called *Volkmann's canals*. The cancellous bone receives its blood supply from vessels that run through the compact or cortical bone. At least one large nutrient artery enters the medullary cavity and branches out to supply the marrow and to anastomose with other arteries from the bony tissue. Large veins accompany arteries, and veins of varying sizes emerge independently from the bones.

Lymphatic vessels are also found in the periosteum and osseous tissue.

Nerves and arteries enter the interior of the bone.

Microscopic Anatomy

A transverse slice of compact bone would reveal a series of circular structures called *haversian systems*. The center of each system is a hole, called a haversian canal, which contains neurovascular structures. Concentric rings of bone matrix encircle each haversian canal and are called *lamellae*. Between the lamellae are little spaces or lacunae that are connected to each other and to the haversian canals by still smaller canals (canaliculi). Each lacuna contains a ma-

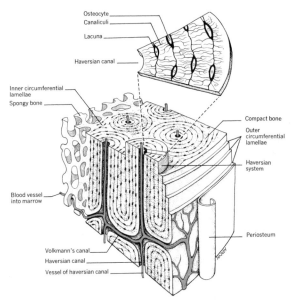

(Chaffee EE, Lytle IM: Basic Physiology and Anatomy, 4th ed. JB Lippincott, 1980)

ture bone cell, or osteocyte. The network of canaliculi between the lacunae and haversian canals is the means by which each haversian system receives nutrients. A longitudinal section of compact bone would demonstrate how haversian canals run parallel to each other up and down the bone and communicate at intervals through Volkmann's canals.

Bone Cells

There are three main types of bone cells. *Osteoblasts*, bone-forming cells, are found on all growing surfaces of bone. *Osteoclasts* are giant cells that tear down bone. The remodeling of bone occurs through the combined efforts of these two types of cells. The osteoblasts deposit newly formed bone, and the osteoclasts resorb bone in a counterbalancing process that determines the strength and size of normal, healthy bone. An *Osteocyte* is a mature bone cell that maintains living bone.

Chemical Composition of Bone

Bone is composed of organic and inorganic matter. The organic constituents of bone are cells, blood vessels, and cartilaginous material; these provide bone with one-third of its total weight. Calcium phosphate is the chief inorganic substance in bone. Calcium carbonate, calcium fluoride, magnesium phosphate, and sodium chloride are present in small percentages. Approximately 99% of the body's calcium supply is stored in the bones.

Development of Bone

Ossification is the formation of bone. There are two kinds of ossification—intramembranous and intracartilaginous.

When a bone develops between membranes of a fibrous connective tissue that will eventually become periosteum, it is called *Intramembranous* ossification. Osteoblasts in the inner and more vascular part of the membrane create small spicules that radiate in all directions. Fibers develop from these spicules and are ossified along with the matrix by the deposition of calcium salts. Some of the osteoblasts are entrapped to form osteocytes in spaces that will become the lacunae. The fibers continue to radiate and ossify, forming more bone spicules into a network of trabeculae. The osteoblasts form layers of bony tissue to increase the thickness of the trabeculae while other layers of bone are being laid down under the periosteum. Osteoclastic activity aids in reorganization of the new bone. The haversian canals are formed when vessels are surrounded by bone. Some sites of this type of ossification are the top and sides of the skull, the sternum, and the flat bones.

In long bones, ossification is preceded by a cartilaginous mass. Blood vessels enter the central shaft (diaphysis) of the cartilage model at what is called a primary center of ossification. As the matrix is mineralized, the cartilage cells, cut off from nutrients, are destroyed. Ossification proceeds toward the ends of the bone. The bone increases in diameter by intramembranous ossification under the periosteum, while the medullary cavity is created by the osteoclasts. Secondary centers of ossification, or epiphyses, develop in the ends of long bones. The epiphysis of a long bone is separated from the shaft by cartilaginous tissue called an *epiphyseal plate*. The cartilage cells in this plate are specialized and organized in rows. Longitudinal growth of the bone occurs as these cells become ossified and are replaced by cell division. This process continues until bone growth is complete. At this time, the end of the long bone is united with the shaft as the epiphyseal plate is replaced by bone.

Nutritional Requirements

Calcium and phosphorus are essential for normal bone growth. These minerals are used by the body for bone growth in the presence of vitamins, specifically vitamin D. Vitamin C is required in the formation and maintenance of the collagenous fibers, which are present in the intercellular substance of bone.

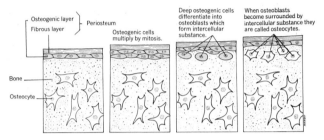

(Chaffee EE, Lytle IM: Basic Physiology and Anatomy, 4th ed. JB Lippincott, 1980)

Hormonal Influence

Hormones play a vital role in the development and function of normal, healthy bone. These hormones include somatotropin (STH), the growth hormone; thyroxin, which is necessary in converting cartilage to bone; glucocorticoids, which influence the metabolism of protein; and parathormone and calcitonin, which work to maintain blood calcium homeostasis. The specific effects of estrogen and testosterone on osteoblastic activity account for the difference in the growth periods for females and males as well as the difference in bone structure. For example, estrogens cause broadening of the female pelvis.

FUNCTIONS OF BONE

The bones of the body form an integrated structure known as the *skeleton*. As a system, the skeleton has six functions.

1. *Provides a framework for the body.* The bones of the skeleton, by their composition and construction, are organs of support that are attached to each other by ligaments. This provides a strong framework for the body, supports surrounding tissues and maintains position, helps to preserve the shape of the body, and allows movement.
2. *Assists the body in movement.* Bones that form movable joints act as levers. When skeletal muscles that are attached to bones of a joint contract, they apply force to these levers; and movement is the result.

3. *Protects vital organs.* Bones form three protective structures—the skull, the rib cage, and the pelvis. These structures enclose or surround vital organs and serve as protection.
4. *Provides storage space for minerals.* The mineral salts that function as part of the body's chemical control mechanism are stored in the bones. Calcium and phosphorus account for the largest percentage of these mineral salts.
5. *Produces blood cells.* Hematopoiesis is the production of blood cells. Erythrocytes and those white blood cells that are granular leukocytes (the neutrophil, eosinophil, and basophil leukocytes) originate in the red marrow of bones.
6. *Remodels or re-forms itself.* The remodeling of bone according to its function is a continuous process carried on by the osteoblasts and osteoclasts.

Bone Disorders Due to Alterations in Structure and Function

Bone structure and function are altered by external or internal factors. Trauma, which results in a fracture, is an external factor. Disorders in other body systems—for example, the digestive or endocrine system—are internal factors that may be responsible for disturbances in the structure and function of bone. These disturbances are often manifested in chronic conditions or disease.

PAGET'S DISEASE

Paget's disease, or *osteitis deformans*, is a slowly progressive condition in which bone plates are laid down around the haversian canals in a completely disorganized pattern because of overactivity of the osteoblasts and osteoclasts. As a result, the bone is not structured to withstand stresses and strains adequately and is, therefore, weaker. On microscopic examination, a bone section will stain in a mosaic pattern that is characteristic of the disease.

The cause of Paget's disease is unknown. It is almost always seen in persons past middle age and may be more common in men.

The number of bones involved in Paget's disease is variable, although the bones most frequently affected are the skull, pelvis, spine, femur, and tibia. The bones enlarge and become broader, thicker, and heavier. They are also weaker than normal bones and are easily fractured. Fractures of these bones heal quickly. The patient may have kyphosis of the thoracic spine, outward bowing of the femurs, outward and forward bowing of the tibias, enlarged feet, an enlarged skull, and pelvic and rib deformities. Compression of nerves may cause symptoms. When the disease is generalized, the patient may be shorter and have a waddling gait. In the advanced stages, respiratory difficulties and cardiovascular diseases are common. This is probably due to skeletal deformities and the fact that cardiac output is increased in Paget's disease.

The only significant laboratory finding is a high serum alkaline phosphatase, which is an index to the amount of new bone being formed. X-ray films show areas of opacity and radiolucency in the affected bones.

The treatment of Paget's disease consists primarily of relieving bone and joint pain. Many patients respond to analgesic and anti-inflammatory drugs. More specific drug therapy may be indicated in cases where pain is intractable. Three drugs that may be considered are mithramycin, calcitonin, and disodium etidronate (EHDP). Mithramycin is a cytotoxic drug that may decrease new bone formation by inhibiting the osteoblasts. Calcitonin inhibits the mobilization of calcium. EHDP is a diphosphonate and is thought to inhibit the formation of hydroxyapatite crystals in bone.

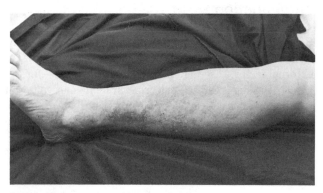

Paget's disease; outward bowing of tibia

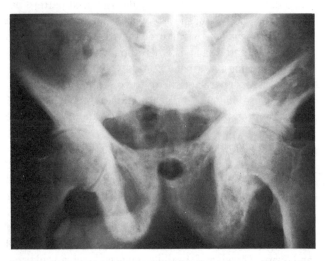

Paget's disease. Note the coarse trabecular pattern and the asymmetry of the pelvis. This patient also has degenerative joint disease in one hip.

HYPERPARATHYROIDISM

Secretion of excessive amounts of parathyroid hormone (parathormone) due to tumors or an enlarged gland will cause demineralization of the skeleton and marked bone destruction. The high serum calcium levels cause soft tissue calcification, hypotonia, and renal calculi.

X-ray films will show a general decrease in long bone mass with cystic areas. Lesions referred to as brown tumors may be seen at the ends of long bones. These tumors are probably caused by the formation of intraosseous hematomas as a result of incomplete fractures. Microscopically there is marked osteoclastic activity and proliferating fibroblastic tissue in place of reabsorbed bone. This process is referred to as *osteitis fibrosa.*

The onset of symptoms is insidious and includes weakness, lethargy, loss of muscle tone, and bone pain. Fractures are common and may result in deformities. Polyuria, polydipsia, and symptoms of renal calculi are evident. Gastrointestinal disorders will eventually result from involvement of the visceral nonstriated muscles.

The treatment of hyperparathyroidism is directed toward the parathyroid gland.

Metabolic Disorders

An overall reduction in bone mass due to a subnormal or abnormal process that is concerned with bone formation may be classified as a metabolic disorder. Such disorders include rickets, osteomalacia, and osteoporosis. Osteoporosis is fairly common in hospitalized orthopedic patients; therefore, the nursing implications for this disease will be discussed in some detail.

RICKETS

Rickets is a disturbance of bone formation during childhood that results from inadequate intake and synthesis of vitamin D, which is necessary for mineral metabolism. As a result, the bones become soft and deformed. Manifestations of rickets include bowing of the extremeties, widening of the ends of the long bones, deformed bones in the cranium and pelvis, and sinking of the middle of the sternum. Microscopically there are large areas of unmineralized bone, an inconsistent alignment of lamellae, and formation of haversian systems.

Nutritional rickets is no longer common in the United States because of the fortification of milk and food products with vitamin D. When the disease is diagnosed in a growing child, it can be halted by the administration of daily required doses of vitamin D and a diet containing liberal amounts of calcium and phosphorus.

Other causes, linked to genetics, kidney defects, and malabsorption syndromes, produce what is known as *resistant rickets,* because high doses of vitamin D are required for treatment.

OSTEOMALACIA

Osteomalacia is essentially an adult form of rickets, since it occurs in mature bones after epiphyseal plates have disappeared. The cause of osteomalacia is an inadequate amount of minerals for normal osteoblastic — osteoclastic activity. Such deficiencies result from many factors, including poor dietary intake, disturbance in vitamin-D or calcium absorption, and excessive loss of serum phosphorus from the kidneys. Microscopically the bone shows a lack of mineral salts, similar to that seen in rickets, in normal osteoid tissue. This disease is relatively rare and often difficult to distinguish from osteoporosis.

OSTEOPOROSIS

Osteoporosis is a condition in which there is a reduction of total skeletal mass or demineralization of bone, to the extent that fractures may occur with minor trauma. Under a microscope, the bone tissue appears normal but decreased in amount, with wide haversian canals, thin trabeculae, and few osteoblasts. X-ray films show thin cortices and few trabeculae, so that the bone has a "washed out" appearance.

Many factors may be involved in causing osteoporosis. The incidence of osteoporosis is highest in postmenopausal women, usually those 60 or older. Men who are afflicted with this condition may be still older. Therefore, it is believed that lack of estrogens and androgens are contributing factors. Osteoporosis may develop as a result of an inadequate diet, endocrine dysfunction, or inactivity.

Back pain is the usual complaint. It may have a sudden or insidious onset and is due to compression fractures of the lumbar spine. Kyphosis and loss of stature may be present as a result of these fractures. Pain will extend along the pathway of an involved nerve and may progress to the pelvis, chest, and shoulders. Many elderly people who sustain hip fractures also suffer from osteoporosis.

The course of treatment varies with the causative factors and clinical features and includes special diets, hormone preparations, and exercise. Prevention of osteoporosis in postmenopausal women is the subject of a considerable amount of discussion. A high-calcium diet along with regular exercise is currently being recommended by many gerontologists. When a high-calcium diet cannot be tolerated, a calcium supplement should be added to the normal diet to bring the daily uptake to 1000–1500 mg.

THE PATIENT WHO HAS OSTEOPOROSIS: NURSING IMPLICATIONS

Patients are not usually admitted to the hospital with a primary diagnosis of osteoporosis. This condition may be noted in the medical history or on the report of an x-ray film taken for the purpose of diagnosing and treating an orthopedic problem such as a fractured hip, fractured humerus, or back pain. When the nurse becomes aware that a patient has osteoporosis, she must make a note of this fact on the Kardex and write orders for specific nursing interventions.

Positioning. In turning or otherwise moving a patient with osteoporosis, the nurse must be extremely careful and gentle. A pillow should be placed between the patient's legs; logrolling is the best method of turning the patient from side to side. In any position, adequate support must be given to the patient's joints. If the patient complains of back pain, Williams' position may be the most comfortable (head of bed raised and knees bent).

Exercise and Ambulation. Promoting and assisting in exercise of the extremities becomes a priority in nursing care because demineralization of bones is increased. The nurse must evaluate the patient's ability and motivation to exercise independently and schedule either active range of motion with supervision or passive range of motion. The physical therapist assists in the exercise program either actively or in a supportive role. Because of the patient's age, orthopedic problem, and general health, *encouragement to exercise* is often what is needed most.

If the patient is ambulating, non-skid slippers or shoes are a necessity. Assistance or assistive devices must be provided if the patient is weak or unsteady.

Nutrition. Careful attention must be given to the patient's eating habits to ensure adequate intake of calcium, vitamin D, and protein. Smaller meals with nourishment in between and at bedtime may be indicated if the patient has a poor appetite. The dietician may be called in to do a nutritional assessment, and menu planning to promote good general health can be initiated.

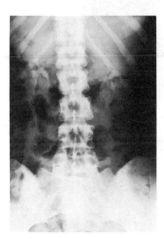 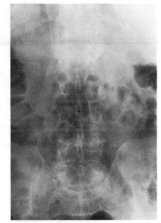

(*Left*) Normal spine. Vertebral bodies are well defined and "white" because of an adequate amount of calcium. (*Right*) Osteoporosis of the spine. The bones have a "washed out" appearance because of mineral loss. Vertebral bodies are somewhat compressed.

Observations. Complaints of pain must be thoroughly evaluated, especially when they are preceded by activity. When the patient has a lack of sensation or decreased sensation, the nurse must also be alert for signs of deformity or an inability on the patient's part to move an extremity.

Patient Education. Suggestions for safety in the home, as discussed on page 194 in discharge planning for a patient who has had a hip pinning, also apply to the patient with osteoporosis. In addition, these patients should be instructed as follows:

1. Keep weight down to decrease the amount of strain on back muscles and help prevent abnormal stresses on the vertebral column.
2. Avoid sudden bending and lifting, such as picking up a child or closing a window sash; these movements may cause vertebral fractures.
3. Sleep on a firm mattress.
4. Wear supportive shoes to reduce muscle fatigue.
5. Avoid walking on ice or snow. (Do not think that a cane will decrease the chance of falling on a slippery surface.)
6. Exercise by walking regularly and often. Bicycle riding and swimming are also excellent forms of exercise. All exercises should be a matter of routine and within the limits of tolerance.

Osteomyelitis

Osteomyelitis is a bone infection and may be acute or chronic. Pathogenic organisms gain access to the bones through the bloodstream by extension from a nearby soft tissue infection or through an open wound such as might occur with a compound fracture. To a large extent, the severity of the disease depends on the virulence of the invading organism.

Hematogenous Osteomyelitis

Bacteria may enter the circulating blood from any source of infection in the body. Examples of such infection include boils, pharyngitis, and infected skin lesions.

The classic patient is a child, and those areas of the body most susceptible to trauma or infection are the ones most commonly involved. Hematogenous osteomyelitis may occur in the adult who has undergone surgery or examination of the genitourinary tract, or whose resistance has been lowered by debilitating illness. In these patients the infection may become localized in a vertebra.

Cause. The organisms most commonly isolated in cases of hematogenous osteomyelitis are *Staphylococcus aureus* and *Streptococcus pyogenes*. Gramnegative bacilli are found in patients with sickle cell anemia, urinary tract infections, and in heroin addicts.

Pathology. Hematogenous osteomyelitis most often occurs in rapidly growing bones on the metaphyseal side of the bone plate. This area is vascular, and the circulation is sluggish. The bacteria become implanted and grow in the bone. The subsequent destruction of these pathogens and the formation of purulent material causes pressure that spreads the infection through the cancellous metaphysis and to the cortical shaft of the bone. The epiphyseal plate usually acts as a barrier, keeping the infection out of the epiphysis. In the hip joint, however, where the epiphyseal plate lies within the joint capsule, the infection may spread from the metaphysis into the joint cavity. Osteomyelitis in a joint is more common in children than in adults.

As the infection breaks through the cortex, it elevates the periosteum and separates the bone from its main source of blood vessels. This stripping of the periosteum also serves as a stimulus to osteoblastic activity, and new immature bone called *involucrum* is laid down. If circulation from the marrow is also cut off, the segment of bone between the involucrum and marrow becomes necrotic and dies. This segment of dead bone is called *sequestrum.* Sequestra may have to be removed surgically when they do not work their way through openings in the involucrum to become draining sinuses. The response of bone tissue to infection is increased osteoblastic — osteoclastic activity. If there is more resorption of bone than there is formation, the bone will be weakened and susceptible to fractures.

Signs and Symptoms. The acute phase of this disease usually begins with malaise, general weakness, and aching. A high fever, chills, and exquisite tenderness over a long bone will follow. There may be a protective muscle spasm, and the child will hold the joint nearest the affected area in a position of flexion. The child will be acutely ill with an

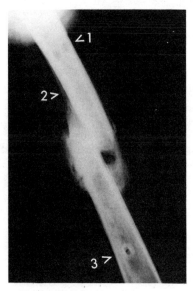

X-ray film of developing osteomyelitis in a femur with a healing fracture: (*1*) sequestra; (*2*) elevated periosteum; (*3*) skeletal pin site (not to be confused with sequestra).

elevated leukocyte count and sedimentation rate. Definite changes in the appearance of the bone may not be visible on x-ray examination for several weeks. Tenderness and pain become localized as the infection advances.

Diagnosis. Blood cultures are frequently positive. However, the diagnosis must often be made on the symptoms and treatment begun to prevent irreparable damage to the bone.

Treatment. *Acute stage.* Large doses of intravenous antibiotics, complete bed rest, and supportive nursing care are indicated. Transfusions are necessary when anemia is present. Surgical drainage of the infected bone is considered when patient response to antibiotic therapy is slow. The limb should be immobilized in a cast or splint. The application of hot, moist dressings may be therapeutic.

Chronic stage. When the patient is no longer acutely ill, the manifestations of osteomyelitis will be low-grade fever, persistent draining sinuses, and recurrent episodes of increased heat, swelling, and pain over the infected area. Antibiotic therapy will be continued based on the results of cultures of the drainage. Sequestra may be surgically removed. If x-ray films show large areas of involved bone, an extensive surgical procedure (saucerization) is considered. A cast is applied to immobilize and support the limb, and the wound is treated through a window.

The treatment of choice for a resistant local infection is closed irrigation and suction of the wound. Two catheters, one for inflowing solutions (detergent or antibiotics) and one for outflowing drainage, are sutured into the closed wound following the removal of diseased bone and sequestra. The irrigation may run continuously, or the drainage tube may be clamped for regular short periods (to allow the wound to fill up with solution) and then opened again. This procedure has a debriding effect. In anaerobic infections, the wound is left open for adequate drainage and allowed to heal by filling in with granulation tissue. Cultures of the drainage are done at intervals; when they are negative, the irrigation is discontinued.

The long-term treatment of patients who have been treated for osteomyelitis may include skin grafting.

Osteomyelitis: Open Wounds

Cause. The most common cause of osteomyelitis in the adult is direct contamination of a bone through an open wound. It may be the result of an open fracture, a surgical procedure, or a puncture or gunshot wound. Whether or not osteomyelitis develops in an open wound depends on the degree of contamination, the nature and number of the invading organisms, the amount of soft tissue damage, and the general resistance of the individual. When a considerable mass of foreign material is introduced into the wound, for example, in joint replacement, that wound becomes more susceptible to infection.

Pathology. When osteomyelitis results from an open wound, the infection generally remains in that part of the bone. Sequestra, sinus formation, and drainage are also usually localized.

Signs and Symptoms. Often the signs and symptoms of infection may become evident 36 to 48 hours after trauma or surgery. The patient will have complaints of pain and pressure in the affected area. Localized swelling, redness, and tenderness are frequently present. An elevated body temperature and malaise are common. Eventually the wound appears inflamed, and the surrounding skin looks "tight and shiny."

Treatment. Immediate opening of the wound is indicated to allow free drainage. Cultures should be taken and appropriate antibiotic therapy should be initiated. These patients are given massive doses of one or more antibiotics. Daily assessment for side effects must be part of the nursing care plan. The extremity should be immobilized in a cast, splint, or traction.

If deep infection persists with recurrence of symptoms and failure of healing, surgical removal of sequestra or saucerization may be necessary. Metal fixation devices or joint prostheses are removed if present. Wounds are left open and packed with petroleum jelly dressings to facilitate drainage, or they are left open or closed over catheters that permit local antibiotic or detergent irrigation. Irrigation is continuous until cultures of the drainage are negative.

Chronic osteomyelitis requires repeated and prolonged hospitalizations and may result in extensive bone and soft tissue loss. Healing is a long process, and skin grafting may be necessary. In any case of osteomyelitis, however, the surgeon's goal in treatment is to overcome the infection with minimal bone loss.

Care of the Patient With Osteomyelitis

Irrigation Systems

There are various methods of setting up closed-wound irrigation systems in the treatment of osteomyelitis. They may involve systems with a wall suction unit or wound drainage containers. Solutions in use include antibiotic solutions and detergents (wetting agents). Furthermore, surgeons often adapt or improvise equipment because of the location and nature of a wound.

Therefore, the first nursing responsibility in the care of a patient with an irrigation system is to understand the mechanics of that system and the problems that may arise in keeping it operational. Frequently a surgeon will anticipate that a system will be difficult to keep going, for instance, because of the position of a catheter. Or for one reason or another, he may choose to regulate the flow of solution so that keeping it from leaking into dressings will be next to

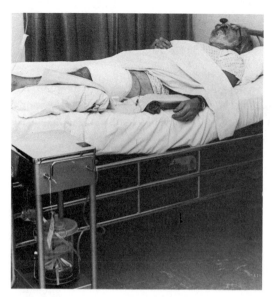

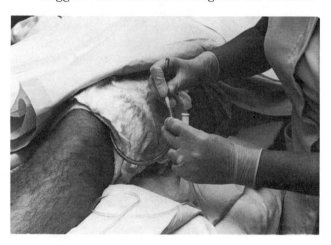

there are no kinks or any evidence of clogging. She must have *explicit* directions from the surgeon about the action to be taken when any tubing *does* become clogged. Which tube can be irrigated and when? Re-

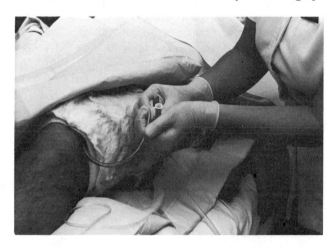

versing the direction of solution flow is sometimes an adequate maneuver when the tubing becomes clogged. The tubing carrying the irrigating solution and the tubing carrying the drainage are removed from their connections to the wound catheters and reversed. This change in the direction of the flow is often enough to release clots in the catheters.

2. The entire system should be kept as sterile as possible. Gloves should be worn when any connecting ap-

impossible. The nurse can save herself time and turmoil if she knows these things when the patient is returned to his room following a surgical insertion of an irrigation system. Then she can take appropriate measures in anticipation of such developments; for example, placing extra pads around the area being irrigated or writing more specific nursing orders about checking the inflow and output.

Some general points in the care of any patient with a wound irrigation system can be made.

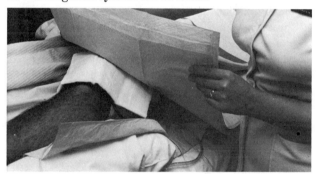

Closed wound irrigation in osteomyelitis; femur.

1. Input and outflow must be maintained at the proper rate. The system must be checked every hour and the flow of solutions noted. The nurse should understand which clamps need adjustment and when. She should also check all tubing and connections to be certain

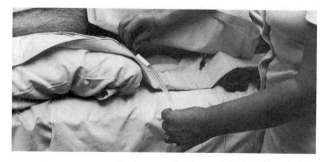

paratus is being handled. Irrigating solutions should be hung and drainage bottles should be switched or emptied as quickly as possible so that the system is not open to the air any longer than is absolutely necessary.

3. Intake and output must be recorded accurately. This requires concise and accurate labeling of irrigating solutions and careful measuring of drainage. The color and character of drainage must also be noted. For the first few days, the drainage solution may be

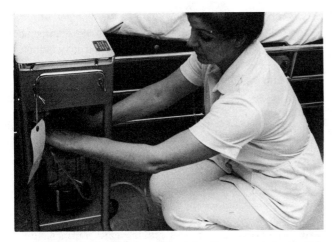

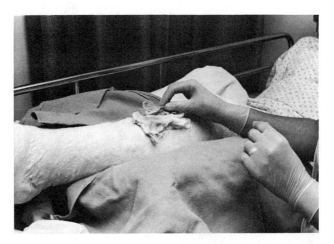

very bloody. It is important for the nurse to know this so that she does not become needlessly alarmed.

4. The nurse should be alert for any reactions to irrigating solutions and report them to the physician.
5. Dressings around catheters must be inspected at least every 3 hours and more often if leakage is present.

At this point, it should be mentioned that leaking of drainage into dressings and cast is a frequent problem. Keeping the bed and the extremity dry can be frustrating for both patient and nurse. This is especially true when the wound is in the leg, because the leg is elevated and drainage may seep down the patient's thigh and into the groin. Placing disposable, plastic-lined pads under the entire leg and

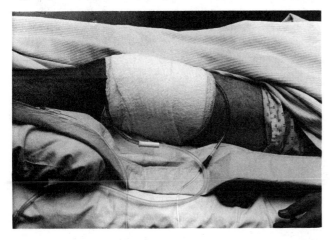

folding the edges toward the leg, all the way around the pads, may be effective in providing a trap for moisture. Another way to trap drainage is to place towel rolls under the edges of disposable drainage pads. The patient needs meticulous skin care of the exposed parts of the extremity. Powders with drying agents should be used in the groin to prevent skin irritation.

Dressings and Cast Care

Any dressing changes must be done using strict sterile technique and extreme gentleness in handling the affected part.

The patient may have a dressing on an open draining wound that is accessible only through the window of a cast. This dressing may be moistened with petroleum jelly or another ointment to provide protection for the wound, to facilitate draining, and to prevent sticking of the gauze. Wet dressings may be used intermittently. Keeping the cast dry is a major challenge. If the wound is irrigated manually or

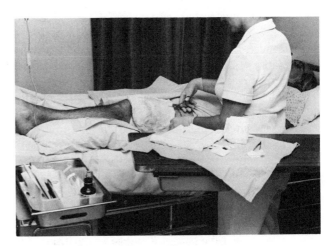

otherwise mositened during dressing changes, it should be done as carefully as possible to avoid wetting the cast unnecessarily. Sterile plastic around the window edge may provide limited cast protection when wound care procedures are being done.

Precautions in Care

Good aseptic technique is imperative in all aspects of wound care, not only to prevent further contamination of the wound but to protect personnel and other patients. Dressings should be cut and removed carefully to keep them intact and out of contact with bed linen. Soiled dressings and compresses should be placed immediately in a plastic bag, and the bag should be tightly closed. Procedures should be planned in advance so that the wound is exposed to the air for a minimal amount of time.

Isolation procedure, according to hospital policy, must be strictly adhered to in handling linen and equipment as well as soiled dressings. Good handwashing at all times is essen-

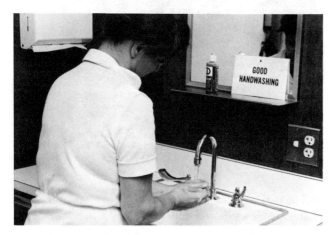

tial. Since osteomyelitis can be both devastating and chronic, patients with infection must be isolated from other patients with orthopedic conditions.

Positioning of the Extremity

Rest of the affected part is a critical factor in the treatment of osteomyelitis. A cast, splint, or traction may be applied to the extremity. Nursing measures must be taken to ensure maintenance of the immobilization apparatus, with attention to the extremity it is supporting. Chapters 2 and 3 give specific details in the nursing care of casted patients or those in traction.

Adequate support must be given to the joints on either side of the infected area since the patient tends to "protect" the painful extremity by positions of flexion. Pillows used for support should be firm. Good overall body alignment on a firm mattress is also essential.

A patient with osteomyelitis has severe pain, and extreme care must be taken when handling the affected extremity. Whenever the patient is turned or repositioned in bed, the involved extremity must be moved so that it remains in the same position in relation to the rest of the body. For example, when a patient with osteomyelitis of the tibia and a long-leg cast is being turned, he should have a pillow

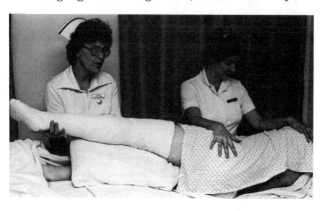

between his legs. One nurse should be "in charge" of handling the leg while the other nurse, or two nurses, assist the patient in turning so that as he moves there is no twisting of either leg or body.

It is impossible to place too much emphasis on the need for gentleness with these patients at all times, not only to prevent pain, but also to prevent pathological fractures due to immature or cystic bone.

Pain Relief and Rest

The patient requires adequate rest to ensure satisfactory healing of the wound and general recovery. Pain medications should be administered as required and their effects evaluated. Special efforts should be made to include scheduled rest periods in between nursing-care routines. Relatives and other visitors must be instructed about the necessity for such intervention.

Nutrition

Fluids should be encouraged every 3 hours. The patient must receive instructions about the importance of a well-balanced diet in his recovery and rehabilitation.

Immobility

The problems of immobility are a potential threat to the patient with osteomyelitis. The prevention of such problems is discussed on pages 94–98.

Psychological Considerations

Not only is osteomyelitis a very serious disease, but the physical effects of the condition and the treatment are unpleasant. Wounds, drainage, and casts become odorous. Fresh air and deodorizing sprays, though beneficial, leave something to be desired. An irrigation system, with all the problems it may entail, is a source of discomfort and aggravation. Pain is usually present to some degree, and the patient suffers from the apprehension of more pain every time he is touched or moved. The prognosis of his disease may be uncertain. His limb may be unsightly.

The self-image is impaired by the prospect of scars, deformity, and limitation of motion. Whatever the patient's overall condition, he can be assured of one fact, and that is, his recovery and rehabilitation will be prolonged and possibly expensive.

The patient with osteomyelitis must have every chance to verbalize his feelings. Tender loving care with extra effort to demonstrate respect for the indidivual and his needs will be appreciated. The nurse must use every opportunity to establish rapport with the person or persons closest to the patient, because supportive care is a major job and an ongoing process after discharge.

Discharge Planning

Home instruction must begin with an evaluation of the patient's understanding of his disease and the importance of self-care in preventing problems and detecting recurrence. Health care agencies should be included in discharge planning if supervision of self-care is required.

Long-term antibiotics are an important part of home treatment. The patient or another member of the family may require instruction on the administration of intravenous antibiotics. Oral antibiotics are certain to be part of home treatment, perhaps for months. The patient and the person responsible for his care must understand the administration of prescribed antibiotics and the importance of watching for side effects.

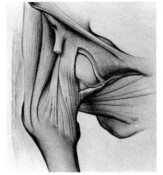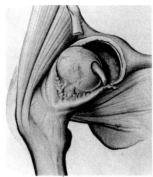

(*Left*) A normal hip. (*Right*) Rheumatoid arthritis in a hip. (Drawings by Robert J. Demarest. Courtesy Eli Lilly and Co)

Arthritis

Definition. Although arthritis means inflammation of a joint, the term is generally used to classify a multitude of conditions that cause pain and aching in joints and connective tissues throughout the body. Not all of these disorders are characterized by inflammation. The major types of arthritis are chronic.

Common Types

There are four types of arthritis that directly involve the joints and are probably more common than other types. Of these, the first two, rheumatoid arthritis and osteoarthritis, are the forms most often encountered by the orthopedic nurse in the hospital. Therefore, they will only be defined here. They are discussed in more detail in later sections of this chapter.

Rheumatoid Arthritis is a chronic systemic disease affecting connective tissue throughout the body. This disease is characterized by inflammatory changes in the linings of synovial joints, which often lead to severe involvement of the joint structures and subsequent destruction.

Osteoarthritis, often called degenerative joint disease, is characterized by the deterioration of joint cartilage and the underlying bone and by the resulting abnormal lateral bone growth, which stems from a physiological attempt to handle normal stress.

Ankylosing Spondylitis, or Marie-Strumpell disease, is a chronic progressive inflammatory disease of the spine and sacroiliac joints that leads to extensive bony ankylosis or scarring within the joint. The disease affects men more often than women, begins in adolescence or early adulthood, and results in a pokerlike spine. The hips and shoulders may also be affected. The common symptoms are pain and stiffness in the back. Treatment involves anti-inflammatory drugs and measures to prevent flexion deformities of the spine, including exercises, positioning, and bracing.

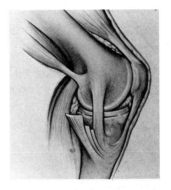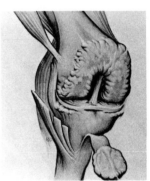

(*Left*) A normal knee. (*Right*) Osteoarthritis in a knee. (Drawings by Robert J. Demarest. Courtesy Eli Lilly and Co)

Gout, or Gouty Arthritis, is a disease in which there is abnormal metabolism of uric acid in the body, evidenced as an increase in uric acid in the bloodstream. The deposition of excessive uric acid as monosodium urate crystals, primarily in the small joints of the body, is believed to trigger an inflammatory response. Accumulations of such crystals in the joints are called *tophi*. Gout classically involves the metatarsophalangeal joint of the big toes. An attack of gout develops suddenly and lasts about 3 to 5 days if not treated. The joint is painful, swollen, and red, and the patient appears ill. Most gout victims suffer recurrent attacks with more and more joint involvement. There is a definite hereditary factor in gout, and it is much more common in males.

An acute attack of gout is treated by colchicine or phenylbutazone, which are anti-inflammatory drugs. Colchicine may also be used in small daily doses to prevent recurrent attacks. Other drugs available for prophylaxis are those that decrease the production of uric acid in the body (allopurinol) or increase the excretion of uric acid by the kidneys (probenecid). Although gout is a disturbance of purine metabolism, the value of restricting foods high in purine is doubtful.

Rheumatoid Arthritis

Incidence

Rheumatoid arthritis is a disease that affects women more often than men. Although it can occur at any age, it is most commonly found in the age group from 20 to 50 years.

Cause

The cause of rheumatoid arthritis is still unknown. One theory currently under investigation holds that rheumatoid arthritis occurs when derangement of the body's immune system, by an internal or external factor, results in the production of antibodies that attack the body's own joints and tissues.

Pathology

Rheumatoid arthritis primarily attacks the linings of the synovial joints. One episode may leave the joint undamaged, but recurrence is likely and some impairment of joint function is common in most patients. In an acute attack, the synovial tissue becomes inflamed and edematous, and fluid accumulates within the joint. Granulation tissue called *pannus* is formed and spreads to the joint, causing destruction of the articular cartilage and eventually of the underlying bone. Involvement of the ligamentous structures results in instability due to laxity, stretching, or rupture of these structures. Severe instability leads to subluxation of the joint. Flexion contractures and ankyloses caused by scarring of the tissues may ultimately immobilize the joint.

Rheumatoid arthritis may also involve other joints, such as the temporomandibular and sternoclavicular joints. Another manifestation of this disease is the appearance of subcutaneous nodules at pressure points in the body, like the elbows. The lungs, pleura, heart, and eyes may be involved in the inflammatory process. Lymphadenopathy and splenomegaly may also be present.

Course of the Disease

The onset of rheumatoid arthritis may be sudden or insidious. It usually begins in one joint or the small joints of the hands or feet, the proximal interphalangeal joints being

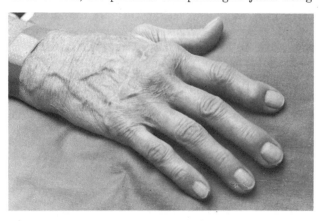

those most commonly affected. This disease is progressive and often spreads to other joints in a symmetrical pattern.

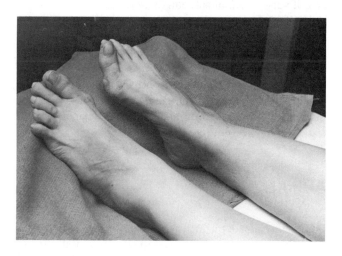

With repeated attacks of rheumatoid arthritis, the patient will develop muscle weakness and atrophy, anemia, and marked weight loss. In most cases, rheumatoid arthritis is characterized by exacerbations and remissions. That is, the

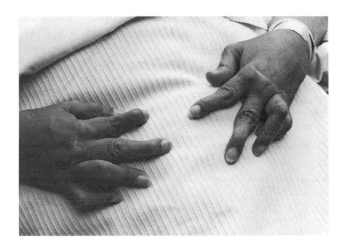

disease seems to "come and go." It is generally unpredictable for each individual, and the amount of disability it causes is also variable.

Clinical Features and Patient History

The patient will present one or more swollen joints that are tender, hot, and red. A major complaint may be that joint discomfort, accompanied by stiffness, is increased upon motion after a period of inactivity; for instance, when rising in the morning. When taking the patient's history, the examiner may learn that malaise, fatigue, and a low-grade fever preceded the onset of joint pain. The patient may also report having had some mild "aches and pains" before the acute attack. Tachycardia may be another symptom.

Diagnostic Tests

An elevated sedimentation rate is the most consistent laboratory finding in patients who have rheumatoid arthritis. There may also be a mild leukocytosis and anemia. The abnormal protein found in the serum (latex agglutination test), called the "rheumatoid factor," is not in itself diagnostic, because this finding is associated with other disease states. C-reactive protein may be positive. Serum protein electrophoresis will show an increase in globulins (see Table 10-1).

Early rheumatoid arthritis may not be apparent on x-ray films. As the disease progresses, however, roentgenograms will show narrowing or absence of joint spaces due to lack of cartilage, loss of subchondral bone, bony spurs, and subluxations.

An analysis of synovial joint fluid may be helpful in conjunction with other tests; for example, if the joint in question is the knee and no phalangeal joints seem to be affected. In this test, the leukocyte count may be elevated, and the fluid will appear cloudy to turbid with decreased viscosity. The complement activity will be low.

In all, however, the diagnostic tests must be correlated with the clinical picture and the patient's history.

Basic Treatment Program

Since rheumatoid arthritis is a chronic disease, treatment is a lifelong process, and self-care and education are of paramount importance. The goal of any treatment program should be to help the patient function as normally and free of pain as possible while preventing unnecessary deformity. The patient and his family need to become involved in this endeavor, which is truly a team effort because it may include members of many professions, specialties, agencies, and organizations, both in and out of the hospital.

Basic considerations in the treatment program for rheumatoid arthritis follow.

Drug Therapy. There is no cure for rheumatoid arthritis. Medications are used in the treatment of this disease to decrease inflammation and relieve pain and stiffness. Table 10-2 lists the drugs currently used in the treatment of rheumatoid arthritis and their side effects and adverse reactions. One drug is often given in combination with another.

Aspirin gr 5, 12 to 16 tablets daily, is still considered to be the most effective medication and is also the cheapest. Many patients cannot tolerate plain aspirin because of the gastric distress that may be a side effect. Taking aspirin with milk or meals may prevent such distress, but some patients need to take buffered or enteric coated aspirin.

Other products that may be substituted for aspirin are added to the market from time to time and have varying degrees of effectiveness in individual patients. It must be noted, however, that many of them also have more severe side effects.

Anti-inflammatory drugs that are sometimes used in place of aspirin include phenylbutazone and indomethacin. In general, propionic-acid derivatives have fewer side effects and are as effective as aspirin, although they cost more.

Favorable results with the use of gold compounds have been reported in a large number of rheumatoid patients for more than 30 years.

Table 10-1. Laboratory Tests: Diagnostic Picture in Chronic Bone and Joint Disease*

Disease	Diagnostic Test	Significant Results
Paget's disease	Phosphatase alkaline	Elevated
Rheumatoid arthritis	Sedimentation rate	Moderately to markedly elevated in acute stage
	Rheumatoid factor	A gamma globulin. Present in most adult cases. May take 6 months to appear
	HLA antigen HLA-DW 4	In about half of the adult cases
	Antinuclear antibodies	Present in about 15% of the cases
	LE factor	Present in about 10% of the cases
	Total serum protein	Globulin increased
		Albumin decreased
	Synovial fluid analysis	Diminished viscosity
		Poor mucin clot
		WBC 75% neutrophils
		Glucose level increased
		RA factor positive
		Complement diminished
Multiple myeloma	Bence-Jones protein (urine)	Positive in about 30% of the cases
	Urine electrophoresis	Elevated for plasma cells
	Total serum protein	Globulin increased
		Albumin decreased
	Bone marrow examination	Positive for plasma cells

* Must be correlated with all clinical findings

Table 10-2.   Some Drugs Currently Used in the Treatment of Rheumatoid Arthritis

Drug	Side Effects
Nonsteroid anti-inflammatory agents	
Aspirin (Acetylsalicylic acid)	At continued high dosage, usually headache, dizziness; tinnitus; difficulty in hearing, seeing; mental confusion; sweating; thirst; gastric bleeding; gastric upset with burning; rash
Phenylbutazone (Pyrazolone derivative)	Nausea; vomiting, epigastric discomfort; diarrhea; skin reactions; peptic ulceration, hemorrhage, perforation. Salt and water retention; ulcerative stomatitis
Indomethacin (Acetic acid derivative)	Headaches; vertigo; mental confusion; gastrointestinal symptoms; abdominal pain; anorexia; peptic ulceration
Sulindac (Derivative of indomethacin)	Constipation; nausea; epigastric pain
Tolmetin (Acetic acid)	Nausea; indigestion; epigastric pain
Alclofenac (Chlorophenylacetic acid)	Skin rash, which may be severe
Diclofenac (Aminophenyl acetic acid)	Gastric upsets; nausea; vomiting; headaches
Propionic acid derivatives Ibuprofen Naproxen Fenoprofen Ketoprofen Flurbiprofen	Side effects in general are epigastric in nature
Flufenamic acid	Diarrhea; nausea; vomiting
Azapropozone (Chemically similar to phenylbutazone)	Epigastric pain; nausea
Specific agents	
Gold	Rash is common and may be severe. The more serious side effects are blood dyscrasias and proteinuria. POTENTIALLY DANGEROUS DRUG.
D-Penicillamine (Degradation product of penicillin)	Loss of taste; anorexia; nausea; rash, proteinuria; thrombocytopenia serious but not as common
Azathioprine (Antimetabolite)	Suppresses bone marrow. Gastrointestinal symptoms and infections, most common
Methotrexate (Antimetabolite)	Gastrointestinal intolerance. Ulcerations in the mouth. Leukopenia; thrombocytopenia; infertility; alopecia; depigmentation
Cyclophosphamide (Immunosuppressive alkylating agent)	Nausea; vomiting; diarrhea; bone marrow suppression; stomatitis; cystitis with hemorrhage; alopecia; infertility; infections
Chlorambucil (Alkylating agent)	Infections; gastrointestinal disturbances; stomatitis; bone marrow suppression
Chloroquine and hydroxychloroquine (Antimalarials)	Due to irreversible retinopathy caused by these drugs, they are only used when other agents are not effective
Corticosteroids and ACTH	
Prednisolone	Side effects are numerous and include Cushing's syndrome, severe gastrointestinal upsets, adrenal insufficiency following withdrawal of therapy, aseptic bone necrosis, impaired carbohydrate metabolism, psychological changes, osteoporosis, fractures, vasculitis neuropathy, myopathy, glaucoma and cataracts, papilledema. Will also facilitate growth and spread of bacteria and viruses
ACTH	Given by injection, this drug causes destructive changes in the joint surfaces after repeated injections

Oral corticosteroids are potent drugs in terms of effectiveness and adverse effects. Their administration requires careful monitoring. They are also expensive. Intra-articular corticosteroid injections are "safe," but their beneficial effect is limited to several weeks.

The antimalarial drug hydroxychloroquine may be considered an additional treatment for some patients, but this medication elicits a slow response that is often not evident for as long as 6 months.

Immunosuppressive drugs, such as methotrexate, are the newest class of agents to be used in the treatment of rheumatoid arthritis, particularly when other drugs do not seem to be halting the progress of the disease. Such drugs require extreme care in administration and close observation for side effects.

Rest. All patients with rheumatoid arthritis require a minimum of 8 hours of sleep each night, with regular rest periods during the day. When the disease is active, even more rest and sleep is beneficial.

Prevention of Deformity. Flexion contractures, especially of the hips and knees, become a grim reality in a very short time in an individual with rheumatoid arthritis. Such a person should always sleep on a firm mattress in proper body alignment. Splints or braces may be required to support specific joints, either at rest or in action. Assistive devices to maintain erect posture become necessary when weight-bearing joints are severely affected.

The importance of exercise to maintain muscle strength and joint motion cannot be overemphasized in the prevention of deformities. Range of motion exercises within the limits of pain and endurance should be a daily activity. Patients with advanced rheumatoid arthritis, especially those who are seriously incapacitated, will need to have some kind of physical therapy program prescribed.

Heat is beneficial in relaxing muscles and decreasing stiffness. Therefore, heat may be helpful, in some form, just before exercise. A hot bath immediately after rising in the morning helps the patient "get started." Paraffin baths are an effective means of applying heat to the hands. Paraffin

wax is melted with a little mineral oil in a double boiler. It is then cooled until a white coating appears on top of the mixture. The hands are dipped quickly, with the fingers slightly separated, in and out of the solution. The hands are allowed to dry, and the procedure is repeated seven or eight times. Next, the patient should have someone wrap his hands in plastic or paper for about 20 minutes. The wax is easily removed and reusable. Hot wet applications can also be applied to the hands.

Adequate Nutrition. Rheumatoid arthritis requires no special dietary management, Individuals with the disease are encouraged to help maintain their health by eating well-balanced diets.

Education. The victim of rheumatoid arthritis needs to know what the disease is all about. He must understand that it is chronic and that the "cures" that are sometimes promised in sensational advertising are false. The nature of the disease renders the patient vulnerable to quackery. A person who is in constant pain is more likely to "try anything once." Should a patient with rheumatoid arthritis go into remission immediately after experimenting with a new "cure," he may be convinced of its value and waste a great deal of money on the cure until he has been convinced of its worthlessness by another attack of the disease. On the other hand, the person with rheumatoid arthritis can be reassured that he has some control over the disability he will suffer and that he can prevent deformities by adhering to his treatment program.

A major component of the educational program for a person with rheumatoid arthritis deals with how to modify the environment to make work easier, thereby allowing him to remain active and independent. The National Arthritis Foundation publishes a tremendous volume of pamphlet literature designed to educate the arthritic in all aspects of the disease. Basic explanations of the disease process, treatment, instructions on self-care, adaptation of the envi-

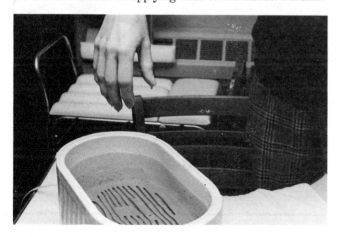

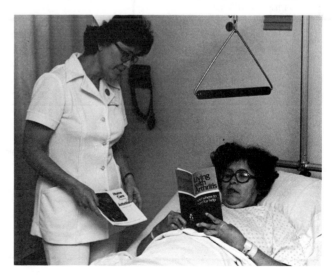

THE "NEW" PATIENT WITH RHEUMATOID ARTHRITIS: SUBJECTIVE DATA WITH IMPLICATIONS FOR NURSING

Significant Data: F. B. is a 44-year-old single female. About 2 years ago she began having episodes of pain and swelling in her right hand. She believed the pain was caused by playing tennis, which she does year round, and did not seek medical attention. A nurse friend told her to take aspirin, which she has been doing for about 6 months. This seemed to help keep her symptoms from becoming too severe until 2 weeks ago when her hand became painful and her joints more swollen. Aspirin brought little relief. Her left hand developed some mild symptoms and she entered the hospital for diagnosis and treatment. She has been told by her physician that she has rheumatoid arthritis. She is fairly well informed about the disease. F. B. has a very successful career as a public-relations director. She has a masters degree in social work and did professional counseling for 5 years. The following information is the result of a frank discussion between patient and nurse, in which problems were identified that could be common to many new rheumatoid arthritis patients. Various approaches to supportive nursing care were identified.

Subjective Data	Problems Identified	Approaches to Supportive Nursing
I'm convinced if I give up tennis, it will go away. That stress seems to bring it on. But I'm not prepared to give up tennis.	Denial of nature of disease	Encourage patient to ask questions about the disease. Provide written information. Concentrate on helping patient formulate solutions to *other* problems. Talk about the "what ifs" and "why nots." Although it may seem that *acceptance* of the disease should facilitate problem solving, the reverse may be true!
It would be a problem if my hands were immobilized, because I am a writer.	Concern over ability to continue to function effectively in a job	Discuss the patient's occupation. Help the patient decide whether or not modification of any manual activities is possible.
I don't think I'll be angry if I have to be hospitalized, but I might. I wouldn't want to get weepy. Crying is a "cop-out." On second thought, I might feel like I want to punch somebody . . . but I wouldn't let that show.	Suppressed anger	Observe for signs of depression and "weepiness." Remind patient whenever necessary that it is "okay" to be angry and that to talk about that anger may be a step toward resolving it.
Exercise and fitness are important to me. I think about that a lot. If I couldn't do needlework, I might read more. I would feel badly about not playing the guitar. But it may be a good manipulating exercise.	Concern over alterations that may have to be made in life-style and "giving up" certain activities	Find out what physical activities are important to the patient and decide which of these will be proper exercise within the limits of pain and fatigue. What are some of the things this person would do if time permitted? Perhaps these are the activities that can be done as substitutes for those that can no longer be tolerated.
My problem is, I'm a physical coward. I don't like pain, and I'd really have to work not to let pain control my life. Besides, pain is fatiguing.	Fear of pain and coping with pain	Discuss prevention and relief of pain and the importance of taking medications as directed and adhering to all aspects of proposed treatment program. Encourage patient to talk about past experiences with pain. What factors contribute psychologically to feelings of pain?

THE "NEW" PATIENT WITH RHEUMATOID ARTHRITIS: SUBJECTIVE DATA WITH IMPLICATIONS FOR NURSING *(Continued)*

Subjective Data	Problems Identified	Approaches to Supportive Nursing
Because I live alone, there are certain things, of necessity, I have to do; and there is no one to do them for me. But given the nature I have, I might be tempted to sit back and let someone take care of me . . . someone whose attention I really want right now. But that would be a conflict for me, too, since I think of myself as coming from strength rather than weakness.	Fear of dependency Fear of acquiring a negative self-image	Both physical and occupational therapists can make suggestions for activities of daily living (ADL) that will relieve stress on joints. The nurse must establish rapport with the patient so that she can ask questions in sensitive areas and make useful suggestions. Include family members in discussions when appropriate. Make them aware that their acceptance of the situation may be critical in helping the patient maintain a positive self-image.

ronment, and quackery are among the subjects covered in pamphlets. The patient can obtain information by writing to: The National Arthritis Foundation, 3400 Peachtree Road, N.E., Suite 1101, Atlanta, GA 30326. State and local groups can often be reached by checking the telephone directory. Such groups not only provide literature but also have meetings designed to educate the arthritic and offer emotional support.

Psychological Support. Throughout a lifetime, the person with rheumatoid arthritis requires support and encouragement from those who are concerned with his welfare. Therefore, these persons must also understand the disease and its ramifications.

Care of the Patient with Rheumatoid Arthritis

Within the hospital setting, the orthopedic nurse will encounter patients with rheumatoid arthritis in several kinds of situations. First, there is the patient who is admitted with "joint aches and pains" for the purpose of diagnosis and initiation of treatment. Nursing priorities in caring for this type of patient are emotional support and education. The second category includes patients who are "old arthritics" suffering from exacerbations of the disease who require intensive treatment and perhaps some adjustment in their current regimen. These patients are probably the greatest nursing frustration in that they show little improvement

during their hospitalization. The third and most common type of patient with rheumatoid arthritis on the orthopedic unit is the one who is there for a surgical procedure to alleviate pain and help restore function; for example, a total knee replacement. Assisting this patient to attain an improved degree of mobility will be a nursing priority along with maintaining his general comfort.

In all cases, the basic aspects of a total treatment program are considered when planning and delivering care. For special considerations in the care of patients with rheumatoid arthritis, see pages 326 and 328.

Planning Care

Formulating a nursing care plan for the patient with rheumatoid arthritis will be done more efficiently and ensure the patient's trust and cooperation, if the nurse remembers and works with these three important points.

1. The rheumatoid patient wakes up with morning stiffness and discomfort. The degree of stiffness and discomfort usually present should be noted on an admission interview and transferred to the Kardex. In other words, how long does it take, in the morning, before the patient is either able to feed himself or is comfortable enough to accept help in eating? Perhaps warm water or a warm wet cloth on the hands a half-hour before breakfast is beneficial. Hygiene routines, bathing, and skin care should be scheduled for when the patient can help himself; for instance, 1 hour after an 8 A.M. dose of aspirin.

PROBLEM SOLVING: RHEUMATOID ARTHRITIS

Significant Data: A. C. is a 48-year old female with severe advanced rheumatoid arthritis, contractures of her knees, hips, and elbows. She has bilateral ulnar deviation but can use her hands, slowly. She walks with crutches. She weighs 150 lb. and is 5'7" tall. Her disease is poorly controlled at present. She is on, and has been on, aspirin and prednisolone for 3 years. She lives with her husband, who helps her get up and dressed every morning before he goes to work. Their daughter is married and lives "30 minutes away." A. C. entered the hospital 3 days ago for a medical workup and possibly a total knee replacement. Yesterday she had a severe flare-up of pain in all of her joints.

Present Nursing Orders

1. Back, buttocks, heel, and elbow care q 3 hr. Rub with lotion, then reposition patient.
2. Convoluted bedpad continuously.
3. Heel and elbow protectors.
4. Arm exercises qid using weight, pulley, and rope setup.
5. Active or passive ROM for lower extremities qid.

Physician Orders

1. Diet as tolerated.
2. Up to bathroom as tolerated with help.
3. Prednisone 5 mg daily with antacid.
4. ASA gr 10 q 4 hr.
5. Nembutal gr iss HS.
6. Demerol 100 mg q 4 hr for severe pain *only,* otherwise give Tylenol #3 tabs. 2.

Data Collection 3:30 P.M.

1. A. C. has had a "bad" day. She refused all care this morning because of severe pain.
2. She ate very little and has needed much encouragement to take fluids.
3. She wanted to go to the bathroom on crutches but had so much pain in her left knee that she had to lie down. When put on the bedpan (fracture pan) she had difficulty staying on it because of hip pain. Has not had a bowel movement for 2 days.
4. Seems to be weak or tired this afternoon.
5. Sometimes she actually screams with hip and knee pain.
6. Refused to do her arm exercises.
7. Has had Demerol twice for pain.
8. Is taking ASA, antacid, and prednisone as scheduled.
9. Physician says he will not do surgery until she has better medical management.
10. Is stiff and says she does not know what to do with herself.

Assessment and Intervention

1. Evaluate pain and stiffness as to exact location. Try to do ROM to see what movements are least painful. Suggest and try to get patient to identify those nursing measures that may increase comfort.
   A. Gentle massage
   B. Hot wet packs to knees and hip at intervals
2. Evaluate effectiveness of ASA and pain medications.
3. Check food and fluid preference. Suggest she ask for nourishment of choice p.r.n.
4. Assess for gastrointestinal distress.
5. Ask dietician to do a nutritional assessment to determine possible cause of weakness and find ways to improve appetite.
6. Recheck initial labwork reports, especially RBC, Hct, Hgb.
7. Order deep breathing and coughing q 4 hr when awake.
8. Order intake and output.
9. Discuss with patient possibility of "total lift" to commode at bedside for bowel movement p.r.n.
10. Is patient concerned about bowels? What is normal pattern of elimination? Does she take laxatives or enemas?
11. Confer with physical therapist. Approach patient together about exercises. Discontinue arm exercises at this time. Evaluate need for splints. Ask physician about order for Hubbard tank daily.
12. Encourage patient to verbalize feelings about postponement of surgery.
13. Discuss your concerns with husband and ask for suggestions.
14. Make note to evaluate (at later date) patient and husband's knowledge of disease and their use of local educational and supportive resources.
15. Ask occupational therapist to make introductory visit.

PROBLEM SOLVING: RHEUMATOID ARTHRITIS *(Continued)*

Potential Nursing Diagnoses

1. Comfort, alterations in: Pain and stiffness: Related to arthritis
2. Respiratory function, alterations in: Related to immobility
3. Impaired gas exchange, potential: Related to hypoventilation
4. Coping, ineffective individual: Related to depression in response to identifiable stressors
5. Self-care deficit: Related to inability to perform activities of daily living
6. Alterations in bowel elimination, potential for: Constipation: Related to immobility, medication, discomfort
7. Mobility, impaired physical: Related to pain and stiffness
8. Nutrition, alterations in: Less than body requirements: Related to pain, depression
9. Noncompliance: Related to impaired ability to perform exercises
10. Urinary elimination, alteration in patterns of, potential for: Related to reduced fluid intake, immobility
11. Injury, potential for: Related to motor deficits
12. Skin integrity, impairment of, potential: Related to immobility
13. Diversional activity deficit: Related to immobility

2. Anticipating needs will enable the nurse to perform tasks and organize objects in the patient's unit in such a way that the patient will feel and actually be less dependent.

This promotes emotional comfort for a patient and saves time for the nurse. If the patient is relatively helpless or uncomfortable, the bedpan should be offered before back care is given and the bottom linen changed. This may save one turning of the patient. The patient should have a glass of water or other liquid within reach. Having several facial tissues folded and tucked under the edge of the pillow or drawsheet is another suggestion. Even the seemingly effortless action of reaching for a tissue can be an ordeal for this person. A small paper bag in which to place used tissues might be taped to the bed rail or bedside stand.

Simple things like asking a patient whether the window shade or blind should be open or closed may mean that the relatively helpless patient does not have to put on the call light 20 minutes after the nurse leaves the room. The call light must not only be within reach, but the patient must have the manual strength and dexterity to use it. Some patients may need to have an alternative call system devised that is extremely sensitive to touch or constructed for ease in handling by either hand or foot.

The task of rearranging the environment should be discussed with the patient and a close family member. The nurse might ask, "What is difficult for you to do? What are you concerned about reaching, or what do you think you might not be able to get when you need it?" This leads to the third and perhaps the most important point in planning care for these patients.

3. Stress apparently plays a role in triggering an exacerbation of the disease or increasing the discomfort of an already present attack.

Obviously, then, when the nurse is planning care for the total knee replacement patient with rheumatoid arthritis whose other joints are "quiet," she must identify and modify or eliminate factors that cause the patient emotional stress. When the patient is in an acute phase of the disease, every effort should be made to learn how that patient "likes things done" and what movements increase pain.

Hygiene

The skin of a patient with rheumatoid arthritis requires special attention because he spends so much time in bed or relatively immobile. Certain soaps may be irritating to his skin, and this should be taken into consideration. Close inspection of bony prominences during the bath routine is imperative. Besides routine back and buttock care, lotion rubs should be frequent wherever pressure points are likely to develop—the elbows, shoulder blades, spinous pro-

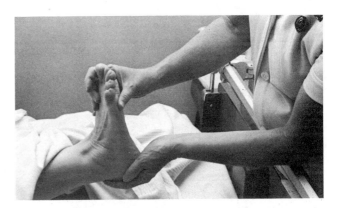

THE PATIENT WITH SEVERE RHEUMATOID ARTHRITIS: SUBJECTIVE DATA AND IMPLICATIONS FOR NURSING

Significant History: B. R. is a 57-year old female who has had rheumatoid arthritis for 19 years. In the last 7 years she has had both hips and knees replaced and is currently walking with a cane. Although she has severe deformities of both hands, she is able to do ADL with the aid of adaptive utensils. Since she is widowed and lives alone, a visiting nurse comes twice a week to help her shower and shampoo her hair. Her three children are married. One year ago she was almost killed in an automobile accident and was hospitalized for 2 months with head and chest injuries and multiple fractures. Her joint replacements and her recovery from a serious accident have made her a person who has positive thoughts and who has finally learned to live with her disease. In an interview at her home she related the history of her disease and identified her major concerns during hospitalization. Subsequent discussion of this data resulted in some insights that should be helpful in nursing management of patients with severe rheumatoid arthritis.

Subjective Data

The last thing the doctor told me when he said I had rheumatoid arthritis was that there would be days when I wished I were dead.

I still feel a lot of guilt about all the years I wouldn't go places with my husband. He's been dead 10 years. He had to spend so much time taking care of me. If he can see me now, I wonder what he thinks of how well I get along. I feel guilty about being bitter those years when my children were growing up. I did not enjoy them as I should have, and they knew it.

Moving was always the worst thing I had to do in the hospital. It was so painful.

I was the most nervous when I had to pivot into a chair. I had to tell who ever was getting me out of bed not to hold their foot against mine because then, when I would stand up, my knees would lock and hurt.

When I was tense, I would feel that tension being transferred to the staff and vice versa. I could always tell when they were tense handling me. Then things never seemed to go well.

Uppermost in my mind, no matter how sick I am, has always been what people think of me and the way I look. That was the reason I never wanted to go anywhere when I was younger. I need to feel I look my best.

Implications for Nursing

The patient who has had rheumatoid arthritis for a long time has undoubtedly suffered emotional trauma that will affect the way in which s/he copes with exacerbations of the disease. The patient's outlook will also be influenced by emotionally traumatic experiences.

It is possible that many patients with severe rheumatoid arthritis not only have days when they wish they were dead but may believe they deserve to be.

Precise and detailed data on what movements are painful, when the patient has the most pain, and what actions seem to be the most helpful in preventing or relieving pain, are essential in planning nursing care.

Every procedure that involves patient movement should be explained and evaluated by both patient and nurse to determine if it is the "best way."

The nurse who cares for the patient with rheumatoid arthritis must be confident in her actions. The patient should be told that it is "all right" to say that s/he feels more secure with certain staff members.

The patient needs to feel accepted and loved. A special effort should be made to have the patient with rheumatoid arthritis groomed before any visits to PT or any other department in the hospital. Positive, frequent comments on appearance and clothing will be appreciated.

cesses, sacrum, coccyx, and heels. If the patient does a considerable amount of side-lying, the shoulder, iliac crests, and malleoli need special attention.

An alternating-pressure mattress, convoluted bedpad, or sheepskin is one more preventive measure against skin breakdown. Heel and elbow protectors should only be used for their softness and not in place of regular skin care. Frequent change of position is the best guarantee against skin problems.

Self-care should be encouraged both to keep the patient as independent as possible and also to provide some exercise.

Bedpan Routine

A fracture bedpan is usually more easily placed than a regular bedpan. However, sitting on a bedpan can be extremely uncomfortable for a patient who has serious deformities or is in severe pain, because he may feel the need to help support himself with his elbows or hands. This is especially true if he is more comfortable in a side-lying position. Frequently these patients maintain better bowel and bladder habits if they can be helped or lifted onto a commode.

Positioning and Comfort

Positions of flexion are the most comfortable for the patient with rheumatoid arthritis but must be avoided and discouraged. He should be repositioned in bed at least every 3 hours. A small flat pillow under the head will create only minimal flexion of the neck. Great care must be taken when

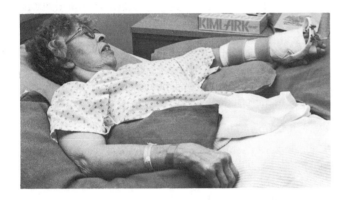

placing any pillows under or around these patients. The fewer pillows used, the better; these patients tend to "bunch" pillows under their knees and lower arms. Small pillows are best for supporting joints. The heels can usually be kept off the bed by placing bath blankets under the calves of the legs. When the patient is lying on his side, a small pillow between the knees will be helpful in preventing adduction deformity of the hip. A trochanter roll positioned along the lateral aspect of the thigh is preferable to a sandbag in maintaining neutral position of the hip joint. Sandbags put pressure on the skin and may also cause the patient to perspire, predisposing him to skin breakdown.

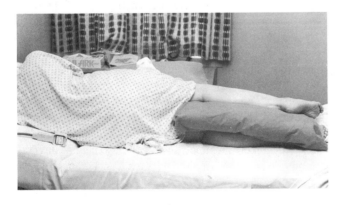

A bed cradle over the lower legs is useful in keeping bedclothes off the feet. Active and passive range-of-motion foot exercises on a regular schedule are better protection against contracture of the Achilles tendon (footdrop) than a footboard. Patients rarely keep their feet against a footboard for any length of time. In addition, the foot does not normally rest at a right angle, and maintaining this position may cause strain in the lower legs.

Time and patience are of the essence in handling the rheumatoid patient with severe pain and deformity. He is often extremely apprehensive about assuming certain positions because of joint pain and may not wish to remain in any one position for longer than a few minutes. All of the communication skills a nurse can muster may be necessary in providing proper body alignment for her rheumatoid arthritis patient.

When the patient is practically unable to stay in any other position but one or two for any length of time, it is essential to increase the frequency of lotion rubs to the area that is being rested on most often. One suggestion for getting a patient off his side or back is to place him on a Stryker frame. Although this maneuver is successful in preventing skin breakdown and further contractures in the rheumatoid arthritis patient, it may be frightening and unacceptable to him without a tremendous amount of emotional support from the entire patient care team.

The patient should always be encouraged to use the trapeze when he is moving himself about in bed because this

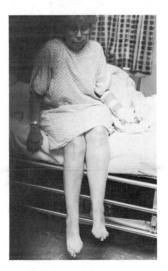 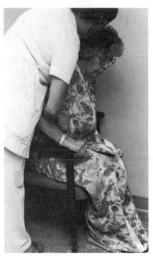

will provide some arm exercise. Since the rheumatoid arthritis patient may have muscle weakness and pain in his legs, the bed should be in a high position when he gets out of bed. This will enable him to slide off the edge without bending or exertion. Likewise, any chair he sits in should have a high enough seat so that he can be assisted in and out of it with a minimum of effort on his part. A chair with arm rests is preferable so that the patient can push himself to a standing position.

Promoting Rest

The orthopedic nurse must remember that the temperature of a room is a factor in keeping the rheumatoid arthritis patient comfortable. Also, as many nursing care routines as possible should be scheduled at the same time so that the patient has rest periods of ample length.

Exercise and Physical Therapy

The patient with acute symptoms cannot exercise his affected joints until pain and swelling subside. However, his other joints need consideration.

The physical therapist and the nurse should evaluate together what the patient is capable of doing in terms of active range of motion and then establish a schedule of active and passive exercises in which both can participate. Rheumatoid arthritis patients are frequently reluctant to exercise, and it will take the combined efforts of both the physical therapist and the nursing staff to keep these patients on an exercise schedule. Establishing a trust relationship becomes extremely critical. Often a patient will become

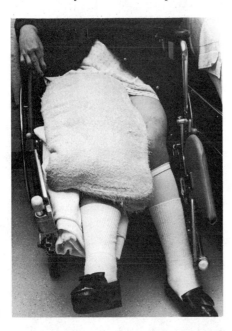

Hot pack

accustomed to working with one therapist and respond much more positively if allowed to exercise with that therapist at all times.

Hot or cold wet applications may be used to help the patient get started with an exercise routine. Paraffin baths are also used by the physical therapy department. Heat will decrease the pain and relax muscles, thereby increasing the patient's ability to move the joints. Cold may be used in place of heat to reduce swelling. The therapist may try both hot and cold applications to determine which is most effective for an individual patient.

In general, the physical therapist initiates and teaches exercises that will strengthen the joints without causing further irritation. Isometric exercises and basic range of motion are the least difficult for a patient to do independently.

Encouraging Independence

Some rheumatoid arthritis patients have extensive hand deformities and need to be cared for completely. Others may require only adaptation of the environment and assistance. Mealtime is a good time to begin evaluating the patient's degree of dependence.

Though it is true that some patients may use adaptive utensils and require only minimal assistance with food placement, it is also true that other rheumatoid arthritis patients would rather be fed than go through the slow, clumsy motions of feeding themselves once they are hospitalized. This is one reason why it is important to know from the beginning what the patient is capable of doing and whether or not feeding himself efficiently is an activity he can learn while hospitalized.

The physical therapist, in consultation with the occupational therapist, should evaluate the severity of the patient's limitations of motion and begin a coordinated exercise regimen to help him maintain his independence or to teach him to become more independent.

Occupational Therapy

The primary goal of the occupational therapist is to encourage function. This may involve proper positioning of the extremity through splinting. (See illustrated guide for making a splint on p. 333.)

Splints made and used by the occupational therapist are designed for resting positions and for function. They are usually made of a lightweight plastic material. When heated to about 150°F. this material becomes very pliable, enabling the therapist to mold it to the joint it must support. After the material is molded into shape, it is cut to the proper fit and then set with ice water or cold spray. The joints most often splinted in the rheumatoid arthritis patient are the joints of the hand, the wrist, or the knee.

The occupational therapist helps the rheumatoid arthritis patient to perform the strengthening exercises initiated by the physical therapist. However, in the occupational therapy department the patient is introduced to coordination exercises designed to facilitate activities of daily living (ADL). For instance, the therapist works with the patient to help him learn a grasp-and-release action. The patient receives instruction and practice in the use of adaptive equipment that will meet his specific needs.

Medications

The patient with newly diagnosed rheumatoid arthritis should know what his medications are for, and he should be instructed about the importance of taking them as directed after he leaves the hospital. Written instructions may be

MAKING A WRIST SPLINT FOR THE RHEUMATOID ARTHRITIS PATIENT

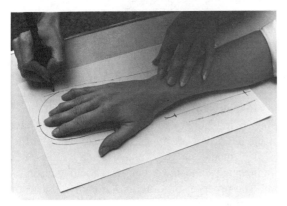

Splints made and used by the occupational therapist are designed for resting positions and for function.

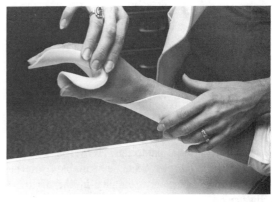

After the material is molded into shape, it is cut to the proper fit.

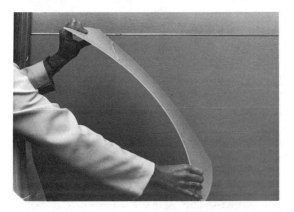

Splints are usually made of a lightweight plastic material.

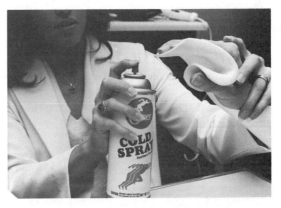

The splint is then set with ice water or cold spray.

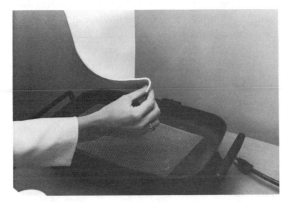

When heated to about 65.5°C (150°F), this material becomes very pliable, enabling the therapist to mold it to the joint it must support.

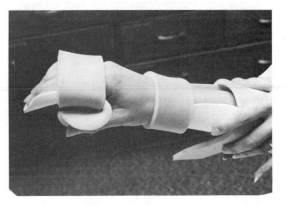

Finished wrist splint in use. The joints most often splinted in the rheumatoid arthritis patient are the joints of the hand, the wrist, or the knee.

necessary. Any change in medications or schedule of administration that is ordered by the physician while an "old arthritic" patient is in the hospital should be explained to the patient immediately so that he does not become upset by the change. The nurse should evaluate *all* rheumatoid arthritis patients' knowledge about medication that has been prescribed for them and ensure that any needed instruction is given.

Sexuality

Body image disturbances, because of impaired mobility and deformity, are common in patients with rheumatoid arthritis. Sexual function may be disrupted by joint contractures and pain. An informational pamphlet, *Arthritis, Living, and Loving: Information About Sex*, is available from the National Arthritis Foundation. Sexuality in the arthritic patient is discussed further in Chapter 11.

Individualizing Patient Care

There are both physical and psychological considerations in individualizing the care of a patient with rheumatoid arthritis.

For the patient who has just learned he has the disease, proper and adequate instruction is a priority. Every instruction and point of information given by the physician must be reinforced by the nurse. The patient should be warned about quackery and reminded that when a cure is discovered, physicians will be the first to know about it.

It is important for the nurse to remember that pain and limitation of motion are major factors in the development of a negative self-image that will adversely affect all of the patient's activities. Providing thorough instruction in the prevention and control of pain and deformity and information on resources available for education and support will go a long way in helping a patient to maintain a healthy self-image. In turn, this will help him adhere to a treatment program, and the whole process can become a positive cycle of action.

Frequently the "new rheumatoid" will leave the hospital in a state of denial. Ample opportunities to discuss the disease and to verbalize his feelings may make acceptance of rheumatoid arthritis less difficult.

Nursing management of the patient who has had rheumatoid arthritis for a long time and bears the signs of treatment, or lack of treatment, is extremely challenging. For example, the patient who has been on corticosteroids for a prolonged period of time is susceptible to infection, and this fact requires special nursing observations and preventive measures. The patient who has not had definite treatment may have skin over atrophied joints that is shiny and tight and requires special care to prevent it from breaking down.

Patients with rheumatoid arthritis often hold convictions that certain ointments, such as those that contain oil of wintergreen, relieve their joint pain and aching muscles.

They have developed rituals that reduce their discomfort and anxiety and attachments for special pillows or blankets. Whatever is important to the patient should be incorporated into the nursing care plan whenever feasible.

The nurse can gain insights into formulating a successful approach to the psychological care of the rheumatoid arthritis patient by considering attitudes that the patient may have toward himself. The patient may have feelings of guilt because of the way his limitations have affected his behavior toward others, or he may feel guilty because he is dependent. Inability to cope with his environment may evoke feelings of inadequacy and hopelessness. He may have fears that his limitations or appearance may cost him the affection of a spouse or loved one. He may consider himself "handicapped" and have concerns about gainful employment. The prospect of a lifetime of pain and discomfort is not easy to face without bitterness. These attitudes may be manifested in a variety of behaviors such as unrealistic dependency (the demanding patient), manipulation, poor communication, or passivity.

Sometimes it is a family member, however, who has the psychological problem; for instance, a need to feel needed. Careful observation of interaction between the patient and his family will help the nurse identify who needs whom or what. For instance, the husband of a patient with rheumatoid arthritis may spend long hours at the bedside assisting in the care of his severely incapacitated wife. Often his help is part of the nursing care plan and greatly appreciated. When this same individual begins doing things for his spouse that she could or should be doing for herself, or when he spends a lot of time roaming through the hospital and visiting with the staff, perhaps he has a need to verbalize his concerns and feelings. Frank discussions of what assistance on his part will benefit his wife, frequent requests for his input into planning care, and acknowledgment by the staff of the value of his participation may be advisable. The husband who feels that his actions are essential to the treatment program designed for his wife may be able to communicate his own thoughts more freely.

Discharge Planning

When considering discharge planning for the patient, the nurse must look at every aspect of the basic treatment program for persons with rheumatoid arthritis, as discussed on pages 323–327.

The entire patient care team will need to confer with the patient and the family. The home environment, as it exists, should be discussed, and adaptations and adjustments should be suggested. Whenever necessary, referrals should be made to home health care agencies. A work simplification program outlined on paper by the occupational therapy department will be extremely beneficial in helping the patient establish routines for activities of daily living. An example of such a program appears on pages 335–337.

GUIDELINES FOR WORK SIMPLIFICATION*

Work simplification is an organized procedure for finding ways to simplify daily tasks. Overwork, overexertion, and strenuous exercise are among the most severe types of stress to which arthritic joints and the cardiopulmonary system can be subjected. These principles of work simplification should be used as guidelines to help you to recognize your work and exercise tolerance levels and at the same time help you to get the most efficient use of your time and energy.

Plan Ahead and Organize and Simplify Your Work

ANALYZE THE JOB

1. *What* is the job and its purpose?
2. *Why* is it necessary?
3. *Where* is the best place to do this job?
4. *When* should the job be done?
5. *How* can I do it in the "best way" for me?
6. *Who* is the best person to do the job or *Who* can help?

DEVELOP NEW AND BETTER METHODS AND SET PRIORITIES

1. Distribute heavy work over longer time periods.
   - Clean one room per day, not all rooms in one day.
   - Split up lawn and outside work (raking, mowing, washing windows) over several days.
2. Eliminate unnecessary details.
   - Let dishes air dry.
   - Fold sheets without pressing.
3. Avoid duplication of activities.
   - Minimize trips to the store by planning weekly menus and shopping lists; keep a running list of needed supplies on the refrigerator.
   - If you have a freezer, cook or bake "double batches," an extra hot dish to pop in the oven when you are tired can seem like a life saver.
4. Use modern labor-saving equipment whenever possible.
   - Electric can opener, electric knife
5. Use fewest possible elements for the job.
   - Select equipment that may be used for more than one job.
   - Use recipes and mixes that emphasize the "one-bowl" method and quick mixing.

Use Your Body Efficiently

MAINTAIN GOOD POSTURE

Your body has three main sections:

Head and neck

Chest and shoulders

Hip and pelvic section

Center these body parts and align them directly over each other. It takes *less* energy to hold your body in this position. Try to keep balanced alignment when you stand, walk, climb stairs, or sit at work or play.

USE STRONGEST MUSCLES AND JOINTS FOR THE JOB

Distribute work over several sets of muscles and use the stronger ones.
- Use both hands and arms to carry objects whenever possible. When lifting heavy objects, lower your body by bending leg joints and keeping back straight. As you return to standing, your leg muscles do the lifting.
- When pushing heavy objects, *lean into* the job and let your legs do the work.

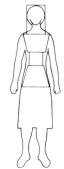

Use smooth, rhythmic, repetitive, larger motions in heavy or tiring work activities.
- Try this in activities such as washing walls, windows, cars, or in raking, gardening, and vacuuming.
- Try working to music (radio, singing), and think pleasant thoughts, feel relaxed, and try to change tasks often.

* Courtesy Occupational Therapy Department, Bellin Memorial Hospital, Green Bay, Wisconsin

GUIDELINES FOR WORK SIMPLIFICATION *(continued)*

AVOID UNNECESSARY MOVEMENTS AND TASKS
BY USING FEWER AND MORE EFFICIENT MOTIONS

1. Sit to work as much as possible.
   - Standing puts more stress on hip joints and uses more energy. Sit *tall!* Remember, though, to sit at tasks that allow you to stay seated without getting up and down often. It is only when you are seated comfortably with work at the right level that you can reduce fatigue. As a general rule, sit for any task that takes longer than 5 minutes; stand and stretch at least every 30 minutes while sitting. For arthritics it is recommended to rest 5–10 minutes of each hour or 10–20 minutes every 2 hours. [Rest means lying down on couch or recliner with eyes closed, body relaxed (no reading, TV, etc.).]
   - Try sitting for jobs such as meal preparation, ironing (adjustable ironing board), painting, working at workbench, gardening (transplanting, weeding, etc.)
   - Have adequate knee room under working surface.
   - Either rest feet flat on floor or on step of chair.
2. Use productive motions.
   - Slide items across counter or floor, instead of lifting and carrying. Use casters or wheels for transporting, and for portable storage or working surface.
   - Let gravity work for you. Drop objects into place rather than placing them. A clothes chute can carry clothes to the basement. Gravity-fed drops for sugar, flour, or feed, or a container below the level of the working surface to catch your work or waste —are all energy savers.

3. Use simultaneous motions with smooth, continuous movements.
   - Dust with both hands or put dishes in cupboard with both hands. Use both hands to wash car or windows or to place objects on shelf.
   - When making bed, smooth as you go, with both arms doing the work. Avoid extra walking. Use fitted sheets for less work. A bed is easier to make if it is away from the walls.
4. Avoid unnecessary bending, stretching, reaching, climbing, and prolonged grip.
   - Use long-handled items such as mop, duster, squeegee, pick-up or reaching tongs, brushes.
   - Store often-used materials within easiest reach (between shoulder height and hip level). Use pegboards, lazy susan, etc.
   - Avoid unnecessary stair climbing. It is one of the most energy-consuming body actions, because it involves lifting and balancing total body weight. Try placing a basket at the bottom of the stairs and putting supplies, laundry, etc., into it and carrying the basket up the steps once rather than making many trips.
   - Use utensils that rest firmly on the table such as a mixmaster or rubber bottomed bowls, or use a rubber mat or octopus suction holder to conserve energy and have both arms free to work.
5. Lay out work areas within normal reach. Try to work in areas that hands overlap and arrange supplies in a semi circle within easy reach.

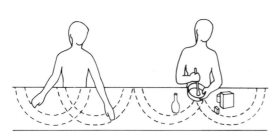

Determining horizontal reaching areas

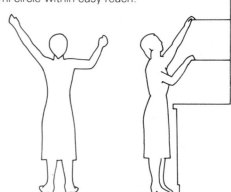

Determining vertical reaching areas

Select and Plan the Proper Work Areas for Your Jobs

HAVE FIXED WORK AREAS, SO SUPPLIES AND
EQUIPMENT MAY BE KEPT THERE READY FOR USE.

PRE-POSITION TOOLS AND EQUIPMENT SO THEY
ARE EASY TO SEE, EASY TO REACH, AND EASY
TO GRASP.

1. Vertical files or partitions are good for high and low storage areas and deep drawers.
2. Use pull-out shelves and lazy susans. Wall panels, pegboards, special hanging devices, and magnetic racks can also be used.
3. Dispose of items that you don't use and increase storage space.

GUIDELINES FOR WORK SIMPLIFICATION *(continued)*

4. If an item is useful in more than one area, buy two and place one in each area to save energy running from one place to another. (Measuring cups, measuring spoons, needle and thread, etc.)

ARRANGE GOOD WORKING CONDITIONS SO THAT YOUR JOB IS MORE PLEASANT AND LESS TIRING.

1. Good lighting helps in reducing eye strain and eye fatigue. Shield bare lamps.
2. Good ventilation is important in removing odors and excessive heat and in providing a change of air. Windows and doors are good for cross-ventilation, but a good fan changes the air quickly.
3. Plan for safety. Locate electrical outlets and switches for easy reach. Choose appliances that are easy to handle.
4. Wear comfortable clothes.

ADJUST WORK HEIGHTS TO THE PERSON AND JOB. PROPER WORK HEIGHTS ENCOURAGE GOOD POSTURE AND REDUCE FATIGUE.

Use work surfaces of different levels for different jobs:
- You should be able to stand straight, but relaxed, and place the palm of your hand (without arm stretching) on a work surface you use when working with short-handled tools. The sink bottom should be the same level for comfortable dishwashing *(A)*.

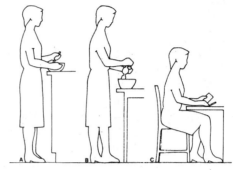

- When using longer tools, see that work surface is at the right height for your hands to be lower than elbows *(B)*.
- A work counter that you sit at to work should be as low as your lap will permit *(C)*.

Pace Yourself—Physically and Emotionally

PREVENT FATIGUE BY MOVING AT A RATE THAT SEEMS EASY AND COMFORTABLE FOR YOU— WITHOUT A FEELING OF HURRY OR PRESSURE.

1. Rest *before* you feel fatigued.
   - Frequent, short rest periods before you are tired are better than a long rest period after you become tired.
   - It is usually best to rest lying down on a firm surface so all parts of your body can rest completely. But remember, a change of activity can also be a rest from what you have been doing.
   - A *slow, steady* rate of work, with short rest periods, will get the job done without doing you in. *Never* work so hard or long that you experience shortness of breath or chest pain.
   - *Never start something that can't be stopped for a rest period when desired.*
2. Control your emotions.
   - Remember, emotional fatigue and stresses can be just as fatiguing as physical ones and place an extra burden on the heart.
   - Learn to control your mind. Be able to "turn it off." Worries, fears, and tensions will prevent you from relaxing during rest.
   - Use your energy to change things you *can* and accept those you can't change. Control your temper and avoid emotional upsets.

LEARN AND PRACTICE RELAXATION

1. First, lie down; tense your whole body; then try to relax each part with the feeling that your body is "sinking" into the floor or couch.
2. You can be relaxed while working, by using muscles properly and relaxing the parts of the body you are not using.

REMEMBER: IT PAYS TO KEEP IN GOOD PHYSICAL CONDITION

1. Use regular, moderate activity to keep in shape.
2. Understand your physical limitations.
3. Continue your activities in a graduated, supervised activity program in order to restore your muscle tone and strength in preparation for "normal" *(for you)* physical activity.

Osteoarthritis

Causative Factors

Osteoarthritis, or degenerative joint disease, is the mechanical "wearing out" of a joint. The causes are unknown, although the disease is associated with the aging process. Osteoarthritis is not systemic and most commonly affects the weightbearing joints of the lower extremities. The causative factors in osteoarthritis of the hip and knee joints are listed on pages 199 and 242. Osteoarthritis may also involve the spine. The disease is relatively common in middle age and old age. Joint destruction varies from person to person but is generally not severely incapacitating.

Signs and Symptoms

The major complaint of a patient with osteoarthritis is of an aching pain upon weight bearing that is relieved by rest. The affected joint may be "stiff," and several minutes of exercise are required before it will "work" again. Crepitus (grating and grinding) may be heard upon movement. Sometimes certain movements of the joint elicit a "creaking" sound. This is especially noticeable in the knee. The joint may appear slightly enlarged, and the patient may complain of intermittent and mild swelling due to effusion. Signs of inflammation are lacking. The patient tends to become tired on exertion.

The patient with osteoarthritis may have increased pain and stiffness in cold, wet weather. Later in the course of the disease there may be contracture of the joint capsule and muscle weakness that will result in considerable limitation of motion and disability. In these cases, pain will tend to be continuous.

Heberden's nodes are a common sign of osteoarthritis; these are bony enlargements in the distal interphalangeal joints of the hands. Since the fingers are nonweightbearing joints, the reason for the development of Heberden's nodes is unknown. They are frequently asymptomatic.

The progress of osteoarthritis is slow, and the severity of the symptoms usually corresponds to the workload placed on the joint.

Diagnosis

Osteoarthritis is diagnosed by x-ray findings and clinical examination. X-ray films will show a narrowed joint space, bony overgrowth, and sclerotic changes.

Treatment

Osteoarthritis is treated medically by drug therapy and physical therapy. Instruction in self-care includes modification of activities to decrease the severity of symptoms.

First of all, it is important to relieve the patient's apprehension about the nature and prognosis of the disease. Although joint damage is irreversible, the patient can be taught that, as a rule, proper care will control the symptoms and that osteoarthritis does not shorten the life span.

Rest is an extremely important feature of a treatment program. The patient should adjust his physical activities to a level that the involved joint is able to tolerate. This may require a change of occupation along with modification of life-style. Simple range-of-motion exercises on a regular schedule will maintain joint mobility and decrease the chance of contractures.

Good nutrition and maintenance of general health will aid the patient in dealing with fatigue, pain, and stiffness. Since obesity aggravates the load on weight-bearing joints, reduction diets are advised for patients with osteoarthritis who are obese.

Aspirin (10 to 15 grains 3 or 4 times daily) may be sufficient to control pain. Other drugs that may be prescribed are indomethacin or phenylbutazone. Joint injections of steroids often provide symptomatic relief.

A physical therapy program may include some form of heat treatment followed by active nonweightbearing exercises to help prevent muscle atrophy. An assistive device such as a cane will often relieve the pain by decreasing the weight placed on the joint. A back brace or corset is sometimes ordered if the patient has osteoarthritis of the spine. In these instances, the patient must be instructed in the proper application and removal of the supportive garment. Severe crippling is not associated with this disease, but occasionally night splints are required to help prevent deformity.

Nursing Implications

In general, the patient with osteoarthritis is treated at home; and the nurse may only have contact with him when he is in the hospital for some type of reconstructive surgery. For this reason, an understanding of the basic features of a treatment program is a nursing responsibility. This will enable the nurse to evaluate the patient's knowledge of the disease and treatment accurately and to provide any needed instruction and psychological support.

1. A review of the principles of good posture may be helpful. The patient with osteoarthritis in the hips or spine should be made to understand that too much sitting is inadvisable because it could lead to flexion contractures and adduction of the hip joints.
2. The patient must be reminded to stand and walk as erect as he can (and this is difficult to remember if he is using an assistive device) in order to decrease the tendency toward dorsal kyphosis.
3. The development of pronated feet is not uncommon in these patients and properly fitting shoes are essential. Before discharge from the hospital the nurse should discuss this fact with the patient and check the condition of the shoes he will be wearing when he goes home.

4. If the patient is recovering from reconstructive surgery that will permit increased function of a joint, he should be instructed that although his activities may be increased, he should still have adequate rest periods each day.

Multiple Myeloma

Definition and Pathology

Multiple myeloma is a plasma cell dyscrasia originating in the bone marrow. The cancellous bone in the ribs, sternum, skull, vertebrae, and proximal ends of long bones is often primarily affected. Multiple myeloma is a rather common, highly malignant, incurable disease most often occurring in the middle-aged or elderly.

Normally, individual units, or clones, of plasma cells synthesize the body's immunoglobulins (Ig) in response to known antigens. In multiple myeloma, there is a neoplastic proliferation of a single clone of plasma cells resulting in excessive production of abnormal globulin, usually gamma globulin (IgG), called hypergammaglobulinemia.

Signs and Symptoms

The clinical manifestations of multiple myeloma are related to (1) the tumor or proliferation of malignant plasma cells with replacement of normal bloodforming marrow and bone destruction, (2) the tumor products (excessive abnormal proteins), and (3) abnormalities in host defense.

The onset of multiple myeloma is insidious. Bone pain resulting from osteolytic lesions is usually dull but not constant months before a diagnosis is established. Pain increases as more plasma cells become deposited in bone marrow. This pain is migratory and similar to arthritic discomfort. Back pain is the most frequent complaint and is due to intraosseous tumor pressure and vertebral collapse. There may be a pathologic fracture of a rib, which will cause pain. The patient may be pale and listless because of the anemia that is produced when bone marrow is destroyed.

Destruction of bone causes the release of excessive calcium, which is excreted in the urine, causing a significant fluid loss. When the renal threshold is exceeded, calcium is accumulated in the bloodstream. Hypercalcemia will result in anorexia, nausea, vomiting, constipation, increased myocardial irritability, lethargy, and confusion. Death occurs when the condition is not treated.

The abnormal proteins (called Bence-Jones proteins, after the man who described them) may precipitate out of the urine and cause a mechanical destruction of the renal tubules and impaired function.

The proliferation of malignant immunoglobulins interferes with normal immunoglobulin production, which means that there will be a decreased level of circulating antibodies in the bloodstream. Therefore, the patient with multiple myeloma may have symptoms of infection.

Laboratory Findings

Besides an elevation in serum calcium and urine calcium, the patient may have elevations of various serum protein levels. Electrophoresis of the urine may demonstrate the presence of Bence-Jones proteins. The blood level of uric acid may rise because of nucleic acid catabolism. Table 10-1, page 323, lists the laboratory tests that may be abnormal and are used in the total diagnosis of multiple myeloma.

X-Ray Findings

On x-ray film, the involved bone will show multiple punched-out areas.

Diagnosis

The diagnosis of multiple myeloma is confirmed when bone marrow aspiration reveals the presence of abnormal plasma cells.

Treatment

The treatment of multiple myeloma is primarily palliative. Radiation therapy is usually prescribed for localized areas of the body. Drug therapy may consist of a combination of an alkylating agent, such as melphalan, to depress bone marrow and retard the growth of malignant cells, and prednisolone to control hypercalcemia. Other combinations of cytotoxic drugs may also be given.

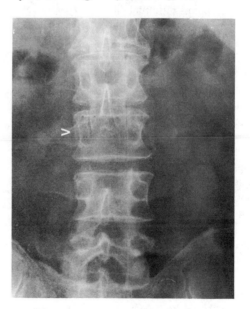

Bone destruction in multiple myeloma. Note absence of spinous process on L3.

Immobilization of a painful back by means of a lumbosacral support or other type of brace is beneficial.

Care of the Patient with Multiple Myeloma

Sometimes the orthopedic nurse only has contact with a patient who has multiple myeloma during the hospitalization period when a diagnosis is made. In a situation such as this, the patient is usually admitted to the unit with a complaint of back pain. Once a diagnosis has been confirmed and the initial treatment is begun, the patient remains in the hospital until a regimen has been established whereby pain is controlled and he has become adjusted to wearing a brace and perhaps to using an assistive device for ambulation. Though the patient may return to the orthopedic unit for reevaluation and alterations in his treatment program, it is just as likely that he will be admitted to a different hospital unit, depending on his condition. Therefore, the orthopedic nurse is a key person in helping the patient and his family adjust to the psychological trauma that occurs when the diagnosis is confirmed. She has a major role to play in the team effort that must be put forth if both patient and family are to succeed in coping with a disease that is painful and incapacitating and has a poor prognosis.

The goals in the nursing management of a patient with multiple myeloma are the following:

1. To prevent problems due to the nature of the disease process, such as infection and pathological fractures.
2. To make observations that will assist in the early diagnosis of conditions due to the advancement of the disease; spinal cord compression, hyperviscosity of the plamsa, and renal failure.
3. To prevent problems of immobility.
4. To help the patient achieve and maintain maximal physical comfort.
5. To detect early signs of side effects of drugs and radiation therapy.
6. To promote patient independence; adaptation to limited mobility.
7. To offer emotional support to patient and family.

Psychological Considerations

The orthopedic nurse must remember that because a diagnosis of multiple myeloma carries with it the certainty of a significantly shortened life span, the patient and the family may well begin the grieving process along with the treatment. She must be prepared for anger, denial, depression, and a host of other feelings associated with death and dying. The patient will need opportunities to verbalize these feelings, as will those who are closest to him.

When the physician informs the patient that he has the disease, the nurse should be present to hear the ensuing discussion. Then she will be able to give direct answers to questions and establish a relationship with the patient and the family that is built on trust. This will be conducive to the expression of feelings and helpful in gaining cooperation in providing the most effective care because the patient's fear of pain and dislike for dependency can best be overcome or modified if he knows that he can trust those who care for him.

Positioning and Movement

Every routine that involves movement of the patient should be done slowly and with extreme gentleness. The patient may experience increased pain and muscle spasm from the slightest jostling. Because ligaments and tendons are attached to the skeleton, even simple twisting and turning puts tension on bones. Pathologic fractures may occur following simple movements if the disease process is far advanced. As much as possible, the patient should be allowed to control his own movements. This will make him less apprehensive and less likely to have increased pain and muscle spasm.

The furniture in the room should be placed so that there is ample space around the bed to allow for free movement by hospital personnel. The nurse must remember to raise and lower bed rails carefully. Both of these measures will reduce the amount of accidental "bumping" against the bed.

The patient with multiple myeloma may lack energy because of anemia and fatigue due to pain, and this fact must also be taken into consideration when planning care.

The patient should have a change of position at least every 4 hours while awake. His joints must always be supported when he is turning or being positioned. A pillow between his legs when he is turned on his side will support

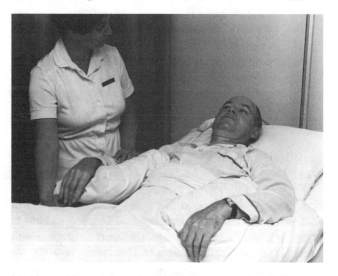

his hip and knee joints. Assisting him in turning "all in one piece," as in logrolling, will prevent twisting of the back muscles. The patient controls this movement by reaching for the bed rail when he begins to turn. The nurse assists by lightly supporting his shoulders and buttocks as he turns toward the opposite side, or toward her, whichever method seems to be most effective. Another nurse may be needed to help, depending on the patient's size and condition. After the patient is repositioned, the placement of pillows will depend on where they will give support and promote comfort. Williams' position may be comfortable when the patient is on his back.

The patient on bed rest should have a fracture bedpan. Positioning the patient on the bedpan must be done carefully. Logrolling may be the preferred procedure.

When the patient is transferred to a stretcher or wheelchair to go to the radiology department for x-ray films or therapy, this maneuver must be done slowly and carefully to avoid bumps and sudden movements. It is a nursing responsibility to inform those who transport the patient with multiple myeloma, such as radiology technicians, about the possibility of causing pathological fractures, pain, and spasm. If necessary, she must instruct them in the best way to get the patient on and off the stretcher, based on what she and the patient have worked out together.

Exercise and Ambulation

Since disuse osteoporosis will further weaken the bones and add still more calcium to the bloodstream, some exercise is necessary for the patient with multiple myeloma. Simple range of motion or isometric exercises, as the patient can tolerate, will have to be part of the nursing care plan if the patient is unable to ambulate.

Pain medication should be given a half-hour before ambulation. Two nurses should be present when the patient gets out of bed. Perhaps only one will be needed to give physical assistance, but the second nurse is necessary for reassurance if the patient is especially weak.

If a lumbosacral support is ordered, the patient should wear it every time he is out of bed. Both the patient and the person who will be responsible for his care at home should be taught the procedure for putting on and removing the corset.

The patient with multiple myeloma, while he is still semi-independent, will quickly establish his routine for getting in

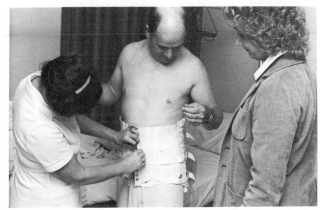

and out of bed with a minimum of pain and effort. For this reason, the nurse must allow him to give the directions or she must ask questions as she is assisting him in this endeavor.

Rest

Rest periods are important. Nursing routines should be scheduled so that the patient has 2 to 3 hours at one time in which to rest or sleep.

Pain

Accurate evaluation of pain is essential from the standpoint of providing adequate relief and in the prevention and early diagnosis of complications.

Back pain will probably be the patient's chief complaint. Analgesics should be administered and their effects noted. Muscle relaxants may be beneficial in reducing spasms.

Leg pain may occur, owing to spinal nerve root compression. However, the nurse and the patient must determine the exact location of all leg pain. Pain or spasm in the calf should alert the nurse to the possibility of thrombophlebitis. In such instances the nurse must inspect the calf for redness and tenderness, and check Homans' sign.

Chest pain and pain in the upper back may be due to pathologic fractures and muscle spasms. But any complaints of chest pain should cause the nurse to suspect pulmonary embolism.

Checking Neurovascular Status

Color, motion, temperature, and sensation (CMTS) of the toes of both feet must be monitored and compared to each other regularly when the patient has any complaints of pain or paresthesia in the lower extremities. Along with checking the neurovascular status of the toes, the nurse should make daily assessments of the legs for numbness. The patient should be asked if his legs feel "heavy" or become excessively tired when he has been walking. These symptoms indicate loss of leg power and may be signs of increased vertebral collapse and spinal cord compression.

Skin Care

Whenever the patient with multiple myeloma is turned on his side, his back should be inspected thoroughly for redness and skin breakdown. If he is receiving radiation therapy, the area undergoing treatment will be designated by indelible

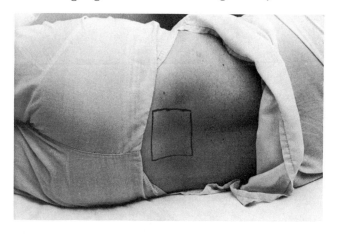

pencil markings. This area is extremely sensitive, and as treatment progresses, the skin will become reddened and scaly. The skin subjected to radiation therapy must not be rubbed or washed with soap. Skin breakdown should be treated according to instruction from the radiologist or attending physician. Protection, in the form of a sheepskin pad or other soft pad, should be provided. The patient must be made aware of the effect of irradiation on his skin. He will then be more conscious of the need for protection of this area and will also recognize the importance of position changes even though turning or other movements are painful.

The buttocks, shoulders, and areas where the skin is not exposed to irradiation require regular gentle lotion rubs. Elbows and heels should be rubbed at the same time.

Stir-up Routine

Deep breathing and coughing should be encouraged every 4 hours while the patient is awake. At this time he should also be asked to move his extremities and exercise his feet. Auscultation of the patient's lungs once a day will be helpful in making judgments about whether or not any additional respiratory support measures are necessary.

Nutrition

Special nutritional needs of the patient with multiple myeloma include foods that will help build blood to combat his anemia. A healthy nutritional state is difficult to maintain in a patient with this disease, however. One reason for this is that he may be anorexic or have nausea and vomiting from medications or radiation therapy or hypercalcemia. He may also be lethargic, and to some extent this will prevent him from eating and drinking adequate amounts. Providing assistance with meals and enough time to eat them will reduce fatigue. Small feedings as desired may be more tolerable. Antiemetics can be helpful in preventing nausea. Good oral hygiene before meals and several times daily will be refreshing and may encourage the patient to "try" all of his meals.

Fluid Intake and Output

Fluids must be encouraged from a nutritional standpoint, to aid in the prevention of kidney damage and to promote urinary excretion of drugs.

The patient should have a small glass of water or a fluid of his choice, with a straw, within easy reach at all times, since a small glass will require less effort to handle. Popsicles are a good source of extra fluid.

The physician may order intravenous fluids, steroids, and diuretics to treat the hypercalcemia. This makes accurate recording of intake and output extremely important.

The Urinary Tract: Specific Observations

Difficulty in voiding, with retention and overflow, may be a sign of spinal cord involvement and should be reported to the physician immediately. Urinary frequency, painful uri-

nation, and hematuria are symptoms of infection as well as hemorrhagic cystitis, which can occur as a side effect of the administration of cyclophosphamide. Checking the specific gravity of voided urine will help monitor alterations in kidney function.

Elimination

When food and fluid intake are not sufficient to maintain regularity in bowel elimination, stool softeners, laxatives, or enemas are advisable. Constipation adds to the patient's gastrointestinal distress and back pain.

Preventing Infection

The patient with multiple myeloma is susceptible to infection and especially pneumonia and urinary tract infections caused by encapsulated organisms. Individuals with signs and symptoms of respiratory infection or any open sores should not be allowed to go into the patient's room. A sign on the door should require visitors to stop at the nursing station before entering the room. The patient and his family should be told about this susceptibility to infection.

Good handwashing with a germicidal solution before doing any nursing care routines is mandatory. Teaching the patient to examine himself for signs of infection is another preventive measure.

The need for oral fluid intake in patients with multiple myeloma cannot be overemphasized.

Early diagnosis of infection is facilitated if the nurse is alert to signs and symptoms and does daily lung auscultations. The nurse should bear in mind the fact that steroids may mask signs of infection. Therefore, she needs to look at the total patient picture when making daily assessments.

Other Observations

To the patient, it often seems as if the treatment is as bad as the disease; and even though he understands this fact, moral support during the course of any treatment is a major nursing effort.

Besides nausea, vomiting, anorexia, and constipation, diarrhea, dryness of the mouth, and stomatitis are among the side effects of antineoplastic drugs. Alopecia (loss of hair) is also common. Drugs and radiation therapy destroy normal cells along with malignant cells. The results of this destruction and bone marrow depression are manifested in reduced platelet counts and white blood counts and more anemia. The patient will have increased fatigue and weakness.

Since followup treatment of patients on chemotherapy and radiation therapy includes blood counts and other lab work, the nurse must conscientiously note results of such tests in order to make observations relative to bleeding tendencies and increased susceptibility to infection.

Toxic manifestations of medications and the effects of radiation therapy should be listed in the Kardex and the appropriate assessments should be made routinely and in response to patient complaints.

Discharge Planning

The patient with multiple myeloma who is going home will need instructions about what he can expect and what he must observe and report. This includes manifestations of the disease or associated problems and the side effects of drugs.

He needs safety reminders specific to his living environment, diet instructions, and points on preventing infection. Good personal hygiene habits are stressed. The family is included in all instruction.

Because this hospitalization may only be the first step toward prolonged and painful death, both the patient and his family need to leave the orthopedic unit feeling as if they have left a whole group of "friends" who will go on caring. This may give them another ounce of inner strength and optimism.

Metastatic Bone Disease

Definition

Metastatic bone lesions are malignant tumors that originate in other organs (primary sites) and involve the skeletal structures of the body. They are also known as secondary tumors. The bloodstream is the route by which most tumor emboli travel to various parts of the skeleton.

Metastases: Pattern and Pathology

Breast carcinoma most often involves the spine, pelvis, upper one-third of the femur, skull, ribs, and humerus.

Carcinoma of the prostate most frequently attacks the vertebrae, femur, pelvis, skull, ribs, and sternum.

From the kidney, a cancer usually spreads to the skull, sternum, spine, humerus, pelvis, ribs, femur, and foot.

Malignancies of the thyroid often affect the skull, ribs, sternum, spine, and humerus.

Lung carcinoma metastasizes most often to the thoracic spine and ribs.

In most cases of metastatic bone disease, the primary tumor is known. Because metastatic lesions are primarily bloodborne, they begin in the bone marrow. These metastases appear as osteoclastic or osteoblastic lesions or a combination of the two.

Signs and Symptoms

The primary clinical manifestations of metastatic bone disease are pain, pathological fractures, and anemia. The characteristics of the pain depend on the bone that is involved. For example, a metastatic lesion in the spine compresses nerve roots and produces symptoms of nerve root compression. In the extremity, a metastatic tumor causes pain, swelling, and tenderness. The onset of pain from a large lesion or lesions, in areas that are subject to pressure, may be sudden and severe. However, small cancerous growths in the ribs and sternum may be asymptomatic or cause only mild transient pain. This type of lesion may be discovered accidentally when the patient is undergoing examinations for other reasons.

X-Ray Findings

These metastases appear as osteoclastic or osteoblastic lesions or a combination of the two. A bone-destroying lesion has decreased density that may or may not be well defined. A tumor that stimulates bone growth will be shown on x-ray film as a dense white area.

Bone Scan

A bone scan is a two-dimensional picture of the skeleton demonstrating the distribution of radioactivity in the bones. The scan is done after the intravenous injection of a radiopharmaceutical. A *radiopharmaceutical*, or bone mineral tracer, is a radioactive element (usually technetium^{99m}Tc) tagged to an inorganic diphosphonate. The tracer accumulates in the skeleton and the blood pool. In the skeleton, the tracer seeks those areas where there is localized reactive or reparative activity. In scanning, these areas are referred to as "hot spots," and they show up as larger dark spots on the scan. The bone scan usually presents a view of the entire skeleton for interpretation in seconds.

A bone scan is helpful in early diagnosis since this examination will reveal an increased uptake of radioactive material in the involved area of a bone before there has been sufficient activity to be visible on x-ray film. See normal bone scan, page 344, and abnormal bone scan, page 345.

Bone Biopsy

A microscopic section of a bone containing suspected tumor cells will confirm a diagnosis made on the basis of past history of malignancy, x-ray films, bone scans, and the patient's subjective symptoms. Bone for this examination is obtained by open or needle biopsy.

Treatment

Metastatic bone disease is usually indicative of an advanced stage of malignant disease. Treatment is directed at halting

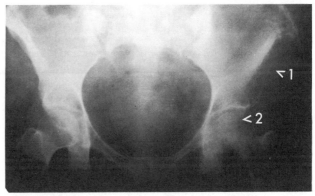

Metastatic bone cancer: (*1*) osteolytic lesion; note also the loss of cortical rim on this side of the pelvis; (*2*) loss of joint space and breakdown of femoral head.

progression of the disease process, relieving pain, and preventing pathological fractures.

Radiation therapy and drug therapy are similar to that prescribed for patients with multiple myeloma. Hormone therapy is indicated for tumors that metastasize from the prostate, breast, thyroid, or kidneys. Surgical management includes internal fixation or other treatment of pathological fractures and amputation.

Laboratory Findings

Laboratory findings are nonspecific in terms of diagnosis. Calcium levels in the blood and urine may be increased, as may the alkaline phosphatase. (See Table 10-1, page 323.)

Nursing Considerations

Nursing management of the patient with metastatic bone disease is essentially the same as the care of the patient with multiple myeloma. Care of the patient who has had an amputation is discussed in Chapter 8. If the patient has had fracture treatment, and depending on the bone that was affected, much of his physical care will be similar to that described in previous chapters.

In many respects, the supportive care of the patient with metastatic bone disease is also comparable to that of the patient with multiple myeloma. However, the patient with this kind of malignancy (unless the primary site is unknown) will usually be at a different level of psychological adjustment.

On the one hand, he and his family have been through the trauma of a diagnosis of cancer. Depending on the malignancy of his primary tumor and given the natural optimism of most human beings, the patient will have built up some hope about his prognosis. On the other hand, and to some degree, he should be emotionally prepared for the possible fatal outcome of his disease. The combination of these two states of mind will present the nurse with a patient who may exhibit few outward signs of further emotional trauma but who may be feeling extremely depressed and more than a little desperate.

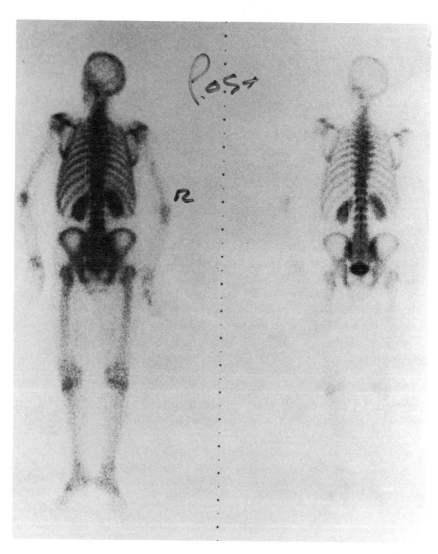

Normal bone scan.

Regardless of his behavior, both the patient and his family have undoubtedly done some thinking about the possibility of his death in the near future. Their attitudes and lifestyles have undergone changes. The role of a nurse as a supportive person has been established in a previous hospitalization. Now the patient and his family have expectations that the orthopedic nurse must identify as soon as possible if she is to be an effective psychological care provider.

Discussion Questions

1. Write nursing orders for the following patient. B. J. is a 50-year-old male patient. He is a history professor at a local university. Eight months ago he began having back pain. The pain became very severe 4 days ago, and he saw his doctor. He was admitted to the hospital and diagnosed yesterday as having multiple myeloma with the possibility of 6 months to 1 year to live. His physician explained the diagnosis to him and his wife. They have discussed it with their 4 teenage children. His treatment will consist of cobalt radiation, medication for pain control, deep heat treatments and physical therapy instruction in learning to use a walker. A lumbosacral support has been ordered. Most of the time he will be on bed rest but may go to the bathroom with help and walker. He moves slowly because of pain. B. J. is a meticulous person who wants to do things for himself. His wife is a nurse who is presently unemployed and will come daily to help him with bath and self-care. Today he has requested some reading material on multiple myeloma and that his visitors be restricted to immediate family. He also asked that no religious personnel or hospice staff visit him at this time.

Consider: His limited mobility because of back pain will be a factor in potential problems. How can his room and routines be adapted and arranged so that he can be as independent as possible? How should he be approached from a communications standpoint? What safety precautions will be necessary? What interaction is necessary with his family in order to plan his care? What observations are necessary?

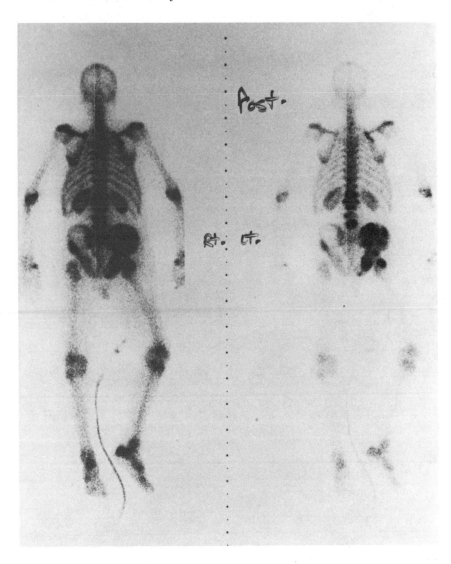

Abnormal bone scan. In checking bone scans, as in checking x-ray films, one looks for signs of asymmetry. Note the asymmetry of uptake and the malignant area in the pelvis. Because tumor metastases are more vascular, localization of isotopes occurs at a faster rate than in the rest of the skeleton. Note "hot spots."

THE PATIENT WITH METASTATIC BONE DISEASE: ASSESSMENT PRIORITIES IN PROBLEM SOLVING

Significant Data: E. P. is a 43-year-old female with metastatic bone disease. Her primary lesion was a breast carcinoma 4 years ago, for which she had a radical mastectomy. She entered the hospital with complaints of pain in her right hip, leg, and back. X-ray films and bone scans revealed metastatic involvement of her pelvis, sacrum, right femoral head, and greater trochanter. She has previously undergone both hormone and steroid therapy. She is 5'2" tall and weighs 180 pounds, much of that weight being fluid retention. She has recently begun chemotherapy. For the past year E. P. has not been able to work outside of her home, but before then she was a high school librarian. Her husband is a salesman and travels out of town for periods of 3 to 4 days at a time. E. P. has two teenagers, a daughter 16 and a son 14. They visit her daily. The daughter is a quiet, mature girl who has been gradually assuming most of the responsibility for maintaining the household.

Nursing Goals

1. Keep patient as comfortable as possible.
2. Prevent pathological fractures.
3. Provide emotional support for patient and family.
4. Report and record side effects of chemotherapy.
5. Prevent problems of immobility
   a. Gastrointestinal problems
   b. Urinary problems
   c. Contractures
   d. Skin breakdown
   e. Pneumonia
   f. Thromobophlebitis
   g. Psychological manifestations, depression, frustration, boredom
   h. Osteoporosis

6 P.M. Patient Complaints

E. P. is unable to get comfortable in spite of repositioning, backrub, and pain medication.

Complains of some shortness of breath.

Had emesis of liquid supper.

States: "I just hate being a bother. I can't stand having to depend on everybody . . . and it's just going to get worse, isn't it? I can accept my illness, but I hate being dependent on everyone."

Assessment Priorities

Check lower extremities for positioning. They must be well supported. Check pressure points, especially ankles, where edema is very evident. Are heels off mattress? Is patient warm or cool enough? Ask patient if she would like to be gotten out of bed into recliner or wheelchair.

Elevate head of bed slightly and check patient response in 15 minutes. Ausculate lungs. Check pulse and respirations. Is patient having *any* chest pain? Is room well ventilated?

Question about symptoms of gastric distress: burning, pain.

Consider all factors (besides disease) that may be causing patient emotional distress . . . absence of husband? Dependence on young daughter? Guilt over daughter having to take adult role at 16? Welfare of teenagers if she dies? Recognize patient may not feel wanted or needed.

Additional Factor in Assessment

This patient needs an opportunity to verbalize her feelings. Sitting at her bedside following assessment actions, taking her hand . . . waiting quietly may be best at this point in time.

2. For the following patient, what nursing observations are necessary to prevent or diagnose problems, and what are those problems? W. L. is a 30-year-old male with recurrent osteomyelitis in the distal femur. The problem originated in a compound fracture 11 years ago. This hospitalization is for incision and drainage of an abscess — his third. He has a closed wound irrigation system. He is on oral antibiotics and has antibiotics in the irrigation solution. His temperature still "spikes" elevations in the evening. He has moderate to severe pain and takes Tylenol #3 almost every 4 hours. This is his seventh postadmission day.

Consider: What are the psychological effects of chronic disease? Problems of wound irrigation due to location of wound? Side effects from antibiotics? Effects of prolonged temperature elevation? Problems of immobility along with length of stay on bed rest.

3. Outline a team approach to the care of the following patient. M.H. is 64 years old with crippling rheumatoid arthritis. She has had both wrists fused and finger joint implants inserted in the last year, and entered the hospital to have her hips and knees replaced. Her first operation is scheduled to be done in 2 days. It will be a total left hip replacement. Today she refuses all care. She cries when anyone moves her or even comes close to her bed. She seems to have more pain and be less cooperative when her husband is visiting. He dotes on her and sits by her bed for hours. The occupational therapist and physical therapist are having the same problems with her that the staff has; she will not let them near her. She has learned to feed herself and refuses. Some members of the nursing staff have requested not to be assigned to take care of her because she is so demanding and they are "tired of her."

Consider: The role of her husband in her rehabilitation and the influence he has on her behavior. Is a team conference advisable as an initial approach, and who should be there? What might be the fears and feelings underlying the patient's behavior?

Bibliography

Acute osteomyelitis. Nurs Mirror 155(15):17, 1982

Alcoff JM: Estrogen replacement therapy. Am Fam Physician 25(6):183, 1982

Algozzine GJ et al: Trolamine salicylate cream in osteoarthritis of the knee. JAMA 247:1311, 1982

Althoff DG: Diagnostic overview: Psoriatic arthritis. Orthop Nurs 2(5):50, 1983

Asterixis can mean salicylate intoxication. Nurs Drug Alert 6:14, 1982

Atherton V, Anwar M: A patient with rheumatoid arthritis and joint tuberculosis. Nurs Times 78:808, 1982

Ball JH, Stephenson V: Rheumatoid arthritis: A systemic disease. Nursing (Oxford) 2:899, 1984

Banwell BF: Exercise and mobility in arthritis. Nurs Clin North Am 19:605, 1984

Banwell BF: The role of the allied health professional in the treatment of arthritis. Primary Care 11:219, 1984

Barzel US: Vitamin D deficiency and osteomalacia in the elderly. Hosp Pract 19(10):129, 1984

Bhardwaj S, Holland JF: Chemotherapy of metastatic cancer in bone. Clin Orthop 169:28, 1982

Black JM: Muscle flaps for chronic osteomyelitis of the lower extremity. Orthop Nurs 2:17, 1983

Blockey NJ: Chronic osteomyelitis. An unusual variant. J Bone Joint Surg (Br) 65:120, 1983

Borrow a drug for gout. Emerg Med 10:106, 1978

Boutaugh M: Arthritis: Myths and realities. Occup Health Nurs 32:346, 1984

Bretherick CA: Physiotherapeutic measures. Nursing (Oxford) 2:922, 1984

Brown-Skeers VM: Rheumatoid arthritis. Crit Care Update 10(4):21, 1983

Carbary L, Carbary C: Ouch! It's gout! J Nurs Care 13(11):13, 1980

Cassady JR: Nursing actions versus arthritis quackery. Rehabil Nurs 19:32, 1985

Cave L: Lowering the uncertainties of arthritis with a nurse-led support group. Orthop Nurs 3(5):39, 1984

Channon H: Nursing care study: Release from pain. Nurs Mirror, 157(13):40, 1983

Chase JA: Spine fractures associated with osteoporosis. Orthop Nurs, 4(3):31, 1985

Chesson S: Social and emotional aspects of rheumatoid arthritis. Nursing (Oxford) 2:914, 1984

Clark CC: Women and arthritis: Holistic/wellness perspectives. Top Clin Nurs, 4(4):45, 1983

Cluca R et al: Passive range of motion exercise. A handbook. Nursing 78(8):59, 1978

Cluca R et al: Active range of motion exercise. A handbook. Nursing 78(8):45, 1978

Cochrane M: Sex and disability. 2. Immaculate infection. Nurs Times, 80(39):31, 1984

Conners VL, Goad SE: Psychosexual development: A model for teaching nursing intervention. J Nurs Educ 23:356, 1984

Conoley S: Arthritis as an iatrogenic disease. Nurs Clin North Am 19:709, 1984

Cunha BA: The use of penicillins in orthopaedic surgery. Clin Orthop 190:36, 1984

Dear MR et al: Promotion of self-care in the employee with rheumatoid arthritis. Occup Health Nurs 30:32, 1982

Dickinson GR: A home-care program for patients with rheumatoid arthritis. Nurs Clin North Am 15:403, 1980

Dickinson G, Gorman T: Adult arthritis. The assessment. Am J Nurs 83:262, 1983

Evans JH: Joint inflexibility: Its relationship to psychological rigidity. Rehab Nurs, 9(4):26, 1984

Faehnrich J: When pathologic fractures threaten. RN 46(11):34, 1983

Fahey J: Current management strategies for rheumatoid and osteoarthritis. Occup Health Nurs, 32:373, 1984

Fish S: Clinical forum, 7. Hormone replacement therapy. Nurs Mirror 157(suppl):i–vii, 1983

Fitzgerald RH et al: Anaerobic septic arthritis. Clin Ortho 164:141, 1982

Fitzsimons VM: Maintaining a positive environment for the older adult. Orthop Nurs 4(3):48, 1985

Gainor BJ, Buchert P: Fracture healing in metastatic bone disease. Clin Orthop 178:297, 1983

Galbraith HJ et al: Paget's disease of bone: A clinical and genetic study. Postgrad Med J 53(615):33, 1977

Gleit CJ, Graham, BA: The role of calcium and estrogen in osteoporosis. Ortho Nurs 4(3):13, 1985

Googe MC: The arthritis foundation. Orthop Nurs 3(5):43, 1984

Gordan GS: Osteoporosis: Early detection, prevention, and treatment. Consultant 20:64, 1980

Gorrie JM: Postmenopausal osteoporosis. JOGN Nurs 11:214, 1982

Grace EM: Gold therapy and rheumatoid arthritis. Can Nurs 79(11):40, 1983

Graham BA, Gleit CJ: Osteoporosis: A major health problem in post-menopausal women. Orthop Nurs 3(6):19, 1984

Gray RG et al: Intra-articular corticosteroids. Clin Orthop 177:235, 1983

Green SA, Ripley MJ: Chronic osteomyelitis in pin tracks. Bone Joint Surg (Am) 66:1092, 1984

Habermann ET et al: The pathology and treatment of metastatic disease of the femur. Clin Orthop 169:70, 1982

Hall BB et al: Anaerobic osteomyelitis. J Bone Joint Surg (Am) 65:30, 1983

Hamblen DL, Carter RL: Sarcoma and joint replacement. J Bone Joint Surg (Br) 66:625, 1984

Hamdy R: The signs and treatment of Paget's disease. Geriatrics 32(6):89, 1977

Hanson B: Outwitting Arthritis. Berkeley, CA, Creative Arts Books, 1980

Hardman M: Multiple myeloma: Suppressing the problem. Nurs Mirror 154(10):47, 1982

Harper A: Initial assessment and management of femoral neck fractures in the elderly. Orthop Nurs 4(3):55, 1985

Harrington KD: New trends in the management of lower extremity metastases. Clin Orthop 169:53, 1982

Harris ED Jr: Pathogenesis of rheumatoid arthritis. Clin Orthop 182:14, 1984

Hart FD: Rheumatology, osteoarthritis and rheumatoid arthritis, part 1. Nurs Mirror 153:ii, 1981

Hawkes KL: Rheumatoid arthritis: A personal account. Nursing (Oxford) 2:918, 1984

Hawley DJ: Nontraditional treatments of arthritis. Nurs Clin North Am 19:663, 1984

Hays K, Rafferty DC: Care of the patient with malignant lymphoma. Nurs Clin North Am 17:677, 1982

Helms CA, Genant HK: Computed tomography in the early detection of skeletal involvement with multiple myeloma. JAMA 248:2886, 1982

Higginson J: When interference can be good: Interferon in the treatment of multiple myeloma. Nurs Mirror 158(2):36, 1984

Hilt N, Cogburn S: Manual of Orthopedics. St Louis, CV Mosby, 1980

Ho G Jr et al: Therapy for septic arthritis. JAMA 247:797, 1982

Holder LE: Radionuclide bone-imaging in the evaluation of bone pain. J Bone Joint Surg (Am) 64:1391, 1982

Hollinshead WH, Rosse C: Textbook of Anatomy, 4th ed. Philadelphia, Harper & Row, 1985

Hosking S: Rheumatoid arthritis: Fundamental nursing care. Nursing (Oxford) 2:900, 1984

Jackson C: Nursing care study: Aching bones. Nurs Times 78:1661, 1982

Jaffe IA: Penicillamine: An alternative to injectable gold. Consultant 22:324, 1982

Jarowski CI, Coleman M: Answers to questions on multiple myeloma. Hosp Med 19(6):33, 38, 1983

Jensen GF: Epidemiology of postmenopausal spinal and long bone fractures. A unifying approach to postmenopausal osteoporosis. Clin Orthop 166:75, 1982

Johnson JA, Repp EC: Non-pharmacologic pain management in arthritis. Nurs Clin North Am 19:583, 1984

Kaplan FS: Glucocorticoid osteopenia. Orthop Nurs 4(3):35, 1985

Karok M: Add exercise to calcium in osteoporosis prevention. JAMA 247:1106, 1112, 1982

Kasner K: Bone metastases. Nursing (Oxford) 2:346, 1983

Kelley W et al: Textbook of rheumatology, 2nd ed. Philadelphia, WB Saunders, 1985

Kilcoyne RF et al: Infections of bones and joints. Nurse Pract 8(3):12, 63, 66, 1983

Klinenberg JR: Hyperuricemia and gout. Med Clin North Am 61:299, 1977

Koerner ME et al: Adult arthritis: A look at some of its forms. Am J Nurs 83:253, 1983

Krutzen P: Living with and adjusting to arthritis. Nurs Clin North Am 19:629, 1984

Kunec JR, Lewis RJ: Closed intramedullary rodding of pathologic fractures with supplemental cement. Clin Orthop 188:183, 1984

Langley LL et al: Dynamic Anatomy and Physiology, 5th ed. New York, McGraw-Hill, 1980

Ledo KM: Ankylosing spondylitis. Orthop Nurs 2(6):39, 1983

LeGallez P: Out-patient nursing, 3. Rheumatology health education. Nurs Mirror 160(3):37, 1985

LeGallez P: Patient education and self-management. Nursing (Oxford) 2:916, 1984

Levy RN et al: Surgical management of metastatic disease of bone at the hip. Clin Orthop 169:62, 1982

Liddel D: An in-depth look at osteoporosis. Orthop Nurs 4(3):23, 1985

Lindenbaum S, Alexander H: Infections simulating bone tumors. A review of subacute osteomyelitis. Clin Orthop 184:193, 1984

Lipson SJ: Rheumatoid arthritis of the cervical spine. Clin Orthop 182:143, 1984

Long MM, Stetts DM: Stress fractures of the femoral neck. Orthop Nurs 4(3):69, 1985

Lorig KR et al: Arthritis self-management: A five-year history of AP patient education program. Nurs Clin North Am 19:637, 1984

Lorig KR: Arthritis self-management: A patient education program. Rehab Nurs, 7(4):16, 1982

Lourie H: Spontaneous osteoporotic fracture of the sacrum. An unrecognized syndrome of the elderly. JAMA 248:715, 1982

Lowery BJ et al: An exploratory investigation of causal thinking of arthritis. Nurs Res: 32:157, 1983

Lukert BP: Osteoporosis: A review and update. Arch Phys Med Rehabil 63:480, 1982

Malek CJ, Brower SA: Rheumatoid arthritis: How does it influence sexuality? Rehabil Nurs 9(6):26, 1984

Mallette LE: Osteoporosis. Approaching treatment with optimism. Postgrad Med 72:271, 1982

Maquet P: The treatment of choice in osteoarthritis of the knee. Clin Orthop 192:108, 1985

Maycock JA: Pain: A different approach. Nursing (Oxford) 2:924, 1984

Mazess RB: An aging bone loss. Clin Orthop 165:239, 1982

McCarty DJ: The management of gout. Hosp Pract 14:75, 1979

Meis M: Loneliness in the elderly. Ortho Nurs 4(3):63, 1985

Mercier LR: Practical Orthopedics. Chicago, Year Book Medical Publishers, 1980

Miller F, Whitehill R: Carcinoma of the breast metastatic to the skeleton. Clin Orthop 184:121, 1984

Mines A: Osteoporosis: A detailed look at the clinical manifestations and goals for nursing care. Can Nurse 81:45, 1985

Mirkin G: Living with arthritis: A few key moves can make a big difference. Health 14:42, 1982

Mooney NE: Coping with chronic pain in rheumatoid arthritis: Patient behaviors and nursing interventions. Orthop Nurs 1:21, 1982

Mooney NE: Coping with chronic pain in rheumatoid arthritis: Patient behaviors and nursing interventions. Rehab Nurs 8(2):20, 1983

Moran-Higgins ME: Perioperative concerns for the patient with osteoporosis. Orthop Nurs 4(3):68, 1985

Morris AJ: Gold salts in the treatment of rheumatoid arthritis. Arthritis Rheum 23:625, 1980

Moskowitz R: Clinical Rheumatology, 2nd ed. Philadelphia, Lea & Febiger, 1982

Neuberger GB: The role of the nurse with arthritis patients on drug therapy. Nurs Clin North Am 19:593, 1984

Nickens HW, Koop CE: Toward a hip fracture prevention project. Orthop Nurs 4(3):52, 1985

Nilsonne U: Limb-preserving radical surgery for malignant bone tumors. Clin Orthop 191:21, 1984

Nowotny ML: If your patient's joints hurt, the reason may be osteoarthritis. Nursing 80, 10(9):39, 1980

Osteosarcoma of the femur. Nurs Mirror 155(18):17, 1982

Palasz J: Management of the patient with renal osteodystrophy. Orthop Nurs 4(3):40, 1985

Palma LF: Family practice grand rounds. Postmenopausal osteoporosis and estrogen therapy: Who should be treated? J Fam Pract 14:355, 1982

Palmason D: Osteoporosis: Catching the silent thief. Can Nurse 81:42, 1985

Patterson DC: Musculoskeletal examination. Occup Health Nurs 32:356, 1984

Patterson DC: The occupational health nurse on the arthritis team. Occup Health Nurs 32:350, 1984

Peasnell IM: Maintaining mobility and independence. Nursing (Oxford) 2:919, 1984

Peasnall IM: Rheumatology nursing. Nurs Mirror 157(5):54, 1983

Perricone N: Overview of joint anatomy and physiology: A basis for understanding and assessing rheumatic conditions. Occup Health Nurs 32:352, 1984

Phillips KF: The use of gold therapy with rheumatoid arthritis. Orthop Nurs 2(4):31, 1983

Pogrund H et al: Osteoarthritis of the hip joint and osteoporosis. Clin Orthop 164:130, 1982

Pugh J et al: Biomechanics of pathologic fractures. Clin Orthop 169:109, 1982

Resnick D: The sclerotic vertebral body. JAMA 249:1761, 1983

Richards M: Osteoporosis. Geriatr Nurs 3:98, 1982

Rickel L: Emotional support for the multiple myeloma patient. Nursing'76 6:76, 1976

Ross DG: Paget's disease. Orthop Nurs 3(3):41, 1984

Schajowicz F: Current trends in the diagnosis and treatment of malignant bone tumors. Clin Orthop 180:220, 1983

Schaller JG: Chronic arthritis in children. Juvenile rheumatoid arthritis. Clin Orthop 182:79, 1984

Schocker JD, Brady LW: Radiation therapy for bone metastasis. Clin Orthop 169:38, 1982

Sherry HS et al: Metastatic disease of bone in orthopedic surgery. Clin Orthop 169:44, 1982

Sim FH, Pritchard DJ: Metastic disease in the upper extremity. Clin Orthop 169:83, 1982

Simon MA: Biopsy of musculoskeletal tumors. J Bone Joint Surg (Am) 64:1253, 1982

Simon MA, Karluk MB: Skeletal metastases of unknown origin. Diagnostic strategy for orthopedic surgeons. Clin Orthop 166:96, 1982

Singer FR, Mills, BG: Evidence for a viral etiology of Paget's disease of bone. Clin Orthop 178:245, 1983

Smith C: Orthopaedics and the elderly. Nurs Times 80(15):46, 1984

Spencer H: Osteoporosis: Goals of therapy. Hosp Pract 17:131, 1982

Spitz PW: The medical, personal, and social costs of rheumatoid arthritis. Nurs Clin North Am 19:575, 1984

Springfield DS: Mechanisms of metastasis. Clin Orthop 169:15, 1982

Stacy-Spencer E: Osteomalacia. Orthop Nurs 3(4):47, 1984

Steffe LA et al: Still's disease in a 70-year-old woman. JAMA 249:2062, 1983

Stephenson V: Occupational therapy and the nurse. Nursing (Oxford) 2(31):912, 1984

Stillwell WT et al: Chrysosporium, a new causative agent in osteomyelitis. A case report. Clin Orthop 184:190, 1984

Sutton JD: The hospitalized patient with arthritis. Nurs Clin North Am 19:617, 1984

Tobiason SJ: The arthritis patient comes to surgery. AORN J 32(4):608, 1980

Wakinshaw M: Diverse rheumatoid disorders. Nursing (Oxford) 2:902, 1984

Webb C: Promoting continence: How would you feel? Community Outlook, p. 45, Feb 1984

Weiland AJ et al: The efficacy of free tissue transfer in the treatment of osteomyelitis. J Bone Joint Surg (Am) 66:181, 1984

Wenger DR: The limping child. Orthop Nurs 1:29, 1982

Wise C: Clinical manifestations of common rheumatic conditions. Occup Health Nurs 32:368, 1984

Wolfe F: Arthritis and musculoskeletal pain. Nurs Clin North Am 19:565, 1984

11

The Fractured Image: Sexuality and the Orthopedic Patient

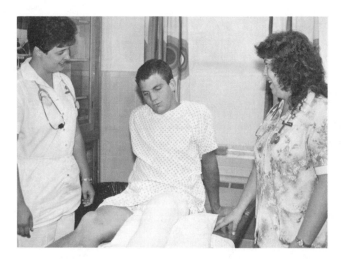

What are little boys made of?
What are little boys made of?
Frogs and snails and puppy-dog tails.
That's what little boys are made of.

What are little girls made of?
What are little girls made of?
Sugar and spice and all that's nice,
That's what little girls are made of.*

Whether one is short or tall, blonde or brunette, young or old, one responds to, or interacts with (for better or for worse) the opposite sex according to an image of self as a male or a female. This is one's sexual image, or sexuality, and it is part of the total self-image. Sexuality is a vital force that creates bonds between human beings, bestows pleasure, and inflicts pain. Thus it follows that sexuality affects health. Caregivers need to consider the sexual concerns of orthopedic patients in the planning and delivery of holistic care.

Shortened periods of hospitalization and modern technology do not necessarily reduce the length of time that a patient with an operated or fractured extremity stays in a cast. Orthopedic disease entities and trauma to any part of the musculoskeletal system result in some degree of immobility. Therefore, the activities of daily living and many aspects of normal human interactions become matters of concern to orthopedic patients. The following scenario exemplifies a concern related to sexuality.

A young male patient who has had surgical repair of torn knee ligaments settles himself for the first time into a wheelchair, with much help from his nurse. Each movement is awkward for his whole body and painful for his casted leg. He asks the question: "How am I going to have any sex with this cast on my leg?"

Whatever the response elicited from the nurse, if any, one thing is certain. This is a difficult question both for the asker and the asked. Very probably it was not the question the patient wanted to ask at all, nor was it meant to be provocative or to be a "proposition."

Although further nursing assessment will provide other nursing diagnoses, at this point, one applicable diagnosis is disturbance in self-concept. The medical, surgical, or traumatic condition related to the possible nursing diagnoses for the orthopedic patient with concerns about sexuality will be referred to in this chapter as *the fractured image*. Insights into the meaning and manifestations of the fractured image, as well as appropriate nursing diagnoses, prevention, and care, will be discussed.

Sexuality and Sexual Image

A sexual image, like an overall self-image, can be positive or negative. A positive sexual image is evident in the person who is comfortable with compliments about his or her appearance. A simple example of the effect on behavior of a negative self-image is that when a young woman sees herself as someone no man would remember, she will act out the part. Her roommate may tell her, "There's a man here to see you," and her reply will be, "I don't know any men."

How does a woman, or man, get that way? What factors influence the formation of a sexual image? Whole books are written on the subject. The following section discusses only basic information that the orthopedic nurse will need as background knowledge to understand the behavior of her patients.

Gender and the Development of a Sexual Image

The development of a sexual image begins, of course, at the beginning. Sex has already been assigned *in utero*, and the first appearance in the world of a new human being is sure

* The Annotated Mother Goose. Baring-Gould WS, Baring-Gould C: New York, Clarkson and Potter, 1962

to invite comments that imply something about society's expectations of that new individual. Typical comments from the physician or a relative include: "Congratulations! You have a big, fine-looking son!" and "Congratulations! You have a nice little girl!" The tone of voice may vary from gruff pride to soft wonder.

The adults of the 1980s, of any age, crawled out of infancy and into childhood socialized in the direction in which they were expected to go. They were dressed and taught their roles. Little girls were, at least for most public appearances, supposed to be pretty, to be little dolls. Their primary social function was to be quiet and "looked at." Little boys were dressed like "little guys," and very soon after learning to walk and talk, the average little boy learned to be tough, flex his muscles, and show Daddy how big he was.

When feelings and curiosities common to any human being entered the life of a growing child, adult reactions were often negative.

"Put that doll down, Jimmy. Do you want to grow up to be a sissy?"

"You're too big to be put to bed. Don't be a mama's boy!"

"Shame on you! Little girls don't get covered with mud."

"Little girls aren't supposed to jump on the furniture!"

Children began learning at a very early age that there were specific behaviors for males and females. Boys were allowed to be "naughty" and aggressive. (Boys will be boys!) Girls were supposed to be more obedient and submissive. (Act like a little lady!) These behaviors extended into sexual expression.

Fortunately, while growing up, the average girl or boy learned, adjusted, resisted, changed, loved and was loved, and became his or her own person. Along the way, however, he or she also learned how to suppress feelings that did not fit traditional male or female roles, and how to feel guilty for having them. Today, more women are truckdrivers and more men do housework. Women may be sexually aggressive, and men find it acceptable. Yet somewhere in most people's psychological makeup the remnants of puppy-dog tails or sugar and spice create anxieties and attitudes that cause problems.

More Anxieties and Attitudes: Cause and Creation

The Age Factor. Some generalizations can be made about the anxieties and attitudes of today's adults. These have to do with how they learned about their own anatomy and sexual functioning and with the accepted morals and behaviors of the era in which they were raised.

Most of today's elderly women were victims of silence on the subject of anatomy and sexual functioning. Menstruation happened to a girl without her prior knowledge. By its nature, the onset of this normal function could be terrifying.

The young girl was further frightened by her mother's embarrassment and reluctance to discuss menstruation beyond referring to it as a "curse" a woman had to endure until she was old.

The average girl in the early 1900s went to her marriage bed either totally ignorant or only vaguely conscious of what to expect, and perhaps having no idea of what a man looked like with his clothes off. Common comments from women in their 80s include: "Nice girls didn't talk about that when I was young," and "When we got married, well, a wife was expected to do her duty."

An elderly man will probably admit that he was encouraged to "sow some wild oats" before marrying; men had sexual freedom if they could find "bad girls." The girls they married, however, frequently went through life refusing to remove their clothing before the bedroom was in darkness, to retain a measure of modesty and "niceness."

Today's middleaged woman, then, most likely had a mother who did not tell her much about anatomy or sex. Sexual awareness, when acquired from the few more liberal mothers or through forbidden reading, was passed along in secret conversations. Any sexual or near-sexual experiences the woman had as a teenager probably added to the guilt she developed as a curious child or learned from her parents. For many such women, the first serious relationship they had with a man resulted in marriage, not infrequently because they were pregnant.

Men who are in their fifties may have had fathers who, if they told them anything, gave them warnings: Be careful of disease; don't get a girl "in trouble." Nocturnal emissions, "wet dreams," may have been mentioned, if at all, only in passing by fathers and with embarrassment by mothers. The double standard was in strict operation: one code of morals for men, and another for women; it was a "man's world."

Many middleaged people remember learning about the differences in female and male anatomy from "playing doctor." Although the children or grandchildren of these generations have grown up in a society where reproductive anatomy and sexual functioning are open subjects and morals and sexual behaviors are a matter of individual preference, they may still be subject to the anxieties and attitudes of their parents and grandparents. A young woman may have arguments with her mother about sunbathing in a string bikini, and her grandmother and her boyfriend's grandmother will be agitated because the young couple want to live together.

Double Messages and Contradictions. The older generations, particularly — made up of those who reached adulthood before or by the early 1950s, — were plagued by double messages, that affect how they relate to each other and to younger people about sexuality.

Sex is dirty . . . save it for the one you love.

It's great to look and act sexy . . . but don't do anything.

Sex is normal . . . but don't talk about it.

These same messages play a part in allowing them to live out contradictions, for although their own attitudes and ideas may be changing, their actions change more slowly. They may openly disapprove of "the way some people live" and yet follow their lives with great interest. This is evident in choice of reading material and in television and movie viewing habits. Young people see their elders saying one thing and doing another. They may accept or reject, then, the values of other generations according to the strength of family attachments and their own needs.

Physical Attributes and Sexuality

In many ways society equates the quality of sexual performance and sex appeal with degree of physical beauty. The sex gods and goddesses of novels, television, and the movies are usually beautiful of face or at least form. How strongly a person believes that physical appearance determines worth as a sexual being also determines the effect his or her physical attributes or shortcomings have on interactions with the opposite sex.

Age and Sexuality

It is a myth that sex is only for the young and that old people are sexless. Yet it is common in all age groups, even the elderly, to regard an older person's interest in sex as inap-

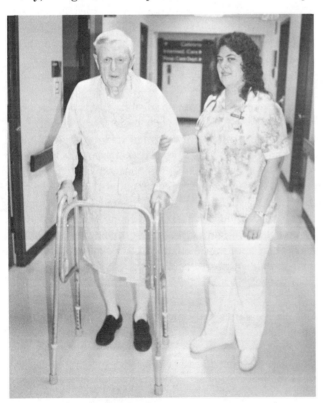

propriate. Although the labels "dirty old man" or "dirty old woman" may be applied with good humor, they are too often the result of ignorance and of perceptions based on a negative sexual image of older people.

The Purpose and Practice of Sex

Whether one believes sex is for procreation or for recreation determines whether one rejects or accepts contraception and pregnancy, which in turn has implications for building anxieties about sex. A sexual image is affected by attitudes about specific sexual acts, homosexuality, and masturbation. Cultural and religious taboos such as incest contribute to our sexuality. Family and social environment, from the happiest of situations to those in which physical and sexual abuse are commonplace, both provide role models and directly affect feelings about sex appeal, sexual capabilities, and sexual acts.

The Sexual Image: General Comments

A sexual image is as individual as its owner, but in general it can be said that:

1. Everyone has a sex drive.
2. "Right" or "wrong" acts of sexual expression are determined by psychological and social forces.
3. Learning and social pressures, such as women's liberation, can greatly modify a person's behavior as a sexual being.
4. A person's sexual identity is affected by life crises such as adolescence, pregnancy, illness, and retirement.

The Fractured Image

What the Fractured Image Is Not

In general, the patient who finds solutions to dilemmas of sexual expression in the hospital does not have an image problem. Examples might be the patient who has succeeded in getting a spouse or significant other into bed with him or her and the patient who engages in masturbation. However, these situations may be problems for the nursing staff. To say "There is a time and a place for everything" is to make a value judgment. In dealing with these behaviors the nurse should strive to respect individual value systems by appropriate actions and communications whenever possible.

Sexual Behavior and Nursing Interventions

When a patient demonstrates the need to fulfill sexual desires—for instance, as mentioned in the preceding examples—the nurse must alert the staff, provide privacy for the patient, and take actions to ensure the emotional comfort of other patients. The nursing care plan may include such interventions as:

1. Instructing the patient to close the door or have the curtain pulled when privacy is desired.
2. Knocking on the door before entering, or calling the patient's name if the curtain is pulled.
3. Providing the patient with a DO NOT DISTURB sign for the door.

The patient may need to be moved to a private room. Considering how readily a patient is transferred when he is disoriented and disturbs a roommate, it is logical to suggest that the same consideration be given to a patient who wants to fulfill sexual needs.

Definition of the Fractured Image

An orthopedic patient who has concerns about sexuality that he or she is unable to deal with is suffering from a fractured image. There are three concerns that may be expressed, one way or another, by a patient with a fractured image. These concerns may be stated as follows:

1. Loss of sex appeal, related to a disturbance in self-concept. The patient feels he or she is unattractive.
2. Loss of ability to function sexually, and fear of inability to function sexually.
3. Fear of causing complications in healing or rehabilitation. (Will I hurt myself?) This can be stated as "fear of the unknown."

Which of these concerns the person has will depend on his or her orthopedic condition; treatment; interactions with caregivers, family, and friends; and, in some instances, sexual image. These concerns are often inseparable in cause and expression. Before they can be described as individual entities or diagnoses, a discussion of factors that contribute to the fractured image is necessary.

Contributing Factors and Nursing Implications

A negative sexual image is not necessarily a contributing factor in the formation of a fractured image. For example, the young woman who does not believe she is attractive to men in the first place may not have concerns about loss of sex appeal when she is wearing a body cast.

Loss of Identity and Loss of Control of the Environment. These feelings begin with the admission procedure and are reinforced throughout the hospitalization period. The necessity for routines often makes the patient feel like a "thing."

Consider the following example: A 56-year-old man is admitted to the orthopedic unit from the emergency room. He has a fractured tibia and fibula. His trousers have been cut and a splint has been applied to his leg. He is in pain and mild shock, apprehensive and upset. The first nursing actions include undressing him, gowning him, and helping him into bed in a semiprivate room next to a total stranger. No matter how kind and gentle the nurses are who perform these actions, they, too, are strangers. This normal procedure may increase the feelings of helplessness invoked by the fact that a fractured leg will temporarily keep him from making all of his own decisions. His clothes and money are taken away. A thorough nursing assessment follows, along with a request for a urine specimen and the question "when was your last bowel movement?" The patient may well feel he has no secrets from the nurse.

Hospital routines—when to wake up, when to bathe, when to eat, and to some extent, when to sleep—contribute to feelings of helplessness.

Two days later, on his way to the physical therapy department in a wheelchair, the patient and the therapist are met in the corridor by a nurse who has "not seen him yet" and so must ask, "Is this 209-2?" The identification band on his arm is the only way everyone will always know his name.

In all of this, some nursing implications are obvious. Choices should be offered whenever possible: When would you like your bath? How early do you want a sleeping pill? Filling out a menu, when appropriate, is an important task for the patient; the selection of food is one decision he can usually make. Individualized meal planning with a dietician should be requested for any patient who lacks appetite or interest in what is offered on the regular menu.

Explanations of routines should be forthcoming so that the patient does not feel "lost in the shuffle." In all likelihood, the average patient does not know that every nurse who checks the identification band before giving a medication or treatment does so as a safety precaution and not because she has forgotten the patient's name. This fact should be called to the attention of every patient early in the hospitalization period.

Problems Due to Condition or Treatment Dependency. The dependency that results from an orthopedic condition or treatment may have a negative effect on the patient's sexual image. The patient who feels he or she is a "bother" will have lowered self-esteem. Requiring assistance with personal care because of an immobilized arm and being unable to get out of bed independently because of an immobilized leg or operated hip, for example, are likely to make the patient acutely aware of being dependent. More specifically, a young male patient with a shoulder repair may find it difficult to feel "like a man" when he has to have his meat cut up by the nurse. The nature of ongoing care as well as the patient's condition reinforces dependency.

Pain medications and immobility cause constipation that demands treatment. The patient becomes dependent on caregivers for relief from this personal problem. Drugs to relieve pain and muscle spasms or to induce sleep and rest increase feelings of helplessness.

Nursing diagnoses related to dependency include potential for anxiety; ineffective individual coping, with frustration or depression; and self-care deficit. A nursing approach

PROBLEM SOLVING: THE PATIENT WITH A FRACTURED IMAGE

Significant Data: T. L. is a 26-year-old policeman who 2 months ago was hit by a speeding automobile while on his motorcycle. His right leg was amputated below the knee. He was home from the hospital only a couple weeks when he developed a necrotic area on the distal stump which is now open and draining serosanguineous material. The physician has ordered whirlpool b.i.d. for the stump as preparation for stump revision. T. L. has no other medical problems. He is a smoker. He is unmarried and lives with his widowed mother and teenage sister. He has one other sister who is married. This is his third day in the hospital.

From 7 A.M. Report	First Nursing Assessment	Data Collected
1. T. L. complains of chest pain this morning, although his vital signs are stable and he does not appear to be in distress.	1. Recheck vital signs. Question about cough. Auscultate lungs. Does pain occur on inspiration, expiration? Deep breathing? Exact location, onset. Does pain radiate? Has he been smoking more? Diaphoretic? Tightness? Gastric distress?	1. b.p. 130/88; T. 98.4°; P. 76; R. 16. Lungs clear. Pain "not bad." Comes and goes across chest. Smoker cough only. Otherwise negative for respiratory complaints.
2. Last night his sister from out of town was here to visit with her new baby. After she left he had a headache and we gave him Tylenol X, which was sufficient.	2. Ask if this was first time he saw baby. How big? Boy or girl? Is headache a problem now?	2. Baby boy, 2 months old. Looks "small." States he dreamt about babies last night but does not remember what.
3. He says he would like to have his hair washed today.	3. Assure him shampoo will be done early, before physical therapy, if that is what he wishes.	3. That will be fine.
4. Dr. S. was in at 4 P.M. and said he would put him on the OR schedule for later this week.	4. Ask what doctor told him about future surgery.	4. Dr. will do revision "probably Friday." Level is unknown at this time. States he would like to "get it over with."
5. His elastic bandage was rewrapped once and there was only a small amount of drainage. No redness. No new areas of necrosis.	5. Check bandage. Rewrap p.r.n. (Will be done routinely after physical therapy.)	5. Bandage is intact and appears dry.

based on patience and empathy will reassure the patient that dependency is a natural side effect of his condition.

Orthopedic problems and treatment and the dependency they entail lead naturally to situations where there is a lack of privacy, violation of modesty, and potential for embarrassment. The application of a body cast necessitates exposing the patient while the torso is being covered or draped. Even positioning a patient for casting the lower extremity may require quick action to prevent the patient from being exposed.

Regular nursing routines related to personal hygiene and elimination violate privacy and modesty to a degree depending on the patient's degree of immobility. The fracture pan is simple to place and remove but also prone to tipping and spilling. Immobile hips and legs force an otherwise able person to sit on a bedside commode. Although a curtain protects him from view, he knows that his roommate and everyone who comes in and out of the room knows that he is

sitting there. This is embarrassing. The nursing attention given to the relief of constipation is also discomforting to a patient. The nursing diagnosis here might be potential for emotional discomfort related to any or all of these things.

Providing privacy, respecting the need for modesty, and understanding that each patient may value them differently is essential. Preventing constipation will reduce the number of humiliating moments the patient must endure. Giving explanations while helping and caring for the patient will decrease the potential for emotional discomfort.

"We are going to put a pad under this fracture pan. They sometimes tip and spill."

"We will keep you covered as best we can while casting."

"It may seem as though you are exposed because your leg is elevated, but the sheet is keeping you well covered."

"Sitting on a commode at the bedside can be awkward, but most patients become less tired than if they tried to get to the bathroom the first time."

PROBLEM SOLVING: THE PATIENT WITH A FRACTURED IMAGE *(Continued)*

Nursing Diagnoses

1. Alteration in comfort: Mild and intermittent chest pain. Related to?
2. Anxiety. Related to actual or perceived threat to biological integrity and body image; potential change in socioeconomic status.

3. Self-concept, disturbance in. Related to loss of body part.

Nursing Orders/Plan

1. Monitor vital signs b.i.d. Check for respiratory distress. Encourage patient to smoke less.
2. Encourage patient to ask physician any questions he might have about surgery—and about prognosis if this is something he wants to know about at this point.
3. Comment on improved appearance of stump.
4. Inquire if patient has need for more or less diversion.
5. Observe visitors: number, who, and when. Establish contact with any peer to determine need for support group. Observe family interactions.
6. Offer patient his own pajamas following bath and shampoo. Check if he has the robe he wants to wear. Make positive comment on his appearance.
7. Seek more information. Set up a team conference, involve physical therapist and M.D. if possible. If not, solicit M.D. input before conference. At team conference introduce (in addition to above plan) the following points for discussion.
   a. Significance, if any, of dream about babies.
   b. Possible concerns about finances. Does he help support his mother and sister?
   c. Is it time to introduce a prosthetist?
   d. How might the traditional image of a policeman be affecting the patient's response to his injury?

Major Concerns: Behaviors, Diagnoses, and Interventions

As pointed out in the preceding discussion, hospital procedures, nursing routines, and various aspects of immobility and dependency render the patient vulnerable to sexual concerns. The following section discusses the factors that seem to be most significant in causing specific concerns. Because the concerns of an orthopedic patient with a fractured image are usually interrelated, and nursing actions may be similar in a wide range of conditions, examples will be used to illustrate behaviors and interventions.

Loss of Sex Appeal

A person's sex appeal is related to how he or she looks to others. The slightest alteration in appearance may cause concern over loss of sex appeal. For instance, the average person who has a red nose and red-rimmed eyes because of a headcold feels unattractive. Orthopedic problems, disease, and trauma involve minor and major alterations in appearance. In combination with the other contributing factors, the effect of such changes can be devastating to a patient's conception of his or her sex appeal.

How does a patient manifest concerns about sex appeal? Inappropriate behaviors that relay messages of: Look at me, don't look at me, touch me, don't touch me, are clues to a disturbance in self-concept related to sex appeal.

A 19-year-old girl enters the hospital to have a Harrington rod inserted for correction of a scoliosis curve. She refuses to take her jeans off to go to bed. Her brother states that the night before, she went to a party with no blouse over her cast. Yet she told the nurse who did her admission interview that she does not want her boyfriend to see her again after surgery until the last brace is off.

In establishing initial rapport, the nurse should acknowledge the patient's concerns about her appearance by asking her to share her feelings about visitors in general.

"We'll be at your bedside often for the first few days, and you will probably rest and sleep in between. But when you start feeling well enough for any visitors outside of your family, we'll talk about who they should be so that you're comfortable."

For this patient, it will be essential from the outset to reinforce the positive aspects of her appearance *now*, and of what the appearance will become after surgery. Patients with scoliosis are often tall and slender.

"Girls like you can find so many clothes. What is the first thing you're going to buy to wear when you're all finished with bracing?"

Sometimes inappropriate behaviors are identified as deviations from what has been perceived as the patient's normal personality. That fact is illustrated in this report: "Mr. J. is a 40-year-old patient with a compound fracture of the left tibia and fibula. He has been here forever; no, only a little over a week. But the last couple of days he has become a problem, becoming more dependent instead of less, insisting today that we do most of his bath. Every time we get him out of bed he exposes himself. He does the same thing in physical therapy."

The patient whose behavior changes in this manner may be the patient who has gradually become less pain-ridden, is beginning to do his own pin site care, and realizes what he looks like to others as a result of his orthopedic condition. A team conference is indicated when behavior such as this develops. Not only is the patient expressing symptoms consistent with the fractured image, but evidently a number of the caregivers are having problems dealing with him. The starting point will be to discuss staff reactions that might elicit a shame response from the patient, and plan to avoid them. Instead the patient needs reassurance that he *is* a male, and that someone notices that he *looks* like one. Nursing actions will include therapeutic communication and acceptable "touch."

"You're getting so good at helping yourself get in and out of bed that we need to be more careful about not exposing you. Perhaps we should think about getting you some shorts to wear all the time so that when you're moving around, especially in P.T. where there are other patients, you won't have to worry about exposing yourself."

"It must be tiresome to bathe in bed as many days as you have had to, even though it is good arm exercise. What if we give you two extra back rubs every day to increase your circulation and make you less tired of it all?"

The care plan for this patient should also include giving special attention to matters of personal appearance. The nurse should offer shampoos, make positive comments when the patient has shaved or combed his hair, and encourage his continued efforts to look his "best." His environment should be kept as orderly as possible. The nurse can note the arrival of get-well cards and gifts and reinforce the idea that many people care about him. The leg in an external fixator is unsightly. Frequent comments on improvements in the appearance of the limb are helpful. As much as possible the nurse should make positive comments when the patient's spouse is present to reassure *her* that progress is being made.

Loss of Ability to Function Sexually

The patient may express feelings of sexual inadequacy (fear of inability to function sexually) when in severe pain, especially on movement, or when motion is so restricted that he or she seems completely helpless. A patient who had recovered from multiple injuries due to a motor vehicle accident was asked if during his hospitalization he had doubts about his ability to function sexually. His response was: "With two broken arms and a broken leg, I didn't give it a thought for awhile. I was *hurting* too much. But when the thought did come, it was like, is *that* broken too?"

If getting on and off a bedpan, or in and out of bed, are consistently difficult and painful, thoughts of sexual inadequacy are very likely to cross the patient's mind. Because trauma patients, in particular, are hospitalized for a long time, it is easy for nurses to become attached to them and so accustomed to doing things for them that the tendency to "baby" them often lingers too long. Frequently, the more stoic a patient is, the more likely the nurse is to be sympathetic and fuss over him or her. These good intentions may reinforce feelings of helplessness.

When the patient makes "poor cripple" jokes or comments about "being a baby," the nurse should be alerted that signs of concern over loss of ability to function sexually may be forthcoming. Measures must be taken to promote sexual integrity. The nurse should try to discover how the patient perceives himself or herself normally.

"Tell me something about yourself, your job, your hobbies. You seem so concerned about being independent."

"Construction work takes a lot of endurance."

"Working outside the home leaves little time for housework, what are your ways of managing?"

The orthopedic patient needs to be reassured that pain as well as dependency is normal, and temporary, and that requiring medication does not mean that he or she is being a "baby."

"No, you are not a baby. Most patients have severe muscle spasms and pain with this kind of knee repair. You *need* hypos now, and sometimes you can't use the urinal. We'll help you stand at the bedside any time you wish. When you feel better you won't have this problem."

There is an element of difficulty in demonstrating an appreciation of the patient's value as an individual while providing reassurance that certain nursing interventions are the routine for many. However, this challenge is one that the orthopedic nurse must meet.

The patient with an exacerbation of crippling rheumatoid arthritis may have a long-standing history of feelings of sexual inadequacy. Patients with this disease should be made aware of the literature available from the National Arthritis Foundation (p. 327) as a matter of routine care. The pertinent pamphlets can be left at the patient's bedside after a simple introduction, which should not be stressful for nurse or patient.

"The National Arthritis Foundation has a variety of pamphlets about arthritis that are easy to read. I'll leave a couple at your bedside for when and if you feel up to reading

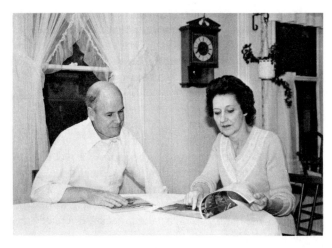

them. There is one on living and loving that talks about special problems when you are in pain.''

Making continuous progress in performing activities of daily living and in ambulation is of utmost importance to the patient who makes ''poor cripple'' or similar jokes about mobility. The nurse should listen for comments about activity being too tiring and for those that are prefaced by ''I can't even . . .'' ''I can't even make the stairs on crutches yet.'' Conferences with the physical therapist and occupational therapist will be helpful in evaluating interactions with the patient and providing the appropriate reinforcement and reassurance.

Statements by the patient that he or she feels like a ''new man'' or a ''new woman'' need a careful reply.

''Making progress can do that for you.''

The nurse should refrain from calling the patient ''new'' to avoid making the implication that the ''old'' was not acceptable.

Fear of the Unknown

The most common concern among patients who suffer from a fractured image is probably related to a basic concept: fear of the unknown. Will I ''hurt'' myself if I have sex? That is, will I complicate healing or rehabilitation? Patients who are embarrassed to talk about sex may ask general questions about activities. For instance:

The woman with rheumatoid arthritis asks, ''Will some exercises make my joints worse? How do I know what I shouldn't do?''

The post-laminectomy patient wonders: ''How soon can I get back to doing all the things I did before surgery, or can't I?''

Some patients make an attempt at humor when they are actually anxious to know what effect the resumption of sexual expression may have on their condition. The approach such patients use may be offensive to the caregiver if she is not aware that fear of the unknown is the underlying

problem. An example of this is the 60-year-old patient with a tibial osteotomy and his leg in a long-leg cast who asks: ''There are supposed to be 100 ways to have sex. Think I can find one, or will I need to come up with the 101st?''

This brings the discussion of fractured image full circle to the young man who asked: ''How am I going to have any sex with this cast on my leg?'' Are these patients asking for sexual counseling? The answer is doubtful. Anyone with a satisfactory sex life will work out the difficulties caused by limited mobility, *if* he or she is aware of which actions will precipitate pain that signals complications or cause complications without pain. The person with an unsatisfactory sex life may be tempted to use an orthopedic condition as an excuse to discontinue sexual relations. This type of patient needs more help, *if* he or she desires it, than orthopedic patient caregivers are equipped to provide. Therefore, patients who ask ''how to'' questions most likely do not want ''how to '' answers. The questions are their way of finding out what kind of activity will precipitate pain and cause complications.

Although the nurse may be surprised by such questions, she must answer them with questions and statements that will allow the patient to comfortably verbalize fears.

''What questions do you have about activities when you go home?''

''If your doctor hasn't told you all you want to know, he may be waiting for you to ask. Writing questions down when you think of them helps you to remember. I'll answer any that I can.''

In general, the nurse can reassure any patient with an immobilized extremity that as long as the mechanism of immobilization is intact and safety is a consideration, no movement will interfere with healing.

For example: ''The cast will hold your leg in a position for healing. You need to be careful about maintaining balance and not falling. The cast will get soft and can be damaged if you get it wet. Otherwise let comfort be a guide to all activities.''

Prevention by early, adequate, and ongoing patient education is the first order of nursing. ''Actually, patients recover from laminectomies quite fast sometimes when they've had a lot of pain for a long time, like you have. Now since you're not having surgery until 2 o'clock, maybe you want to start thinking of questions about what you can do after surgery. Write them down, and then when you feel up to it, you can start asking your doctor what you want to know. I'll help clarify in any way I can.''

Prevention, as well as treatment, of the fractured image includes helping the patient maintain self-esteem during periods of dependency. ''Let's put this blue robe on you when you go to P.T. It's so pretty more people ought to *see* you in it.''

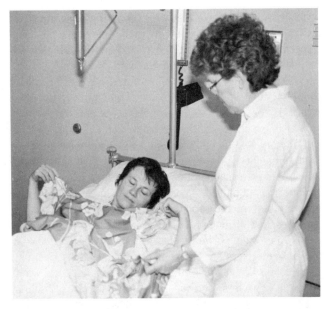

Another measure that helps prevent the fractured image is reassuring patients that pain tends to make everything else seem unimportant or impossible and that, yes, it too will pass. When the nurse reviews preoperative instruction with patients who are to have total hip replacement, she should point out that the do's and don't's of the exercise program will alert the patient to proper positions for any activity, and that they will be in written form. This kind of discussion may prompt patients to think about sexual concerns and help them to formulate questions. Patients, like other learners, forget much of what they learn. Therefore the nurse should evaluate instruction at regular intervals.

The Nurse: Psychological Considerations

Understanding the nature and expression of the fractured image should alleviate guilt feelings on the part of the nurse: What did *I* do? Why would he ask *me* that? Why is he suddenly doing this to *me*? Caring for the patient with a fractured image can be a challenge to the nurse's value system. However, holistic orthopedic patient care demands the integration of measures for prevention, diagnosis, and treatment of this condition in patient care planning. The nurse who is uncomfortable with the subject of sexuality should seek peer support whenever necessary.

Discussion Questions

1 What further nursing assessment is necessary after the following report? Mrs. R. is a 48-year-old patient with chronic back pain. She was supposed to be measured for her brace today, but the woman from the orthotics company who was going to do it was off, and the patient said she'd rather wait for *her*.

Consider: What is the procedure in measuring for a back brace? Did the patient have feelings about a man doing the measuring? How might other aspects of her treatment be affecting her modesty. Privacy?

2 Discuss a nursing approach to this patient. C. M. is a 19-year-old male patient with a fractured femur. He is going into a cast brace tomorrow. We are all glad because he has been in traction too long! The staff feels that he is getting a little fresh. And this morning he was calling "Nurse, nurse! I need a nurse!" When someone would go to his room, he wouldn't say anything, he would just look at his roommate and they would laugh and laugh.

Consider: Who has problems? What clarification and assessment will identify specific patient needs? Is a team conference needed?

Bibliography

Alexander B: Sexual problems: Now that they're "out of the closet" how can you help? Consultant 24(6):217, 221, 1984

Anderson ML: Talking about sex—with less anxiety. J Psychiatr Nurs 18:10, 1980

Assey JL et al: Who is the seductive patient? Am J Nurs, 83:530, 1984

Baird S: Development of a nursing assessment tool to diagnose altered body image in immobilized patients. Orthop Nurs 4:47, 1985

Bartscher PW: Human sexuality and implications for nursing intervention: A format for teaching. J Nurs Educ 22:123, 1983

Birchall J: Coping with sexuality: "In a private place". . . the mentally handicapped patient . . . masturbation. Nurs Times 80(50):31, 34, 1984

Boyer G: Sexuality and aging. Nurs Clin North Am 17:421, 1982

Byer JP: Sexuality and the elderly. Geriatr Nurs 4:293, 1983

Carolan C: Sex and disability: Bridging the gap, part 3. Nurs Times 80(40):49, 1984

Carolan C: Sex and disability: "Handicap—less important than loving", part 1. Nurs Times 80(39):28, 1984

Cochrane M: Sex and disability: "Immaculate infection". . . those with rheumatoid arthritis, part 2. Nurs Times 80(39):31, 1984

Damrosch SP: Graduate nursing students' attitudes toward sexually active older persons. Gerontologist 24:299, 1984

Davies M: Coping with sexuality: Unspoken anxieties, part 1. Nurs Times 80(50):29, 1984

Dawson-Shepherd R: Sex and disability: Why the carpet is no longer big enough, part 3. Nurs Times 80(39):33, 1984

Fuentes RJ et al: Sexual side effects: What to tell your patients . . . what not to say . . . commonly prescribed drugs, part 1. RN 46(2):34, 1983

Hampton PJ: Coping with the male patient's sexuality. Nurs Forum 18:304, 1979

Hobson KG: The effects of aging on sexuality. Health Soc Work 9:25, 1984

Leonard C: Understanding sexuality: Talking through a taboo. Nurs Mirror 153:19, 1981

Levitt R: Sex and physical disability. J Neurosurg Nurs 13:127, 1981

Llewelyn S et al: Sex: More than the facts; the contribution of psychology to an understanding of sexual behavior. Nurs Mirror 156(11):38, 1983

Masters W, Johnson V: Human Sexual Response. Boston, Little, Brown & Co, 1966

McCary JL: McCary's Human Sexuality, 3rd ed. New York, Van Nostrand Co, 1978

McIntosh D: Sexual attitudes in a group of older women. Issues Mental Health Nurs 3:109, 1981

Marks RG: Sexual side effects: How drugs can change fertility. RN 46(5):61, 1983

Meredith L: Some thoughts on teaching student nurses human sexuality. LAMP, p. 21, Mar 1984

Miller S: Recognizing the sexual health care needs of hospitalized patients. Can Nurse 80(3):43, 1984

Nelson WC: Lowering the bedrail: Helping people remain intimate while in the hospital. J Christ Nurs 1:17, 1984

Professional attitudes of RN's to human sexuality. Aust Nurs J 11:51, 1981

Race A, Leecraft J, Crist T: The Sex Scene. Understanding Sexuality. Hagerstown, Harper & Row, 1975

Reinstein L: Sexual adjustment after lower extremity amputation. Arch Phys Med Rehabil 59:501, 1978

Rosenzweig N, Pearsall FP: Sex Education for the Health Professional. New York, Grune & Stratton, 1978

Semmers JP et al: Sexual problems in middle age. Consultant 20:226, 1980

Sex and aging: A game people play. Geriatr Nurs 3:263, 1982

Weinberg JS: Human sexuality and spinal cord injury. Nurs Clin North Am 17:407, 1982

Whipple B: A holistic view of sexuality: Education for the health professional. Top Clin Nurs 1:91, 1980

Woods NF: Human Sexuality in Health and Illness, 3rd ed. St. Louis, Mosby, 1985

Yoselle H: Sexuality in the later years. Top Clin Nurs 3:59, 1981

Yoshino S: Sexual problems of women with rheumatoid arthritis. Arch Phys Med Rehabil 62:122, 1981

Zola IK: Denial of emotional needs to people with handicaps. Arch Phys Med Rehabil 63:68, 1982

Appendix: Fractures: A Discussion of Classic Types

The purpose of this discussion is to provide (1) general statements about fractures in particular anatomic locations and (2) descriptions of the more common classic types of fractures and their treatment.

Although fractures have "names" given to them in literature, orthopedic surgeons do not all necessarily refer to these names when making a diagnosis.

In using this section as a reference, it is important to remember (as frequently pointed out throughout the text) that the treatment of choice for any orthopedic condition depends not only on the nature of the injury or disease but also on the surgeon's familiarity and success with a particular type of treatment. Physicians may also differ (due to experience) in opinions about the length of time required for certain fractures to unite.

The Upper Extremity

THE HAND

Some sources indicate that fractures of the phalanges and metacarpals are the most frequently encountered of all fractures. Whether or not a fracture of the hand is reduced at all prior to immobilization depends on the location of the fracture and how acceptable deformity is in relation to function. Stiffness, malunion, and rotational malalignment are complications following phalangeal or metacarpal fractures.

Mallet Finger

One cause of this deformity is an avulsion fracture of the dorsal articular surface of the distal phalanx, in which the extensor tendon attached to the fracture fragment is unable to extend the distal joint. The fracture fragment may be tilted and malrotated.

Treatment. Open reduction with insertion of Kirschner wires may be necessary. The proximal interphalangeal joint is immobilized in 60 degrees of flexion. Motion of this joint,

to prevent stiffness, may be started at 3 weeks. Bony union at the fracture site may take as long as 10 weeks.

Boxer's Fracture

Also called *fighter's fracture*, this fracture is the most frequent of all metacarpal neck fractures and involves the fifth metacarpal.

Treatment. The amount of angulation determines whether or not the fracture is reduced. A plaster splint, which immobilizes the fingers in some degree of flexion and extends from the distal interphalangeal joint of the ring and little fingers to the upper forearm, may be applied following reduction. The splint may be removed in 2 to 3 weeks, and gentle motion begun.

Bennett's Fracture

In this fracture, often sustained in a fist fight, a small volar lip fragment is broken off the base of the thumb metacarpal. The fracture is intra-articular, and bony union may be slower than in a shaft fracture.

Treatment. Closed manipulation with percutaneous (through the skin) pinning may be successful. Otherwise, open reduction with internal fixation is indicated. A thumb spica cast may be worn for 4 to 6 weeks. Percutaneous wires may be left in place for 8 weeks. Active motion is begun at the surgeon's discretion.

THE WRIST

Because most of the soft tissue structures that pass through the wrist are in rigid compartments and close to bones and joints, they are subject to injury when a fracture is sustained. This includes the nerves and blood vessels supplying the carpal bones. The carpal bones are also extensively covered with cartilage, which means that their normal blood supply is limited, and union of the fracture may take a long time.

The scaphoid bone, because it forms the radial portion of *both* rows of carpals, is the most frequently fractured of all carpal bones. Most scaphoid fractures heal, but in general, fractures in this bone have a higher incidence of nonunion than those in most other bones. Probably the main reason for this is impairment of the blood supply to one of the fragments. A gauntlet type cast (p. 52) is usually applied for 2 to 3 months.

Colles' Fracture (Fracture of the Distal Radius)

Colles' fracture, as described by Abraham Colles 160 years ago, is quite common. In this fracture the distal end of the radius is broken off and displaced posteriorly. A fracture of the styloid process of the ulna is often associated with this injury.

The deformity is classic in appearance. The forearm appears shortened. Posteriorly, there is a depression about one and one-half inches from the wrist, with a posterior angulation of the hand and wrist and radial deviation. On the anterior side, the wrist appears very full.

Treatment. Closed reduction, under some form of anesthesia, is the treatment of choice. The surgeon applies manual traction in line with the deformity by grasping the injured hand. Countertraction is provided on the humerus with the elbow flexed. After muscle spasm has been relieved and the bone ends disimpacted, the distal fragment of the fracture is positioned in alignment with the proximal fragment, while the hand is held in slight palmar flexion and ulnar deviation. Reduction of a Colles' fracture restores the length of the radius and brings the distal radial joint surface forward.

A long arm cast is usually applied with the forearm in slight pronation and the wrist in slight flexion and ulnar deviation. Occasionally, if there is extensive comminution, impaction of articular fragments, or impingement of the median nerve, an open reduction may be done.

X-ray films must be taken immediately after reduction and again after immobilization. When there is minimal displacement, some surgeons prefer to use plaster splints instead of a cast. The cast may be on as long as 8 weeks.

THE FOREARM

The muscles that connect the radius and ulna and control pronation and supination cause strong deforming forces when fractures occur. For this reason closed reduction is difficult, and general anesthesia is usually required. When such fractures are reduced, longitudinal and rotational alignment must be corrected. Solitary fractures are more common in the ulna than in the radius. Compartment syndrome (pp. 57–59) is a possibility in forearm fractures and may result an ischemic contracture.

Ulnar Fractures

Fractures in the shaft of the ulna are commonly caused by a direct blow.

Treatment. Treatment depends on the site of the fracture and the amount of displacement. Those fractures that occur in the distal half usually unite following immobilization in a long arm cast. Since there is more soft tissue in the proximal forearm, a cast may not provide the desired stabilization. Therefore, fractures in this location may require open reduction and internal fixation. Bony union occurs in about 3 months.

Monteggia's Fracture

Generally speaking, Monteggia's fracture is a fracture of the *proximal third of the ulna,* with dislocation of the radial head.

Treatment. While there is controversy over the most appropriate method of treatment for this fracture, many surgeons recommend open reduction with compression plate fixation of the ulna. The radial head may usually be reduced by closed means. A long arm cast is applied. Follow-up x-ray films are necessary at 2 and 6 weeks to determine if reduction is being maintained.

Galeazzi's Fracture

This fairly common fracture of the forearm occurs at the junction of the *middle and distal thirds of the shaft of the radius.* Subluxation of the radioulnar joint may accompany this fracture or may occur gradually as it is being treated.

Treatment. Because there is a risk of subluxation of the radioulnar joint with this treatment, closed reduction is not considered satisfactory by many authorities. Open reduction with fixation by a compression plate is the most successful in regaining and maintaining the alignment necessary for restoring proper function. A cast or plaster splint may be applied to incorporate elbow and wrist to prevent rotation of the forearm. After approximately 6 weeks the splint or cast may be removed and active exercises begun to restore pronation and supination.

THE ELBOW

The elbow joint is actually composed of three joints: the humeroradial, the humeroulnar, and the radioulnar. The articulation of the ulna with the humerus provides the basic hinge action of the elbow. The two joints involving the radius are important in providing manual dexterity. The radial and median nerves run anterior to the elbow, and the ulnar nerve runs posterior to the elbow. Numerous blood vessels also pass over and around the elbow articulations. Swelling about the elbow when fracture occurs compresses the nerves and blood vessels and causes irreversible damage in a matter of hours. For the first 48 hours following injury it is imperative that hourly observation of neurovascular status be carried out.

Treatment. Treatment of the elbow fractures depends on the location and the extent of the fracture. Open reduction is often required because of the complex anatomical structure of the elbow. Motion of the joint may be started within 3 to 6 weeks after treatment. Complete motion in the elbow joint may not be possible for 3 to 6 months, although in some cases a fracture will heal in about 8 weeks.

Complications. A rare disease, myositis ossificans, or the formation of bone tissue in or adjacent to muscle, may follow a fracture. This complication is thought to be due to many factors, including some aspects of treatment. In the past, the elbow was one of the most frequent locations of this disease. Although improved techniques in the management of elbow fractures have greatly reduced the incidence of myositis ossificans, it should still be considered a possibility.

FRACTURES OF THE HUMERUS

The Shaft of the Humerus

Muscle action on the shaft of the humerus frequently causes overriding and displacement of fragments when a fracture is sustained. The proximity of the radial nerve to the humerus makes it accessible to injury also.

Treatment. Closed reduction with maintenance of alignment by a hanging cast (p. 50), an arm sling, or some form of arm traction (pp. 124 – 126) is generally considered to be the best form of treatment.

Following reduction of the fracture, it is very important to encourage the patient to do shoulder and finger exercises as soon as he can tolerate them in order to prevent stiffness. To perform pendulum and circumduction exercises of the shoulder the patient should lean forward with the cast or sling hanging free.

Elbow motion is begun when there is enough union at the fracture site to permit it. Complete healing may take 3 months or longer depending on the fracture pattern determining the contact between the ends of the fragments.

Complications. Complications of this fracture include radial nerve damage, which is evidenced by wrist drop, and nonunion.

The Proximal Humerus (Neck)

Fractures of the upper end of the humerus are fairly common and occur most often in the elderly. In these fractures, the pectoralis major muscle tends to pull the distal fragment or the shaft of the humerus medially and anteriorly. The deltoid muscle will pull it upward. Aseptic necrosis may develop in displaced neck fractures since the blood supply to the head of the humerus is interrupted.

Treatment. The goal in the treatment of fractures of the proximal humerus is to restore function of the shoulder and prevent adhesions.

Initial immobilization for fractures with minimal displacement is best accomplished by a sling or immobilizer. The fragments are held in place by periosteum and the rotator cuff. Consequently gentle active assistive exercises may be permitted as soon as enough healing has occurred to allow the head and shaft to rotate in unison.

Fractures of the proximal humerus in which there is more than minimal displacement require open reduction.

The technique of internal fixation that is used depends on the pattern of the fracture, the degree of displacement, and extent of injury to the muscles. Exercise programs are initiated and increased as healing permits.

Proximal fractures of the humerus may heal in 2 to 3 months, but stiffness and discomfort following motion and function may persist for months.

THE SHOULDER AREA

The Clavicle (Collar Bone)

The clavicle is an S-shaped bone that may be fractured at any point. These fractures are more common in children. If the fracture is displaced, the shoulder will slump downward and inward, and the deformity may be palpable. The patient will hold his arm against his chest in a protective maneuver. The undisplaced clavicular fracture may be overlooked.

Treatment. When displacement is minimal and the ligaments are not torn, a sling may be a satisfactory form of treatment. In displaced fractures the shoulder must be maintained in an upward and backward position to allow the fracture to heal in alignment. In a child, the figure-eight dressing is usually adequate. In an adult, this dressing may not be wholly successful and some deformity will be present after healing. Some authorities advise the use of a Velpeau dressing for 10 days to 2 weeks prior to the application of a figure-eight or a shoulder spica. Open reduction is only considered in complicated cases. The healing time for fractures of the clavicle is generally considered to be about 8 weeks.

The Scapula

Although the scapula, because of its location, may be fractured in many different sites, fractures of this bone are uncommon. Factors largely responsible for this are the protective muscles covering the bone, and the scapula's ability to move along the chest wall. Great force, either direct or indirect, is required to fracture the scapula, and the extent of associated injuries frequently obscures an initial diagnosis. When a patient has a fractured scapula, he may hold his arm in adduction.

Treatment. Methods of treatment of scapular fractures vary greatly according to location of the fracture site.

The Acromioclavicular Joint

Fractures associated with dislocation of the acromioclavicular joint occur in the acromion, the clavicle, or the coracoid process. The most frequent cause of this injury is a fall on the point of the shoulder with the arm in adduction.

Treatment. Whether the most desirable form of treatment is open or closed reduction seems to be a subject of controversy.

The Spine

A fracture of the spine may occur as a separate injury but is often associated with multiple injuries and damage to the spinal cord.

Stable fractures of the spine include compression fractures of the vertebral bodies without dislocation or comminution. A spinal fracture is considered unstable if the spinal cord is threatened by the possibility of shifting fracture fragments. Instability of the spine may be progressive over a period of months or years and is more likely to occur where there has been disruption of a number of structural elements of the spine.

In order to determine the type of treatment ot be instituted, the surgeon must know the type and the degree of neurologic involvement.

THE CERVICAL SPINE

Treatment. A stable fracture of the cervical spine may be treated with a cervical orthosis and exercise. Where there is an unstable fracture of the cervical spine with no neurologic deficit, the patient will tolerate bed rest in cervical traction for 8 to 10 weeks (p. 100). When ambulation is permitted, a neck brace is applied. Patients with severe spinal cord injuries tolerate bed rest poorly because of paralysis and impaired body functions. Death often results from metabolic complications.

Cervical spine fractures may be treated by the application of a halo body cast or by surgical fusion.

THE THORACOLUMBAR SPINE

Most fractures of the spine are in the distal thoracic or lumbar area, and are stable.

Treatment. Generally, reduction of such fractures is not attempted because it is difficult both to accomplish and to maintain. Furthermore, many sources feel that prolonged immobility in extension, which is necessary to maintain reduction of these fractures, causes more pain and stiffness than it eliminates. The treatment of choice is usually a period of bed rest followed by application of a corset brace or a cast, and a program of exercise. Low back pain may persist for years after treatment.

The Pelvis

Although there are numerous classifications of pelvic fractures, such fractures are rare. The most important thing about pelvic fractures is the fact that they are so often associated with intra-abdominal injury (pp. 103–104).

Treatment. The treatment is bed rest in or out of pelvic sling traction (pp. 103–106).

THE COCCYGEAL AREA

Fractures in the coccygeal area are more common in women, probably beause of the construction of their pelvises. A week of bed rest and hot sitz baths may be sufficient treatment for this fracture. The muscle forces in this part of the body may cause pain and spasm for weeks following this injury.

The Lower Extremity

THE HIP

Fractures of the hip are discussed in Chapter 5.

THE SHAFT OF THE FEMUR

The femur is the longest bone in the body. Because of the stress it must endure, it is also the strongest bone in the body. Powerful muscles surrounding this bone provide it with an unlimited blood supply so that it has a great ability to heal fractures. In fractures of the femoral shaft, problems arise more often in restoring the bone to functional capacity in a reasonable time, than in healing.

Subtrochanteric fractures or those of the proximal femur are subject to the deforming forces of the abductor muscles and the hip flexors.

In fractures of the *mid-shaft,* although the adductor muscles tend to create varus deformity, the lateral thigh muscles counteract this force and act to stabilize these fractures.

Treatment. Skeletal traction is the most common type of traction used to reduce and immobilize femoral fractures until they are either satisfactorily reduced for an internal fixation procedure or sticky enough for application of a hip spica or cast brace. In deciding whether or not to do internal fixation of a subtrochanteric fracture, the surgeon considers the severity of the fracture, the stress factor, and the age and condition of the patient. A plate and screw device that extends into the neck of the femur, such as a hip nail, may be used for internal fixation.

Following traction, midshaft fractures are commonly treated by intramedullary rods, unless there is a high degree of comminution or the fracture is open. In some cases percutaneous pins and a plaster cast (pins and plaster) may be indicated.

Complete union of a femoral shaft fracture takes about 6 months.

Complications. Delayed union is the most frequent complication of femoral fractures.

Distal Shaft of the Femur (Supracondylar)

Those fractures that occur at the distal end of the femur or in the supracondylar area are displaced by the pull of the thigh muscles as well as by the force exerted by the gastrocnemius muscle.

Treatment. Recommended treatment of this type of fracture is skeletal traction. With a pin in the proximal tibia, the leg is placed in suspension traction with the knee flexed. The length of time the patient spends in traction will depend on whether or not the surgeon intends to apply a hip spica or a cast brace.

Many surgeons advocate knee movement while the patient is in traction to prevent adhesions involving the quadriceps and to hasten healing.

Open reduction of supracondylar fractures is generally considered undesirable. One reason for this is the difficulty encountered in proper insertion of a fixation device on the contours of this part of the femur.

Bony union is to be expected in 3 to 4 months.

THE KNEE JOINT

Fractures that extend into the knee joint involve the femoral condyles or the articular surfaces of the tibial plateau, or both. Such fractures seriously impair the function of the knee joint, and reduction must be accurate. However, even meticulous reduction does not ensure complete restoration of proper joint function. Joint incongruity can result from irregularities that develop during the healing process. Traumatic arthritis is not an uncommon development in patients with knee joint fractures.

Traction. Skeletal traction through the tibia may be an effective means of reduction for a fracture that is not displaced. Open reduction and internal fixation by screws and bolts is often necessary in order to restore joint surfaces. Since the knee is a complex weightbearing joint, the amount of ligamentous injury that is incurred with a fracture must be considered when the method of treatment is being chosen. One advantage of open reduction is that early motion of the knee joint is possible.

Although fractures in the knee joint heal rapidly, they are not stable enough for full weight bearing for 3 to 4 months.

Bumper or Fender Fractures

Fractures of the tibial condyles are often referred to in literature as "bumper" or "fender" fractures, since they often happen to the pedestrian who is struck by an automobile. Falls from heights, especially twisting falls, are also responsible for this type of injury.

Treatment. The methods of treatment include casting, traction, and open reduction.

The Patella

The patella is located in the quadriceps tendon. This sesamoid bone serves as protection for the femoral condyles and provides leverage for the quadriceps.

Treatment. Fractures of the patella are treated by nonoperative methods when the fragments are undisplaced and there is no comminution. A long leg cylinder cast is applied and quadriceps exercises are initiated a few days after injury. Physicians differ in how soon they will allow weight bearing and removal of the cast.

Wire sutures may be used in internal fixation of patellar fractures, whereas a patellectomy is indicated when there is extensive comminution.

THE TIBIA

Fractures of the tibial shaft are quite common. Its anatomical location and the fact that it is covered only by a thin layer of subcutaneous tissue and skin make the tibia susceptible to injury. These same factors make the bone accessible to the surgeon when open reduction of fractures is required. The blood supply to the tibia is somewhat limited since the anterior surface of the bone is not covered by muscles.

The tibia is fractured by direct violence, such as occurs in a motor vehicle accident, or by the indirect violence of a twisting force. Angulation and rotation are the deformities that are likely to be present following the injury.

Because the anterior compartment of the leg is enclosed by an inelastic sheath, it is vulnerable to compartment syndrome when the tibia is fractured (pp. 57–59).

Treatment. Most sources recommend closed reduction of tibial fractures. A long leg cast may be applied, and the patient is allowed full weight bearing in 2 to 4 weeks. Some surgeons advocate a below-knee, patellar-tendon-bearing cast after several weeks in a long leg cast. Open reduction when necessary is accomplished by a compression plate.

In all methods of treatment of tibial fractures, maintenance of quadriceps strength is stressed. The healing period is about 4 months. Delayed union is a common complication.

THE FIBULA

Fractures of the fibula by itself are rare. They usually occur with tibial fractures.

Treatment. Since the fibula is a nonweightbearing bone, fracture fragments are likely to remain in good alignment. As a general rule fibular fractures require no reduction. However, the leg is usually immobilized in a cast.

THE ANKLE

The ankle, a modified hinge joint, is composed of the distal ends of both the tibia and fibula and the talus. The talus fits into a slot, or mortise, formed by the lower end of the tibia and the lateral (fibular) and medial (tibial) malleoli.

The mechanism of ankle injuries are external rotation, abduction, adduction, and vertical compression. Extensive tearing of ligaments may occur with fracture.

The objective in the treatment of all ankle fractures is relocation of the talus in the mortise and restoration of smooth, correct joint function.

Fractures of the ankle involve one malleolus or are bimalleolar (Pott's). A trimalleolar fracture includes the posterior lip of the tibia, and may be termed *Cotton's fracture.*

Treatment. Stable ankle fractures are immobilized in splints until swelling subsides, after which a short leg walking cast is applied for about 1 month. Displaced fractures are reduced surgically if the talus cannot be repositioned by closed reduction. Screws are frequently used for internal fixation. A cast is applied following surgery, and full weight bearing on a walking cast may begin after the sutures are removed. The ankle is immobilized for 2 to 3 months.

THE FOOT

The hindpart of the foot is composed of the talus, calcaneus, or heel bone and the navicular, cuboid, and three cuneiform bones. The talus and calcaneus are the most commonly fractured bones of the foot. The forepart of the foot is made up of five metatarsals and the phalanges of the five toes.

Talus Fractures

There are several important factors to be considered in reducing fractures of the talus. The talus is part of a joint. Its superior surface bears tremendous weight for the size of its surface area. Also, much of the talus is covered with articular cartilage, and consequently the number of points of entry for blood vessels is limited. Accurate realignment of fractures of the talus is imperative for the joint to function properly and for re-establishment of circulation to the bone.

Treatment. Undisplaced fractures of the talus may be treated by immobilization in short leg casts. Unstable fractures require open reduction and pinning. Arthrodesis may be indicated where there is severe comminution. Healing is slow and may take 3 months. Weight bearing is delayed until sufficient bony union is present.

Calcaneal Fractures

The calcaneus is fractured more often than any other tarsal bone. If the subtalar joint is involved, particular attention must be paid to accurate reduction. Pressure dressings or short casts are used. Open reduction is not usually indicated.

The amount of weight bearing that is allowed depends on the segment of the calcaneus that was fractured and its stability. The healing period is about 8 weeks.

Metatarsal and Phalangeal Fractures

Fractures of the metatarsals and phalanges are usually caused by crushing injuries and therefore there may be extensive soft tissue injury. Such fractures are usually immobilized by casts or splinting. They heal in about 4 weeks.

Jones' Fracture

This fracture occurs at the base of the fifth metatarsal and is the most common type of metatarsal fracture. The application of a snug dressing or adhesive strapping is usually all that is required for treatment. The patient is allowed partial weight bearing with the aid of crutches. Immobilization of the fracture continues for approximately 6 weeks.

Bibliography

Adams JC: Outline of Fractures, 8th ed. New York, Churchill Livingstone, 1983

Barton NJ: Fractures of the hand. J Bone Joint Surg (Br) 66(2):159, 1984

Betts-Symonds GW: A biomechanical approach to the treatment of phalangeal fractures, part 6. Nurs Times 78:2083, 1982

Betts-Symonds GW: Functional bracing of femoral shaft fractures, part 8. Nurs Times 78:2127, 1982

Betts-Symonds GW: Functional bracing of fractures of the tibia and fibula, part 7. Nurs Times 78:2123, 1982

Betts-Symonds GW, Bell AP: Functional bracing of Bennett's fracture, part 1. Nurs Times 28:1995, 1982

Betts-Symonds GW, Hodgkinson V: The treatment of forearm fractures: Functional bracing, part 4. Nurs Times 78:2026, 1982

Betts-Symonds GW et al: Functional bracing of humeral fractures, part 2. Nurs Times 78:1998, 1982

Betts-Symonds GW et al: Functional bracing of metacarpal fractures: An original way of treating metacarpal fractures, part 3. Nurs Times 78:2023, 1982

Blackburn N et al: Correction of the malunited forearm fracture. Clin Orthop 188:54, 1984

Breen TF Jr et al: Fractures of the femoral shaft in a regional hospital setting. J Trauma 23:483, 1983

Briscoe S: Fractured femur. Nurs Mirror 156(26):50, 1983

Chaffee E, and Lytle IM: Basic Physiology and Anatomy, 4th ed. Philadelphia, JB Lippincott, 1980

Clancey GJ et al: Nonunion of the tibia treated with Kuntscher intramedullary nailing. Clin Orthop 167:191, 1982

Connolly JF: The pelvis: Fracture pitfalls. Emerg Med 15:183, 1983

Connolly JF: The thoracic and lumbar spine: Fracture pitfalls. Emerg Med 15(1):183, 1983

Crenshaw AH (ed): Campbell's Operative Orthopaedics, 6th ed. St Louis CV Mosby, 1980

Dabezies EJ et al: Fractures of the femoral shaft treated by external fixation with the Wagner device. J Bone Joint Surg (Am) 66(3):360, 1984

Davis P: A break from the bottle. An elderly alcoholic man with a fractured femur: Nursing care study. Nurs Mirror 156(2):40, 1983

Evers JA, Werpachowski D: Dealing with fractures. RN 47(11):53, 1984

Fink RJ, Katz GI: Reduction of medial malleolar fractures. Clin Orthop 178:214, 1983

Fisk GR: The wrist. J Bone Joint Surg (Br) 66(3):396, 1984

Flanders J: Pott's luck. Nurs Mirror 158(16):29, 1984

Fractures. Nurs Mirror 156(1): inside back cover, 1983

Friedenberg ZB: Update on fractures. Fracture repair: Conflicts and consensus. Selected abstracts, part 2. Orthop Nurs, 3(6):43, 1984

Hardegger FH et al: The operative treatment of scapular fractures. J Bone Joint Surg (Br) 66(5):725, 1984

Healy WL, Brooker AF, Jr: Distal femoral fractures: Comparison of open and closed methods of treatment. Clin Orthop 174:166, 1983

Heppenstall R: Fracture Treatment and Healing. Philadelphia, WB Saunders, 1980

Hollinshead WH: Textbook of Anatomy, 3rd ed. Hagerstown, Harper & Row, 1974

Hunter SG: The closed treatment of fractures of the humeral shaft. Clin Orthop 164:192, 1982

Joseph FR: Evaluation of the Zickel supracondylar fixation device. Clin Orthop 169:190, 1982

Langley LL et al: Textbook of Anatomy, 3rd ed. Hagerstown, Harper & Row, 1974

Larson C, Gould M: Orthopedic Nursing, 9th ed. St. Louis, CV Mosby, 1978

Larsson K, van der Linden W: Open tibial shaft fractures. Clin Orthop 180:63, 1983

Ma YZ et al: Treatment of fractures of the patella with percutaneous suture. Clin Orthop 191:235, 1984

Mercier LR: Practical Orthopedics. Chicago, Year Book Medical Publishers, 1980

Moed BR et al: Screw fixation of closed oblique and spiral fractures of the tibial shaft. Clin Orthop 177:196, 1983

Perry CR et al: A new surgical approach to fractures of the lateral tibial plateau. J Bone Joint Surg (Am) 66(8):1236, 1984

Pinczewski L et al: Hangman's fracture: Nonoperative management with the halocast. Aust NZ J Surg, 53(1):71, 1983

Pollock FH et al: The isolated fracture of the ulnar shaft. Treatment without immobilization. J Bone Joint Surg (Am), 65(3):339, 1983

Pozo JL et al: The long-term results of conservative management of severely displaced fractures of the calcaneus. J Bone Joint Surg (Br) 66(3):386, 1984

Pritchett JW: Supracondylar fracture of the femur. Clin Orthop 184:173, 1984

Raney RB, Brashear HR: Shand's Handbook of Orthopaedic Surgery, 9th ed. St. Louis, CV Mosby, 1978

Richter-Davies L et al: Emergency management of lower extremity fractures. Assessment and Fracture Management of the Lower Extremities, pp 38–44, 1984

Roberts RS: Surgical treatment of displaced ankle fractures. Clin Orthop 172:164, 1983

Robinson JE, Marx LO: Nail-safe method. Am J Nurs 85(2):158, 1985

Rockwood CA, Green DP: Fractures. Philadelphia, JB Lippincott, 1975

Santavirta S et al: Fractures of the talus. J Trauma 24(11):986, 1984

Sarmiento A et al: The role of soft tissue in the stabilization of tibial fractures. Clin Orthop 105:116, 1974

Schmidt A, Rorabeck CH: Fractures of the tibia treated by flexible external fixation. Clin Orthop 178:162, 1983

Stearns CM: Surgical implants used for fractures of the lower extremity. Assessment and Fracture Management of the Lower Extremities, pp 54–59, 1984

Stearns HC III: Principles of lower extremity fracture management. Assessment and Fracture Management of the Lower Extremities, pp 45–53, 1984

Stern PJ, Drury WJ: Complications of plate fixation of forearm fractures. Clin Orthop 175:25, 1983

Stern PJ et al: Intramedullary fixation of humeral shaft fractures. J Bone Joint Surg (Am) 66(5):639, 1984

Update on fractures. Fracture repair: Conflicts and consensus. Selected abstracts, part 1. Orthop Nurs 3(5):25, 1984

Wehbe MA, Schneider LH: Mallet fractures. J Bone Joint Surg (Am) 66(5):658, 1984

Weseley MS et al: Rush pin intramedullary fixation for fractures of the proximal humerus. J Trauma 17(1):29, 1977

Zickel RE et al: A new intramedullary fixation device for the distal third of the femur. Clin Orthop 125:185, 1977

Italicized page numbers indicate illustrations; page numbers followed by the letter *t* indicate tabular material.

Index

after chemonucleolysis, 145
after laminectomy, 140
in leg casts, 70
in rheumatoid arthritis, 331
in spinal fusion, 149
in traction, 97
balanced skeletal, 121
Buck's, 114
with Crutchfield tongs, 127
in intervertebral disk herniation, 133
with pelvic belt, 107–108
with pelvic sling, 103, 104
Russell's, 116
Bence-Jones protein, urinary, in multiple myeloma, 323t, 339
Bennett's fracture, 360
Biceps brachii muscle, nursing assessment of, 4t, 11t
Biopsy of bone, in metastatic disease, 343
Blanching sign of nails, 9t, 17t
in casts, 59
in injuries, 27
Bleeding
in knee repair, postoperative, 245, 246t, 249
in lower extremity amputation, postoperative, 271
nursing assessment and management of, 24, 28
Blisters, in casted fractures, 61
Blood pressure, measurement of, 26t
Blood vessels
assessment of. *See* Neurovascular assessment
of bone, 312
and avascular necrosis in fractures, 48, 176, 177, 362
and hematogenous osteomyelitis, 316–317
of knee, 227, *227*
Body cast, 52
in scoliosis, 159–160, 161, 166–167, 167t
in spinal fusion, 152
Body image. *See* Self-image
Body-powered arm prosthesis, 290–291
Bones. *See also specific bones*
anatomy of, 311, *311*, 312, *312*
biopsy of, in metastatic disease, 343
blood supply of, 312
and avascular necrosis in fractures, 48, 176, 177, 362
and hematogenous osteomyelitis, 316–317

cancellous, 311
fracture of, 43
cells in, 312
in fracture healing, 46, *46*
chemical composition of, 312
chronic disease of, 311–349
compact, 311
fracture of, 43
cortex of, 311
definition of, 311
development of, 312–313
fractures of, 42–89. *See also* Fracture(s)
functions of, 313
hormonal influence on, 313
in hyperparathyroidism, 314
marrow of, 311
in multiple myeloma, 323t, 339
in metabolic disorders, 314–315
nutritional requirements of, 313
and osteomalacia, 315
and osteoporosis, 315
and rickets, 314
Paget's disease of, 36t, 313–314, *314*, 323t
radionuclide scan of
in metastatic bone disease, 343, *345*
normal, *344*
remodeling of, 47, *47*, 312, 313
tumors of
brown, 314
laboratory findings in, 36t
metastatic, 36t, 343–345
Boredom of patients
in balanced skeletal traction, 121
in spinal fusion, 150
Boxer's fracture of hand, 360
Braces
in fractures, 45–46
vertebral, 170
leg, with cast, 80–82
in scoliosis, 156–158
after cast removal, 167
Milwaukee, 156, 157, *157*, *158*
in spinal fusion, 151
Brachioradialis reflex, testing of, 12t
Bristow shoulder repair, 304, *304*
Brown tumors of bone, 314
Buck's traction, 109–114
application of, 109–111
in hip fractures, 175, 179–180
in hip reconstruction, 203
indications for, 109
nursing assessment in, 93
tape used in, 109–110
irritation from, 111–112

wrapping bandages in, 110–111
problems from, 112–113
Bumper fractures, 364
Bunion, 296, 298t–299t
formation of, *295*
Bunionectomy, 296, *296*, 298t–299t
problem-solving approach in, 298t–299t
Bursae of knee, 227

Calcaneus, fractures of, 365
Calcium
in bones, 312
dietary
and bone growth, 313
in osteoporosis, 315
serum and urine levels of, 36t
in metastatic bone disease, 36t, 344
in multiple myeloma, 36t, 339
Callus formation, in fracture healing, 47, *47*
Cancellous bone, 311
fracture of, 43
Cardiorespiratory system, nursing assessment of, 30t
Carpal bones, fracture of, 360
Carpal tunnel syndrome, *301*, 301–302
Cart
cast, 52, *52*
traction, 91, *91*
Cartilage, semilunar, of knee, 226, *226*
injuries of, 228, 229–230, *230*
McMurray's test of, 228, *228*
Cast(s), 50–83
application of, 52–55
steps in, *53*, 53–54, *54*
arm, 50, *50*, *51*, 65–69. *See also* Arm, casts on
bivalved, 61–62
body, 52
in scoliosis, 159–160, 161, 166–167, 167t
in spinal fusion, 152
cleaning of, 55, 57
in closed reduction of fracture, 44
compartment syndrome in, 57–59
drainage in, 62–63
drying of, 56, 75, 77, 81, 160
exercise in, 64–65, 68–69, 70, 71, 79, 82, 83
finishing edges of, 56–57
in foot surgery, 298–299
general discomfort in, 65
green, 56